DECODING THE CODES

A Comprehensive Guide to ICD, CPT & HCPCS Coding Systems

DISCLAIMER

ICD listings at the category and subcategory levels and all CPT or HCPCS headings, subheadings, and listings in this textbook are italicized. The italicized CPT codes and descriptors used or applied as examples are subject to the copyright of the American Medical Association (AMA) and are adapted only for instructional purposes. Any additional utilization of the CPT codes and descriptors is prohibited without the explicit consent of the AMA. The clinical scenarios in this book are adaptations of the clinical supplements circulated by the AMA.

The clinical documentation used as examples in this manual was excerpted from authentic patient records. The names of physicians, patients, and facilities were changed to fictitious appellations to ensure confidentiality. Similarities to actual persons or institutions are merely coincidental.

DECODING THE CODES

A Comprehensive Guide to ICD, CPT & HCPCS Coding Systems

ALEX TOTH, CMA, CCS, CPC

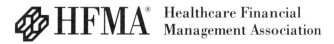

HFMA® Healthcare Financial
Management Association

Educational Foundation

McGraw-Hill

New York   San Francisco   Washington, D.C.   Auckland   Bogotá
Caracas   Lisbon   London   Madrid   Mexico City   Milan
Montreal   New Delhi   San Juan   Singapore
Sydney   Tokyo   Toronto

Library of Congress Cataloging-in-Publication Data

Toth, Alex
    Decoding the codes : a comprehensive guide to ICD, CPT & HCPCS
coding systems / Alex Toth.
      p.   cm.
    Includes index.
    ISBN 0–7863–1246–7
    1. Nosology—Code numbers. 2. Medicine—Terminology—Code
numbers. I. Title.
RB115.T68 1997
610′.1′48—dc21
                              97-38713
                                   CIP

McGraw-Hill

A Division of The McGraw·Hill Companies

1 2 3 4 5 6 7 8 9 0 BKM/BKM 9 0 9 8 7

ISBN 0-7863-1246-7

Printed and bound by Book-Mart Press, Inc.

This publication is designed to provide accurate and authoritative information
in regard to the subject matter covered. It is sold with the understanding that
neither the author nor the publisher is engaged in rendering legal, accounting,
or other professional service. If legal advice or other expert assistance is
required, the services of a competent professional person should be sought.

    *—From a Declaration of Principles jointly adopted by a Committee of
    the American Bar Association and a Committee of Publishers.*

McGraw-Hill books are available at special quantity discounts to use as
premiums and sales promotions, or for use in corporate training programs. For
more information, please write to the Director of Special Sales, McGraw-Hill,
11 West 19th Street, New York, NY 10011. Or contact your local bookstore.

CONTENTS

Chapter 12

CPT Coding: Evaluation and Management Services   310

Chapter 13

CPT Coding: Anesthesia and Surgery   357

Chapter 14

CPT Coding: Radiology, Pathology and Laboratory, and Medicine   426

LIST OF TABLES

P R E F A C E

This publication fulfills the objective of supplying a comprehensive textbook on coding by using both ICD and CPT. Principles in this manual range from basic concepts to advanced techniques designed to provide clinical coding instruction. Primarily aimed at skills necessary in the workplace, the content of this book is geared to all persons who utilize this classification system. These include, but are not limited to, the staff employed in hospitals and other healthcare facilities or agencies, in physicians' offices, and in insurance firms.

The numerous examples and questions in this manuscript present a general pedagogical course on ICD coding and CPT coding in the preparation or training of health information managers, medical record administrators and technicians, patient account supervisors and clerks, medical secretaries, medical office assistants, and insurance claims processors and examiners. This textbook has a widespread focus to appeal to a broad spectrum of the healthcare industry.

Certain coding instructional manuals are planned primarily for hospital personnel whereas other coding instructional manuals are intended primarily for physicians' office personnel. This textbook targets formal edification in coding toward any and all who need to understand and comprehend the classification systems.

This coding textbook does not attempt to incorporate either medical and surgical terminology or anatomical and physiological principles into the coding instruction. Based upon past teaching experiences, the author asserts that instruction in clinical terminology, anatomy, and physiology should be acquired from a separate textbook or obtained in a separate course or courses apart from genuine coding instruction. A singular subject in a vocational school, a technical college, or a university, realistically and practically, cannot encompass concepts and techniques from several disciplines due to the continually increasing scope of academic content within each of the disciplines.

The ICD coding system is provided through the World Health Organization. Two federal agencies, the National Center for Health Statistics and the Health Care Financing Adminstration, update the ICD volumes annually. The CPT coding system is also updated annually by the American Medical Association. Periodic updates of this textbook also are planned in order to perpetuate its usefulness as an instructional manual for learning to code with the most current volumes of ICD and CPT.

ORGANIZATION OF THE CHAPTERS
Learning objectives precede the text of each of the sixteen chapters. These sets of learning objectives are primarily predicated upon the three lowest levels in the cognitive domain of Bloom's taxonomy, although the task of coding does necessitate cognitive activity at the problem-solving level, and analysis is needed for application of coding principles. Each individual set of learning objectives is generally sequenced in an ascending order of complexity.

The textual content of each chapter is replete with examples to facilitate teaching and to expedite learning, without the use of overly simplistic analogies. However, if the coding instructor chooses to present this subject matter in a rudimentary form, this instructional manual allows such presentation.

The subject matter is delineated into sections. If a particular section is deemed as unessential or inconsequential for a certain class of students, the instructor may opt to omit that section. Likewise, any of the extensive review exercises presented at the conclusion of each chapter may be omitted at the discretion of the instructor.

Significant terms and significant phrases are grouped under the label of key concepts and placed immediately subsequent to the text of each of the chapters. Definitions of the key concepts enable either self-evaluation for the learner or class exercises. Completion of definitions or explanations for the key concepts may require the learner to reference sources other than the textbook, such as the coding volumes, a medical dictionary, or a standard English dictionary.

The review exercises at the culmination of each chapter generally parallel the progression of the subject matter within that chapter. Blank lines allow flexibility for the textbook to be utilized as a workbook. Abundant questions and problems permit their distribution among students to deter collusion. The clinical documentation at the end of selected chapters is designed to enhance applied coding skills.

Instructors should forewarn students that many healthcare providers and many third-party payors formulate and specify unique coding or reporting policies. Although the established guidelines should be followed, employers or insurance carriers may deviate or digress from the uniform and consistent rules of coding and reporting. Therefore, application of these principles in the classroom might contrast with application of these principles of coding and reporting in the workplace.

R E V I E W E R S

We at McGraw-Hill Healthcare Education Group would like to acknowledge and thank the following Healthcare Financial Management Association members for reviewing this manuscript.

Patricia Turner
Patient Accounts Manager
Hood River Memorial Hospital
13th & May Streets
Hood River, OR 97031

Daniel Remington
Manager of Patient Business Services
Kaiser Permanente
7201 North Interstate Avenue
Portland, OR 97217

1

CHAPTER

Coding and Coding Systems

LEARNING OBJECTIVES

Upon completion of this chapter the learner should be able to:

1. State at least three specific coding systems currently in use throughout the United States.
2. Report the three major elements of the HCPCS coding system.
3. Define the concept of a code and discuss its characteristics.
4. Define the concept of a classification system and explain its basic features.
5. Define the concept of a nomenclature and discuss its fundamental attributes.
6. Define the concept of a third-party payor.
7. Express at least three examples of the usage of numeric identifiers for distinct entities.
8. Explain at least three differences among the variations in diagnostic coding and procedural coding in different healthcare settings.
9. Discuss the historical evolution of both the ICD coding system and the CPT coding system.
10. Explain the process of updating both the ICD coding system and the CPT coding system.
11. Discuss the association between code number and descriptor.
12. Explain the distinction between fee-for-service insurance coverage and prepaid insurance coverage.
13. State the leading third-party payors in both the public sector and the private sector.
14. Explain the utility of coding systems as a medium of communication within the healthcare industry.

THE CODING PROCESS

Coding is the process of selecting preestablished numerals or alphabetic characters called digits to represent an individual or an entity (a specific activity or particular item) among distinct and dissimilar individuals or entities. For example, an identification number (analogous to a social security number) is a form of code that represents and symbolizes the person who was allocated or assigned that unique number. Comparably, the numbers or letters or combination of numbers or letters that comprise the digits of a code enable activities and items to be placed into absolute and definite categories or groupings. Thus, a code can distinguish and classify an element like a diagnosis (such as hernia or ulcer), or a symptom (such as fever or chest pain), or a procedure (such as an appendectomy), or a service (such as psychotherapy), or a supply (such as a bandage). These identifying and symbolizing codes can be arranged and positioned in a distribution or classification of associated and related elements (such as categories of diseases, types of tissues, groups of procedures, or varieties of supplies). The consequence of this distribution and classification of elements like diagnoses or procedures accords and imparts the development of a scheme that is labeled or entitled as a coding system.

In the healthcare field diverse codes specify each of the varying disorders, injuries, operations, tests, equipment, and all other clinical entities. Therefore, separate and unique codes are used to signify each diagnosis, such as a diagnosis of viral pneumonia or a diagnosis of intrinsic asthma, and to indicate each procedure such as a chest x-ray or a bronchoscopy. Each and every diagnostic code is a unique and exclusive form of representation to precisely delineate a disorder or a symptom; each and every procedural code is a unique and exclusive form of representation to accurately depict a component activity or service performed or rendered in the assessment or therapy of a patient.

CLINICAL CODING SYSTEMS

Throughout the preceding decades, a multitude of coding and classification systems were formulated and developed for various applications in the healthcare field. These included generic coding systems such as the Systematized Nomenclature of Medicine (SNOMED) and specific coding systems such as the Diagnostic and Statistical Manual of Mental Disorders (DSM-IV) outlined and devised for the specialty of psychiatry. Scores of coding and classification systems associated with medical care and surgical care, both generic or universal systems as well as specific or limited systems, were contrived and circulated. Several of these specialized systems for coding and classification remain in contemporary use in the healthcare field, including those systems that are functional in tumor registries and trauma registries. However, many of these coding and classification systems are now defunct. Currently in the United States, only two systems, the International Classification of Diseases, Ninth Edition, Clinical Modification (ICD-9-CM) and Physicians' Current Procedural Terminology (CPT) prevail in general usage by most clinical specialties and by third-party payors. These payors ordinarily are insurance carriers, with the exception of sporadic organizations that self-insure their associates.

ICD-9-CM is a three volume coding and classification system originally designed for statistical compilation of morbidity and adapted much later as a reimbursement mechanism. This classification is based upon the official version of the International Classification of Diseases (ICD) promulgated by the World Health Organization in Geneva, Switzerland. Volume I of ICD-9-CM contains tabular listings of diseases, Volume II is an index to the tabular listings of the first volume, and Volume III contains tabular listings of procedures used in clinical patient care as well as an index to the tabular listings of these procedures. CPT is a single volume compendium and coding system for procedures and services rendered in patient care and was drafted at its inception to facilitate reimbursement and research. The CPT coding system is also enmeshed within the framework of the Health Care Financing Administration Common Procedure Coding System (HCPCS), a coding system predominantly for ancillary healthcare services and clinical supplies. The substance of this textbook focuses exclusively on teaching and learning the ICD-9 diagnostic and therapeutic coding system, the CPT procedural coding system, and the more comprehensive HCPCS coding system utilized for reporting data concerning services, pharmaceuticals, equipment, and supplies.

Every ICD-9 code describes and denotes a different diagnosis, symptom, service, or procedure. Each ICD-9 diagnostic code consists of at least three numeric digits, most of which are followed by a decimal point and one or two additional numeric digits. Thus, ICD-9 code number 540.9 delineates acute appendicitis and ICD-9 code number 824.8 delineates a fracture of the ankle.

Special sections of the ICD-9 diagnostic classification feature an alphabetic character preceding the numeric digits. Alphabetic characters are not used with the ICD-9 procedure codes.

Each ICD-9 procedural code consists of a least two numeric digits, which are followed by a decimal point and one or two additional numeric digits. Thus, ICD-9 code number 47.0 delineates an appendectomy and ICD-9 code number 79.06 delineates a closed reduction of a fractured ankle.

The CPT coding system lists procedures and services, and enables a method to catalog and tally variations of procedures and services. Each CPT code consists of five numeric digits and represents a different procedure, service, or supply. Thus, CPT code number *29840* denotes a diagnostic arthroscopy of the wrist, whereas CPT code number *29870* denotes a diagnostic arthroscopy of the knee. Moreover, CPT code number *27330* designates an arthrotomy of the knee, whereas CPT code number *27437* designates an arthroplasty of the knee.

NOMENCLATURE AND TERMINOLOGY

The term "nomenclature" refers to the vocabulary used in conjunction with any classification system. A nomenclature is a scheme of names given to entities within the categories or groupings that comprise the classification system. Nomenclature is synonymous with terminology.

The term "osteoarthritis," for example, describes an inflammation of a bone joint, such as the hip, knee, or ankle. The term "rheumatoid arthritis" describes another condition affecting joints. A medical nomenclature groups various joint disorders into a clinical classification by etiology (cause of the disorder) or by topography (body location), or perhaps by both.

The word "arthroscopy," for instance, in accepted medical terminology is utilized to describe the process of visualizing a joint by means of a special device. The word "arthrotomy" is similarly a standard medical term utilized to describe the incision of a joint. And likewise the word "arthrectomy" is a conventional medical term utilized to describe the excision of a joint. A medical nomenclature might place these disparate and discrete joint procedures into separate categories or groupings and might further itemize these procedures by anatomic site (such as hip, knee, or ankle).

INTERNATIONAL CLASSIFICATION OF DISEASES

The International Classification of Diseases (ICD) as a coding system lists diagnoses, symptoms, services, and procedures and was designed for statistical compilation of morbidity and mortality. ICD-9 facilitates the indexing of patient health records by disease or operation and expedites the storage retrieval of clinical patient care data. In 1950, the United States Public Health Service began utilizing the ICD classification system for statistical indexing applications. Soon thereafter, Columbia Presbyterian Medical Center in New York City started to index all medical records using ICD. Other healthcare facilities likewise adopted this practice, and several years later the Commission on Professional and Hospital Activities, located in Ann Arbor, Michigan, initiated composite indexing of patient care statistics from multiple participating hospitals.

A cooperative study conducted in 1956 by the American Hospital Association and the American Association of Medical Record Librarians disclosed that the International

Classification of Diseases provided a suitable and efficient framework for indexing medical records. A clinical adaptation of diagnostic coding with the ICD system was prepared by 1959, and certain procedural coding with ICD was also included. Although international accord on the innovative procedure classification of ICD was not achieved, an ancillary procedural classification was implemented by 1962. Clinical indexing of patient care was a prime consideration in the formulation of the eighth revision of ICD in 1966, and therefore further detail was included in the classification for this application. The American Hospital Association in conjunction with the United States Public Health Service developed the necessary modifications and submitted them to the World Health Organization. ICD-8 was released in 1968, and became the official statistical classification for morbidity and mortality in the United States. That year also witnessed the publication of the hospital adaptation of ICD, known as H-ICD-A, by the Commission on Professional and Hospital Activities, which five years later, in 1973, reissued the manual as H-ICDA-2.

International conferences sponsored by the World Health Organization between 1971 and 1975 gradually resulted in a universally accepted tabular list and alphabetic index for procedures. Initially, the rudimentary procedure classification was separated into clinical specialties, with listing developed and grouped into supplementary documents termed fascicles. There was a fascicle for surgical procedures, a fascicle for radiological procedures, a fascicle for laboratory procedures, and so forth. These fascicles were regarded as an adjunct to, rather than a part of, the ICD coding system. Revision and release of the fascicles was separate and distinct from, and not coordinated with, the revision and release of the disease classification. Primary input for the ongoing development of the fascicles by the World Health Organization came through physicians from the United States. Eventually, these fascicles were merged, increased detail was incorporated with expanded rubrics for coding (rubrics are directives or guidelines), and a composite procedural classification became standardized as Volume 3 of the coding system with the release of ICD-9. Approximately eighty percent of the procedural classification refers to surgical procedures, with approximately twenty percent remaining devoted to diagnostic procedures or nonsurgical therapeutic procedures.

In 1977, a steering committee was convened by the National Center for Health Statistics to develop and revise the ICD coding system to reflect advances in clinical care. Organizations represented on this steering committee included the American Association of Health Data Systems, the American Hospital Association, the American Medical Record Association, the Association for Health Records, the Council on Clinical Classifications, the Health Care Financing Administration, the Commission on Professional and Hospital Activities, and the World Health Organization. A revised publication, International Classification of Diseases, Ninth Revision, Clinical Modification (ICD-9-CM) was released officially effective January 1, 1979.

The term "clinical" was intended to convey that the modification was designed for the indexing of patient care data and health statistics. ICD-9-CM was updated periodically in its initial years of utility, but in 1985, the Department of Health and Human Services established the ICD-9-CM Coordination and Maintenance Committee to develop and implement annual revisions to this three-volume coding system that is published in several configurations such as the consolidation of three volumes in one book or binder.

The combined total of entries in ICD-9 contained within the tabular list of Volume 1, the alphabetic index of Volume 2, and the tabular list and alphabetic index of Volume 3 far exceeded that of predecessor volumes of this classification system. The disease listings were expanded to encompass health-related conditions and to allow for greater specificity of detail at the fifth digit level. Appendices to the disease tabular were enhanced to provide reference resources for coders.

The alphabetic index was revised to include many diagnostic terms synonymous with those in Volume 1, but that do not appear within the disease tabular listings. Volume 3 was expanded to render increased clinical specificity for operative procedures that were not accommodated in predecessor revisions of this classification. Rubrics in Volume 3 were expanded to four digits for most of the codes, and the number of listings for diagnostic procedures and therapeutic procedures was increased. Responsibility for Volume 3 modifications was transferred to the Health Care Financing Administration (HCFA) effective with the third edition of ICD-9-CM.

The clinical modification of ICD-9 in usage throughout the United States is completely compatible with the parent ICD-9 classification used elsewhere throughout the world. Therefore, morbidity statistics and mortality statistics can be compared or contrasted on an international level.

The format of ICD-9-CM is slightly revised from that of ICD-9. Inclusion terms are indented beneath the code titles, and code numbers not used for primary tabulation are printed in italics. A dual classification in ICD-9 was modified through the deletion of duplicate rubrics and their substitution with manifestation categories represented by italicized code numbers and titles. Also, American spelling of words is used throughout the ICD-9-CM volumes.

Sequential arrangement of the three-digit category rubrics in ICD-9-CM remains unchanged from that of ICD-9, and no additional three-digit category rubrics were inserted. However, many unsubdivided three-digit category rubrics were separated into subcategories in order to provide either for additional clinical detail or for additional clinical accuracy. Furthermore, through the use of fifth digits, designated listings were generated to provide for increased detail and greater accuracy.

Actually, only twenty-eight categories of the ICD-9 coding system were substantially affected by the American modification of the system. The majority of affected categories are located in the Mental Disorders chapter. A special symbol (the lozenge ▱) indicates the categories that were clinically modified.

PHYSICIANS' CURRENT PROCEDURAL TERMINOLOGY

CDT is an acronym that symbolizes Physicians' Current Procedural Terminology (the initial letter "P" is dropped from the acronym). The CPT coding system is based on a derivative of the California Relative Value System, which was developed and originally published by the California Medical Association in 1956. A relative value system accounts for or rationalizes the duration of time, the cognitive and technical skill, and the overhead expense imperative to perform a specific procedure or to render a particular service.

The American Medical Association (AMA), which is headquartered in Chicago, Illinois, crafted and disseminated the premier edition of CPT in 1966, ten years after the debut of the prototype California Relative Value System. The original edition of CPT also included diagnostic codes.

Initially, major revisions of the CPT coding system were forestalled and a new edition of Physicians' Current Procedural Terminology was promulgated only upon intervals of several years' duration. Consequently in 1970, the AMA published CPT-2, the second edition of CPT, which surpassed by seventy percent the number of procedural entries in the first edition. CPT-3, the third edition of CPT, was released in 1973, and CPT-4, the fourth edition of CPT, was released in 1977.

Due to the rapid modifications in scientific and clinical technology and also to the swift alterations in third-party payor regulations throughout the past decades, revisions to the

TABLE 1-1

Computerized Versions of the CPT Coding System

Type	Function
CPT full procedure magnetic tape	Exact replication of CPT codes and descriptors
CPT short procedure magnetic tape	Nontechnical abridgment of CPT codes and descriptors
CPT floppy diskettes	Exact replication of, or nontechnical abridgment of, CPT codes and descriptors

CPT coding system became more extensive and therefore more frequent. The fourth edition, CPT-4, was revised four times in the span of seven years, and subsequently since 1984, the CPT manual has undergone significant updating each year. The title of the CPT manual, termed a volume, reflects the year of publication. Thus, the volume presently in use is entitled CPT-(year), and is available in a choice of a standard edition (spiral bound or soft bound), or professional edition (spiral bound or three-ring looseleaf).

Each year the AMA also publishes and circulates a soft-bound Hospital Outpatient Services version of the CPT volume. This manual is basically the standard text of CPT with the inclusion of an account of procedures reportable as ambulatory surgery, as well as annotations for endoscopic procedures and reportable radiology codes.

To reiterate, the CPT coding system is revamped and published annually by the American Medical Association. Only the most recent volume is valid for the numerous contemporary uses of the manual.

The AMA also produces the CPT coding system in four computerized formats: the CPT full procedure magnetic tape; the CPT short procedure magnetic tape; and the CPT floppy diskette with either the short description or the long description. This diskette is double sided and double density, and is available in both 3 and 1/2 inch and 5 and 1/4 inch sizes (Table 1–1). The CPT full procedure and service description tape exactly replicates the code number and narrative text contained in the CPT manual, utilizing a maximum of eighty characters on a single line. The CPT short procedure and service description tape duplicates the code number but condenses the narrative text of the CPT manual into concise statements using nontechnical laymens' terms and utilizing a maximum of twenty-eight characters on a single line. The format and content of the CPT floppy diskette is identical with either that of the CPT long or short procedure and service description tape.

VOLUME UPDATES

Scientific and clinical research continually modify the recognized diagnostic entities extant within Volume 1 and Volume 2 and the procedural entities extant within Volume 3 of ICD-9 (Table 1–2). Modifications to the coding system are proposed by various practitioners, agencies, or societies.

Principal responsibility for updating Volume 1 and Volume 2 of ICD-9 is vested with the National Center for Health Statistics. Principal responsibility for updating Volume 3 of ICD-9 is vested with the Health Care Financing Administration.

Each of these governmental departments conducts open hearings on proposed updates to the ICD-9 coding system. Upon conclusion of a formalized decision-making process, official authorized addenda to ICD-9 are released each year effective on October 1.

TABLE 1-2

ICD Coding System Updating Process

1. Suggestion (regarding diagnostic classification) is submitted to Task Force on Classification of the Council on Clinical Classifications or to the Steering Committee of the National Center for Health Statistics, or suggestion (regarding procedure classification) is submitted to the Coordination and Maintenance Committee of the Health Care Financing Administration.

2. Task Force, Steering Committee, or Coordination and Maintenance Committee agrees to review suggestion. **yes** or **no**

3. If **yes,** quarterly process of suggestion review begins.
   If **no,** process ends without further action.

4. Task Force, Steering Committee, or Coordination and Maintenance Committee reviews suggestion and formulates recommendation or decision.

5. Task Force, Steering Committee, or Coordination and Maintenance Committee approves recommendation or decision affirmatively.   **yes** or **no**

6. If **yes,** determination regarding suggestion is reflected in the forthcoming volume.
   If **no,** process ends without further action.

Codes and descriptors listed in the current CPT system are customarily in conformity with contemporary medical practice as actuated by practitioners in healthcare settings throughout the nation. Therefore, the substance and content of each CPT volume are reviewed annually for the following:

1. Procedures and services may become outmoded and obsolete;
2. Procedures and services may undergo modifications to accommodate changes in the standards for clinical patient care;
3. Procedures and services that are innovative may be developed.

Every year the American Medical Association evaluates and surveys the most recent CPT volume with the assistance of suggestions and recommendations from an Editorial Panel that convenes quarterly and is comprised of physician members from the AMA as well as physician representatives of major insurance carriers. The fourteen physician members of the CPT Editorial Panel consist of ten associates of the American Medical Association, one delegate from Blue Cross and Blue Shield, one delegate from the Health Insurance Association of America, one delegate from the Health Care Financing Administration, and one delegate from the American Hospital Association.

In addition, the collaborative endeavors of a support staff uniting ancillary personnel from within the AMA and from both the healthcare industry and the insurance industry are employed. An Advisory Committee comprised of representatives from assorted specialties of clinical practice, including seventy-six physician representatives and nine nonphysician representatives of professional healthcare associations or organizations, are consulted for pertinent and relevant advice and counsel when additions, revisions, or deletions are proposed for approval by various practitioners, associations, or organizations (Table 1-3).

Research under the auspices of the CPT Editorial Panel is conducted and guided by utilization of information from current clinical periodicals and clinical textbooks along with the AMA's Diagnostic and Therapeutic Technology Assessment Program (DATTA) as well as supplemental technology assessment panels. Outcomes of this research are appraised and discussed in open forum prior to a formal vote by the CPT Editorial Panel with respect to an

T A B L E 1–3

CPT Coding System Updating Process

1. Suggestion is submitted to CPT Editorial Panel.
2. CPT Editorial Panel agrees to review suggestion. **yes** or **no**
3. If **yes,** suggestion is fowarded to CPT Advisory Committee.
   If **no,** process ends without further action.
4. CPT Advisory Committee reviews suggestion.
5. CPT Advisory Committee recommendation is transmitted to CPT Editorial Panel.
6. CPT Editorial Panel approves recommendation. **yes** or **no**
7. If **yes,** determination regarding suggestion is reflected in the forthcoming volume.
   If **no,** process ends without further action.

addition, a revision, or a deletion to the CPT coding system. Ordinarily about three hundred topics, based on the recommendations and suggestions, are studied and deliberated by the CPT Editorial Panel within a fiscal year.

CODES AND TITLES OR DESCRIPTORS

The ICD-9 volumes encompass tabular listings of more than twenty-five thousand codes. The CPT volume comprises a sequential listing of more than eight thousand numeric codes. Each code in either the ICD-9 volumes or the CPT volume is accompanied by an explanatory narrative statement termed a "title" in ICD or a "descriptor" in CPT.

To exemplify, ICD-9 code 055.2 represents the diagnosis title *Postmeasles otitis media* and ICD-9 code 280.9 represents the diagnosis title *Iron deficiency anemia,* unspecified. The ICD-9 code 13.11 represents the procedure Intracapsular cataract extraction of lens by temporal inferior route. Likewise, the CPT code *50920* denotes the descriptor for *Closure of ureterocutaneous fistula,* and CPT code *99238* denotes the descriptor for *Hospital discharge day management.*

Each code and its associated narrative title or descriptor are characteristically self-definitive with only a solitary meaning and significance. Furthermore, each code and associated narrative title or descriptor are mutually exclusive of every other code and associated narrative title or descriptor.

Codes and titles or descriptors are used to report and account for established or potential diagnoses as well as clinical procedures and services rendered by physicians or by auxiliary healthcare professionals working subordinate to the directives of physicians within the extent permitted and allowed by state and federal laws and statutes. Thus, physician assistants and registered nurses or nurse practitioners perform some of the procedures contained in the volumes.

Studies published in nursing journals indicated and disclosed the purview or extent to which registered nurses and other non-physician practitioners including physician assistants routinely render procedures and services listed in the coding manuals. In these studies, the authors inferred or concluded that registered nurses in specialty care units frequently administer (with marginal or no supervision from a physician) procedures or services (such as cardiopulmonary resuscitation and blood or blood component transfusion) that are delineated by procedural codes and descriptors.

These nomenclature and classification systems provide an established and consistent technical language to precisely and succinctly communicate disease conditions or diagnostic and therapeutic procedures and services performed by all qualified healthcare practitioners in clinical environments. These code numbers denote and indicate diagnoses and services and thereby provide an effective and efficient mechanism for valid and reliable nationwide communication among healthcare providers (facilities and physicians). Coding systems also facilitate communication with other health industry personnel, including the employees of the approximately fifteen hundred associations and organizations that provide health insurance coverage.

The translation of verbal descriptions of diseases, injuries, health conditions, and procedures into coded numerical designations is a complex activity, and constitutes both an art and a science. To code accurately and precisely, a coder must be versed in medical terminology. Lack of knowledge of the language of medicine precludes accurate and precise coding. The task of coding was originally designed to index, for research purposes, certain clinical information contained in patient medical records. In the contemporary healthcare industry, however, greater emphasis is placed on coding as a means of financial reimbursement rather than a facilitation of research endeavors.

Data generated by coding is also utilized for healthcare planning and review of utilization patterns as well as for quality of care monitoring. To produce meaningful statistics, coding must be performed with diligent effort and concentration. Coders should not assign codes haphazardly or through guesswork. In situations of uncertainty, appropriate resources should be consulted, such as determining facts through a medical reference publication or ascertaining information from a physician.

REPORTING TO THIRD-PARTY PAYORS

Insurance carriers are designated as third-party payors, with patients comprising the first party and healthcare providers comprising the second party. Payments or reimbursement from insurance carriers are categorized as either direct or indirect. Direct insurance payments are sent from the third-party payor to the healthcare provider. Indirect insurance payments, however, are sent from the third-party payor to the patient.

In the United States, health insurance coverage is offered through many alternative plans. The plans encompass both the standard fee-for-service health insurance coverage arrangements as well as the prepaid health insurance coverage arrangements.

Through fee-for-service plan provisions or contractual agreements, the insurer pays the provider for each covered service rendered. These fee-for-service plans include individual policyholder indemnity insurance in which each singular person purchases his or her coverage from an insurance firm, and group policyholder indemnity insurance (a group healthcare plan) in which an employer or an association purchases coverage for an entire group from an insurance firm.

Through prepaid plan provisions or contractual agreements, the insurer pays the provider a fixed or predetermined sum (termed a capitation) for contingent services accessible to each person (termed a member) insured, regardless of the actual services rendered to each plan member. These prepaid plans include the health maintenance organization (HMO) in which the aggregate of services rendered to each member patient is directed by a primary care physician, the preferred provider organization (PPO) in which the services rendered to each member patient are opted from within a network of providers (physicians and facilities), and the individual practice association (IPA) in which the services rendered to each member patient are opted from among individual healthcare providers.

In the public sector of the United States, the largest third-party payor of reimbursement for healthcare services is the federal Medicare program, consisting of Medicare Part A for reimbursement of hospital and other inpatient services and Medicare Part B for reimbursement of physician and other outpatient services. Healthcare providers under an incentive agreement with Medicare are entitled participating providers; healthcare providers not under an agreement with Medicare are entitled non-participating providers.

Third-party payors in the public sector also include the state Medicaid programs of public assistance; the Civilian Health and Medical Program of the Uniformed Services (CHAMPUS); the Civilian Health and Medical Program of the Veterans Administration (CHAMPVA); and workers' compensation for job-related injuries and illnesses. Federal law mandates that each state maintain a workers' compensation fund.

In the private sector of the United States, third-party payors of reimbursement for healthcare services include not-for-profit organizations and for-profit organizations. The preeminent among such non-profit organizations is Blue Cross and Blue Shield, with its diverse variations of basic and supplemental coverage for reimbursement of hospital or other inpatient services and physician and other outpatient services. Healthcare providers who contract with Blue Cross and Blue Shield are labeled participating providers; healthcare providers who do not contract with Blue Cross and Blue Shield are labeled non-participating providers. The multitude of commercial insurance carriers are for-profit enterprises such as General American or Prudential. Employers may devise self-insurance plans to bestow coverage to their employee members without the involvement of an established insurance carrier.

Claims submitted to third-party payors for reimbursement contain confidential patient information (codes for diagnoses and procedures). Therefore, each patient (or his or her legal representative) must sign an authorization to release this information to the insurance carrier. Healthcare facilities regularly include a clause for this information release in the general consent form signed during the admitting process. Physician providers typically use a separate authorization form for the release of claims information to insurance carriers, and this authorization must be renewed at least annually to uphold its validity.

The Health Care Financing Administration, which oversees the Medicare program and most Medicaid programs of public assistance under the auspices of state governments, mandates the utilization of CPT codes and descriptors for reporting procedures and services rendered by physicians. Since 1987, HCFA and Medicare demand the utilization of CPT codes

TABLE 1–4

Utilization of Coding Systems by Healthcare Facility

Facility	Diagnostic Coding	Procedural Coding
Physician office	ICD-9-CM	CPT-4
Ambulatory care clinic	ICD-9-CM	CPT-4
Mental health clinic	DSM-IV	CPT-4
Nursing facility	ICD-9-CM	CPT-4
Outpatient hospital	ICD-9-CM	CPT-4
Acute care hospital	ICD-9-CM	ICD-9-CM
Tertiary care hospital	ICD-9-CM	ICD-9-CM
Pediatric hospital	ICD-9-CM	ICD-9-CM
Psychiatric hospital	DSM-IV	CPT-4
Tumor registry	ICD-0	
Trauma registry	ICD-9-CM	ICD-9-CM

and descriptors for all hospital outpatient surgical procedures and services including such procedures and services rendered in psychiatric hospitals and rehabilitation hospitals. Hospital inpatient procedures and services are reported with codes from Volume 3 of ICD-9-CM, a manual employed almost exclusively by hospital personnel in medical record departments and utilization review departments (Table 1–4).

A myriad of the commercial insurance carriers also require ICD-9 and CPT codes and descriptors with the submitted billing charges of practitioners and facilities, and frequently these commercial insurance carriers adapt the ICD-9 and CPT nomenclature and classification systems to their unique internal administrative rules and interpretations.

Codes represent the associated narrative descriptors, which sometimes entail complex clinical procedural terminology and may avert the task of entering these narrative descriptors on the claims forms. Consequently, the codes foster the establishment of uniformity and avail the simplification of claims submitted to governmental and commercial healthcare insurance carriers. The coding system sustains its utility for healthcare education and healthcare research, for patient care outcome analysis or reviews, for clinical quality assurance or quality improvement surveys, and for actuarial and statistical purposes.

KEY CONCEPTS

alphabetic code _____

alpha-numeric code _____

classification _____

classification system _____

clinical specialty _____

code _____

coding system _____

CPT _____

descriptor _____

diagnosis _____

digit _____

edition _____

fascicle _____

fee-for-service health insurance plan _____

group indemnity insurance _____

HCPCS _____

health maintenance organization _____

ICD _____

ICD-9-CM _____

individual indemnity insurance _____

individual practice association _____

mutual exclusion _____

narrative _____

nomenclature _____

numeric code _____

preferred provider organization _____

prepaid health insurance plan _____

procedure _____

rubric _____

service _____

symptom _____

terminology _____

third-party payor _____

title _____

trauma registry _____

tumor regisrty _____

volume _____

REVIEW EXERCISES

1. Describe numeric identifiers for persons (driver's license numbers, medical record numbers, and so forth), for places (zip codes, apartment numbers, and so on), and for things (catalog numbers for merchandise such as auto parts or office equipment). _____

_____

_____

2. Which coding system is the most extensively used in the United States at the present time to code diagnoses and symptoms? _____

_____

_____

3. What is the meaning of the word "nomenclature"? Identify nomenclature in use in occupations (as in auto mechanics or cosmetology), or in avocations (as in baseball or numismatics).

_____

_____

4. Discuss the historical evolvement of the ICD coding system. _____

_____

_____

5. Describe the differences between ICD-9 and ICD-9-CM. _____

_____

_____

6. Discuss the historical evolution of the CPT coding system. _____

_____

7. Differentiate between an edition and a volume of the ICD coding system. _____

_____

_____

8. Differentiate between an edition and a volume of the CPT coding system. _____

_____

_____

9. Describe the supplementary information imparted in the Hospital Outpatient Services version of the CPT volume. _____

_____

_____

10. Explain and detail the computerized formats of the CPT coding system. _____

_____

_____

11. Express the decision-making process entailed in implementation of additions, revisions, or deletions to the ICD coding system. _____

_____

_____

12. Express the decision-making process entailed in implementation of additions, revisions, or deletions to the CPT coding system. _____

_____

_____

13. Define "mutually exclusive" and demonstrate the significance of this term in a classification system. _____

_____

_____

14. Clarify the distinction between fee-for-service health insurance plans and prepaid health insurance plans. _____

_____

_____

15. State the pre-eminent third-party payors in the public sector and the pre-eminent third-party payors in the private sector at the present time in the United States. _____

_____

_____

16. Explain the fundamental utility of each volume of the ICD-9 coding system. _____

_____

_____

17. Clarify which nomenclature and classification systems are utilized to code procedures in the hospital setting. Distinguish between systems in use for hospital procedural coding and those in use for office or clinic procedural coding. _____

_____

_____

18. Discuss the utility of the HCPCS coding system. _____

_____

_____

19. Identify major users of data generated by both the ICD coding system and the CPT coding system. _____

_____

_____

20. How and why do the ICD coding system and the CPT coding system enable and facilitate a means of communication among healthcare practitioners and healthcare providers? _____

_____

_____

21. Do the bureaucratic regulations of the Health Care Financing Administration impact the usage of either the ICD coding system or the CPT coding system? What effect did HCFA produce on the utility of the ICD coding system and the CPT coding system? _____

_____

_____

22. Does interpretation of coding policies and procedures vary among third-party payors? Do insurance carriers vary with respect to implementation of regulations about coding? Discuss situations in which billing problems affect or impact the utility of the ICD coding system and the CPT coding system. _____

_____

_____

2 CHAPTER

Format and Content of the ICD-9 Coding System

LEARNING OBJECTIVES

Upon completion of this chapter the learner should be able to:

1. Explain the basic format of ICD-9.
2. Describe the fundamental hierarchy within the ICD-9 coding system.
3. Discuss the association between the common segment of a narrative title and subsequent listings.
4. Explain and interpret the abbreviations among the listings of the ICD-9 coding system.
5. Explain and interpret the symbols (including punctuation) among the listings of the ICD-9 coding system.
6. Define the concept of a modifier in ICD-9.
7. Discuss the usefulness of modifiers within the ICD-9 coding system.
8. Express the potential variations in the format of modifiers.
9. Distinguish between essential modifiers and nonessential modifiers in the ICD-9 coding system.
10. Explain and interpret the types of instructional notations used in the ICD-9 coding system.
11. Explain and interpret the types of cross-references used in the ICD-9 coding system.
12. Report upon the similarities and dissimilarities among the various sections of the ICD-9 coding system.
13. State the content of each of the appendices in the ICD-9 volumes.
14. Discuss the utility, the format, and the content of the guidelines and instructional notations in the ICD-9 volumes.
15. Demonstrate knowledge of the proper index search sequence by correctly assigning code numbers from the ICD-9 volumes for narrative statements of procedures and services.
16. Describe and discuss the process of selection of a principal diagnosis.
17. Describe and discuss the process of selection of a principal procedure.

ORGANIZATION OF ICD-9

The <u>International Classification of Diseases</u> (ICD-9) is maintained by the World Health Organization. In the United States, this coding system is adapted by the National Center for Health Statistics and the Health Care Financing Administration. The consequent adaptation, the clinically modified edition, ICD-9-CM, is disseminated annually from the United States Government Printing Office (GPO).

Volume 1 of ICD-9-CM is comprised of a lengthy and comprehensive Classification of Diseases and Injuries, and two supplementary classifications, the Classification of Factors Influencing Health Status and Contact with Health Service and the Classification of External Causes of Injury and Poisoning. Volume 2 of ICD-9-CM is comprised of alphabetical indices as well as specialized tabular indices to the listings contained within each of the classifications in Volume 1.

Five appendices also are incorporated into the generic Volume 1 of ICD-9-CM that emanates from the GPO. These appendices are: Appendix A, the Morphology of Neoplasms; Appendix B, the Glossary of Mental Disorders; Appendix C, the Classification of Drugs by American Hospital Formulary Service List Number and Their ICD-9-CM Equivalents; Appendix D, the Classification of Industrial Accidents According to Agency; and Appendix E, the List of Three-Digit Categories.

Several of the United States commercial publishers of ICD-9-CM modify the sequence of these appendices. Certain editions among these adaptations of ICD-9-CM augment Volume 1 with additional appendices. These supplementary appendices do not affect code and title selection, but instead, the supplements contain data such as complications and comorbidities or unacceptable diagnoses that impact reimbursement under the Medicare prospective payment system.

Distinctive editions released by commercial publishers of ICD-9-CM incorporate information from the appendices into the Classification of Diseases and Injuries. Additional innovations found among certain of these publications include anatomical diagrams and bibliographical references to enhance comprehension and understanding of the classification, as well as unique color schemes to indicate the reimbursement potential inherent in various entities.

Volume 1 of ICD-9-CM contains a table of contents and an introduction. The introduction section presents general explanations and directions concerning the format and content of this volume as well as several broad guidelines for its utilization. Brief and condensed instructions regarding the abbreviations and symbols used in ICD-9-CM are also stated in the introduction.

The main tabular portion of Volume 1, the Classification of Diseases and Injuries, is comprised of sequential numerical listings of code numbers and narrative titles for a multitude of diagnoses. Not all three-digit categories are used in the ICD-9-CM diagnostic classification; gaps exist both within and between several of these category ranges. This tabular listing is divided into seventeen chapters with the following ranges of categories and codes:

1. Infectious and Parasitic Diseases (category range 001–139; code range 001.0–139.8)
2. Neoplasms (category range 140–239; code range 140.0–239.9)
3. Endocrine, Nutritional, and Metabolic Diseases, and Immunity Disorders (category range 240–279; code range 240.0–279.9)
4. Diseases of the Blood and Blood-Forming Organs (category range 280–289; code range 280.0–289.9)
5. Mental Disorders (category range 290–319; code range 290.0–319)

6. Diseases of the Nervous System and Sense Organs (category range 320–389; code range 320.0–389.9)

7. Diseases of the Circulatory System (category range 390–459; code range 390–459.9)

8. Diseases of the Respiratory System (category range 460–519; code range 460–519.9)

9. Diseases of the Digestive System (category range 520–579; code range 520.0–579.9)

10. Diseases of the Genitourinary System (category range 580–629; code range 580.0–629.9)

11. Complications of Pregnancy, Childbirth, and the Puerperium (category range 630–677; code range 630–677)

12. Diseases of the Skin and Subcutaneous Tissue (category range 680–709; code range 680.0–709.9)

13. Diseases of the Musculoskeletal System and Connective Tissue (category range 710–739; code range 710.0–739.9)

14. Congenital Anomalies (category range 740–759; code range 740.0–759.9)

15. Certain Conditions Originating in the Perinatal Period (category range 760–779; code range 760.0–779.9)

16. Symptoms, Signs, and Ill-Defined Conditions (category range 780–799; code range 780.01–799.9)

17. Injury and Poisoning (category range 800–899; code range 800.00–999.9)

Within most of these seventeen chapters (which are discussed in more detail in subsequent pages), a framework of sections is devised with section headings that generally are either anatomic terms (such as Disorders of the Eye and Adnexa 360–379) or diagnostic terms (such as Arthropathies and Related Disorders 710–719). Throughout Volume 1, each chapter heading is identified with all uppercase letters and boldface type, and each section heading is identified in all uppercase letters and normal typeface.

Certain sections in several chapters of Volume 1 are partitioned into subsections (for instance, Chapter 5 is divided into subsections). The sections and subsections are comprised of three-digit categories. Category titles are printed in boldface type and are usually titled with either anatomic terms (such as category *527, Diseases of the salivary glands,* and category *743, Congenital anomalies of eye*); or with diagnostic terms (such as category *426, Conduction disorders,* and category *653, Disproportion*).

Most categories encompass several subcategories. These subcategories are indented beneath the categories and are also printed in boldface type. Subcategories are ordinarily titled with either anatomic terms (such as subcategory *151.1, Pylorus,* and subcategory *682.5, Buttock*), or with diagnostic terms (such as subcategory *373.11, Hordeolum externum,* and subcategory *787.4, Visible peristalsis*).

Volume 3 of ICD-9 encompasses both the tabular list and the alphabetic index for diagnostic and therapeutic operations, procedures, and services. Unlike the diagnostic classification of ICD-9, the tabular list and alphabetic index are unified into one volume. Location of the tabular list precedes the alphabetic index in the generic edition of ICD-9-CM, but is reversed in the editions of certain commercial publishers.

The ICD-9 procedure classification was developed from a modification of Fascicle V entitled "Surgical Procedures," of the former ICD Classification of Procedures in Medicine, which was promulgated by the World Health Organization. All three-digit rubrics in the category range 01–86 are maintained as they appear in Fascicle V to the extent feasible. Nonsurgical procedures are segregated from the surgical procedures and confined to category rubrics 87–99 to the extent feasible. Selected detail contained in the remaining fascicles of the ICD Classification of Procedures in Medicine was accommodated wherever possible, but compatibility was not maintained whenever a different axis was deemed more clinically appropriate.

The structure of the ICD-9-CM procedure classification is based upon anatomy rather than surgical specialty (unlike the CPT coding system which is based on surgical specialty). The codes in the procedure classification of ICD-9-CM are strictly numeric; no alphabetic characters are utilized. The procedure classification is developed with a two-digit structure with one decimal digit and often two decimal digits placed where necessary.

The main tabular portion of Volume 3, the Procedure Classification, contains sequential numerical listings of numerous procedures and services. For no apparent reason, category 17 is the only two-digit category that is not utilized in the ICD-9-CM procedural classification. The procedural tabular is divided into sixteen chapters with the following ranges of categories and codes:

1. Operations on the Nervous System (category range 01–05; code range 01.01–05.9)
2. Operations on the Endocrine System (category range 06–07; code range 06.01–07.99)
3. Operations on the Eye (category range 08–16; code range 08.01–16.99)
4. Operations on the Ear (category range 18–20; code range 18.01–20.99)
5. Operations on the Nose, Mouth, and Pharynx (category range 21–29; code range 21.00–29.99)
6. Operations on the Respiratory System (category range 30–34; code range 30.01–34.99)
7. Operations on the Cardiovascular System (category range 35–39; code range 35.00–39.99)
8. Operations on the Hemic and Lymphatic System (category range 40–41; code range 40.0–41.99)
9. Operations on the Digestive System (category range 42–54; code range 42.01–54.99)
10. Operations on the Urinary System (category range 55–59; code range 55.01–59.99)
11. Operations on the Male Genital Organs (category range 60–64; code range 60.0–64.99)
12. Operations on the Female Genital Organs (category range 65–71; code range 65.01–71.99)
13. Obstetrical Procedures (category range 72–75; code range 72.0–75.99)
14. Operations on the Musculoskeletal System (category range 76–84; code range 76.01–84.99)
15. Operations on the Integumentary System (category range 85–86; code range 85.0–86.99)
16. Miscellaneous Diagnostic and Therapeutic Procedures (category range 87–99; code range 87.01–99.99)

Within these sixteen chapters (which are discussed in more detail in subsequent pages), there is no subdivision into sections. The chapter headings are printed in boldface type in all uppercase letters. A framework of categories and subcategories comprises the hierarchical structure of the individual chapters of Volume 3 in similar format to that of Volume 1.

The category titles in Volume 3 are printed in boldface type and are usually titled with either anatomic terms (such as category *29, Operations on pharynx,* and category *77, Incision, excision, and division of other bones*); with diagnostic terms (such as category *79, Reduction of fracture and dislocation*); or with procedural terms (such as category *72, Forceps, vacuum, and breech delivery,* and category *92, Nuclear medicine*).

The subcategories in Volume 3 are indented beneath the categories and are also printed in boldface type. Subcategories are ordinarily titled with either anatomic terms (such as subcategory *25.0, Diagnostic procedures on tongue,* and subcategory *60.7, Operations on seminal vesicles*); with diagnostic terms (such as subcategory *21.0, Control of epistaxis,* and subcategory *58.5, Release of urethral stricture*); or with procedural terms (such as subcategory *31.2, Permanent tracheostomy,* and subcategory *97.0, Nonoperative replacement of gastrointestinal appliance*).

HIERARCHY AND STRUCTURE OF ICD-9

The overwhelming abundance of codes and narrative titles listed in the volumes of ICD-9-CM are validated and supported by a format of guidelines, notations, and symbols. The comprehensive ICD-9-CM classification follows a definite hierarchical structure comprised of five levels for diagnostic entities and four levels for procedural entities (Table 2–1 and Table 2–2). These levels, placed in descending order of size and scope, are the previously discussed chapters, sections (and subsections), three-digit categories, four-digit subcategories, and five-digit listings.

The most complete listings are the individually distinctive five-digit codes and narrative titles that constitute the lowest level of the ICD-9-CM hierarchy. Nonetheless, not every code and narrative title can be identified with five distinct levels of the hierarchy of the ICD-9-CM coding system. Many codes and narrative titles are presented in their entirety at the subcategory level, and a few are presented in their entirety even at the category level.

For example, subcategory *276.8, Hypokalemia,* and subcategory *564.0, Constipation,* are complete at the fourth hierarchical level, the lowest level for those entities. Three-digit category *600, Benign prostatic hypertrophy,* and three-digit category *267, Ascorbic acid deficiency,* are complete at the third hierarchical level, which in these instances is not further subdivided. Therefore, certain three-digit categories comprise a fully accurate and precise code and narrative title at merely the third level in the hierarchical structure of ICD-9-CM.

This hierarchical structure maintained in the ICD-9-CM volumes can also be explained in an increasing order of size and scope. For example, in Volume 1, the specific five-digit code and narrative title listing *692.71, Sunburn,* is included within subcategory *692.7, Due to solar radiation.* This subcategory, *Due to solar radiation,* is included within category *692, Contact dermatitis and other eczema.* This category, *Contact dermatitis and other eczema,* is contained

TABLE 2–1

Hierarchical Structure of the ICD-9 Diagnostic Tabular

Chapter
Section
Category
Subcategory
Listing

TABLE 2–2

Hierarchical Structure of the ICD-9 Procedural Tabular

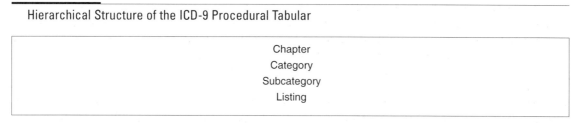

Chapter
Category
Subcategory
Listing

with the section entitled, Other Inflammatory Conditions of Skin and Subcutaneous Tissue. And finally, the section, Other Inflammatory Conditions of Skin and Subcutaneous Tissue, is contained within the chapter, Diseases of the Skin and Subcutaneous Tissue.

The most complete listings are the individually distinctive five-digit codes and narrative titles that constitute the lowest level of the ICD-9-CM hierarchy. Nonetheless, not every code and narrative title can be identified with five distinct levels of the hierarchy of the ICD-9-CM coding system. Many codes and narrative titles are presented in their entirety at the subcategory level, and a few are presented in their entirety even at the category level.

For example, subcategory *276.8, Hypokalemia,* and subcategory *564.0, Constipation,* are complete at the fourth hierarchical level, the lowest level for those entities. Three-digit category *600, Benign prostatic hypertrophy,* and three-digit category *267, Ascorbic acid deficiency,* are complete at the third hierarchical level, which in these instances is not further subdivided. Therefore, certain three-digit categories comprise a fully accurate and precise code and narrative title at merely the third level in the hierarchical structure of ICD-9-CM.

Exclusive listing of an individual diagnosis or service in a specific chapter or section of an ICD-9-CM volume does not restrict, limit, or confine its use to any specific type of facility or specialty group of physicians. Any designated facility or qualified physician practice, regardless of specialty, may report diagnoses and services rendered with applicable codes and narrative titles located anywhere within the ICD-9-CM volumes. For example, code *173.1, Malignant neoplasm of skin of eyelid,* might be reported by an oncologist, a dermatologist, or an ophthalmologist.

The primary bulk of the ICD-9-CM diagnostic tabular volume, the seventeen chapters, encompasses thousands upon thousands of listings of individual codes and narrative titles, presented in serial or sequential numeric order. Several chapters of Volume 1 (such as Chapter 1 and Chapter 17) are very extensive and encompass many entities. Other chapters (such as Chapter 4 and Chapter 15) are more circumscribed and narrower in scope.

Each section within the chapters of the ICD-9-CM diagnostic tabular volume is divided into categories arranged accordingly by etiology (causation) or by topography (site). Subcategories likewise are normally partitioned into listings organized and classified either by etiology or by topography.

Sequentially, the last subcategories (within a category) are residuals reserved for other related diagnoses not specifically classified or for vague and nonspecific diagnoses. For instance, subcategory *111.8, Other specified dermatomycoses,* and subcategory *568.9, Unspecified disorder of peritoneum,* exemplify residual subcategories.

The preponderance of listings in the ICD-9-CM volumes are self-contained and do not directly correspond with any specific prior or following listing in the classification. However, certain listings in the ICD-9-CM volumes maintain an established format in which a portion of the narrative title of the category relates and connects with subsequent narrative titles of subcategories.

Instead of reiterating repetitious and redundant information within categories or sub-categories of codes and narrative title listings, the narrative title listed within that group contains a common narrative expression (the part of the title that is not repeated) and this part of the narrative title is implicitly implied for the remaining subcategories. Code numbers and narrative titles listed below that listing understandably refer back to the common narrative expression for each of these dependent or subordinate narrative titles of subcategories. As examples, the clinical diagnosis represented by code *534.01, Acute with hemorrhage with obstruction,* is actually, *Gastrojejunal ulcer, acute with hemorrhage with obstruction,* and the clinical diagnosis represented by code *551.03, Bilateral, recurrent,* is actually, *Femoral hernia with gangrene, bilateral, recurrent.*

Volume 3 procedure listings, however, generally repeat the applicable portion of the category title within the subcategory title. As examples, the clinical procedure represented by code *22.02, Aspiration or lavage of nasal sinus through natural ostium,* is contained in subcategory *22.0, Aspiration and lavage of nasal sinus;* and the clinical procedure represented by code *76.74, Open reduction of maxillary fracture,* is contained in subcategory *76.7, Reduction of facial fracture.*

In several isolated instances, the diagnostic tabular of Volume 1 also follows this format. Note the title in the listing for code *375.21, Epiphora due to excess lacrimation.* The subcategory title in this example is merely, *Epiphora.*

Thus, all of the narrative descriptors for diagnoses, services, and procedures listed in the diagnostic tabular listings of the ICD-9-CM coding system are not necessarily printed in entirety. Instead, certain indented narrative titles refer to the aforementioned common narrative expression of the category title or subcategory title listed prior to the series of indented listings. Terminology in the indented diagnostic narrative title listing always assumes or warrants a subordinate position or status to the title listing at the next higher level in the structure of the coding system.

Conversely, this format is not generally adhered to in the tabular list for procedures. Listings within the subcategories contain titles more specific than the subcategory title. Nonetheless, terminology in the indented procedural narrative title still assumes or warrants a subordinate position or status to the title listing at the next higher level in the structure of the coding system.

ABBREVIATIONS IN ICD-9

Abbreviations, symbols, and other notations are sometimes referred to by the term "conventions." Two abbreviations are frequently utilized in ICD-9-CM: NEC for "not elsewhere classifiable," and NOS for "not otherwise specified" (Table 2–3).

"Not Elsewhere Classifiable," abbreviated as NEC, is used for two purposes that can only be distinguished by reference to the tabular listings in Volume 1. The first purpose is a warning that specified forms of the condition are classified differently when vaguely

T A B L E 2–3

Abbreviations Used in the ICD-9 Coding System

Abbreviation	Message
NEC	Not elsewhere classifiable (used for other entities)
NOS	Not otherwise specified (used for unspecified entities)

defined terms are stated in the documentation. The codes provided for such ambiguous terms should be used only if more precise information is not available. Note the subterm "leg NEC" under the index entry "Inflammation . . . ," and the subterm "in intestine NEC" under the index entry, "Worm."

The second purpose of the NEC abbreviation is to facilitate code assignment with explicitly stated terms for which a more specific category is not provided in the tabular listings of Volume 1. In such instances, no amount of additional information will alter the selection of the code, simply because the existing classification system was not designed to accommodate such specificity.

The abbreviation NEC guides the coder in situations where patient care documentation indicated a condition not specifically mentioned in the index and not specifically classified in the tabular. The coder is warned and alerted by this abbreviation to search for specified index entries that may be differently classified. However, for many vague and ambiguous terms, as well as for many innovative and unique terms, a definitive classification is not provided in the tabular list. Thus, additional information does not alter the selection and assignment of the code.

The NEC convention is a feature of the alphabetic index, such as demonstrated in entries for: "Fasciitis, traumatic NEC" or "Lactation, mastitis NEC," and "Histoplasmosis, American, with specified manifestation NEC." In the latter example, the NEC abbreviation is utilized only if specific classification is possible with the listed subterms "with endocarditis," "with meningitis," "with pericarditis," "with pneumonia," or with "retinitis."

The abbreviation NOS guides the coder in situations where patient care documentation indicated a condition lacking enough specificity and detail to be classified in the existing structure of a particular portion of the coding system. The NOS convention is a feature of the tabular list, such as exemplified in entries for *389.9 Unspecified hearing loss* (subtitled: *Deafness NOS*) and *698.9 Unspecified pruritic disorder* (subtitled: *Itch NOS,* Pruritus NOS).

These abbreviations are utilized in the alphabetic index to Volume 3 of ICD-9-CM. NEC, or not elsewhere classifiable, appears frequently. The code number for the term including NEC is to be reported only when the coder lacks the information necessary to code the term to a more specific category. For instance, the index entries "Application . . . cast 93.53", "Repair liver NEC 50.69," and "Irrigation, trachea," exemplify the Volume 3 usage of this convention with nonspecific documentation.

NOS or not otherwise specified, as an abbreviation is the equivalent of "unspecified." Examples of this abbreviation in the tabular list of Volume 3 are found under subcategory *51.04, Other cholecystotomy,* in the entry, "Cholelithotomy NOS" and under subcategory *85.54, Bilateral breast implant,* in the entry "Breast implant NOS."

SYMBOLS IN ICD-9

A symbol is a conventional printed sign that represents a quantity or quality. Classification systems, including ICD-9-CM, CPT, and HCPCS, customarily use symbols to signify certain characteristics or attributes pertaining to particular codes. ICD-9-CM symbolizes attributes and characteristics with symbols commonly used in grammatical punctuation. Six symbols—brackets, parentheses, braces, the colon, the lozenge, and the section mark—appear throughout the listings of the ICD-9-CM volumes (Table 2–4).

Brackets [ ] are used to enclose synonyms, alternative terms, or explanatory phrases. To exemplify, category title *120, Schistosomiasis,* is followed by the alternative term [bilharziasis] in brackets, and the entry under listing *747.41, Total anomalous pulmonary venous return,* is followed by the synonymous abbreviation [TAPVR] in brackets.

TABLE 2–4

Symbols Used in the ICD-9 Coding System

Symbol	Message
Brackets [ ]	Synonyms, alternative wordings, and explanatory phrases.
Parentheses ( )	Supplementary words that do not affect code assignment.
Colon :	Incomplete term which needs modification.
Braces { }	Enclose a series of terms that is modified by the statement appearing at the right of the brace.
Lozenge ⌑	Denotes a four-digit rubric that is unique to ICD-9-CM (as compared with ICD-9).
Section Mark §	Denotes the placement of a footnote which applies to all subdivisions in that code range.

Parentheses ( ) are used to enclose supplementary words that may be present or absent in the statement of a disease or in the statement of a procedure without affecting the code number assignment. As examples, the first entry under subcategory *421.0, Endocarditis (acute) (chronic) (subacute),* contains three parenthetical expressions, and subcategory *680.0* utilizes both brackets and parentheses in the entry, *Ear [any part], Face [any part, except eye], Nose (septum), Temple (region).*

In the alphabetic index, parentheses serve a similar function. Note the parenthetical expressions following the index entry "Examination." That term is followed by four words each enclosed in parentheses: (general); (routine); (of); and (for). To further exemplify, note the terms in parentheses following the index entry "Myotonia"; the terms (acquisita) and (intermittens) are enclosed within parentheses.

The colon : is used in the tabular list of Volume 1 after an incomplete term that needs one or more of the modifiers that follow in order to facilitate code assignment to a specific category. Subcategory *257.1, Postablative testicular hypofunction,* contains the entry, Testicular hypofunction: iatrogenic, postirradiation, postsurgical. Subcategory *596.8, Other specified disorders of bladder,* contains two entries with colons, Bladder: calcified, contracted, and Bladder: hemorrhage, hypertrophy, and listing *786.52, Painful respiration,* contains the entry Pain: anterior chest wall, pleuritic.

Braces { } are used in Volume 1 to enclose a series of terms, each of which is modified by the statement appearing at the right of the brace. Subcategory *230.2, Stomach,* contains the entry, Body, Cardia, Fundus} of stomach, and subcategory *429.0, Myocarditis, unspecified,* contains the entry, Myocarditis: NOS, chronic (interstitial), fibroid, senile} (with mention of arteriosclerosis). Subcategory *642.0, Benign essential hypertension complicating pregnancy, childbirth, and the puerperium,* contains the entry, Hypertension: benign essential, chronic NOS, essential, pre-existing NOS} specified as complicating, or as a reason for obstetric care during pregnancy, childbirth, or the puerperium. Note that in the second of these three examples, the conventions of colon and parentheses were also utilized. The second and third examples also encompassed the abbreviation NOS.

The lozenge symbol ⌑ printed in the left margin of the tabular preceding the diagnostic code denotes a four-digit rubric unique to ICD-9-CM. The contents of these rubrics are not the same as those in ICD-9. The lozenge symbol is used only in Volume 1. Examples of the use of the lozenge are: ⌑ *250.2, Diabetes with hyperosmolarity,* ⌑ *296.0, Manic disorder, single episode,* and ⌑ *312.2, Socialized conduct disorder.* Fifteen three-digit categories contain subcategories that are denoted by the lozenge. Those categories are:

013	800
015	801
016	803
017	804
250	813
296	823
312	851
	852

The section mark symbol § preceding a code denotes the placement of a footnote at the bottom of the page. Information in that footnote is applicable to all subdivisions in that category or subcategory. Examples of the use of the section mark are in category *§342 Hemiplegia and hemiparesis,* and in category *§666 Postpartum hemorrhage.* One hundred and sixty-nine three-digit categories in Volume 1 are denoted by this symbol. The categories denoted with a section mark are:

010	312	645	672	814	E800	E824
011	342	646	673	815	E801	E825
012	345	647	674	816	E802	E826
013	346	648	675	823	E803	E827
014	403	651	676	831	E804	E828
015	404	652	711	832	E805	E829
016	410	653	712	833	E806	E830
017	433	654	715	834	E807	E831
200	434	655	716	835	E810	E832
201	531	656	718	838	E811	E833
202	532	657	719	851	E812	E834
203	533	658	730	852	E813	E835
204	534	659	741	853	E814	E836
205	535	660	764	854	E815	E837
206	550	661	765	864	E816	E838
207	574	662	789	865	E817	E839
208	634	663	800	866	E818	E840
242	635	664	801	868	E819	E841
250	636	665	802	881	E820	E842
295	637	666	803	941	E821	E843
296	640	667	804	942	E822	E844
299	641	668	805	943	E823	E845
303	642	669	807	944		
304	643	670	810	945		
305	644	671	811	948		

Similar punctuation is utilized as symbols in Volume 3 of ICD-9-CM. These symbols include brackets, parentheses, colons, braces, and the section mark.

Brackets [ ] are used to enclose synonyms, alternative wordings, or explanatory phrases. Listing *41.32* in the tabular list of Volume 3, *Closed [aspiration] [percutaneous] biopsy of spleen,* and listing *95.24, Electronystagmogram [ENG]* exemplify the use of this convention.

Parentheses ( ) are used to enclose supplementary words that may be present or absent in the statement of a procedure without affecting code number selection or assignment. For instance, the second example under listing *22.42, Obliteration of frontal sinus (with fat),* encloses the last two words in a parenthetical expression, but these two modifying words do not affect code number selection or assignment.

The entries in the alphabetic index to Volume 3 frequently include parenthetical expressions. Note for example, the index entry, "Curettage," which is followed by parenthetical expressions (with packing) and (with secondary closure). Such parenthetical expressions modify the entry but do not affect code number selection or assignment.

Colons : are used in the tabular list of Volume 3 after an incomplete term that needs to be augmented by one or more of the modifiers that follow, in order to ascertain assignment to a designated category. To exemplify, listing *33.42, Closure of bronchial fistula,* contains the entry, "Fistulectomy: bronchocutaneous, bronchoesophageal, bronchovisceral." Likewise, subcategory *53.9, Other hernia repair,* contains the entry, "Repair of hernia: ischiatic, ischiorectal, lumbar, obturator, omental, retroperitoneal, sciatic."

Braces { } are used to include a series of terms, each of which is modified by the statement appearing at the right of the brace. As examples, under subcategory *56.0, Transurethral removal of obstruction from ureter and renal pelvis,* is the entry, Removal of: blood clot, calculus, foreign body} from ureter or renal pelvis without incision. Under subcategory *99.1, Injection or infusion of therapeutic or prophylactic substance,* is the inclusion note, Includes injection or infusion given: hypodermically, intramuscularly, intravenously} acting locally or systemically. Notice in these examples the usage of other symbols; the colon is used in both, and the latter example comprises an inclusion note (a convention discussed in the next section of this chapter).

The section mark symbol § is used in Volume 3 of ICD-9-CM. The section mark symbol preceding a category number denotes the placement of a footnote at the bottom of the page. Information in that footnote is applicable to each subcategory indicated. Subcategory *78.0, Bone graft,* is denoted with a section mark that refers to the explanatory footnote at the bottom of the page. Fifty-one subcategories in Volume 3 are denoted by this symbol. The subcategories denoted with a section mark are:

38.0	77.0	78.0	79.0	80.0	90.0
38.1	77.1	78.1	79.1	80.1	90.1
38.3	77.2	78.2	79.2	80.2	91.1
38.5	77.3	78.3	79.3	80.3	91.2
38.6	77.4	78.4	79.4	80.4	91.3
38.8	77.6	78.5	79.5	80.7	91.4
	77.7	78.6	79.6	80.8	91.5
	77.8	78.7		80.9	91.6
	77.9	78.8			91.7
		78.9			91.8
					91.9

INSTRUCTIONAL NOTATIONS IN ICD-9

Four instructional notations are frequently utilized in ICD-9-CM. These are: "includes"; "excludes"; "use additional code, if desired"; and "code also underlying disease" (Table 2–5).

TABLE 2-5

Instructional Notations Used in the ICD-9 Coding System

Notation	Message
includes	Encompasses the listed entities within the grouping at that level of the hierarchy.
excludes	Refers code selection to another portion of the classification system.
use additional code	Directs the assignment of another code to supplement and further specify the reported entity.
code also	Directs the assignment of codes to report other components of an entity.

The "includes" notation may appear below a section title, as indicated by, Organic Psychotic Conditions 290–294, Includes: psychotic organic brain syndrome; or this notation may appear below a category title, as indicated under category *676*, Includes: the listed condition during pregnancy, the puerperium, or lactation. The "includes" notation further defines the title or exemplifies the contents of the entity at that level by providing synonyms or variants for the entity described by the title associated with that heading or listing.

The "excludes" notation also may appear: below a chapter title, such as that under the title of Chapter 3; below a section title, as indicated under, Other Diseases of Skin and Subcutaneous Tissue 700–709; below a category title, such as the exclusion note indicated under category *368, Visual disturbances;* below a subcategory title, such as the exclusion note below the entries in subcategory *521.7;* or below the title of an individual listing, such as that below the listing for code number *825.29*.

The "excludes" notation directs the coder to another portion of the classification if certain specified entities are to be coded. For instance, in the last example of the preceding paragraph, this exclusion note refers the coder to the subcategory listing *825.0*.

Italicized typeface is used for all exclusion notes. This italicization should not be confused, however, with the italicizing utilized to identify those rubrics that should not be used for primary tabulations of disease.

The "use additional code, if desired" notation actually translates to "use additional code." This notation implies that an additional code should be selected in order to fully report the diagnostic condition or the procedural service. The notation to "use additional code" also directs the assignment of a code to identify a manifestation.

Location and placement of this instructional notation vary. Note for example the use of this convention under category title *331, Other cerebral degenerations*. The instructional notation directs the coder to use an additional code to report any associated mental disorder. Likewise, under category title *506, Respiratory conditions due to chemical fumes and vapors,* the coder is directed to use an E code to report the external cause of the respiratory condition.

The "code also underlying disease" notation, used only in the tabular list of Volume 1, implies that another code should be selected for primary reporting of the disease. With this notation, the code and its associated title appear in italics, and represent a manifestation of an underlying disease condition.

The underlying disease condition should be sequenced first and the manifestation should be sequenced afterwards. As examples, subcategory title *359.5, Myopathy in endocrine diseases classified elsewhere,* is followed by a direction to code the underlying disease, and the same notation is utilized in subcategory *711.3, Postdysenteric arthropathy*.

The fifty-one following diagnostic categories contain one or more italicized codes and titles:

320	372	590
321	373	595
323	376	598
330	420	601
331	421	604
334	422	608
336	424	616
337	456	628
357	484	711
358	516	712
359	517	713
362	567	720
364	573	727
365	580	730
366	581	731
370	582	737
371	583	774

Several instructional notations appear in Volume 3 of ICD-9-CM. The notation of "includes:" appears immediately under a two-digit category title or a three-digit subcategory title to further define, or to present examples of, the contents of that category or subcategory. To exemplify, an inclusion note appears under category title *06, Operations on thyroid and parathyroid glands,* and an inclusion note appears under subcategory title *86.6, Free skin graft.*

The notation of "excludes:" appears at various levels in the classification and indicates entities to be coded and reported elsewhere as indicated in each situation. An exclusion note appears under the two-digit category title *12, Operations on iris, ciliary body, sclera, and anterior chamber,* under the three-digit subcategory title *54.0, Incision of abdominal wall,* and an inclusion note appears under the four-digit listing *35.62, Repair of ventricular septal defect with tissue graft.*

The notation "code also:" appears in the tabular list for two purposes. This notation serves as an instruction to code each component of a procedure when these components are accomplished in the same session. For example, "code also anastomosis other than end-to-end," indicated under subcategory *56.4,* and "code also any mention of external fixator device . . . ," indicated under category *79,* direct the selection and assignment of an additional code.

This instruction, "code also," appears as a notice to code the use of special adjunctive procedures or equipment. For example, "code also cardiopulmonary bypass . . . ," denoted under category *35,* and "code also any associated forceps extraction," denoted under subcategory *72.4,* direct the selection and assignment of an additional code.

CROSS-REFERENCES IN ICD-9

Cross-references direct the coder to review additional information and provide the coder with possible modifiers for a term or its synonyms. There are three types of cross-references used in the alphabetic index: "see," "see also," and "see category" (Table 2–6).

The cross-reference "see" is an explicit direction to look elsewhere, and is utilized primarily with synonyms, eponyms, and abbreviations. This convention is frequently used in

TABLE 2–6

Cross-References Used in the ICD-9 Coding System

Cross-Reference	Message
see	Direction to search elsewhere in the index.
see also	Direction to first search under that main term entry and then to search elsewhere in the index.
see category	Direction to search in the tabular list.

reference to anatomical sites, and for direction with many general adjectival modifiers not normally used in the alphabetic index.

As a cross-reference, "see" guides reference to the appropriate main term, under which is located all modifying information concerning that entity. To exemplify, under the main term index entry, "Neuritis" is the subterm, "general" with the cross-reference "see Polyneuropathy" and under the main term index entry "Choledocholith" is the cross-reference "see Choledocholithiasis" referring to the sucessive main term entry.

The cross-reference "see also" directs the coder to look under another main term if all the modifying information that is sought cannot be located by searching under the main term entry and its subterms. For example, under the main term index entry, "Pressure," appears the subterm "area, skin ulcer," followed the cross reference (see also Decubitus). And likewise, the main term index entry "Mouse, joint" is followed by the cross-reference (see also Loose, body, joint).

The cross-reference "see category" directs the coder to Volume 1 for important information governing the use of the specific code in the entry. For example, the index entry "Syringomyelitis, late effect, see category 326," guides code selection and assignment to a specific category of the tabular list of Volume 1.

Cross-references also provide the coder with possible modifiers for a procedural term or its synonyms. There are three types of cross-references used in Volume 3, cross-references identical to those used with the diagnostic classification.

The cross-reference "see" is an explicit direction to look elsewhere. This notation is used with terms that do not define the type of procedure performed. To exemplify, the main term "Kineplasty" is followed by the cross-reference "see Cineplasty."

The cross-reference "see also" directs the coder to search under another main term if all of the information sought cannot be located under the first main term entry. For instance, the main term "Excision" is followed by numerous subterms including "aneurysm (arteriovenous)." The cross-reference notation after this entry directs the coder to "see also Aneurysmectomy."

The cross-reference "see category" directs the coder to the tabular list for further information or specific site references. For example, the index entry "Apheresis, therapeutic, see category 99.7" guides code selection and assignment to a specific category (technically a specific subcategory) of the tabular list of Volume 3.

The alphabetic index for diseases and the alphabetic index for procedures are organized by main terms printed in boldface type and are followed for ease of reference by indented subterms printed in normal type. In the first section of the alphabetic index for diseases, the main terms usually identify disease conditions such as "Empyema," or "Splenomegaly." However, there are several exceptions to this general rule. Obstetric conditions are found under "Delivery," "Pregnancy," and "Puerperal." Complications of medical care and complications from surgical procedure are indexed under "Complications." Late effects of diseases and injuries are found under the entry "Late effects." The V Codes from the Supplementary Classifications of Factors Influencing Health Status and Contacts with Health Services are found under such main term references as: "Admission" or "Status."

A main term may be followed by a series of terms, called nonessential modifiers, which are placed in parentheses. The presence or absence of these modifying parenthetical terms in the diagnosis has no effect upon the selection of the code listed in the main term. Examples of nonessential modifiers following the term "Eczema" are: (acute) (allergic) (chronic) (erythematous) (fissum) (occupational) (rubrum) (squamous).

A main term in the index may also be followed by a list of subterms, called essential modifiers, which do have an effect upon the selection and assignment of an appropriate code for a stated diagnosis. These subterms form individual line entries and describe essential differences in site, etiology, or clinical type. In the preceding example, the subterms "asteatotic" and "atopic" are essential modifiers in code selection and assignment.

General adjectives, such as acute, chronic, or hereditary, and references to anatomic site appear as main terms, but these adjectives have only a "see condition" reference. Note the entry "Bulbar" is followed by this notation as is the entry "Medulla."

Many index entries in Volume 2 are not cross-referenced; they are unexpected and usually located perchance. Note entries for: "Divorce V61.0"; "Drinking, habitual 303.9"; "Dropped, dead 798.1"; and "Dysfunction, psychosexual with inhibited sexual excitement 302.72."

Certain main terms are followed by referencing notes that are used to define terms and to provide coding instructions. For instance, note the instructions in the box under the main term "Injury," and the instructions in the box under the nonessential modifiers below the main term "Wound." Instructional cross-reference notes are also used to list the fifth-digit subclassifications for those groups of categories, all of which use the same fifth-digits, as in the instructions in the box below the nonessential modifiers under the main term "Diabetes, diabetic." In these instances, only the four-digit code is stated for the individual subterm entry. Therefore, the coder must refer to the note following the main term to obtain the appropriate fifth-digit subclassification.

Notes are also used in Volume 3 to reference fourth-digit subclassifications for those categories that use the same fourth-digit subdivisions. In these cases, only the three-digit code is provided for the individual entry. The coder must refer to the note following the main term to obtain the appropriate fourth-digit subclassification. Such an instructional notation appears in the box following the subterm "microscopic (specimen) (of)" among the various subterms under the main term index entry "Examination."

Eponyms (diseases named for persons) are listed both as main terms in their appropriate alphabetic sequence and under the main terms "Disease" or "Syndrome." A description of the disease or syndrome is usually included in parentheses following the eponym. Common examples of such eponyms are Hodgkin's disease and Downs syndrome.

Operations named for persons are listed both as main terms in their appropriate alphabetic sequence and under the main term "Operation." A description of the procedure or anatomic site affected usually follows the eponym. Common examples of eponyms for surgical procedures are the Caldwell-Luc operation (maxillary sinusotomy), and the Oscar Miller operation (midtarsal arthrodesis).

APPENDICES IN ICD-9

Volume 1 of ICD-9-CM includes five appendices to supplement the volume (Table 2–7). Appendix A classifies neoplasms by morphology codes, commonly known as the M codes. The

TABLE 2–7

Appendices in ICD-9

Appendix	Content
Appendix A	Morphology codes for neoplasms, often called M codes
Appendix B	Glossary with definitions of mental disorders
Appendix C	Classification of drugs by formulary list
Appendix D	Classification for industrial accidents
Appendix E	Listing of three digit ICD-9 categories

M codes are utilized by tumor registries and by pathology departments. Appendix B comprises a glossary with clinical definitions of mental disorders. This glossary is primarily utilized by clinicians in psychiatry and behavioral medicine. Neither Appendix A nor Appendix B are ordinarily used by coders and neither appendix affects reimbursement.

Appendix C classifies pharmaceuticals in accordance with the American Hospital Formulary Service List. Coders sometimes refer to Appendix C to categorize new drugs not listed in the Table of Drugs and Chemicals. Appendix D comprises a classification of industrial accidents; this appendix is used by trauma registries and by clinicians in occupational medicine, but is seldom used by coders and does not affect reimbursement.

As a reference for use by researchers and to maintain comparability with its parent ICD-9 classification system, a list of three-digit categories is given in Appendix E. Although these categories form natural statistical groupings, they cannot substitute for the required five-digit ICD-9-CM code.

INDICES IN ICD-9

Volume 2 of ICD-9-CM serves as the comprehensive reference index to Volume 1 of ICD-9-CM. Three indexes are present in the second volume. The first section of Volume 2 is comprised of the Index to Diseases and Injuries. The second section is comprised of the Table of Drugs and Chemicals, and the third section is comprised of the Index to External Causes of Injuries and Poisonings.

The alphabetic index in Volume 2 is an important supplement to the tabular listings because it contains many diagnostic terms that do not appear in Volume 1. Terms listed in the categories of the tabular listings are not meant to be exhaustive. Rather, they serve as examples of the content of the category. The alphabetic index, however, includes most diagnostic terms currently in use in the United States.

A competent coder should never select codes directly from the alphabetic index. After locating a code in the index, the coder should always refer to that code in the tabular listings for important instructions. These directives are in the form of: instructional notes and cross-references suggesting or requiring the use of additional codes, inclusion notes that confirm and verify code selection; and exclusion notes that guide code assignment elsewhere in the tabular listings.

In accordance with of A Chicago Manual of Style by The University of Chicago Press, letter-by-letter alphabetizing is used throughout the alphabetic index of Volume 2. This method of alphabetizing disregards single spaces and single hyphens, and produces sequences, for example, that would place the index entry "sickle cell trait" before the index entry "sick sinus syndrome."

Numbers, whether Arabic or Roman, or the adjective version of the number (first, second, third, fourth) are placed in the index in numerical sequence. For instance, "Disorder, factor, coagulation . . . VII . . . IX," exemplifies Roman numerals in sequential order in the index. "Disorder, nerve, cranial," lists sub-subterms in sequential order . . . "seventh . . . eighth . . . ninth," and so on.

References using the word "with" immediately follow the main term to which they refer. When multiple "with" references are present, they are indented under "with" and listed in alphabetical sequence. Note the entries following "with" under the index main term entry "Pyelitis." These subterms are arranged in alphabetical order.

The first section of Volume 2, the Index to Diseases and Injuries, contains alphabetical entries of terms referring to the conditions listed in the main classification of Volume 1. This section also encompasses index entries for the Supplementary Classification of Factors Influencing Health Status and Contact with Health Services (the V codes) as well as the morphology of neoplasms (commonly referred to as the M codes).

The second section of the alphabetic index in Volume 2, the Table of Drugs and Chemicals, contains an extensive, but not exhaustive, listing of drugs and other chemical substances and toxic agents. However, manifestations of poisoning or adverse effects of drugs and chemicals are found in the disease and injury index in the first section, and are listed under the specific symptom or disease.

In Volume 2, the Table of Drugs and Chemicals identifies the following types of poisoning by drugs and nonmedicinal chemical substances as the external cause of adverse effects: accidental poisoning; assault; misadventure in therapeutic use; suicide attempt; and undetermined cause. Each of the substances is assigned a code in the poisoning section of the classification. The appropriate codes from the supplementary External Cause of Injury and Poisoning Classification classify the nature of the poisoning.

This drug and chemical tabular also contains the American Hospital Formulary Service list numbers. These numbers are keyed to the American Hospital Formulary Service classification, which is continually updated and amended and can be used to categorize new drugs not listed in the table by name. The Formulary Service list numbers are found in the Table of Drugs and Chemicals under the main term "Drug." These list numbers and their ICD-9-CM equivalents are also found in Appendix C of Volume 1.

The third section of the alphabetic index in Volume 2 contains the Index to External Causes of Injuries and Poisonings (the E codes). The terms in this index are not medical diagnoses, but instead describe the circumstances under which an accident or act of violence occurred. These entries classify the underlying cause or means of injury.

The main terms in this third section of Volume 2, terms such as "Burning, burns" or "Fall, falling" usually represent the type of accident or violent activity, with the specific agent or other circumstance listed below the main term. Many of the entries in this section are distinctive and perhaps unexpected as exemplified by the main term entry "Cat" followed by subterm entries "bite" and "scratch."

The hypertension table, found in Volume 2 under the main term "Hypertension," contains a complete listing of all conditions due to or associated with hypertension and classifies them according to malignant, benign, and unspecified. For example, note the subterm "cardiorenal" (disease)" in the hypertension table and the specified code numbers for that entry.

Neoplasms are listed in the alphabetic index in two ways: by anatomic site and by morphology. A comprehensive list of anatomic sites is found in a table under the main term, "Neoplasm." The neoplasm table contains six columns: malignant primary; malignant secondary; malignant carcinoma in situ; benign; uncertain behavior; and unspecified. Histological terms for neoplasms such as carcinoma and adenoma, are listed as main terms in the appropriate alphabetic sequence and are usually followed by a cross-reference to the neoplasm table.

Each morphological term appears with its morphology code from ICD-0 as in "Cystoma M8440/0," or "Hepatoma (malignant) M8170/3." These morphology codes are used to supplement the appropriate ICD-9-CM neoplasm code, which indicates the site of the neoplasm. A complete listing of ICD-0 morphology codes is found in Appendix A of Volume 1.

For certain conditions, it is important to record both the etiology and the manifestation of the disease. In many cases, this is accomplished with the use of a single five-digit code. As examples, listing *377.03 Papilledema associated with retinal disorder,* and listing *482.81 [Pneumonia due to] Anaerobes,* include a manifestation within a single code number and title listing.

For some conditions, it is not possible to provide specific fifth-digit subclassifications that encompass both etiology and manifestation. In such cases, the two facets of the disease are coded individually, and the alphabetic index lists both codes. Both codes should be recorded to indicate the etiology and the manifestation of the disease in the same sequence as that used in the alphabetic index. Note the main term entry "Varix" followed by many subterm entries. Locate the subterm "esophagus" under the main term "Varix." The subterm "esophagus" includes the sub-subterm "bleeding in cirrhosis of liver" and two code numbers. The first code number, *571.5* represents the etiology, and the code number in brackets *[456.20],* represents the manifestation.

The alphabetic index of Volume 3 is an important supplement to the tabular list of that volume because it contains many procedural terms that do not appear in the classification. Terms listed in the categories of the tabular list are not meant to be exhaustive, but instead serve as examples of the content of the category. The alphabetic index to Volume 3, however, includes most of the procedural terms currently in use in the United States.

An entry in the alphabetical index of Volume 3 may refer the coder to the tabular list for important instructions. These guidelines are in the form of: instructional notes or cross-references suggesting or requiring the use of additional codes; inclusion notes that confirm or verify code selection; and exclusion notes that direct code assignment elsewhere.

Letter-by-letter alphabetizing is used throughout the alphabetic index to procedures in similar manner to that used in the diagnostic index of Volume 2. Letter by letter alphabetizing disregards single spaces and single hyphens and produces sequences for example, that place the index entry "Ziegler operation" before the index entry "Z-plasty."

The prepositions "as," "by," and "with" immediately follow the main term to which they refer. When multiple prepositional references are present, they are listed in alphabetic sequence. For instance, the subterm entries under the main term entry "Graft, grafting" include the subterm "bone." Beneath the nonessential modifiers for the subterm, "bone," are several sub-subterms following the preposition "with." These sub-subterms are arranged in alphabetical order.

CODING GUIDELINES FOR ICD-9

Both the alphabetic index and the tabular list should be used when locating and assigning a code. Reliance on only the alphabetic index or on only the tabular list can lead to errors in code assignment and to less specificity in code selection.

Locate each term by using the alphabetic index and verify the code selected by using the tabular list. Read and be guided by instructional notations that appear in either the alphabetic index or the tabular list.

Both the alphabetic index to the diagnostic classification and the alphabetic index to the procedure classification of ICD-9-CM are comprised of nominative entries of terms designated as main terms. These main terms are printed in bold type, and frequently are followed by entries designated as subterms that are printed in normal type. These subterms are often followed by indented entries called sub-subterms that refer to the antecedent subterm.

The entries are guides or directives to the correlating code numbers. For example, "Snow blindness 370.24," in the alphabetic index to Volume 1, and, "Ileotomy 45.02," in the alphabetic index to Volume 3, direct appropriate code selection and assignment.

Main term entries are of several varieties:

- A name of the diagnosis or symptom in Volume 2 or the name of the procedure or service in Volume 3 (examples from Volume 2: Kyphosis; Stricture; or Pain and examples from Volume 3: Biopsy; or Reconstruction).

- A synonym of the stipulated term (examples from Volume 2: Inanition; Melancholia; or Paresthesia and examples from Volume 3: Encircling procedure; or Take-down).

- An eponym of the stipulated term (examples from Volume 2: Devic's disease; Hong Kong ear; or Pendred's syndrome and examples from Volume 3: Bobb operation; or Masters' stress test).

- An abbreviation or abridgment of the stipulated term (examples: from Volume 2: HIV infection; or RDS and examples from Volume 3: ERCP; MAST; or UFR).

A main term in the alphabetical index of an ICD-9-CM volume may be an unaccompanied entry, such as "Decompression sickness," in the alphabetic index to Volume 1, and "Vaginoplasty" in the alphabetic index to Volume 3. Or the main term entry may be followed by a number of subterms that annotate or modify the main term and consequently influence code selection, such as, "Dermatitis" in the alphabetic index to Volume 1, and, "Laryngectomy," in the alphabetic index to Volume 3.

Whenever subterms appear under main term index entries, each subterm must be carefully reviewed to insure accurate code number selection. Certain subterms could be misleading. For instance, the procedural index entries "Cardiectomy" and "Cardioplasty" refer to the cardia of the stomach and not to the heart.

An indented entry under a subterm is called a sub-subterm. The entry, "superficial," beneath the subterm, "sclera," below the main term, "Injury," exemplifies a sub-subterm in Volume 2. The entry, "ileal," beneath the subterm, "conduit," below the main term, "Formation," exemplifies a sub-subterm in the index of Volume 3.

For certain generic main term index entries, more than one ICD-9-CM code number appears to be applicable. These seemingly appropriate code numbers may or may not be numerically sequential.

If these code numbers constitute a numeric sequence, the first code number and the last code number of the sequence are indicated, each of which is separated with a hyphen. For instance, the entry in the alphabetic index for Volume 1, "Perforation, bladder, with ectopic pregnancy," offers a cross-reference to a sequence of codes, 633.0–633.9. This type of numeric entry is referred to as a "code range."

To diminish the size of the alphabetical reference index and to accord a space-saving convention to the ICD-9-CM volumes, certain words in the index entries are merely implied, with their actual intent inferred from the context of the other terms in that entry. The predominant usage of this convention is with procedures and services denoted in subterm entries. To exemplify, the lengthy itemization of subterm entries under the main term, "Excision," in Volume 3 implies the use of the word "of" or "by" in many instances.

All diagnostic codes and all procedure codes should be used and reported at their highest level of specificity. Three-digit diagnostic codes should be assigned only if there are no four-digit codes within that code category. Four-digit diagnostic codes should be assigned only if there is no fifth-digit subclassification for that category. Fifth-digit diagnostic subclassification codes should be assigned for those categories where such rubrics exist. Three-digit procedural codes should be assigned only if there are no four-digit procedural codes within that subcategory.

Codes labeled "other specified" (NEC—not elsewhere classified) or "unspecified" (NOS—not otherwise specified) should be used only when neither the diagnostic or procedural statement nor a thorough review of the patient care documentation provides adequate information to permit the assignment of a more specific code. The code assignment for "other" or NEC should be used when the information documented specifies a condition or service, but no separate code for that condition or service is provided. The code assignment for "unspecified" or (NOS) should be used when the information documented does not permit either a more specific or "other" code assignment.

If the alphabetic index guides code assignment to a category labeled "other (NEC)" or labeled "unspecified (NOS)," the coder should refer to the tabular list and review the titles and inclusion terms in the subdivisions under that particular category (or subcategory), to determine if the information available can justify assignment of an entity to a more specific code.

If the same condition is described in the patient care documentation as both acute (or subacute) and chronic, and separate subentries exist in the alphabetic index at the same indentation level, both conditions should be coded and reported and the acute (or subacute) condition code should be sequenced before the chronic condition code. For example, acute cystitis should be sequenced before chronic cystitis.

A single code used to classify two diagnoses, either a diagnosis with an associated secondary manifestation or an associated complication is called a "combination code." Combination codes are identified by referring to subterm entries in the alphabetic index and by reading the inclusion and exclusion notes in the tabular list. For example, code number *404.92* is a combination code for hypertensive heart and renal disease with renal failure. Code selection is accessed first through the hypertension table entry in the alphabetic index and then through the category in the tabular listings.

A combination code should only be assigned if that code fully identifies the diagnostic conditions involved or if the alphabetic index directs combination coding. Multiple coding should not be used if the classification provides a combination code that clearly identifies all of the elements documented in the diagnosis. If the combination code lacks the necessary specificity in describing the manifestation or the complication, an additional code may be reported as a secondary code. To exemplify, cryptococcal meningitis is reported with two code numbers: *117.5* and *321.0.*

Multiple coding is required for certain conditions not subject to the rules for combination codes. Instructions for conditions requiring multiple coding appear in the alphabetic index and in the tabular list. For instance, category *813* of the diagnostic tabular encompasses fractures of the radius and ulna, meaning that this category is utilized to code fractures of either bone or fractures of both.

Codes for both the etiology and the manifestations of a disease appear following the subentry term. The secondary code is italicized and placed in slanted brackets. The codes for manifestations that appear in italicized print cannot be designated and reported as a principal diagnosis. Both codes should be assigned in the same sequence in which they appear in the alphabetic index. Instructional terms in the tabular list, such as "code also . . . ," "use additional code for any . . . ," and "note . . . ," generally indicate appropriate circumstances to use more than one code to report the etiology and the manifestation of a condition.

Multiple coding instructions should be applied throughout the classification if appropriate, whether or not multiple coding directions appear in the alphabetic index or the tabular list.

However, indiscriminate multiple coding or the coding and reporting of irrelevant information, such as symptoms or signs characteristic of the diagnosis, should always be avoided. To exemplify, even with specific documentation, abdominal pain would not be reported with a diagnosis such as acute gastric ulcer, nor would chest pain be reported with a diagnosis of hiatal hernia.

A late effect is a residual effect (produced by a condition) after the termination of the acute phase of an illness or injury. There is no definite time limit that determines when a late effect code can be used. The residual may be apparent early, such as hemiplegia or aphasia in cerebrovascular accident cases, or it may occur months or years later, such as internal derangement of a joint due to a previous sports injury.

Coding of late effects requires two codes: one for the residual condition, and one for the cause of the late effect, which is sequenced before the other code, except in those few instances in which the code for late effect is followed by a manifestation code identified in the tabular list as an italicized code. The code for the acute phase of the illness or injury that produced the late effect should never be reported with a code for the cause of the late effect.

If a diagnosis documented at the time of an inpatient discharge is qualified as probable, suspected, likely, questionable, possible, or to be ruled out, the condition should be coded and reported as if the problem existed or was established. Of course, the coder must peruse the patient record and ascertain that the stated condition is consistent with the diagnostic workup and the plans for further observation, and that the therapeutic approach corresponded closely with the potential diagnosis. Thus, after reviewing the documentation, for example, probable urinary tract infection should be coded as urinary tract infection on the report of an inpatient admission.

This guideline for coding and reporting suspected conditions is not applicable to outpatient episodes of care, however. For instance, a presenting symptom such as polyuria should be coded and reported for the outpatient encounter, even though the clinician may suspect the underlying cause to be a urinary tract infection.

Any condition described at the time of discharge as impending or threatened should be coded and reported as a confirmed diagnosis if the condition did occur. If the condition did not occur, the alphabetic index should be referenced to determine if the index entry for that condition is followed by a subentry term for impending or threatened. Additionally, the coder should review main term entries for "Impending" and "Threatened." If applicable subterms are listed, the designated code should be selected and assigned. If applicable subterms are not listed, the existing forerunner condition, and not the condition described as impending or threatened, should be coded and reported.

The alphabetic index to Volume 1 and the alphabetic index to Volume 3, both organized by main terms which are printed in boldface type, usually base reference upon the condition or service, rather than upon the anatomic site involved. A main term ordinarily may be followed by a series of terms known as modifiers. As in grammar, a modifier (adjective or adverb) limits or restricts the meaning of a term. A descriptive word such as "chronic" modifies a noun naming a condition such as "sinusitis." A descriptive word such as "completely" modifies a verb naming an action such as "excised."

The presence or absence of modifiers placed within parentheses in the tabular list or alphabetical index has no effect upon the selection or assignment of the code listed for the main term. These modifiers in parenthetical expressions are called nonessential modifiers. For instance in Volume 2, the term (ischemic) following the index entry, "Necrosis, necrotic," is a nonessential modifier. In Volume 3, the main term index entry, "Casting," is followed by the nonessential modifier (for immobilization).

A main term may also be followed by a list of subterms. These subterms are enclosed within parentheses and consequently do affect the selection and assignment of an appropriate code for a stated entity. These subterms form individual line entries and describe essential differences in etiology or topography or in procedural technique. These subterms are called essential modifiers. For instance, in Volume 2, the subterms, "cirrhotic" and "congenital," beneath the main term index entry, "Splenomegaly," are essential modifiers that determine code selection and assignment. And in Volume 3, the main term index entry, "Epilation," followed by the subterm, "eyebrow," is subsequently followed by two sub-subterms, "cryosurgical" and "electrosurgical." These two sub-subterms are essential modifiers for the process of code selection and assignment.

Terms that identify incisions are listed as main terms in the alphabetic index of Volume 3. If the incision was made only for the purpose of performing further surgery, the instruction "omit code" is provided. Note the entry "as operative approach—omit code" beneath the main term entry, "Laminotomy."

With certain operative procedures, the individual components of the procedure are generally reported. In these instances, the alphabetic index lists both codes. Note the entry, "Anastomosis," in Volume 3. Following this main term entry are numerous subterms including "bladder," and sub-subterm "with . . . ileum." Two code numbers, *57.87* and *45.51,* are listed for this entry.

To proficiently utilize the ICD-9-CM coding system for code number selection, the alphabetical index to the appropriate ICD-9-CM volume should be utilized in the subsequent prescribed search sequence (Table 2–8). First and foremost, the index should be scanned to locate a main term either for the diagnosis or symptom (or for the procedure or service rendered).

If this initial search is ineffective or unproductive, the index should be scanned to locate a main term for the disease or injury diagnosed or treated or for any synonyms, eponyms, or abbreviations associated with the main term. The attending physician should be consulted if a suitable index entry still cannot be located.

Second, after the location of the appropriate main term, the coder should survey all subterms and all sub-subterms indicated beneath that main term and should observe any cross-reference notations related to that entry. Third, the applicable code number or code range should be chosen.

Fourth and lastly, code number selection should be finalized through verification of the code number in the tabular code number and narrative descriptor listings. If necessary, to

TABLE 2–8

ICD-9-CM Index Search Sequence

1. Locate main term for diagnosis or symptom (or for procedure or service). **yes** or **no**
   If **yes**, then to #5; if **no**, then to #2
2. Locate main term for organ or anatomic site diagnosed or treated. **yes** or **no**
   If **yes**, then to #5; if **no**, then to #3
3. Locate main term for disease or injury diagnosed or treated. **yes** or **no**
   If **yes**, then to #5; if **no**, then to #4
4. Contact physician for clarification of procedure or service rendered and selection of appropriate main term.
5. Survey all subterms and all sub-subterms denoted beneath the main term and observe any cross-references and instructional notations related to that entry.
6. Choose a suitable and warranted code number, code range, or code series.
7. Affirm code number, code range, or code series in the tabular listings of code numbers and narrative titles.
8. Analyze the applicable narrative title and finalize code selection and assignment.

determine a precise code number from within a code range, the coder should thoroughly review all of the code number and narrative title listings within the range to discern the most specifically applicable code number and narrative title.

In summary, there are several basic elements in coding diagnoses and procedures with ICD-9-CM. The searching process should always begin with the alphabetic index. All coding conventions, cross-references, and instructional notations should be closely reviewed and should guide and direct the code search process. All subentry terms should be scanned for specificity in code selection, and the selected code should be verified in the appropriate tabular list of ICD-9-CM, prior to finalizing code assignment.

As with every coding system, ICD-9-CM code number selection must absolutely never be accomplished solely by utilizing the alphabetic index to the volume. Even if only one code number is printed in the main term index entry for the diagnosis or symptom (or for the procedure or service) being reported, the code number must be verified in the numerical tabular listings in order to guarantee accurate and precise code number and narrative title selection.

SELECTION OF PRINCIPAL DIAGNOSIS

The principal diagnosis is defined in the Uniform Hospital Discharge Data Set (UHDDS) as "that condition established after study to be chiefly responsible for occasioning the admission of the patient to the hospital for care." The circumstance of the patient healthcare encounter always influence the selection of the principal diagnosis for that encounter, nonetheless.

In determining the principal diagnosis, the coding directives in the ICD-9-CM manuals take precedence over all other coding guidelines. Consistent and complete documentation in the patient health record facilitates clear determination of the principal diagnosis. With multiple ailments or multiple injuries, adequate patient care documentation should denote the severity of each condition and indicate that which is most responsible for occasioning the episode of care.

Without such definitive documentation, and unfortunately deficient patient care documentation is a common problem, the application of coding guidelines and the determination of a principal diagnosis may become a difficult, and perhaps impossible, task. Comprehensive coding guidelines incorporate and further define sequencing rules. Such guidelines are published in Coding Clinic to expedite the selection of a principal diagnosis.

Codes for symptoms, signs, and diagnostic findings from Chapter 16, Volume 1, of ICD-9-CM should not be reported as a principal diagnosis if a related definitive diagnosis was established in that episode of care. If a documented sign or symptom is followed by contrasting/comparative diagnoses, the sign or symptom code is sequenced first; and thus, a sign or symptom potentially could be reported as a principal diagnosis in particular situations.

All of the contrasting or comparative diagnoses following the sign or symptom designated as a principal diagnosis should be coded and reported secondarily, although these entities are suspected but unconfirmed conditions. For example, if a diagnosis were rendered as, "leg pain due to either tendonitis or fasciitis," the principal diagnosis coded and reported is simply, "leg pain." The tendonitis and the fasciitis are suspected and unconfirmed conditions, but are nevertheless reported as secondary diagnoses.

In those instances in which two or more contrasting or comparative diagnoses are concurrently documented as "either/or" (or with similar terminology) without the designation of a predominant sign or symptom, both conditions are coded and reported as if the diagnoses were confirmed. These diagnoses are sequenced according to the circumstances of the admission in order to ascertain the principal diagnosis.

If no further determination can be made as to which of two documented diagnoses should be designated as the principal diagnosis, either diagnosis may be sequenced first. For instance, an uncertain diagnosis of tendonitis versus fasciitis could be coded and reported either with tendonitis as the principal diagnosis and fasciitis as a secondary diagnosis or with fasciitis as the principal diagnosis and tendonitis as a secondary diagnosis.

Likewise, if two or more interrelated conditions, such as diseases within a single ICD-9-CM category, or manifestations characteristically associated with a certain disease, potentially fulfill the criteria defining a principal diagnosis, either condition may be sequenced first. For instance, acute viral sinusitis and acute viral pharyngitis are fairly comparable in terms of resource intensity relating to treatment and care. Therefore, for a patient concurrently afflicted with both ailments, either of these two conditions could be coded and reported as the principal diagnosis.

To further exemplify this guideline, consider the reporting of codes for the episode of care of an elderly patient admitted with shortness of breath. If this patient was found to be both in decompensated congestive heart failure and in acute exacerbation of chronic obstructive lung disease, either diagnosis could be sequenced as the principal diagnosis. The presenting complaint, shortness of breath, is symptomatic of both conditions. For reimbursement purposes, especially in an inpatient setting, the diagnosis with the highest potential for reimbursement could be sequenced as the principal diagnosis.

This sequencing guideline is routinely applicable to principal diagnosis selection, unless the circumstances of the admission, the treatment provided, the tabular list, or the alphabetic index indicate otherwise. However, italicized codes in the tabular listings, which are also the codes in slanted brackets in the alphabetic index, should never be sequenced as a principal diagnosis, and should always be reported as secondary codes.

Similarly, if the same condition is described as both acute (or subacute) and chronic, the acute condition has sequencing priority. Thus, if both acute cystitis and chronic cystitis are documented, chronic cystitis could not be designated as the principal diagnosis.

Moreover, a residual condition or the nature of the late effect has sequencing priority over the late effect code for the cause of the residual condition, except in the specific instances in which the alphabetic index otherwise directs code selection and assignment. For example, contracture as a late effect of burns is the principal diagnosis if care and treatment of the patient encounter is directed at the contracture.

Codes from the observation series are assigned as principal diagnoses for: outpatient encounters or inpatient admissions to evaluate evidence indicating an abnormal condition; or following an accident or other incident that ordinarily resulted in a health problem. Observation codes should be reported for the principal diagnosis if no supporting evidence for the suspected condition was found and no treatment was required in that episode of care. This guideline is applicable even though the patient may be scheduled for continuing observation in the office or clinic setting following discharge.

The general guideline defining the principal diagnosis as the condition that after study occasioned the healthcare encounter remains in effect even in situations in which treatment was not carried out due to unforeseen circumstances. For example, in an episode of care for a patient admitted for inguinal hernia repair but discharged before surgery because of urgent business problems, the principal diagnosis is the inguinal hernia. If this patient was admitted for inguinal hernia repair but the surgery was canceled because the patient suffered a myocardial infarction, the principal diagnosis would still be the inguinal hernia, because that condition was responsible for the episode of care.

The circumstances and resource intensity of care and treatment should determine the sequence of additionally reported diagnoses. If the documentation in the patient record does not allow a definitive sequence of diagnoses to be ascertained, then any recognized comorbidity or complication could be granted sequencing priority for coding and reporting purposes.

Reimbursement considerations, if applicable, influence the selection of recognized comorbidities and complications as high priority secondary diagnoses.

SELECTION OF PRINCIPAL PROCEDURE

The principal procedure is defined in the Uniform Hospital Discharge Data Set (UHDDS) as "the procedure most closely related to the principal diagnosis." This standard guideline is subject, however, to the circumstances of the healthcare encounter.

In determining the principal procedure in an episode of care, the coding directives in the ICD-9-CM manuals take precedence over all other coding guidelines. Adequate documentation in the patient health record is crucial to ensure clear determination of a principal procedure when multiple surgical operations are performed within a single healthcare encounter. Comprehensive procedural coding guidelines are incorporated and sequencing rules are defined in the publication Coding Clinic.

In general, therapeutic procedures have sequencing priority over diagnostic procedures. Therefore, if multiple procedures, both diagnostic and therapeutic, are performed, the principal procedure reported should be a therapeutic procedure. For instance, ligation of external hemorrhoids should receive priority over a colonoscopy if both were rendered in one episode of care, and likewise, the excision of a keratotic lesion of the thigh should receive priority over a concurrent skin biopsy of the same site.

Procedures referred to by the instructional notation "code also" are regarded as secondary procedures, and not intended for primary tabulation as a principal procedure. For instance, procedure listing *42.19, Other external fistualization of esophagus,* is supplemented with an instructional notation, "code also any resection." The resection is considered as a secondary procedure for sequencing purposes.

If two or more interrelated conditions are treated with operative procedures, the principal procedure is that procedure posing the most serious risk to the patient's health status. For example, a cancer patient rendered an operative procedure on an organ vital for life such as the liver might concurrently be rendered an operative procedure on a segment of the colon. The procedure performed on the liver would, of course, be reported as the principal procedure.

If clinical acumen cannot ascertain which procedure poses the greatest threat to health status, the procedure that is the most resource intensive may be designated as the principal procedure. Reimbursement considerations, if applicable, would guide the selection of a principal procedure in these situations.

In those unusual instances in which unforeseen complications or unexpected incidents occurred, and thereby necessitated the rendering of procedures unrelated to the initial reason for the encounter or visit, the principal procedure is the most resource intensive procedure rendered. To exemplify, if a patient was admitted for overnight observation following extensive liposuction, and if that patient accidentally sustained a fractured mandible when a lighting fixture fell from the ceiling, repair of the mandibular fracture could become the principal procedure reported for that healthcare encounter.

KEY CONCEPTS

abbreviations _____   category _____

anatomic term _____   chapter _____

appendices _____   classification _____

braces _____   code also _____

brackets _____   code also underlying disease _____

code and narrative title _____

colon _____

combination code _____

common narrative expression _____

conventions _____

cross-reference _____

diagnostic term _____

eponym _____

essential modifier _____

etiology _____

excludes notation _____

hierarchical level _____

hierarchical structure _____

includes notation _____

indented code and title _____

instructional notation _____

italicized code and title _____

listing _____

lozenge _____

main term _____

manifestation _____

multiple coding _____

nonessential modifier _____

parentheses _____

principal diagnosis _____

principal procedure _____

procedural term _____

punctuation _____

resource intensity _____

section _____

section mark _____

see _____

see also _____

see category _____

subcategory _____

subentry term _____

sub-subterm _____

subterm _____

supplementary classification _____

symbols _____

topography _____

use additional code if desired _____

REVIEW EXERCISES

1. What terms define the separation of the ICD-9-CM coding system into hierarchical levels?

   _____

   _____

2. What variations or distinctions specify the titles ascribed to chapters, sections, categories, and subcategories? _____

   _____

   _____

3. Specify the hierarchical level of each of the subsequent designations:

   A. 523, Gingival and Periodontal Diseases _____

   B. 785.51, Cardiogenic shock _____

   C. 600–608, Diseases of Male Genital Organs _____

   D. 593.0, Nephroptosis _____

   E. 802.0, Fracture of nasal bones, closed _____

   F. 740–759, Congenital Anomalies _____

   G. 550.00, Inguinal hernia, with gangrene_____

4. What criteria determines the chapter or section from which a facility or a physician is permitted or entitled to select codes for reporting billed charges? _____

_____

_____

5. Choose any two chapters of the ICD-9-CM volumes and itemize each section enumerating the range of corresponding code numbers contained within those chapters. _____

_____

_____

6. Choose any section of the ICD-9-CM volumes and itemize each category as well as each subcategory included within (if applicable). Enumerate the range of corresponding code numbers for each category and subcategory itemized. _____

_____

_____

7. What intent is conveyed by a colon following a narrative term under a category title or a subcategory title? What intent is conveyed by an indented code number and narrative title listing? _____

_____

_____

8. Write the full diagnosis, service, or procedure title for the following code numbers from the ICD-9-CM diagnostic tabular list:

A. 112.4 _____

B. 512.8 _____

C. 297.1 _____

D. 172.0 _____

E. 437.3 _____

F. 276.3 _____

G. 365.13 _____

9. Write the full diagnosis, service, or procedure title for the following code numbers from the ICD-9-CM procedural tabular list:

A. 52.09 _____

B. 45.01 _____

C. 39.27 _____

D. 34.22 _____

E. 27.54 _____

F. 16.0 _____

G. 07.3 _____

10. Identify the abbreviation used to indicate "not elsewhere classifiable" in the diagnostic tabular list. Scan the ICD-9-CM Volume 2 and list at least ten entries that denote "not elsewhere classifiable."

11. Identify the abbreviation used to indicate "not elsewhere classifiable" in the procedural tabular list. Scan the ICD-9-CM Volume 3 alphabetic index and list at least ten entries that denote "not elsewhere classifiable."

12. Identify the symbol used to indicate "not otherwise specified" in the diagnostic tabular list. Scan the ICD-9-CM Volume 1 and list at least ten entries that denote "not otherwise specified."

13. Identify the symbol used to indicate synonyms, alternative wordings, or explanatory phrases. Scan the ICD-9-CM volumes and list at least ten entries that denote such terms.

14. Identify the symbol used to indicate supplementary words that do not affect code determination. Scan the ICD-9-CM volumes and list at least ten entries that denote such words.

15. Identify the symbol used to indicate an incomplete term that requires modification. Scan the ICD-9-CM volumes and list at least ten entries that contain an incomplete term.

_____   _____
_____   _____
_____   _____
_____   _____
_____   _____

16. Identify the symbol used to indicate a series of terms modified by the statement printed at the right of the symbol. Scan the ICD-9-CM volumes and list at least ten entries that denote such modification.

_____   _____
_____   _____
_____   _____
_____   _____
_____   _____

17. Identify the symbol used to indicate a four-digit rubric unique to ICD-9-CM. Scan the ICD-9-CM volumes and list at least ten entries that contain this rubric.

_____   _____
_____   _____
_____   _____
_____   _____
_____   _____

18. Identify the symbol used to indicate the placement of a footnote applicable to all subdivisions in that code range. Scan the ICD-9-CM volumes and list at least ten entries denoting that message.

_____   _____
_____   _____
_____   _____
_____   _____
_____   _____

19. Identify and explain the instructional notations utilized in Volume 1 of the ICD-9-CM coding system. _____
_____
_____

20. Identify and explain the instructional notations utilized in Volume 2 of the ICD-9-CM coding system. _____
_____
_____

21. Identify and explain the instructional notations utilized in Volume 3 of the ICD-9-CM coding system. _____
_____
_____

22. Indicate whether the listed word is a noun (commonly a main term index entry), an adjective (usually a modifier), a verb (not ordinarily an indexed term), or an adverb (also not ordinarily an indexed term).

A. surgery _____   K. benign _____
B. psychiatric _____   L. instability _____
C. acute _____   M. surgically _____
D. syndrome _____   N. atrophic _____
E. operative _____   O. malignancy _____
F. labile_____   P. clinical_____
G. medical _____   Q. severely _____
H. therapeutic _____   R. operation _____
I. hypertrophy _____   S. procedure _____
J. pulmonary _____   T. dysfunction _____

23. Indicate whether the listed term is an essential modifier or a non-essential modifier.

A. The subterm "spontaneous" beneath the main term index entry "Pseudofracture"_____
_____

B. The subterm "visual" beneath the main term index entry "Discomfort"_____
_____

C. The sub-subterm "complicated" under the subterm "forehead" beneath the main term index entry "Wound"_____

D. The sub-subterm "blastic" under the subterm "lymphoid" beneath the main term index entry "Leukemia" _____

E. The sub-subterm "trigone" under the subterm "bladder" beneath the main term index entry "Anomaly" _____

F. The sub-subterm "congenital" under the subterm "syphilitic" beneath the main term index entry "Synovitis" _____

G. The sub-subterm "acquired" under the subterm "joint" beneath the main term index entry "Hypermobility" _____

H. The sub-subterm "endoscopic" under the subterm "gallbladder" beneath the main term index entry "Lithotripsy" _____

I. The sub-subterm "hand" under the subterm "tendon" beneath the main term index entry "Recession" _____

J. The sub-subterm "gland" under the subterm "thymus" beneath the main term index entry "Exploration" _____

24. Describe the proper techniques for ascertaining correct ICD-9-CM code number selection by using the alphabetical reference index to the ICD-9-CM tabular volume._____
_____
_____

25. Scan the alphabetical reference index to the ICD-9-CM tabular volume and list a minimum of ten main terms for which cross-reference notations are designated.

_____   _____
_____   _____
_____   _____
_____   _____
_____   _____
_____   _____

26. Locate within the alphabetical reference index to the ICD-9-CM tabular volume and list at least ten main terms for which a code range (instead of a specific code number) is enumerated.

_____   _____
_____   _____
_____   _____
_____   _____
_____   _____
_____   _____

27. Scan the alphabetical reference index to the ICD-9-CM tabular volume and list a minimum of ten subterm entries with implied meanings through omitted words.

_____   _____
_____   _____
_____   _____
_____   _____
_____   _____
_____   _____

28. Through utilization of the alphabetical index to the ICD-9-CM tabular volume, select accurate and precise code numbers for the following diagnoses.

A. angina pectoris _____
B. chronic bronchitis _____
C. benign prostatic hypertrophy _____
D. abdominal pain _____
E. hiatal hernia _____
F. fracture of two ribs _____
G. congestive heart failure _____
H. viral gastroenteritis _____
I. neuromyelitis optica _____
J. portal hypertension _____
K. erosive gastritis _____
L. contusion of chest _____
M. lichen planus _____
N. vulvovaginitis _____
O. cardiogenic shock _____
P. acute periodontitis _____
Q. congenital alopecia _____
R. postconcussion syndrome _____
S. rubella _____
T. Parkinson's disease _____
U. arteriosclerotic heart disease _____
V. rheumatoid arthritis _____
W. toxic myocarditis_____
X. cerebrovascular accident _____
Y. idiopathic corneal edema _____
Z. persistent vegetative state _____

3 CHAPTER

Format and Content of the CPT Coding System

LEARNING OBJECTIVES

Upon completion of this chapter the learner should be able to:

1. Explain the fundamental format of the CPT volume.
2. Describe the basic hierarchy within the CPT coding system.
3. Discuss the association between the common segment of a descriptor and its alternative options.
4. Interpret and explain the symbols among the listings of the CPT coding system.
5. Report upon the similarities and dissimilarities among the sections of the CPT coding system.
6. State the content of each of the appendices in the CPT volume.
7. Define the concept of a modifier in CPT.
8. Define and explain the concept of a code range.
9. Define and explain the concept of a code series.
10. Report the types of cross references used in the index of the CPT volume.
11. Express the potential variations in the format of modifiers.
12. Discuss the usefulness of modifiers within the CPT coding system.
13. Demonstrate knowledge of the proper index search sequence by correctly assigning code numbers from the CPT volume for narrative statements of procedures and services.
14. Discuss the utility, format, and content of the section guidelines in the CPT volume.
15. Discuss the utility, format, and content of the special report prepared to coincide with the reporting of unlisted procedure codes or unlisted service codes.

HIERARCHY AND LEVELS OF CPT

The multitude of codes listed in each CPT volume are supported and validated by a format of guidelines, notations, and symbols. The comprehensive CPT classification and coding system maintains a strict hierarchical structure that consists of five levels in the hierarchy (Table 3–1). These levels, placed in descending order of size and scope, are termed: sections;

TABLE 3–1

Hierarchical Levels in the CPT Coding System

Section
Subsection (Category)
Heading (Subcategory)
Subheading
Listing

subsections, which are divisions of sections and are labeled as categories in the Evaluation and Management Services section; headings, which are divisions of subsections that are comprised of relatively larger groups of code numbers and related descriptors, in the Evaluation and Management Services section these are divisions of categories and are called subcategories; subheadings, which are divisions of headings that are comprised of relatively smaller groups of code numbers and related descriptors, subheadings may be further divided into sub-subheadings; and listings, which are each of the individual code numbers and its descriptor.

This hierarchical structure maintained in the CPT volume can also be explained in an increasing order of size and scope. For example, the specific code number *10040* is included within the subheading *Incision and Drainage*. This subheading, *Incision and Drainage*, is included within the heading *Skin, Subcutaneous and Accessory Structures*. This heading, *Skin, Subcutaneous and Accessory Structures*, is encompassed within the subsection *Integumentary System*, and the subsection is encompassed within the *Surgery* section.

However, not every code number and descriptor can be identified with five distinct or decisive levels of the hierarchy of the CPT coding system. As examples, the *Anesthesia* section is not divided into subsections but is partitioned directly into headings; the *Pathology and Laboratory* section in general also does not distribute its listings into subheadings.

The main segment of the CPT volume is divided into six sections:

1. Anesthesia (codes *00100* through *01999*)
2. Surgery (codes *10040* through *69979*)
3. Radiology (codes *70010* through *79999*)
4. Pathology and Laboratory (codes *80002* through *89399*)
5. Medicine (codes *90700* through *99199*)
6. Evaluation and Management (codes *99201* through *99499*)

Within most of these six sections (which are discussed in more detail in subsequent pages of this chapter), a framework of subsections is devised with titles that generally are either anatomic terms (as *Mediastinum and Diaphragm*) or procedural terms (as *Chemotherapy Administration*). Throughout the CPT volume, the section title is identified adjacent to the page number at the bottom of each even-numbered page of the manual (example: / *Surgery*) and also identified at the top of every page along with the first code number and the last code number listed on that specific page.

The headings are printed in blank font and are usually titled with either anatomic terms (examples: *Trachea and Bronchi; Abdomen, Peritoneum, and Omentum; Anterior Segment; Gastrointestinal Tract*), or with procedural terms (examples: *Application of Casts and Strapping; Medical Radiation Physics* . . .)

The subheadings are printed in blank font and separated from the preceding text with a line. The subheadings are ordinarily also titled with either anatomic terms (examples: *Tricuspid Valve; Hematopoietic, Reticuloendothelial, and Lymphatic System*), or with procedural terms (examples: *Free Skin Grafts, Hernioplasty, Herniorrhaphy, Herniotomy; Cesarean Delivery; Ophthalmoscopy*), and titled less frequently with diagnostic terms (examples: *Pressure Ulcers (Decubitus Ulcers); or Thoracic Aortic Aneurysm*).

SECTIONS IN CPT

Exclusive listing of an individual procedure or service code number and descriptor in a specific section or subsection of the CPT volume does not restrict, limit, or confine its use to any specific specialty group of physicians. Any qualified physician, regardless of specialty, may report procedures and services rendered with applicable code numbers and descriptors located anywhere within the CPT volume (for example, excisions of a herniated disk are performed by neurosurgeons and by orthopedic surgeons, and hair transplants are performed by plastic surgeons as well as by physicians in other specialties).

The primary bulk of the CPT volume and the preponderant and paramount portion of the CPT volume consists of the six sections comprising thousands of individual code number and descriptor listings. These listings are presented in serial or sequential numeric order with the exception of the code numbers and descriptors incorporated in the *Evaluation and Management Services* section. The *Evaluation and Management Services* section is the initial section of the CPT volume because these code numbers and descriptors are utilized by all practicing physicians and are the most frequently reported.

The next section, the *Anesthesia* section, contains code number and descriptor listings for anesthesia services and is the shortest (most concise) section of the CPT volume, followed sequentially by the longest and most technically complex section of the CPT coding system, the *Surgery* section.

The *Surgery* section of the CPT volume is divided into seventeen separate subsections categorized and aligned primarily by body systems: *Integumentary System; Musculoskeletal System; Respiratory System; Cardiovascular System; Hemic and Lymphatic Systems; Mediastinum and Diaphragm; Digestive System; Urinary System; Male Genital System; Intersex Surgery; Laparoscopy/Hysteroscopy; Female Genital System; Maternity Care and Delivery; Endocrine System; Nervous System; Eye and Ocular Adnexa*; and *Auditory System*.

Each subsection encompassed within the *Surgery* section of the CPT volume (examples: *Cardiovascular System* or *Nervous System*) normally is further divided into headings arranged accordingly by organs or anatomical sites (examples: *Heart and Pericardium,* in the *Cardiovascular System* subsection of the *Surgery* section; and *Spine and Spinal Cord,* in the *Nervous System* subsection of the *Surgery* section). These headings generally are subsequently subdivided into clusters of procedures organized in congruence with surgical processes such as incision, excision, repair, removal, and so forth (examples: the heading of *Kidney,* in the *Urinary System* subsection of the *Surgery* section is parceled into subheadings for *Incision, Excision, Renal Transplantation, Introduction, Repair, Endoscopy,* and *Other Procedures;* and the heading of *Conjunctiva,* in the *Eye and Ocular Adnexa* subsection of the *Surgery* section is parceled into subheadings for *Incision and Drainage, Excision and/or Destruction, Injection, Conjunctivoplasty,* and *Other Procedures*).

The succeeding section of the CPT volume, the *Radiology* section, is designated for radiological procedures and services. This section is partitioned into four subsections: *Diagnostic Radiology (Diagnostic Imaging); Diagnostic Ultrasound; Radiation Oncology;* and *Nuclear Medicine*. Within each subsection of the *Radiology* section (examples: *Diagnostic Radiology;*

or *Diagnostic Ultrasound*) the headings as well as certain subheadings are principally assorted in congruence with organs or anatomical sites (examples: *Head and Neck, Chest, Spine and Pelvis, Upper Extremities, Lower Extremities, Abdomen, Gastrointestinal Tract, Urinary Tract, Gynecological and Obstetrical, Heart,* and *Veins and Lymphatics* in the *Diagnostic Radiology* subsection of the *Radiology* section; and *Head and Neck, Chest, Abdomen and Retroperitoneum, Spinal Canal, Pelvis, Genitalia, Extremities, Vascular Studies,* and *Ultrasonic Guidance Procedures* in the *Diagnostic Ultrasound* subsection of the *Radiology* section).

The next section of the CPT volume, the *Pathology and Laboratory* section, is partitioned into fifteen subsections that are apportioned for listings of code numbers and descriptors for laboratory procedures and services performed either in physician offices or healthcare facilities, or in external reference laboratories. These subsections are: *Automated, Multichannel Tests; Organ or Disease Oriented Panels; Drug Testing; Therapeutic Drug Assays; Evocative/Suppression Testing; Consultations (Clinical Pathology); Urinalysis; Chemistry; Hematology and Coagulation; Immunology; Transfusion Medicine; Microbiology; Anatomic Pathology; Surgical Pathology;* and *Other Procedures.*

The final and concluding section of the CPT volume is the *Medicine* section, which is comprised of twenty-one subsections: *Immunization Injections; Therapeutic or Diagnostic Infusions; Therapeutic or Diagnostic Injections; Psychiatry; Biofeedback; Dialysis; Gastroenterology; Ophthalmology; Special Otorhinolaryngologic Services; Cardiovascular; Non-Invasive Vascular Diagnostic Studies; Pulmonary; Allergy and Clinical Immunology; Neurology and Neuromuscular Procedures; Central Nervous System Assessments/Tests; Chemotherapy Administration; Special Dermatological Procedures; Physical Medicine and Rehabilitation; Osteopathic Manipulative Treatment; Chiropractic Manipulative Treatment;* and *Special Services and Reports.*

Each subsection bounded within the *Medicine* section normally coincides with a clinical specialty or a clinical service and contains typically dissimilar titles for the headings and the subheadings in that particular subsection (examples: the *Dialysis* subsection of the *Medicine* section includes headings for *End Stage Renal Disease Services, Hemodialysis, Peritoneal Dialysis,* and *Miscellaneous Dialysis Procedures;* and the *Allergy and Clinical Immunology* subsection of the *Medicine* section includes headings for *Allergy Testing* and *Allergen Immunotherapy*).

LISTINGS IN CPT

The lowest level in the hierarchical structure of the CPT coding system is the solitary and distinctive listing of an individual code number and its descriptor. The majority of the listings in the CPT volume are self-contained and do not directly relate to any specific prior or subsequent listing. However, numerous listings in the CPT volume maintain a differently established format in which a portion of a descriptor correlates and connects with subsequent descriptors.

Rather than reiterate repetitious and redundant information within groups of code number and descriptor listings, the first descriptor listed within that group encompasses a common narrative expression (the part of the descriptor that is not repeated or reiterated), which is printed once and is followed by a semicolon. Code numbers and descriptors listed below the first descriptor refer back to the common narrative expression (which is the descriptor followed by the semicolon) and each of these dependent or subordinate descriptors is indented. As examples, the procedure represented by code number *24366* is *Arthroplasty, radial head,* the procedure represented by code number *45307* is *Proctosigmoidoscopy, rigid; with removal of foreign body;* the procedure represented by code number *69511* is *Mastoidectomy, radical;* and the service represented by code number *88045* is *Necropsy (autopsy); forensic examination coroner's call.* Terminology in an indented descriptor listing beneath a semicolon always warrants or assumes a subordinate position or status to the descriptor listing immediately before the semicolon.

SYMBOLS IN CPT

A symbol is a conventional printed sign that represents a quality or quantity. Classification systems, including ICD-9-CM, CPT, and HCPCS, customarily use symbols to signify particular attributes or characteristics pertaining to certain codes. Three symbols, the circle or bullet (○), the triangle or delta or pyramid (Δ), and the star or asterisk (*), frequently appear throughout the listings of the CPT volume (see Table 3–2). Hundreds of code numbers and descriptors are added, revised, or deleted preceding the annual dissemination of the updated CPT volume. These additions, revisions, and deletions are indicated by means of symbols.

A newly added CPT code number is symbolized with a small black circle or bullet (○) printed to the left of the code number. Examples of recently added code numbers are ○*15758* and ○*43496.* This distinguishing identification of an added code number appears only in the CPT volume in which this specific code number debuts. In the subsequently published CPT volume, this added code number is listed without the symbol. For instance, recently added code numbers ○*15756* and ○*49906* are symbolized with the circle or bullet, but this symbol will not be retained in the new printing of the CPT volume.

A newly revised CPT code descriptor (a revision includes any modification of the narrative expression or any alteration of a definition) is symbolized with a small black triangle or delta or pyramid (Δ) printed to the left of the corresponding code number. Examples of code numbers with recently revised descriptors are Δ*26121* and Δ*75555.* This distinguishing identification of a revised descriptor appears only in the CPT volume in which this revised descriptor debuts. In the subsequently published CPT volume, the revised descriptor will be listed without the symbol. For instance, recently revised descriptors for code numbers Δ*25332* and Δ*52340* are symbolized with the triangle or delta or pyramid, but this symbol will not be retained in the new printing of the CPT volume.

A newly deleted CPT code number is symbolized by enclosure within parentheses, alongside a cross reference notation to an equivalent replacement code number. Examples of recently deleted code numbers are *(60555)* and *(76949).* This distinctive identification of a deleted code number appears not only in the volume from which the particular code number is deleted, but also in the subsequently published CPT volume. Reference to the deleted code number or descriptor is retained in the new printing of the CPT volume. For instance,

TABLE 3–2

Symbols Used in the CPT Coding System

Symbol	Message
Circle or bullet ○	Added code
Triangle or pyramid or delta Δ	Revised descriptor
Parentheses ( )	Deleted code
Star or asterisk *	Surgical package not applicable

previously deleted code numbers *(46920)* and *(83040)* remain enclosed within parentheses in the current CPT volume and newly deleted code numbers *(27611)* and *(61051)* shall remain enclosed within parentheses in subsequent volumes of CPT.

A relatively minor surgical procedure that involves variable preoperative or postoperative services (these terms are explained in Chapter 13) is symbolized with a small black star or asterisk (*) printed to the right of the code number. This star or asterisk denotes that the "surgical package concept" is not applicable for this procedure due to the indefinite nature of preoperative and postoperative services. The surgical package concept simply designates that preoperative and postoperative care are included in the reported procedure code (this concept is also thoroughly discussed in Chapter 13). Examples of code numbers followed by the star or asterisk and often referred to as "starred procedures" in the CPT volume are *46050** and *57452**.

The version of CPT for Hospital Outpatient Services uses additional symbols to signify particular characteristics or attributes pertaining to certain codes. Five symbols, the section mark (§), the clover (♣), the checkmark (✓), the lozenge (□), and the diamond (◊) appear throughout the listings of this version of the CPT volume (see Table 3–3). If one of these special symbols in the Hospital Outpatient Services version of CPT is applicable to a listing that is symbolized with a circle or a triangle, then the special symbol is printed at the left of the circle or the triangle. The section mark (§), the clover (♣), the checkmark (✓), and the lozenge (□) are utilized solely in the *Surgery* section of the CPT volume. The diamond (◊) is utilized solely in the *Radiology* section of this adapted CPT volume.

A code number and descriptor listing for an ambulatory surgery center procedure is symbolized with a section mark (§) printed at the left of the code number (example: §*31020 Sinusotomy, maxillary (antrotomy); intranasal*). An ambulatory surgery center procedure is a diagnostic or therapeutic service appropriately performed on an outpatient basis.

The code number and descriptor listing for a potential ambulatory surgery center procedure is symbolized with a clover (♣) printed at the left of the code number (example: ♣*27245 Open treatment of intertrochanteric, pertrochanteric, or subtrochanteric femoral fracture; with intramedullary implant,* . . .). Recognition of the ambulatory surgery or outpatient surgery status of a procedure denoted with the clover symbol is (for Medicare patients only) contingent upon and pending the approval of the Health Care Financing Administration (HCFA). The clover symbol generally is retained in merely one or two subsequent volumes of CPT; authorization by HCFA automatically transforms the clover symbol into the section mark symbol.

The code number and descriptor listing for a potentially non-covered procedure is symbolized with a checkmark (✓) printed at the left of the code number (example: ✓*15781*

T A B L E 3–3

Additional Symbols Used in the Hospital Outpatient Services Version of the CPT Coding System

Symbol	Message
Section Mark §	Ambulatory surgery center procedure
Clover ♣	Potential ambulatory surgery center procedure
Checkmark ✓	Potentially non-covered procedure
Lozenge □	Non-covered procedure
Diamond ◊	Reportable radiology code

Dermabrasion; segmental, face). Recognition of the ambulatory surgery or outpatient surgery status of a procedure denoted with the checkmark symbol is (for Medicare patients only) in jeopardy, conditional upon or pending the decision of the Health Care Financing Administration (HCFA). The checkmark symbol is also generally retained in only one or two subsequent volumes of CPT. Revocation by HCFA automatically removes the checkmark symbol from the listing.

A code number and descriptor listing for a non-covered procedure is symbolized with a lozenge (□) printed at the left of the code number (example: □*58301 Removal of intrauterine device (IUD)*. A non-covered procedure is a diagnostic or therapeutic service that is more appropriately rendered in an office or clinic setting, and not in the ambulatory surgery center or hospital environment.

A listing of a reportable radiology code is symbolized with a diamond (◊) printed at the left of the code number (example: ◊*74455 Urethrocystography, voiding, radiological supervision and interpretation*). A reportable radiology code may be submitted by a hospital to Medicare with a claim for reimbursement.

CODING GUIDELINES FOR CPT

The bulk of each CPT volume is committed to the six sections that comprise the sequential numerical listings of code numbers and descriptors for a multitude of procedures and services. Nevertheless, every CPT volume additionally contains a table of contents, an introduction, six sets of guidelines (a set of guidelines at the beginning of each of the six sections), four appendices, and an alphabetical reference index to the individual listings in each publication.

The introduction to the CPT volume presents general information with explanations and directions concerning its format and presents several broad guidelines for its utilization. Brief and condensed instructions regarding modifiers, special reports, unlisted procedures, and unlisted services are also included. For example, the CPT manual states that an unlisted procedure (for instance, the Baxter operation) or an unlisted service (for instance, an intraoperative consultation) may require the submission of a special report to the third-party payor. Also, any procedure or any service that is unusual, variable, or new, may require the submission of a special report to the third-party payor.

The special report should include, if applicable, an explanation of the complexity of the symptoms, the pertinent physical findings, the diagnoses or concurrent problems, the diagnostic and therapeutic procedures and services performed, and the plans for follow-up care. If applicable, the special report should also include a clarification of and justification for the clinical appropriateness of the procedure or the service, including a reasonable and proper description of the nature, extent, time, staff, and equipment necessary to render the procedure or the service.

Guidelines are placed at the beginning of each of the six sections of the CPT volume. These guidelines define terms and concepts essential to understanding and comprehension for the appropriate coding and reporting of the procedures and services listed in that designated section of the CPT manual. As examples, the guidelines presented in the CPT volume define terms such as "established patient" and "concurrent care"; and define the modifiers applicable to codes in the various sections of the manual.

APPENDICES IN CPT

The CPT volume includes four appendices to supplement the volume (Table 3–4). A comprehensive itemization of every current CPT modifier along with an accompanying definition

TABLE 3–4

Appendices in CPT

Appendix	Content
Appendix A	Comprehensive itemization of all current CPT modifiers
Appendix B	Summary of all additions, revisions, and deletions included in the updated CPT
Appendix C	Summary of all additions, revisions, and deletions included in the computerized short procedure version
Appendix D	Clinical examples that typify patient encounters for evaluation and management services

comprises the content of Appendix A. A summarization (in numerical order) of all additions, revisions, and deletions incorporated in the current, updated volume of the CPT coding system comprises the content of Appendix B. A synopsis of all additions, revisions, and deletions encompassed within the current, updated, computerized (magnetic tape or diskette) version of the CPT abridged procedure and service description comprises the content of Appendix C. Sketches of clinical scenarios (the Clinical Examples Supplement) that typify patient encounters for evaluation and management services are found in Appendix D.

MODIFIERS IN CPT

A modifier limits or restricts meaning. An adjective such as "acute" modifies a noun naming a condition such as "cystitis." An adverb such as "copiously" modifies a verb naming an action such as "irrigate." The CPT coding system contains thirty numeric modifiers. A list of these modifiers with definitions is itemized and located in Appendix A of the CPT volume. CPT code modifiers are used to augment the reporting of procedures and services rendered by physicians, but should not be reported by hospitals in billing charges submitted to third-party payors.

Each of the thirty CPT code modifiers may be utilized as appendages, two numeric digits attached to a procedure or service code, and followed by a hyphen (examples: 14001-22 and 65850-52). These modifiers may also be utilized as supplements, an entire five-digit code (*099* plus the two digits of the modifier) reported in addition to a procedure or service code (examples: *14001* with *09922;* and *65850* with *09952*). A five-digit modifier code number may also be appended with certain two-digit modifiers to convey significant facts about the procedure or service rendered.

The CPT code modifiers represent a narrative description that supplements the listed code descriptor with qualifying information. For instance, modifier *-66 (09966)* can alter the descriptor for code number *33400* by signifying the involvement of a surgical team, and modifier *-55 (09955)* can alter the descriptor for code number *67036* by signifying postoperative management only. Modifiers relevant to physician-rendered procedures and services listed in a particular section of the CPT volume are presented in the guidelines at the beginning of that section, and are discussed and explained more thoroughly in the subsequent chapters of this text (which relate to the specific sections of the CPT manual).

To reiterate, a CPT code modifier furnishes a mechanism to annotate the reporting of a procedure or a service rendered by a physician. The modifier signifies that the procedure or the service was influenced by special circumstances (examples: modifier *-23,* unusual anesthesia; modifier *-32,* mandated services), although this procedure or service was not essentially changed in definition.

If pertinent, multiple modifiers may augment a single code by either of two methods. The first method incorporates repeated entries of the code number that denote the procedure or service provided, appended with a hyphen followed by the applicable modifier. For example, code *56633-82* may be reported with code *56633-47*. The second method incorporates separately reporting the modifiers as five-digit modifier codes, supplementing the code number that denotes the procedure or service provided. For example, code *56633* reported with both modifier code *09982* and modifier code *09947*.

If multiple modifiers are listed to augment a single code, modifier *-99* should be used to indicate the reporting of an individual code with multiple modifiers. For example, code *56633-99* should be reported with code *56633-82* and code *56633-47*. Modifier *-99* should be listed preceding any other modifier, and the supplementary modifiers should be listed in descending numerical order. For instance, modifier *-82* should precede modifier *-47*, and so on.

Justification to third-party payors for the utilization of certain modifiers may necessitate the preparation of a special report (or perhaps simply a brief explanatory note) containing factual details with respect to the special circumstances regarding the procedure or service rendered. Accurate and precise utilization of modifiers is imperative for proper and adequate CPT coding.

INDEX IN CPT

A comprehensive alphabetical reference index to the listings of the CPT coding system is located in the back of each CPT volume. The index is comprised of nominative entries of terms designated as main terms, which are printed in bold type and are frequently followed by entries designated as subterms, which are printed in normal type. These subterms are often followed by indented entries called sub-subterms that refer to the antecedent subterm.

The index entries are guides or directives to the correlating code numbers (examples: Binocular Microscopy 92504; Exercise Therapy 97110; Inguinal Orchiopexy 54640). Entries of main terms are of several varieties:

- The name of procedure or service (examples: Angiography or Urinalysis).
- The name of the organ or anatomic site (examples: Epididymis; Spine).
- The name of the disease or injury condition diagnosed or treated (examples: Cataract; Rubella).
- A synonym of the stipulated term (examples: Drill Hole; Intensive Care).
- An eponym of the stipulated term (examples: Denis Browne Splint; Mayo Procedure).
- An abbreviation or abridgment of the stipulated term (examples: CAT Scan; HTLV-II).

A main term in the alphabetical index of the CPT volume may be an unaccompanied entry (examples of a main term without a subterm: Fibrinogen; Ureterostomy), or may be followed by a number of subterms that annotate or modify the main term and consequently influence code selection (examples of a main term with subterms: Cytopathology; Incision).

If subterms appear under main term index entries each subterm must be carefully reviewed to insure accurate code number selection (examples of a main term with subterms of divergent meanings: Diaphragm; Repositioning). An indented entry under a subterm is called a sub-subterm (examples of a sub-subterm: Endoscopic indented under the subterm Bile Duct Stone, a subterm of the main term Lithotripsy; and Percutaneous Fixation indented under the subterm Fracture, a subterm of the main term Thumb).

For certain generic main term index entries, more than one CPT code number appears to be applicable. These seemingly appropriate code numbers may or may not be numerically sequential. If these code numbers constitute a numeric sequence, the first and the last code numbers of the sequence are indicated, each of which is separated with a hyphen (examples: After Hours Medical Services; Neurorrhaphy). This type of numeric entry is referred to as a "code range." If these code numbers do not form a numeric sequence, each code number is indicated (in numerical order) and is separated with a comma from the foregoing code number (examples: Dacryoadenectomy; Occult Blood). This type of numeric entry is referred to as a "code series."

Notations in the CPT volume labeled as cross-references direct those using the CPT coding system to review additional information. Two styles of cross-references are functional in the alphabetical index to the listings of the CPT manual. The cross-reference "see" (used primarily with synonyms, eponyms, and abbreviations) leads code number searches to the term printed behind the word (examples: Bed Sore, see Pressure Ulcer; IPPB, see Intermittent Positive Pressure Breathing). The cross-reference "see also" leads code number searches to another main term if a procedure or a service is not included in the index entries either as a main term or among subterm entries under a main term (examples: Endoscopy, see also Arthroscopy; Spinal Cord, see also Cauda Equina and see also Nerve Root).

To diminish the size of the alphabetical reference index and to accord a space-saving convention to the CPT volume, certain words in the index entries are merely implied, and their intent inferred from the context of the other terms in that entry. The predominant usage of this convention is with procedures and services denoted in subterm entries (examples: main term Abdomen, subterm Hernia Repair, sub-subterm Anesthesia implies anesthesia for hernia repair; main term Opiates implies chemical examination of a specimen for opiates).

To proficiently utilize the CPT coding system for code number selection, the alphabetical index to the CPT volume should always be used in the subsequent prescribed search sequence (Table 3–5). First and foremost, the index should be scanned to locate a main term either for the procedure or service rendered or for the organ or anatomic site diagnosed or treated. If this initial searching is ineffective or unproductive, the index should be scanned to locate a main term for the disease or injury diagnosed or treated, or for any synonyms, eponyms, or

TABLE 3–5

CPT Index Search Sequence

1. Locate main term for procedure or service.   **yes** or **no**
   If yes, then go to #5; if no, then go to #2.
2. Locate main term for organ or anatomic site diagnosed or treated.   **yes** or **no**
   If yes, then go to #5; if no, then go to #3.
3. Locate main term for disease or injury diagnosed or treated.   **yes** or **no**
   If yes, then go to #5; if no, then go to #4.
4. Contact physician for clarification of procedure or service rendered and selection of appropriate main term.
5. Survey all subterms and all sub-subterms denoted beneath the main term and survey any cross-references related to it.
6. Choose a suitable and warranted code number, code range, or code series.
7. Affirm code number, code range, or code series in the numerical section listings of code numbers and descriptors.
8. Analyze the applicable descriptor and finalize code selection.

abbreviations associated with the main term. The attending physician should be consulted if a suitable entry still cannot be located.

Second, after the location of the appropriate main term, the coder should survey all sub-terms and all sub-subterms indicated beneath that main term and should observe any cross-reference notations related to that entry. Third, the applicable and warranted code number, code range, or code series should be chosen. Fourth and lastly, code number selection should be finalized through verification of the code number in the numerical section code number and descriptor listings. If necessary, all of the code number and descriptor listings within a stated range or series should be thoroughly reviewed to discern the most accurate code number and descriptor selection.

As with the ICD-9-CM diagnostic coding system (and every coding system), CPT code number selection must absolutely never be accomplished solely by utilizing the alphabetic index to the volume. Even if only one code number is printed in the main term index entry for the procedure or service being reported, that code number must be verified in the numerical section listings in order to guarantee accurate and precise code number and descriptor selection.

KEY CONCEPTS

abbreviation _____	modifier _____
anatomic term _____	parentheses _____
appendix _____	procedural term _____
category _____	section _____
circles _____	section title _____
code and descriptor _____	semicolon following descriptor _____
code range _____	special report _____
code series _____	starred procedure _____
common narrative expression _____	stars _____
cross-reference _____	subcategory _____
diagnostic term _____	subheading _____
eponym _____	subsection _____
five-digit modifier _____	subsection title _____
guideline _____	sub-subheading _____
heading	sub-subterm _____
hierarchical level _____	subterm _____
hierarchical structure _____	symbols _____
hierarchy _____	synonym _____
indented code and descriptor _____	triangles _____
index _____	two-digit modifier _____
listing _____	unlisted procedure _____
mainterm _____	unlisted service _____

REVIEW EXERCISES

1. What terms define the separation of the CPT coding system into hierarchical levels? _____

_____

_____

2. What variations or distinctions specify the titles ascribed to subsections, headings, and sub-headings? _____

   _____

   _____

3. Specify the hierarchical level of each of the subsequent designations:
   A. *Arthrodesis* _____

   _____

   B. *Sinus of Valsalva* _____

   _____

   C. *Ureter* _____

   _____

   D. *Middle Ear* _____

   _____

   E. *Immunology* _____

   _____

   F. *Cardiography* _____

   _____

   G. *Tests and Measurements* _____

   _____

4. What criteria determine the section or subsection from which a physician is permitted or entitled to select codes for reporting billed charges? _____

   _____

   _____

5. Choose any two sections of the CPT volume and itemize each subsection or category (enumerating the range of corresponding code numbers) contained within those subsections or categories. _____

   _____

   _____

6. Choose any subsection or category in the CPT volume and itemize each heading as well as each subheading included within that subsection or category (if applicable). Enumerate the range of corresponding code numbers for each heading and subheading itemized. _____

   _____

   _____

7. What intent is conveyed by a semicolon following a descriptor listing? What intent is conveyed by an indented code number and descriptor listing? _____

   _____

   _____

8. Write the full procedure descriptor or the full service descriptor for the following code numbers in the CPT volume:
   A. 21386 _____

   _____

   B. 33513 _____

   _____

   C. 52204 _____

   _____

   D. 66625 _____

   _____

E. 78001 _____

_____

F. 86906 _____

_____

G. 92990 _____

_____

9. Identify the symbol used to indicate an added code appearing in a new volume of CPT. Scan the CPT volume and list at least ten newly added code numbers.

_____   _____

_____   _____

_____   _____

_____   _____

_____   _____

10. Identify the symbol used to indicate a revised descriptor appearing in a new volume of CPT. Scan the CPT volume and list at least ten code numbers with revised descriptors.

_____   _____

_____   _____

_____   _____

_____   _____

_____   _____

11. Identify the symbol used to indicate a code deleted from a new volume of CPT. Scan the CPT volume and list at least ten newly deleted code numbers.

_____   _____

_____   _____

_____   _____

_____   _____

_____   _____

12. Identify the symbol used to indicate a listing for a surgical procedure not bounded by the surgical package concept. Scan the CPT volume and list code numbers for at least ten procedures that are not bounded by the surgical package concept.

_____   _____

_____   _____

_____   _____

_____   _____

_____   _____

13. As a rule, what symbol utilized in the CPT coding system will be retained adjacent to a specific code number in later CPT volumes? _____

_____

_____

14. What is the standard content of the special report submitted to third-party payors with the utilization of a code number for an unlisted procedure or an unlisted service? _____

_____

_____

15. Select two sections of the CPT volume. Compare and contrast the contents of the set of guidelines for both of the chosen sections. Write a brief synopsis of the similarities and differences between the two sets of guidelines. _____

_____

_____

16. Summarize the content of each of the four appendices in the current CPT volume. _____

_____

_____

17. What are the advantages and disadvantages of the use of modifiers in a coding system? __

_____

_____

18. Scan the comprehensive list of code modifiers in the CPT volume. Which of the modifiers must never be used concurrently to report special circumstances involving the rendering of a procedure or service? _____

_____

_____

19. In what sequence should multiple modifiers used concurrently be reported? _____

_____

_____

20. What potential problems can occur with the overuse of modifiers in the CPT coding system? _____

_____

_____

21. Describe the proper technique for ascertaining correct CPT code number selection by using the alphabetical reference index to the CPT volume. _____

_____

_____

22. Scan the alphabetical reference index to the CPT volume and list a minimum of ten main terms for which cross-reference notations are designated.

_____   _____

_____   _____

_____   _____

_____   _____

_____   _____

23. Locate within the alphabetical reference index to the CPT volume at least ten main terms for which a code range (instead of a specific code number) is enumerated.

_____   _____

_____   _____

_____   _____

_____   _____

_____   _____

24. Locate within the alphabetical reference index to the CPT volume at least ten main terms for which a code series (instead of a specific code number) is enumerated.

_____	_____
_____	_____
_____	_____
_____	_____
_____	_____
_____	_____

25. Scan the alphabetical reference index to the CPT volume and list a minimum of ten subterm entries with implied meanings through omitted words.

_____	_____
_____	_____
_____	_____
_____	_____
_____	_____
_____	_____

26. Use the alphabetical index to the CPT volume to select accurate and precise code numbers for the following procedures or services:
    A. otoplasty _____
    B. diphtheria antibody _____
    C. sensorimotor exam _____
    D. ankle fusion _____
    E. spleen repair _____
    F. exploration of breast _____
    G. omental flap _____
    H. range-of-motion test of hand _____
    I. vaginal cyst excision _____
    J. myelography of brain _____
    K. chest artery ligation _____
    L. gentimicin assay _____
    M. ocular implant removal _____
    N. replacement of pulmonary valve _____
    O. enterolysis _____
    P. lacrimal sac biopsy _____
    Q. Unna paste boot removal _____
    R. hemograft of skin _____
    S. mitral valve replacement _____
    T. removal of cranial tongs _____
    U. cystoplasty _____
    V. heel spur excision _____
    W. mastopexy _____
    X. phrenic nerve avulsion _____
    Y. Stamey procedure _____
    Z. Kasai procedure _____

4

CHAPTER

ICD Coding: Infectious Diseases; Neoplasms; Endocrine, Nutritional, Metabolic, and Blood Disorders

LEARNING OBJECTIVES

Upon completion of this chapter the learner should be able to:

1. Describe the parameters for coding and reporting conditions regarded as manifestations of disease.
2. Describe the parameters for coding and reporting conditions regarded as late effects.
3. Describe the parameters for coding and reporting primary neoplasms.
4. Describe the parameters for coding and reporting secondary neoplasms.
5. Describe the parameters for coding and reporting neoplasms of uncertain behavior in contrast to those for neoplasms of unspecified nature.
6. Explain the proper usage of the table for coding neoplasms.
7. Describe the parameters for coding and reporting complications of diabetes.
8. Describe the parameters for coding and reporting anemia.
9. Discuss the impact of comorbidities and complications on billing and reimbursement for diagnoses and procedures involving infectious, parasitic, neoplastic, endocrine, nutritional, metabolic, or blood diseases.
10. Apply knowledge of coding principles by assigning accurate and precise codes to report diagnoses of infectious or parasitic disease.
11. Apply knowledge of coding principles by assigning accurate and precise codes to report diagnoses of neoplasms.
12. Apply knowledge of coding principles by assigning accurate and precise codes to report diagnoses and procedures pertaining to endocrine, nutritional, metabolic, and immunity diseases or disorders.
13. Apply knowledge of coding principles by assigning accurate and precise codes to report diagnoses and procedures pertaining to the blood and blood-forming organs.

ICD CODING OF INFECTIOUS AND PARASITIC DISEASES

Chapter 1 of the ICD-9-CM diagnostic tabular volume contains listings of codes for infectious diseases and parasitic diseases, and is the longest and most obscure chapter of Volume 1. This chapter, extending from category 001 through category 139, includes diseases generally recognized as communicable or transmissible as well as diseases of unknown but possibly infectious origin. The chapter consists of sixteen sections (Table 4–1).

The first section on intestinal infectious diseases includes cholera, typhoid fever, salmonella infections, bacillary dysentery, bacterial food poisonings, and amebiasis. The second section on tuberculosis encompasses tubucular infections (human and bovine) that are pulmonary, respiratory, meningeal, intestinal, peritoneal, mesenteric, musculoskeletal, and genitourinary, as well as tuberculosis of other organs. The codes in this section are applicable to tuberculosis that is disseminated, generalized, or miliary, and are applicable whether the disease affects a single site, multiple sites, or an unspecified site.

Zoonotic bacterial diseases in the third section include plague, tularemia, anthrax, brucellosis, glanders, melioidosis, and other diseases. The fourth section lists other bacterial diseases, including leprosy, diphtheria, whooping cough, strep throat, scarlet fever, erysipelas, tetanus, septicemia, and actinomycotic infections. Category 041 provides additional codes and narrative titles to be used to identify the bacterial agent in diseases classified elsewhere. Entries in this category are also used to classify bacterial infections of an unspecified nature or an unspecified site.

If the diagnosis of septicemia with shock or the diagnosis of general sepsis with septic shock is documented, the septicemia condition should be sequenced first and the septic shock should be sequenced as a secondary condition. The septicemia code assignment should

---

TABLE 4–1

Sections and Subsections in Chapter 1, Volume 1 of ICD-9-CM

1. Intestinal Infectious Diseases (category range 001–009)
2. Tuberculosis (category range 010–018)
3. Zoonotic Bacterial Diseases (category range 020–027)
4. Other Bacterial Diseases (category range 030–041)
5. Human Immunodeficiency Virus (HIV) Infection (category range 042–044)
6. Poliomyelitis and Other Non-Arthropod Borne Viral Diseases of the Central Nervous System (category range 045–049)
7. Viral Diseases Accompanied by Exanthem (category range 050–057)
8. Arthropod-Borne Viral Diseases (category range 060–066)
9. Other Diseases due to Viruses and Chlamydiae (category range 070–079)
10. Rickettsioses and Other Arthropod-Borne Diseases (category range 080–088)
11. Syphillis and Other Venereal Diseases (category range 090–099)
12. Other Spirochetal Diseases (category range 100–104)
13. Mycoses (category range 110–118)
14. Helminthiases (category range 120–129)
15. Other Infectious and Parasitic Diseases (category range 130–136)
16. Late Effects of Infectious and Parasitic Diseases (category range 137–139)

identify the type of bacteria, if the organism was identified. As examples, sepsis produced by *Pseudomonas* would be coded and reported as 041.7; sepsis produced by *Klebsiella* would be coded and reported as 041.3. Negative or inconclusive blood cultures do not preclude a diagnosis of septicemia in patients with clinical evidence of this condition.

The fifth section on human immunodeficiency virus includes other specified conditions, including AIDS-like syndrome and AIDS-related complex. Previous printings of ICD-9-CM provided a table for coding human immunodeficiency virus depending on its presence with other diseases or its causative effect in the etiology of other disorders. This table was, however, deleted from the classification.

Non-arthropod borne viral diseases in the sixth section include meningitis and poliomyelitis. In the seventh section, viral diseases accompanied by exanthem include smallpox, cowpox, chickenpox, herpes zoster, herpes simplex, measles (including rubeola), and rubella (including German measles). An additional code should be used to report any associated meningitis.

Arthropod-borne viral diseases in the eighth section include yellow fever, dengue, viral encephalitis (tick-borne and mosquito-borne), and arthropod-borne hemorrhagic fever. Other viral diseases grouped in the ninth section include viral hepatitis, rabies, mumps, ornithosis, infectious mononucleosis, and trachoma. Category 079 provides listings of additional codes and narrative titles to be used to identify the viral agent in diseases classifiable elsewhere. Codes in this category should also be used to classify a virus infection of an unspecified nature or an unspecified site.

Rickettsioses in the tenth section include typhus, malaria, leishmaniasis, and trypanosomiasis. In the eleventh section, venereal diseases include syphilis of various specifications, including congenital syphilis, early syphilis, late syphilis, cardiovascular syphilis, and neurosyphilis. Gonococcal infections also are classified in this section. Categories 092 and 096 both provide a code and narrative title to report syphilis without clinical manifestations, with positive serological reaction and negative spinal fluid test, less than two years after infection. An additional code and narrative title should be utilized to report any associated mental disorder.

Spirochetal diseases in the twelfth section include leptospirosis, yaws, and pinta. In the thirteenth section, mycoses include dermatophytosis, dermatomycosis, candidiasis, coccidioidomycosis, histoplasmosis, as well as blastomycotic infections. An additional code and narrative title should be used to identify and report any additional clinical manifestation. Opportunistic mycoses include infections of the skin, subcutaneous tissues, and/or organs by a wide variety of fungi, generally considered to be pathogenic by compromised hosts only.

Helminthiases in the fourteenth section include schistosomiasis and other trematode infections, echinococcosis and other cestode infections, trichinosis, filiarial infection, ancylostomiasis, and unspecified intestinal parasitism. The fifteenth section is a residual section that encompasses diseases such as toxoplasmosis, trichomoniasis, pediculosis, acariasis, and sarcoidosis. The sixteenth and final section of Chapter 1 classifies late effects of infectious and parasitic diseases.

Category *137 Late effects of tuberculosis* is used to indicate conditions classifiable in categories 010–018 as the cause of late effects, which are classified elsewhere. The late effects include those specified as sequelae, due to old or inactive tuberculosis, without evidence of active disease.

Category *138 Late effects of acute poliomyelitis* is used to indicate conditions classifiable in category 045 as the cause of late effects, which are classified elsewhere. The "late effects" include conditions specified as sequelae that are present after the onset of the acute poliomyelitis.

Category *139 Late effects of other infectious and parasitic diseases* is used to indicate conditions classifiable in categories 001–009, to categories 020–041, or to categories 046–136 as the cause of late effects, which are classified elsewhere. These late effects include conditions specified as such, but also include sequelae of diseases classifiable in the above categories if there is evidence that the disease itself is no longer present.

ICD CODING OF NEOPLASMS

Chapter 2 of the ICD-9-CM diagnostic tabular volume, designated for listings of neoplasms, classifies all tumors, including those that are functionally inactive. This chapter, extending from category 140 through category 239, includes malignant and benign neoplasias as well as carcinoma in situ and neoplasms of uncertain or unspecified morphology.

An additional code from Chapter 3 may be used to identify functional activity associated with any neoplasm. To identify the histological type of a neoplasm, a comprehensive coded nomenclature that comprises the morphology rubrics of ICD-0 is contained in Appendix A.

Categories 140 through 195 inclusive are for the classification of primary malignant neoplasms according to their point of origin. A malignant neoplasm with an undetermined point of origin that is classifiable in two or more subcategories within a three-digit rubric and whose point of origin cannot be determined should be classified in the subcategory .8 (examples: code number 140.8 for contiguous or overlapping sites of the lip; code number 157.8 for contiguous or overlapping sites of the pancreas)

Three subcategories (*149.8, 159.8,* and *165.8*) are provided for malignant neoplasms that overlap the boundaries of three-digit rubrics within certain systems. Overlapping malignant neoplasms that cannot be classified as indicated above should be assigned to the appropriate subcategory of category 195.

The neoplasm chapter (Chapter 2) consists of eleven sections listed in Table 4–2.

Categories 235 through 238 classify by site certain histomorphologically well-defined neoplasms, the subsequent behavior of which cannot be predicted from the present appearance. Category 239 classifies by site neoplasms of unspecified morphology and behavior, including growth, not otherwise specified, or tumor, not otherwise specified. The term "mass" unless otherwise stated, should not be regarded as a neoplasm. Additional codes and narrative titles should be used to identify and report any functional activity due to the neoplasm.

If primary treatment in the episode of care is directed at the malignancy as the principal diagnosis, the malignant condition should be designated except if the purpose of the outpatient encounter or inpatient admission was for a radiotherapy or chemotherapy session. In such cases, the malignancy should be coded and sequenced secondarily. For example, reporting code numbers on a claim for a patient who was status post bilateral oophorectomy for ovarian carcinoma and who was admitted for chemotherapy, necessitates the sequencing of code number *V58.1* as the principal diagnosis code and the reporting of code number *183.0* as a secondary diagnosis code.

If a patient was admitted for the purpose of radiotherapy or chemotherapy and develops complications such as uncontrolled nausea and vomiting or dehydration, the principal diagnosis should be admission for radiotherapy *V58.0*, or admission for chemotherapy *V58.1*. If this patient experienced severe vomiting and consequent dehydration as a result of the chemotherapy, code number *V58.1* would still be reported as the principal diagnosis code, by reason that chemotherapy was the cause for admission. The vomiting (code number *787.0*) and the dehydration (code number *276.5*) should be reported as secondary diagnosis codes.

If an episode of inpatient care involved surgical removal of a primary site malignancy or a secondary site malignancy followed by adjunct chemotherapy or radiotherapy, the

T A B L E 4–2

Sections in Chapter 2, Volume 1 of ICD-9-CM

1. Malignant Neoplasm of Lip, Oral Cavity, and Pharynx (category range 140–149) with designated categories for lip, tongue, salivary organs, gum, mouth, oropharynx, nasopharynx, and hypopharynx.
2. Malignant Neoplasm of Digestive Organs and Peritoneum (category range 150–159) with designated categories for esophagus, stomach, small intestine, colon, rectum and anus, liver, gallbladder, pancreas, and peritoneum.
3. Malignant Neoplasm of Respiratory and Intrathoracic Organs (category range 160–165) with designated categories for nasal cavities and accessory sinuses, larynx, trachea, bronchus and lung, pleura, thymus, heart, and mediastinum.
4. Malignant Neoplasm of Bone, Connective Tissue, Skin, and Breast (category range 170–175) with designated categories for bone and articular cartilage, connective and soft tissue (including blood vessel, bursa, fascia, fat, ligament, muscle, nerves and ganglia, synovia, tendons, and sweat glands), female breast, male breast, and malignant melanoma.
5. Malignant Neoplasm of Genitourinary Organs (category range 179–189) with designated categories for cervix, placenta, uterus, ovary and uterine adnexa, prostate, testis, penis, bladder, and kidney.
6. Malignant Neoplasm of Other and Unspecified Sites (category range 190–199) with designated categories for eye, brain, thyroid gland, other endocrine glands, and lymph nodes. Category 195 provides a listing of codes and narrative titles for malignant neoplasms of contiguous sites whose point of origin cannot be determined.
7. Malignant Neoplasm of Lymphatic and Hematopoietic Tissue (category range 200–208) with designated categories for lymphosarcoma and reticulosarcoma, Hodgkin's disease, multiple myeloma, lymphoid leukemia, myeloid leukemia, and monocytic leukemia.
8. Benign Neoplasms (category range 210–229) with designated categories for mouth and pharynx, digestive system, intrathoracic organs, bone and articular cartilage, lipoma, connective and soft tissue, skin, breast, uterine leiomyoma, ovary, other female genital organs, male genital organs, kidney and other urinary organs, eye, brain and nervous system, thyroid glands, other endocrine glands, hemangioma and lymphangioma.
9. Carcinoma in Situ (category range 230–234) with designated categories for digestive organs, respiratory system, skin, breast, and genitourinary system.
10. Neoplasm of Uncertain Behavior (category range 235–238) with designated categories for digestive and respiratory systems, genitourinary organs, or endocrine glands and nervous system.
11. Neoplasm of Unspecified Nature (category 239).

malignancy should be coded as the principal diagnosis, using codes in the 140–198 series of categories, or if appropriate, codes in the 200–203 series of categories. To exemplify, the principal diagnosis for a patient admitted to receive a modified radical mastectomy for carcinoma of the central portion of the breast should be reported with code number *174.1*. Even though chemotherapy was administered during the same episode of care, the principal diagnosis (and reason for admission) was the malignancy, which required the administration of chemotherapy.

If the reason for admission was to determine the extent of the malignancy, or for a procedure such as paracentesis or thoracentesis, the primary malignancy or appropriate metastatic site should be designated as the principal diagnosis, even though chemotherapy or radiotherapy was administered. In the event of any diagnostic workup for the malignancy or its metastases, the malignancy should be regarded as the principal diagnosis.

If the primary malignancy was previously excised or eradicated from its site and there was no adjunct treatment directed to that site and no evidence of any remaining malignancy at the primary site, an appropriate code from the V10 category should be used to indicate the former site of the primary malignancy. Any mention of extension, invasion, or metastasis to a nearby organ or to a distant site should be coded as a secondary malignant neoplasm to that site and may be the principal diagnosis in the absence of treatment directed to the primary site. Reporting diagnoses of liver metastases from a previously excised carcinoma of the colon, therefore, requires the use of code number *197.7* as the principal diagnosis to represent the metastatic condition and the use of code number *V10.05* to represent the history of colonic carcinoma.

If a patient was admitted because of a primary neoplasm with metastasis, and treatment was directed toward the secondary site only, the secondary neoplasm should be designated as the principal diagnosis even though the primary malignancy is still present. For example, brain metastases (code number *198.3*) should be reported as the principal diagnosis if a patient were admitted for brain imaging, even though the metastatic condition resulted from oat cell carcinoma of the lower lobe of the lung, which is still present. The lung malignancy (code number *162.5*) should be reported as a secondary diagnosis code in this example.

Symptoms, signs, and vaguely defined conditions listed in Chapter 16 that are characteristic of, or associated with, an existing primary or secondary site malignancy cannot be reported to supercede the malignancy code for the principal diagnosis, regardless of the number of admissions or encounters for treatment and care of the neoplasm. For instance, abdominal pain from gastric carcinoma, even if severe and requiring pain management, should not be coded and reported as the reason for admission. The gastric carcinoma (code number *151.9*) should be coded and reported as the principal diagnosis in such cases.

If the patient admission was for management of an anemia associated with a malignancy, and the treatment was only for anemia, the anemia should be designated as the principal diagnosis and should be reported with an appropriate code for the malignancy. Thus, sideroblastic anemia resulting from treatment of pancreatic duct cancer (code number *285.0*) should be coded and reported as the principal diagnosis if treatment for the anemia necessitated the episode of care. The pancreatic malignancy (code number *157.3*) should be reported as a secondary diagnosis code.

If the admission was for management of an anemia associated with chemotherapy or radiotherapy and the only treatment rendered was for the anemia, the anemia should be designated as the principal diagnosis and the appropriate codes for the malignancy are reported secondarily. Thus, hemolytic anemia resulting from chemotherapy (code number *283.0*) should be coded and reported as the principal diagnosis if treatment for the anemia necessitated the episode of care. The code numbers for the malignancy should be reported as secondary diagnosis codes.

If the patient admission was for management of dehydration due to a malignancy, the chemotherapy, or a combination of both, and only the dehydration was treated (by intravenous rehydration, for instance), the dehydration should be designated as the principal diagnosis, and the codes for the malignancy should be reported secondarily. Thus, dehydration (code number *276.5*) resulting from adenocarcinoma of the bladder neck (code number *188.5*) should be coded and reported as the principal diagnosis if treatment for the dehydration necessitated the episode of care. The condition of adenocarcinoma of the bladder should be coded and reported as a secondary diagnosis code.

If the admission was for treatment of a complication resulting from a surgical procedure such as a colon resection performed for the treatment of an intestinal malignancy, the complication should be designated as the principal diagnosis if treatment was directed at resolving the complication. For instance, if a postoperative infection developed and required additional care and a subsequent admission, the postoperative infection (code number *998.59*) should be reported as the principal diagnosis because that condition necessitated the readmission of the patient.

ICD CODING OF ENDOCRINE DISEASES AND OPERATIONS, NUTRITIONAL AND METABOLIC DISEASES, IMMUNITY DISORDERS, AND BLOOD DISEASES

Chapter 3 of the ICD-9-CM diagnostic tabular volume is designated for listings of endocrine, nutritional, metabolic, as well as immunity disorders, and classifies these maladies in categories 240 through 279. All neoplasms, whether or not functionally active, are classified in Chapter 2. However, codes from Chapter 3 should be used to identify functional activity associated with any neoplasm or with ectopic endocrine tissue. Chapter 3 consists of four sections (Table 4–3).

Thyroid disorders in the first section include goiter (simple and nodular), thyrotoxicosis, hypothyroidism (congenital and acquired), and thyroiditis. Additional codes should be utilized to identify any associated mental retardation or to identify causative drugs, if applicable.

An additional code should be utilized to identify the manifestation of diabetes and other disorders of pancreatic internal secretion. The fifth-digit subclassification for diabetes reports the presence or absence of insulin dependency. Other endocrine disorders classified in this second section include disorders of the parathyroid glands, disorders of the pituitary gland and its hypothalamic control, diseases of the thymus gland, disorders of the adrenal glands (pituitary induced or drug induced), ovarian dysfunction, testicular dysfunction, and polyglandular dysfunction.

Categories of listings in Volume 3 of ICD-9-CM are established for surgical procedures on the various components of the endocrine system. These include category range 06–07 for: operations on the thyroid and parathyroid glands as well as operations on certain other endocrine glands including the adrenals, the pineal gland, the pituitary gland, and the thymus.

Nutritional deficiencies in the third section include protein calorie malnutrition; vitamin deficiencies; deficiencies of thiamine, niacin, or ascorbic acid; and other dietary deficits. Metabolic disorders in the fourth section include disorders of amino acid transport and metabolism; disorders of carbohydrate transport and metabolism; disorders of lipoid metabolism; disorders of plasma protein metabolism; gout; disorders of mineral metabolism; disorders of fluid, electrolyte, and acid-base balance; obesity; and hyperalimentation. An additional code should be utilized to identify any associated mental retardation.

Chapter 4 of Volume 1 of ICD-9-CM, listing hematologic disorders and diseases, consists of a single section, Diseases of Blood and Blood-Forming Organs (category range 280–289). This chapter of the diagnostic tabular excludes listings of anemias complicating pregnancy or the puerperium. These listings in Chapter 4 do include iron-deficiency anemias, hereditary hemolytic anemias, acquired hemolytic anemias, aplastic anemia, coagulation defects, purpura and other hemorrhagic conditions, and diseases of the white blood cells (excluding leukemia).

Categories of listings in Volume 3 of ICD-9-CM are established for surgical procedures on the various components of the hemic and lymphatic systems. These include category range 40–41 for operations on the lymphatic system and operations on the bone marrow and spleen.

TABLE 4–3

Sections in Chapter 3, Volume 1 of ICD-9-CM

1. Disorders of Thyroid Gland (category range 240–246)
2. Diseases of Other Endocrine Glands (category range 250–259)
3. Nutritional Deficiencies (category range 260–269)
4. Other Metabolic and Immunity Disorders (category range 270–279)

INFECTIOUS DISEASES REPORTING FOR BILLING

Billing of third-party payors involves the submission of diagnostic and procedural data with the claim. Ordinarily, the reporting of the principal diagnosis and/or principal procedure impacts the amount of reimbursement received by the healthcare provider.

The principal diagnosis is defined as the condition responsible for the admission of the patient to the health service encounter or episode of care. The principal procedure is defined as the procedure most closely associated with the patient's principal diagnosis for that specific admission, encounter, or episode of care.

Generally, the diagnosis or procedure posing the greatest risk to the patient is the most resource intensive diagnosis or procedure. However, under exceptional circumstances, especially those involving an inpatient in an acute care facility, the most resource intensive diagnosis or procedure, or the condition or treatment presenting the greatest risk to the patient, may be unrelated to the criteria establishing the patient's principal diagnosis. Such a situation may occur if a patient is admitted for a relatively minor problem and major complications occur unexpectedly. For instance, a patient might be admitted for bacterial food poisoning and develop staphylococcal septicemia during the hospital stay.

Insurance carriers ordinarily mandate and limit coding and reporting to diagnoses specifically assessed or treated and to procedures actually rendered during that particular admission, encounter, or episode of care. The principal diagnosis and principal procedure are sequenced first and all other relevant diagnoses and procedures are reported in descending order of clinical significance and resource intensity. For instance, a severe condition such as gas gangrene would be sequenced before a less severe condition such as viral gastroenteritis. These acute conditions would likewise precede a chronic condition such as late latent syphilis.

Reporting of code numbers for nonspecific (unspecified) infectious or parasitic diseases should be avoided if possible. Personnel responsible for coding and billing should attempt to ascertain the most specific code not only for reimbursement purposes, but also to generate meaningful data for statistical and research purposes. Accurate and complete documentation by physicians in the patient health record, as well as the timely placement of laboratory reports in that record, may alleviate the necessity of reporting codes for unspecified infectious or parasitic diseases.

Designated ICD-9-CM codes are recognized as comorbidities by certain third-party payors, especially Medicare. For inpatient admissions, these comorbid conditions may increase the amount of reimbursement received by the provider. Comorbidities among the infectious and parasitic diseases are represented by the following code numbers:

011.00	011.01	011.02
011.03	011.04	011.05
011.06	011.10	011.11
011.12	011.13	011.14
011.15	011.16	011.20
011.21	011.22	011.23
011.24	011.25	011.26
011.30	011.31	011.32
011.33	011.34	011.35
011.36	011.40	011.41
011.42	011.43	011.44
011.45	011.46	011.50
011.51	011.52	011.53
011.54	011.55	011.56
011.60	011.61	011.62

011.63	011.64	011.65
011.66	011.70	011.71
011.72	011.73	011.74
011.75	011.76	011.80
011.81	011.82	011.83
011.84	011.85	011.86
011.90	011.91	011.92
011.93	011.94	011.95
011.96	012.00	012.01
012.02	012.03	012.04
012.05	012.06	012.10
012.11	012.12	012.13
012.14	012.15	012.16
013.00	013.01	013.02
013.03	013.04	013.05
013.06	013.10	013.11
013.12	013.13	013.14
013.15	013.16	013.20
013.21	013.22	013.23
013.24	013.25	013.26
013.30	013.31	013.33
013.34	013.35	013.36
013.40	013.41	013.42
013.43	013.45	013.46
013.50	013.51	013.52
013.53	013.56	013.60
013.60	013.62	013.63
013.64	013.65	013.66
013.80	013.81	013.82
013.83	013.84	013.85
013.86	013.90	013.91
013.92	013.93	013.94
013.95	013.96	014.00
014.01	014.02	014.03
014.04	014.05	014.06
014.80	014.81	014.82
014.83	014.84	014.85
014.86	016.00	016.01
016.02	016.03	016.04
016.05	016.06	016.10
016.11	016.12	016.13
016.14	016.15	016.16
016.20	016.21	016.22
016.23	016.24	016.25
016.26	016.30	016.31
016.32	016.35	016.36
016.40	016.41	016.42
016.43	016.44	016.45
016.46	016.50	016.51
016.52	016.53	016.54

016.55	016.56	016.60
016.61	016.62	016.63
016.64	016.65	016.66
016.70	016.71	016.72
016.73	016.74	016.75
016.76	016.90	016.91
016.92	016.93	016.94
016.95	016.96	017.20
017.21	017.22	017.23
017.24	017.25	017.26
017.30	017.31	017.32
017.33	017.34	017.35
017.36	017.40	017.41
017.42	017.43	017.44
017.45	017.46	017.50
017.51	017.52	017.53
017.54	017.55	017.56
017.60	017.61	017.62
017.63	017.64	017.65
017.66	017.70	017.71
017.72	017.73	017.74
017.75	017.76	017.80
017.81	017.82	017.83
017.84	017.85	017.86
017.90	017.91	017.92
017.93	017.94	017.95
017.96	018.01	018.02
018.03	018.04	018.05
018.06	018.80	018.81
018.82	018.83	018.84
018.85	018.86	018.90
018.91	018.92	018.93
018.94	018.95	018.96
031.0	036.0	036.1
036.2	036.3	036.40
036.41	036.42	036.43
036.81	036.82	036.89
037.0	038.0	038.1
038.2	038.3	038.40
038.41	038.42	038.43
038.44	038.49	038.8
038.9	040.0	042.0
046.2	052.0	052.1
052.7	052.8	052.9
053.0	053.10	053.11
053.12	053.13	053.19
053.79	053.8	054.3
054.5	054.71	054.72
054.79	054.8	055.0
055.1	055.2	055.71

055.79	055.8	056.00
056.01	056.09	056.71
056.79	056.8	070.20
070.21	070.22	070.23
070.30	070.31	070.32
070.33	070.41	070.42
070.43	070.44	070.49
070.51	070.52	070.53
070.54	070.59	070.6
070.9	072.0	072.1
072.2	072.3	072.71
072.72	072.79	072.8
086.0	090.40	090.41
090.42	090.49	093.0
093.1	093.21	093.22
093.23	093.24	093.81
093.82	093.89	093.9
094.0	094.1	094.2
094.3	094.81	094.87
094.89	094.9	098.0
098.10	098.11	098.12
098.13	098.14	098.15
098.16	098.17	098.19
112.0	112.4	112.5
112.81	112.83	112.84
112.85	114.0	114.2
114.3	114.9	115.00
115.01	115.02	115.03
115.04	115.05	115.10
115.11	115.12	115.13
115.14	115.15	115.19
115.90	115.91	115.92
115.93	115.94	115.95
115.99	116.0	116.1
117.3	117.4	117.5
117.6	117.7	118
130.0	130.1	130.2
130.3	130.4	130.5
130.7	130.8	135
136.3	137.0	137.1
137.2	138	

The Medicare prospective payment system is predicated upon diagnosis related groups (DRG's) that are determined by the ICD-9-CM code numbers, which are reported on the claim submitted by the healthcare provider to the payor. These DRG's are distributed into major diagnostic categories (MDC's). The DRG's pertinent to infectious and parasitic diseases are distributed into MDC 18, Infectious and Parasitic Diseases, Systemic or Unspecified Sites

TABLE 4-4

Diagnosis Related Groups for Infectious and Parasitic Diseases

DRG 415, Operating Room Procedure for Infectious and Parasitic Diseases
DRG 416, Septicemia, Age Greater than 17
DRG 417, Septicemia, Age 0–17
DRG 418, Postoperative and Posttraumatic Infections
DRG 419, Fever of Unknown Origin, Age Greater than 17 with Comorbidity or Complication
DRG 420, Fever of Unknown Origin, Age Greater than 17 without Comorbidity or Complication
DRG 421, Viral Illness, Age Greater than 17
DRG 422, Viral Illness and Fever of Unknown Origin, Age 0–17
DRG 423, Other Infectious and Parasitic Diseases Diagnoses

(Table 4–4). The DRG's relevant to human immunodeficiency virus are distributed into MDC 25, Human Immunodeficiency Virus Infections (Table 4–5).

ONCOLOGY AND HEMATOLOGY REPORTING FOR BILLING

In this chapter, the prior section on coding of neoplasms explained the guidelines for reporting the principal diagnosis for services relating to oncology or hematology. The coder should be aware that the principal diagnosis is always the condition responsible for the admission of the patient to the health service admission, encounter, or episode of service.

As previously explained, the diagnosis presenting the most significant risk to the patient is usually the most resource intensive diagnosis. Nonetheless, under exceptional circumstances, especially those involving a patient in an acute care facility, the most resource intensive diagnosis may not fulfill the criteria for a principal diagnosis. These circumstances might occur when a patient was admitted for treatment of a benign tumor and further diagnostic examination revealed a malignancy.

Insurance carriers usually require that only active diagnoses be reported on the claim. Active diagnoses are specifically investigated or treated during the reported admission, encounter, or episode of care. The principal diagnosis, sequenced first, is followed by relevant secondary diagnoses in descending order of clinical significance and resource intensity. For example, the code number representing a primary site malignancy should precede the code number representing a metastatic site, provided that care and treatment is still directed toward the primary neoplasm.

The reporting of code numbers for nonspecific sites of neoplasms (.9 in the classification of Chapter 2, Volume 1) should be avoided. Coders should attempt to determine the most

TABLE 4-5

Diagnosis Related Groups for Human Immunodeficiency Virus

DRG 488, Human Immunodeficiency Virus with Extensive Operating Room Procedure
DRG 489, Human Immunodeficiency Virus with Major Related Condition
DRG 490, Human Immunodeficiency Virus with or without Other Related Condition

specific tumor site and assign the code number accordingly, not only for reimbursement purposes, but also to generate meaningful data for statistics, for research, and for cancer registries. Likewise, the reporting of nonspecific codes for anemia (.9 in the classification of Chapter 4, Volume 1) should also be avoided. Accurate, complete, and timely documentation in the patient care record by healthcare practitioners might preclude the need to report codes for nonspecific neoplasms.

Certain codes for neoplastic conditions are recognized as comorbidities by many third-party payors, notably Medicare. For inpatient admissions, these comorbid conditions may increase the amount of reimbursement received by the healthcare provider. Comorbidities among the various neoplastic conditions are represented by the following ICD-9-CM code numbers:

150.0	150.1	150.2
150.3	150.4	150.5
150.8	150.9	151.0
151.1	151.2	151.3
151.4	151.5	151.6
151.8	151.9	152.0
152.1	152.2	152.3
152.8	152.9	153.0
153.1	153.2	153.3
153.4	153.5	153.6
153.7	153.8	153.9
154.0	154.1	154.2
154.3	154.8	155.1
155.1	155.2	156.0
156.1	156.2	156.8
156.9	157.0	157.1
157.2	157.3	157.6
157.8	157.9	162.2
162.3	162.4	162.5
162.8	162.9	163.0
163.1	163.8	163.9
164.0	164.1	164.2
164.3	164.8	164.9
176.4	176.5	189.0
189.1	189.2	191.0
191.1	191.2	191.3
191.4	191.5	191.6
191.7	191.8	191.9
192.0	192.1	192.2
192.3	192.8	196.0
196.1	196.2	196.3
196.5	196.6	196.8
196.9	197.0	197.1
197.2	197.3	197.4
197.5	197.6	197.7
197.8	198.0	198.1
198.2	198.3	198.4

198.5	198.6	198.7
198.81	198.82	198.89
199.0	200.00	200.01
200.02	200.03	200.04
200.05	200.06	200.07
200.08	200.10	200.11
200.12	200.13	200.14
200.15	200.16	200.17
200.18	200.20	200.21
200.22	200.23	200.24
200.25	200.26	200.27
200.28	200.80	200.81
200.82	200.83	200.84
200.85	200.86	200.87
200.88	201.00	201.02
201.03	201.04	201.05
201.06	201.07	201.08
201.10	201.11	201.12
201.13	201.14	201.15
201.16	201.17	201.18
201.20	201.21	201.22
201.23	201.24	201.25
201.26	201.27	201.28
201.40	201.41	201.42
201.43	201.44	201.45
201.46	201.47	201.48
201.50	201.51	201.52
201.53	201.54	201.55
201.56	201.57	201.58
201.60	201.61	201.62
201.63	201.64	201.65
201.66	201.67	201.68
201.70	201.71	201.72
201.73	201.74	201.75
201.76	201.77	201.78
201.90	201.91	201.92
201.93	201.94	201.95
201.96	201.97	201.98
202.00	202.01	202.02
202.03	202.04	202.05
202.06	202.07	202.08
202.10	202.11	202.12
202.13	202.14	202.15
202.16	202.17	202.18
202.20	202.21	202.22
202.23	202.24	202.25
202.26	202.27	202.28
202.30	202.31	202.32
202.33	202.34	202.35

202.36	202.37	202.38
202.40	202.41	202.42
202.43	202.44	202.45
202.46	202.47	202.48
202.50	202.51	202.52
202.53	202.54	202.55
202.56	202.57	202.58
202.60	202.61	202.62
202.63	202.64	202.65
202.66	202.67	202.68
202.80	202.81	202.82
202.83	202.84	202.85
202.86	202.87	202.88
202.90	202.91	202.92
202.93	202.94	202.95
202.96	202.97	202.98
203.00	203.01	203.10
203.11	203.80	203.81
204.00	204.01	204.10
204.11	204.20	204.21
204.80	204.81	204.90
204.91	205.00	205.01
205.10	205.11	205.20
205.21	205.30	205.31
205.80	205.81	205.90
205.91	206.00	206.01
206.10	206.11	206.20
206.21	206.80	206.81
206.90	206.91	207.00
207.01	207.10	207.11
207.20	207.21	207.80
207.81	208.00	208.01
208.10	208.11	208.20
208.21	208.80	208.81
208.90	208.91	

Comorbidities among the various hematological conditions are represented by the following ICD-9-CM code numbers:

280.0	281.4	281.8
282.4	282.60	282.61
282.62	282.63	282.69
283.0	283.10	283.11
283.19	283.2	283.9
284.0	284.8	284.9
285.0	285.1	286.0
286.1	286.2	286.3
286.4	286.5	286.6
286.7	286.9	287.0

287.1	287.2	287.3
287.4	287.5	287.8
287.9	288.0	288.1

Certain DRG's pertinent to oncological conditions are assigned to MDC 17, Myeloproliferative Disease and Disorders, and Poorly Differentiated Neoplasms; however, many DRG's associated with other major diagnostic categories also relate to neoplastic conditions (Table 4–6). The DRG's relevant to hematological conditions are distributed into MDC 16, Diseases and Disorders of the Blood and Blood-Forming Organs and Immunological Disorders (Table 4–7).

TABLE 4-6

Diagnosis Related Groups for Neoplasms

DRG 10, Nervous System Neoplasms with Comorbidity or Complication (MDC 1)

DRG 11, Nervous System Neoplasms without Comorbidity or Complication (MDC 1)

DRG 64, Ear, Nose, Mouth, and Throat Malignancy (MDC 3)

DRG 82, Respiratory Neoplasms (MDC 4)

DRG 172, Digestive Malignancy with Comorbidity or Complication (MDC 6)

DRG 173, Digestive Malignancy without Comorbidity or Complication (MDC 6)

DRG 199, Hepatobiliary Diagnostic Procedure for Malignancy (MDC 7)

DRG 203, Malignancy of Hepatobiliary System or Pancreas (MDC 7)

DRG 239, Pathological Fractures and Musculoskeletal and Connective Tissue Malignancy (MDC 8)

DRG 257, Total Mastectomy for Malignancy with Comorbidity or Complication (MDC 9)

DRG 258, Total Mastectomy for Malignancy without Comorbidity or Complication (MDC 9)

DRG 259, Subtotal Mastectomy for Malignancy with Comorbidity or Complication (MDC 9)

DRG 260, Subtotal Mastectomy for Malignancy without Comorbidity or Complication (MDC 9)

DRG 274, Malignant Breast Disorders with Comorbidity or Complication (MDC 9)

DRG 275, Malignant Breast Disorders without Comorbidity or Complication (MDC 9)

DRG 303, Kidney, Ureter, and Major Bladder Procedures for Neoplasm (MDC 11)

DRG 318, Kidney and Urinary Tract Neoplasms with Comorbidity or Complication (MDC 11)

DRG 319, Kidney and Urinary Tract Neoplasms without Comorbidity or Complication (MDC 11)

DRG 338, Testes Procedures for Malignancy (MDC 12)

DRG 344, Other Male Reproductive System Operating Room Procedures for Malignancy (MDC 12)

DRG 346, Malignancy of Male Reproductive System with Comorbidity or Complication (MDC 12)

DRG 347, Malignancy of Male Reproductive System without Comorbidity or Complication (MDC 12)

DRG 354, Uterine and Adnexa Procedures for Non-Ovarian/Adnexal Malignancy with Comorbidity or Complication (MDC 13)

DRG 355, Uterine and Adnexa Procedures for Non-Ovarian/Adnexal Malignancy without Comorbidity or Complication (MDC 13)

DRG 357, Uterine and Adnexa Procedures for Ovarian or Adnexal Malignancy (MDC 13)

DRG 363, Dilatation and Curettage, Conization, and Radioimplant for Malignancy (MDC 13)

DRG 366, Malignancy of Female Reproductive System with Comorbidity or Complication (MDC 13)

DRG 367, Malignancy of Female Reproductive System without Comorbidity or Complication (MDC 13)

DRG 400, Lymphoma and Leukemia with Major Operating Room Procedures (MDC 17)

DRG 401, Lymphoma and Nonacute Leukemia with Other Operating Room Procedure with Comorbidity or Complication (MDC 17)

T A B L E 4–6

Diagnosis Related Groups for Neoplasms—cont'd

DRG 402, Lymphoma and Nonacute Leukemia with Other Operating Room Procedure without Comorbidity or Complication (MDC 17)

DRG 403, Lymphoma and Nonacute Leukemia with Comorbidity or Complication (MDC 17)

DRG 404, Lymphoma and Nonacute Leukemia without Comorbidity or Complication (MDC 17)

DRG 405, Acute Leukemia without Major Operating Room Procedure, Age 0–17 (MDC 17)

DRG 406, Myeloproliferative Disorders or Poorly Differentiated Neoplasms with Major Operating Room Procedures with Comorbidity or Complication (MDC 17)

DRG 407, Myeloproliferative Disorders or Poorly Differentiated Neoplasms with Major Operating Room Procedures without Comorbidity or Complication (MDC 17)

DRG 408, Myeloproliferative Disorders or Poorly Differentiated Neoplasms with Other Operating Room Procedures (MDC 17)

DRG 409, Radiotherapy (MDC 17)

DRG 410, Chemotherapy without Acute Leukemia as Secondary Diagnosis (MDC 17)

DRG 411, History of Malignancy without Endoscopy (MDC 17)

DRG 412, History of Malignancy with Endoscopy (MDC 17)

DRG 413, Other Myeloproliferative Disorders or Poorly Differentiated Neoplasm Diagnoses with Comorbidity or Complication (MDC 17)

DRG 414, Other Myeloproliferative Disorders or Poorly Differentiated Neoplasm Diagnoses without Comorbidity or Complication (MDC 17)

DRG 473, Acute Leukemia without Major Operating Room Procedure, Age Greater than 17 (MDC 17)

DRG 481, Bone Marrow Transplant (MDC 0)

DRG 492, Chemotherapy with Acute Leukemia as Secondary Diagnosis (MDC 17)

T A B L E 4–7

Diagnosis Related Groups for Diseases of the Blood and Blood-Forming Organs

DRG 392, Splenectomy, Age Greater than 17

DRG 393, Splenectomy, Age 0–17

DRG 394, Other Operating Room Procedures of the Blood and Blood-Forming Organs

DRG 395, Red Blood Cell Disorders, Age Greater than 17

DRG 396, Red Blood Cell Disorders, Age 0–17

DRG 397, Coagulation Disorders

DRG 398, Reticuloendothelial and Immunity Disorders with Comorbidity or Complication

DRG 399, Reticuloendothelial and Immunity Disorders without Comorbidity or Complication

ENDOCRINOLOGY AND IMMUNOLOGY REPORTING FOR BILLING

The sequencing rules discussed in the two preceding sections are also applicable to the reporting of code numbers for endocrine, nutritional, and metabolic diseases, as well as for immunity disorders. However, not every code and narrative title in the ICD-9-CM diagnostic classification represents an entity that may be reported as a principal diagnosis.

Specific ICD-9-CM codes are commonly considered as an unacceptable principal diagnosis by a majority of third-party payors including Medicare and Medicaid. Unacceptable principal or primary diagnoses for endocrine, nutritional, and metabolic conditions are:

250.00	250.01	250.02
250.03	278.00	278.01

Reporting of code numbers for nonspecific (unspecified) endocrine, nutritional, or metabolic diagnoses should be avoided if possible. The personnel responsible for coding and billing should attempt to report the most specific code that is provided in the classification. The fifth-digit subclassification should be utilized for commonly reported conditions such as diabetes and obesity. Adequate patient healthcare documentation expedites reimbursement to the healthcare provider and facilitates statistical research in the healthcare industry.

Comorbidities among the various endocrinological conditions are represented by the following ICD-9-CM code numbers:

242.00	242.01	242.10
242.11	242.20	242.21
242.30	242.31	242.40
242.41	242.80	242.81
242.90	242.91	250.01
250.02	250.03	250.11
250.12	250.13	250.21
250.22	250.23	250.31
250.32	250.33	250.41
250.42	250.43	250.51
250.52	250.53	250.61
250.62	250.63	250.71
250.73	250.81	250.82
250.83	250.91	250.92
250.93	251.0	251.3
252.1	253.2	253.5
254.1	255.0	255.3
255.4	255.5	255.6
258.0	258.1	258.8
258.9	259.2	

Comorbidities among the various nutritional conditions are represented by the following ICD-9-CM code numbers:

260	261	262
263.0	263.1	263.2
263.8	263.9	269.0

Comorbidities among the various metabolic conditions are represented by the following ICD-9-CM code numbers:

273.3	276.0	276.1
276.2	276.3	276.4
276.5	276.6	276.7
276.8	276.9	277.00
277.01		

Comorbidities among the various immunological conditions are represented by the following ICD-9-CM code numbers:

279.02	279.03	279.04
279.05	279.06	279.09
279.10	279.11	279.12
279.13	279.19	279.2
279.3	279.4	279.8
279.9		

The DRG's pertinent to endocrine, nutritional, and metabolic conditions are distributed into a single major diagnostic category: MDC 10, Endocrine, Nutritional, and Metabolic Diseases and Disorders (Table 4–8).

TABLE 4–8

Diagnosis Related Groups for Endocrine, Nutritional, and Metabolic Diseases

DRG 285, Amputation of Lower Limb for Endocrine, Nutritional, and Metabolic Disorders

DRG 286, Adrenal and Pituitary Procedures

DRG 287, Skin Grafts and Wound Debridement for Endocrine, Nutritional, and Metabolic Disorders

DRG 288, Operating Room Procedures for Obesity

DRG 289, Parathyroid Procedures

DRG 290, Thyroid Procedures

DRG 291, Thyroglossal Procedures

DRG 292, Other Endocrine, Nutritional, and Metabolic Operating Room Procedures with Comorbidity or Complication

DRG 293, Other Endocrine, Nutritional, and Metabolic Operating Room Procedures without Comorbidity or Complication

DRG 294, Diabetes, Age Greater than 35

DRG 295, Diabetes, Age 0–35

DRG 296, Nutritional and Miscellaneous Metabolic Disorders, Age Greater than 17 with Comorbidity or Complication

DRG 297, Nutritional and Miscellaneous Metabolic Disorders, Age Greater than 17 without Comorbidity or Complication

DRG 298, Nutritional and Miscellaneous Metabolic Disorders, Age 0–17

DRG 299, Inborn Errors of Metabolism

DRG 300, Endocrine Disorders with Comorbidity or Complication

DRG 301, Endocrine Disorders without Comorbidity or Complication

KEY CONCEPTS

comorbidity _____

complication _____

diagnosis related group _____

etiology _____

functional activity _____

in situ _____

late effect _____

major diagnostic category _____

manifestation _____

metastases _____

morphology _____

neoplasm _____

neoplasm table _____

related complex _____

syndrome _____

unacceptable diagnosis _____

uncertain behavior _____

underlying disease _____

REVIEW EXERCISES

1. Describe the purpose of the fifth-digit subclassification for the coding of tuberculosis. _____

   _____

   _____

2. Explain the use of a secondary code in the coding and reporting of septicemia. _____

   _____

   _____

3. Explain the use of a secondary code in the coding and reporting of a clinical manifestation. __

   _____

   _____

4. Explain the use of a secondary code in the coding and reporting of a late effect of disease. ___

   _____

   _____

5. Discuss the proper usage of each of the six columns of the table in the alphabetic index for the coding of neoplasms. _____

   _____

   _____

6. Differentiate a neoplasm of uncertain behavior from a neoplasm of unspecified behavior. ____

   _____

   _____

7. Explain the circumstances when a code number for a secondary neoplasm may be reported as a principal diagnosis. _____

   _____

   _____

8. Describe the purpose of the fifth digit subclassification for the coding of diabetes. _____

   _____

   _____

9. Prioritize (rank in order for reporting purposes) the following clusters of diagnoses:
   A. intestinal trichomoniasis, botulism, gastroenteritis _____

   _____

   B. hypertension, viral warts, pulmonary tuberculosis _____

   _____

C. contact dermatitis, typhoid fever, convulsions, hallucinations _____

D. salmonella gastroenteritis, malaise, insomnia, rubella _____

E. abnormal lung scan, adenocarcinoma of colon, benign neoplasm of thoracic cavity _____

F. squamous cell carcinoma of mouth, blue nevus of forearm, urinary tract infection _____

G. anxiety depression, malignant melanoma, splenomegaly _____

H. diabetes with ketoacidosis, kyphosis, nasopharyngitis _____

I. constipation, pseudofolliculitis barbae, sickle cell anemia _____

J. viral gastroenteritis, late latent syphilis, carcinoma in situ of cervix _____

10. Identify at least ten codes and narrative titles that represent infectious or parasitic disease conditions which are recognized by Medicare as complications or comorbidities.

    _____   _____
    _____   _____
    _____   _____
    _____   _____
    _____   _____
    _____   _____

11. Identify at least ten codes and narrative titles that represent neoplastic conditions which are recognized by Medicare as complications or comorbidities.

    _____   _____
    _____   _____
    _____   _____
    _____   _____
    _____   _____
    _____   _____

12. Identify at least five codes and narrative titles that represent endocrine system conditions which are recognized by Medicare as complications or comorbidities. _____

13. Identify at least ten codes and narrative titles that represent hematologic conditions which are recognized by Medicare as complications or comorbidities. _____

14. Assign precise, accurate code numbers from the ICD-9-CM volume for the following infectious and parasitic diseases:
    A.   cholera due to *Vibrio cholerae* _____

    B.   congenital syphilis with encephalitis _____

C. athlete's foot _____

D. food poisoning due to *Clostridium botulinum* _____

E. tuberculosis of the large intestine _____

F. late nodular ulcerated yaws _____

G. meningo-eruptive syndrome _____

H. swimming pool conjunctivitis _____

I. louse-borne relapsing fever _____

J. bubonic plague _____

K. urban yellow fever _____

L. pneumococcal septicemia _____

M. pneumonia due to *Pneumocystis carinii* _____

N. geniculate herpes zoster _____

O. tapeworm infection _____

P. pneumonitis due to toxoplasmosis _____

Q. Bazin's disease _____

R. guinea worm infection _____

S. tinea blanca _____

T. rat-bite fever _____

U. nonvenereal endemic syphilis _____

V. faucial diphtheria _____

W. gonococcal arthritis _____

X. blindness due to AIDS _____

Y. algid malaria _____

Z. arthritis due to rubella _____

AA. Pfeiffer's disease _____

_____

BB. Eastern equine encephalitis _____

_____

CC. chronic amebic diarrhea _____

_____

DD. Norwegian scabies _____

_____

EE. tuberculosis of glottis _____

_____

FF. infection by pinworms _____

_____

GG. gastrointestinal anthrax _____

_____

HH. infection by Zopfia Senegalensis _____

_____

II. scarlet fever _____

_____

JJ. achromic and hyperchromic lesions of pinta _____

_____

KK. subacute spongiform encephalopathy _____

_____

LL. syphilitic meningitis _____

_____

MM. rubeola _____

_____

NN. Siberian tick typhus _____

_____

OO. Colorado tick fever _____

_____

PP. mumps hepatitis _____

_____

QQ. lupoid of Boeck _____

_____

RR. viral enteritis _____

_____

SS. Katayama disease _____

_____

TT. tuberculoma of spinal cord _____

_____

UU. primary cutaneous coccidioidomycosis _____

_____

VV. glanders _____

_____

WW. leptospiral meningitis _____

_____

XX. Hansen's disease _____

_____

15. Assign precise, accurate code numbers from the ICD-9-CM volume for the following neoplasms:
    A. squamous cell carcinoma of commissure of lip _____

    B. neoplasm of uncertain behavior in the brain _____

    C. adenocarcinoma of Meckel's diverticulum _____

    D. benign neoplasm of parathyroid gland _____

    E. malignant neoplasm of visceral pleura _____

    F. benign tumor of abdominal wall _____

    G. malignancy of bone of wrist _____

    H. lymphogranulomatosis _____

    I. adenocarcinoma of labia majora _____

    J. carcinoma of lacrimal duct _____

    K. squamous cell carcinoma of base of tongue _____

    L. adenocarcinoma of the esophagus _____

    M. malignancy of thoracic esophagus _____

    N. benign neoplasm of spinal meninges _____

    O. malignant neoplasm of supraglottis _____

    P. leiomyoma of uterus _____

    Q. carcinoma of the pinna _____

    R. subacute leukemia _____

    S. adenocarcinoma of uterine fundus _____

    T. malignant tumor of groin _____

    U. squamous cell carcinoma of lateral aspect of floor of mouth _____

    V. unspecified neoplasm of the respiratory system _____

    W. malignant tumor of intestinal tract _____

    X. congenital lymphangioma _____

Y.   malignant neoplasm of upper respiratory tract _____

Z.   benign tumor of mediastinum _____

AA.   adenocarcinoma of the uterus _____

BB.   Brill-Symmers disease _____

CC.   malignant neoplasm of corpus cavernosum _____

DD.   metastatic tumor of the kidney _____

EE.   squamous cell carcinoma of the lateral wall of the nasopharynx _____

FF.   carcinoma of the trachea _____

GG.   malignant tumor of the pancreas _____

HH.   benign prostatic tumor _____

II.   malignancy of the thymus _____

JJ.   benign neoplasm of the frenulum labii _____

KK.   malignant neoplasm of the male breast _____

LL.   Kahler's disease _____

MM.   malignant growth of the renal calyces _____

NN.   malignant tumor of the cauda equina _____

OO.   adenocarcinoma of the pharynx _____

PP.   malignant melanoma of the face _____

QQ.   malignant growth of the liver _____

RR.   benign neoplasm of the cornea _____

SS.   malignancy of the frontal sinus _____

TT.   benign growth of the nipple _____

UU.   malignant melanoma of the thigh _____

VV.   Burkitt's tumor _____

WW. malignant neoplasm of the cervical stump _____

XX. malignant tumor of the parathyroid gland _____

16. Assign precise, accurate code numbers from the ICD-9-CM volume for the following endocrine, nutritional, and metabolic diseases and immunity disorders:
   A. multinodular nontoxic goiter _____

   B. diabetic coma _____

   C. kwashiorkor _____

   D. congenital X-linked agammaglobulinemia _____

   E. Basedow's disease _____

   F. carcinoid syndrome _____

   G. zinc deficiency _____

   H. hyperkalemia _____

   I. cyst of thyroid _____

   J. insulin coma _____

   K. severe calorie deficiency _____

   L. exogenous obesity _____

   M. simple goiter _____

   N. Lloyd's syndrome _____

   O. active rickets _____

   P. glycogenosis _____

   Q. chronic fibrous thyroiditis _____

   R. hyperparathyroidism _____

   S. nutritional dwarfism _____

   T. Barraquer-Simons disease _____

   U. congenital thyroid insufficiency _____

    V. testicular hypofunction _____

    W. ascorbic acid deficiency _____

    X. macroglobulinemia _____

    Y. pituitary hypothroidism _____

17. Assign precise, accurate code numbers from the ICD-9-CM volume for the following operations on the endocrine system:

    A. suture of the thyroid gland _____

    B. repair of adrenal gland _____

    C. substernal thyroidectomy _____

    D. partial excision of thymus _____

    E. excision of lesion of thyroid _____

    F. unilateral exploration of adrenal field _____

    G. biopsy of parathyroid gland _____

    H. hypophysectomy _____

    I.   reopening of wound of thyroid field for removal of hematoma _____

    J. bilateral adrenalectomy _____

    K. excision of thyroglossal duct _____

    L. aspiration of Rathke's pouch _____

    M. hemithyroidectomy _____

    N. biopsy of pituitary gland, transsphenoidal approach _____

    O. excision of thyroid by transoral route _____

    P. incision of pineal gland _____

    Q. complete thyroidectomy _____

    R. transplantation of thymus _____

    S. complete parathyroidectomy _____

T. partial adrenalectomy _____

U. autotransplantation of parathyroid tissue _____

V. total excision of pituitary gland, transsphenoidal approach _____

W. aspiration biopsy of thyroid _____

X. division of nerves of adrenal glands _____

Y. complete substernal thyroidectomy _____

18. Assign precise, accurate code numbers from the ICD-9-CM volume for the following diseases of the blood and blood-forming organs:

A. Paterson-Kelly syndrome _____

B. Stokes' disease _____

C. vegan's anemia _____

D. Jordan's anomaly _____

E. hereditary leptocytosis anemia _____

F. vascular pseudohemophilia _____

G. acquired hemolytic anemia _____

H. angiohemophilia _____

I. aplastic anemia due to drugs _____

J. Von Jaksch's anemia _____

K. iron deficiency anemia _____

L. acquired polycythemia _____

M. scorbutic anemia _____

N. hereditary eosinophilia _____

O. sickle cell anemia _____

P. thrombocytasthenia _____

Q. acquired hemolytic anemia with hemoglobinuria _____

R. acquired hypoprothrombinemia _____

_____

S. constitutional aplastic anemia _____

_____

T. acquired sideroblastic anemia _____

_____

U. normocytic anemia due to blood loss _____

_____

V. hypersplenism _____

_____

W. amino acid deficiency anemia _____

_____

X. infantile genetic agranulocytosis _____

_____

Y. hereditary hemolytic anemia _____

_____

19. Assign precise, accurate code numbers from the ICD-9-CM volume for the following operations
on the hemic and lymphatic systems:

A. bone marrow transplant _____

_____

B. extended regional lymph node excision _____

_____

C. aspiration of bone marrow for transplant _____

_____

D. biopsy of lymphatic structure _____

_____

E. excision of deep cervical lymph node _____

_____

F. radical neck dissection _____

_____

G. dilation of peripheral lymphatics _____

_____

H. simple lymphadenectomy _____

_____

I. puncture of spleen _____

_____

J. cannulation of thoracic duct _____

_____

K. transplantation of spleen _____

_____

L. plastic repair of spleen _____

_____

M. ligation of thoracic duct _____

_____

N. allograft of bone marrow _____

_____

O. partial splenectomy _____

_____

P. excision of axillary lymph node _____

Q. splenotomy _____

R. total splenectomy _____

S. radical groin dissection _____

T. incision of lymphatic structure _____

U. open biopsy of spleen _____

V. bilateral radical neck dissection _____

W. marsupialization of splenic cyst _____

X. radical excision of periaortic lymph nodes _____

Y. biopsy of bone marrow _____

CODING OF CLINICAL DOCUMENTATION

Read the following clinical reports and assign precise, accurate diagnostic and procedural code numbers from the appropriate sections of the ICD-9-CM volumes.

PATIENT: Goodman, Robert   **MR#:** 99-04-01

SURGEONS: Thompson & Fox   **ASSISTANTS:** Lemanski & McNamara

Preoperative Diagnosis:
Pituitary adenoma.

Postoperative Diagnosis:
Pituitary adenoma.

Operation:
Excision of pituitary adenoma by sublabial transsphenoidal transseptal approach.

Procedure:
The patient had been previously anesthetized and placed in the neurosurgical head holder. The anterior nares were inspected and two neurosurgical Cottonoids impregnated with a 4% Cocaine solution were placed into the anterior nasal chambers bilaterally. The anterior nasal septum, floor of the nose, and premaxillary area were infiltrated with approximately 8 cc of 2% Xylocaine with Epinephrine 1:100000. The face and abdomen were then prepped and draped in the usual manner. A left anterior hemitransfixion incision was performed and an anteroposterior mucoperichondrial and mucoperiosteal tunnel were created on the left. There was marked dislocation of the quadrilateral cartilage with fragmentation and multiple dense adhesions along the floor of the nose and anteriorly along the previous septal fracture line. Using blunt and sharp dissection, the adhesions were lysed. Several small fenestrae were created along the inferior ridge and anteriorly. A right posterior mucoperiosteal tunnel was created after disarticulating the quadrilateral cartilage. An inferior floor of the nose tunnel on the left was created using a Freer elevator. Due to the extreme deformity of the nasal cartilage, essentially submucous resection of quadrilateral cartilage and radical bony septectomy were performed. Thereafter, the remaining quadrilateral cartilage could be displaced from the maxillary crest into the right nasal chamber. A retrograde dissection was performed and an inferior tunnel on the right created. There was a large maxillary crest spur that was removed with a chisel. The face of the maxilla was then dissected beneath the piriform aperture. The anterior nasal spine was identified and removed with a Jansen-Middleton. Attention was turned to the anterior gingival labial sulcus. Incision was performed from the left canine fossa to the contralateral canine fossa. Mucoperiosteum overlying the premaxilla was incised and the previously encountered dissection plane was found. Then the Hardy was placed sublabially and used to visualize the face of the sphenoid. The mucoperiosteum was cleaned off of the face of the sphenoid. The sphenoid sinus ostea was identified and small anterior fenestrae were created in the face of the sphenoid. Thereafter, Dr. Fox enlarged the sphenotomy and completed his portion of the procedure to be dictated separately. Following removal of the adenoma and packing of the sphenoid sinus, the wound was closed. Several fenestra of the mucoperichondrial tunnel were closed with interrupted sutures of 3-0 chromic. The septum was quilted with interrupted sutures of 4-0 chromic. Then two interrupted sutures of Vicryl were placed in the columella and lateral alar areas to prevent collapse of the nose on the face

of the premaxilla. The sublabial incision was then closed with interrupted sutures of 3-0 chromic and bilateral intranasal trumpets were placed along with Telfa packing. The patient was uneventfully awakened from general anesthesia and removed to the recovery room in stable condition.

Codes: _____

PATIENT: Gebhardt, Ruth   **MR#:** 99-04-02

SURGEONS: Kelly   **ASSISTANTS:** Shapiro

Preoperative Diagnosis:
Diffuse lymphadenopathy, unknown etiology.

Postoperative Diagnosis:
Lymphoma, pathology pending.

Operation:
Biopsy of right supraclavicular lymph node.

Brief Clinical History:
The patient is a 61-year-old white female who presents with a 1-month history of diffuse lymphadenopathy, most prominent in the cervical and supraclavicular areas.

Operative Note:
The patient was brought to the OR and placed in the supine position on the operating room table in the usual manner. She was then prepped and draped in sterile fashion over the right supraclavicular area.

Procedure:
The superficial lymph node just above the right clavicle was chosen for biopsy. 1% Lidocaine was used to infuse over the lymph node and a #15 blade was used to make an approximately 3-cm incision over the node. Then the #15 blade was used to dissect down to the subcutaneous tissue and a Bovie was used for hemostasis. Dissection was carried down through the platysma muscle and tenotomy scissors were used to dissect above the lymph node. The lymph node was then pulled up into the wound with a pair of DeBakey forceps. After this was completed, a mosquito was used to grip down under the base of the lymph node, and tenotomy scissors were used to cut down on top of the mosquito. This was repeated three times until the lymph node was removed out of the wound and sent to pathology for sectioning. Next the pedicle of the lymph node was tied off with 3-0 silk. The wound was then copiously irrigated and hemostasis was maintained with electrocautery. The wound was closed with 3-0 Vicryl times three simple sutures, and the skin was closed with a running 4-0 Vicryl subcuticular. Steri-strips and a sterile dressing were then applied. The patient tolerated the procedure without complications and was transferred to the post-anesthesia recovery area in stable condition. Blood loss was minimal and no fluids were administered.

Codes: _____

PATIENT: Kramer, Dennis   **MR#:** 99-04-03

SURGEON: Owens

Specimens:
A: Right spermatic cord lipoma.
B: Right inguinal node.

Gross Examination:
A: Received is a fragment of fibromembranous and fatty tissue that measures 4.4 cm ×
3.0 cm × 2.0 cm. On cut section most of the tissue appears to be fat, which is circumscribed
and appears to be partially encapsulated. One representative section is submitted.
B: Received is a fragment of yellow fatty tissue measuring 1.5 cm × 1.4 cm × 0.8 cm. On cut
section all of the tissue appears to be fat and appears to be partially encapsulated. No evident lymph node structure is identified grossly. One representative section is submitted.

Microscopic Diagnoses:
A: Hernia sac and lipoma.
B: Lymph node showing fatty replacement.

Codes: _____

PATIENT: Moran, William   **MR#:** 99-04-04

SURGEON: Reed

Clinical Diagnosis:
Mass of left cheek, inner aspect of left side of mouth.

Postoperative Diagnosis:
Same.

Operative Procedure:
Excision of mass of left mouth

Specimen:
Lesion from inner left aspect of mouth

Gross:
The specimen labeled "cyst from left side of mouth" consists of a piece of soft tissue that is irregular in shape, measuring approximately 2.0 cm × 1.5 cm × 1.2 cm in maximum dimensions. In cut section almost the entire specimen is made up of a whitish gray, slightly firm
mass with somewhat glistening and mucoid lobulated appearance in the cut surface. Small
amount of pinkish red soft tissue consistent with the skeletal muscle is focally noted in the periphery of the lesion. The entire surgical margin is labeled with green ink. The specimen is serially sectioned and totally submitted as Block A and Block B.

Microscopic:

The sections show a low-grade mucoepidermoid carcinoma made up primarily of glandular or cystic spaces lined by goblet cells containing large amounts of intracytoplasmic mucin. Cystic dilation of the glands containing large amounts of mucin in the lumen are also frequently seen. Extravasation of mucin into the interstitial tissue, between collagen and skeletal muscle fibers, carries with it nests and groups of tumor cells. Small groups and nests of intermediate and poorly differentiated squamous cells are occasionally seen next to mucin-producing cells lining the glandular and cystic spaces. The stroma shows fairly dense fibrosis containing foci of chronic inflammatory cell infiltrates, predominantly plasma cells. The tumor involves surgical margins labeled with green ink at multiple points.

Diagnosis:
Low-grade mucoepidermoid carcinoma.

Codes: _____

PATIENT: Valentino, Billy   **MR#:** 99-04-05

SURGEON: Moss

Clinical Diagnosis:
Right cervical lymphadenopathy.

Postoperative Diagnosis:
Right cervical lymphadenopathy.

Operative Procedure:
Excisional biopsy of right cervical lymph node.

Specimen:
Right cervical lymph node.

Gross:
The specimen is labeled as "right cervical lymph node" and consists of an irregular mass of tissue that is 1.3 cm × 1.1 cm in greatest dimensions. A lymph node is identified. On cut sections it is pale white in appearance. It is bisected, totally submitted, labeled as Block A and Block B.

Microscopic:
The section of the cervical lymph node shows partial loss of normal architecture and infiltration by polymorphous cellular infiltrate typical of Hodgkin's lymphoma. The infiltrate is mostly comprised of eosinophils, lymphocytes, and histiocytes. Several typical lacunar and multilobated giant cells are also included. Many of the cells are multilobated and have smudgy nuclei; however, several typical binucleated Reed-Sternberg cells are also identified. One lymph node included also shows increased fibrosis with tendency to nodule formation. The pattern is consistent with the nodular sclerosing type of Hodgkin's lymphoma.

Diagnosis:
Hodgkin's lymphoma, nodular sclerosing type.

Codes: _____

PATIENT: Blair, Henry   **MR#:** 99-04-06

ATTENDING PHYSICIAN: Osborn

Reason for Admission:

The patient is a 68-year-old black male with a history of recently diagnosed squamous cell esophageal cancer who presented with a complaint of nausea and vomiting since the day prior to admission. One week ago, he had a previous food impaction secondary to esophageal narrowing that required esophagogastroduodenoscopy with balloon dilation. He was doing well until yesterday, when nausea and vomiting occurred with ingestion of pureed food as well as with drinking liquids. The patient admits to eating cheese curls the prior evening. He has no fever, cough, hematemesis, or melena. His last bowel movement was the morning of the day prior to admission.

Past Medical History:

The patient's history is significant for esophageal cancer without evidence of metastases. The patient refused surgery and had radiation therapy, which he currently also refuses. The tumor is located at the gastroesophageal junction and the patient has required multiple dilations as an outpatient to restore esophageal patency. Last month, a G-tube was placed through which the patient receives medications as well as four or five cans of Ensure daily. The patient has non–insulin-dependent diabetes mellitus and a history of myocardial infarction in 1988. Echocardiogram obtained last month revealed right ventricular enlargement and right atrial enlargement with normal left ventricular function. The patient has a history of hypertension and a history of peptic ulcer disease. He has no known drug allergies.

Medications on Admission:

Cardizem 30 mg q.i.d.; Digoxin 0.125 mg q.d.; Tagamet 300 mg liquid q. h.s.; Nitrol Paste 1 inch q. 6 hours p.r.n.; Reglan 250 mg q. a.m.; Compazine 10 mg p.r.n.; Tylenol 3 p.r.n.; and Easy-Lax 2 mg p.r.n.

Family History:

Not significant.

Social History:

The patient lives by himself. He has a sixty pack per year history of smoking.

Review of Systems:

The patient has noticed a ten pound weight loss within the past two months and has increased coughing while eating.

Physical Examination:

The patient is an emaciated, elderly black male in no acute distress.

Vital Signs: Temp 36.5; BP 108/64; Pulse 75. There were no orthostatic changes.

HEENT: Examination showed temporal wasting. Pupils are equal, round, and reactive to light; bilateral arcus senilis present. Oropharynx is pink and moist without lesions. The neck is supple with no adenopathy.

Lungs: Clear to auscultation.

Heart: Regular rate and rhythm; 3/6 systolic ejection murmur at the left sternal border; no rubs or gallops.

Abdomen: Scaphoid with minimal tenderness to palpation in the right upper quadrant; decreased bowel sounds; clean, dry dressing over his G-tube.

Extremities: 2+ pulses; thin, bony extremities; no cyanosis or edema.

Rectal: Heme negative.

Neurological: Nonfocal.

Laboratory Data:

Sodium 132; potassium 4.7; chloride 93; bicarbonate 26; BUN 17; creatinine 0.8; glucose 204; amylase 48; total bilirubin 0.2; AST 930; WBC 16300; hemoglobin 8.0; hematocrit 26.7; platelet count 102400; PT 14.7; PTT 28.1; abdominal x-ray showed no air fluid levels.

Condition on Discharge:

Stable.

Discharge Medications:

Tagamet 300 mg q. 8 hours; Compazine p.r.n.; Lanoxin 0.125 mg b.i.d.; Nitrol Paste one inch q 6 p.r.n.; Jevity 5 to 6 cans per day via G-tube.

Discharge Diet:

Jevity 6 cans per day and pureed foods; the patient was told to avoid solid foods.

Follow-up:

Seven to ten days in GI Clinic.

Final Diagnoses:

Esophageal stricture secondary to squamous cell carcinoma.

Peptic ulcer disease.

Non–insulin-dependent diabetes mellitus.

History of hypertension.

History of myocardial infarction.

Codes: _____

PATIENT: Smith, Christopher   **MR#:** 99-04-07

ATTENDING PHYSICIAN: Wilson   **CONSULTANT:** Hsaio

History of Present Illness:

The patient is a 40-year-old white male who was diagnosed with AIDS three years ago. He was recently discharged from this hospital four days prior to this admission. During this prior admission, he had an extensive workup for intractable nausea, vomiting, and diarrhea. He underwent endoscopy and biopsy, which revealed *Cryptosporidium* in the duodenal area. Since the patient was discharged four days ago, he has been extremely weak and has been nauseated and experiencing intermittent diarrhea. He became short of breath on exertion and so light-headed that he could not walk from his bedroom to his bathroom. These complaints necessitated that the patient return to the emergency room.

Past Medical History:

Acquired immunodeficiency syndrome with *Cryptosporidium* infection causing diarrhea. *Staphylococcus* in right kidney. This patient was admitted multiple times in the past for nausea, vomiting, diarrhea, and dehydration.

Medications on Admission:

AZT 100 mg p.o. five times a day; Tagamet 300 mg b.i.d.; Lomotil one tablet p.o. t.i.d.; Reglan 10 mg q. a.c. and q. h.s.; Amitriptyline 35 mg p.o. t.i.d.; Erythromycin 200 mg q.i.d.

Social History:

The patient is a homosexual and has a history of mild tobacco and alcohol use.

Physical Examination:
General: Cachetic without acute distress.
Vital Signs: Temp 35.6; Pulse 122; Resp 24; BP 92/70 standing, 100/70 sitting, showing orthostasis.
HEENT: Bitemporal wasting; pupils equal, round, and reactive to light and accommodation.
Neck: Supple, no lymph nodes.
Lungs: Clear.
Cardiovascular: Regular rhythm; S-1 and S-2, no murmurs.
Abdomen: Soft; bowel sounds positive; no tenderness; and no organomegaly.
Rectal: Laxed tone; guaiac positive; liquid stools of brown color.
Extremities: No edema; no cyanosis; muscular wasting.
Skin: Rash on abdomen with maculopapular characteristics.

Laboratory Data:
WBC 6000; hemoglobin 14; hematocrit 32; platelets 456000; arterial blood gases, pH 7.47, PCO2 25, PO2 128; bicarbonate 21; oxygen saturation 98%; sodium 128; potassium 2.7; chloride 93; CO2 18; BUN 44; creatinine 2.1; glucose 116; AST 65; ALT 34; total bilirubin 1; amylase 4; magnesium 1.2; calcium 9.4; phosphate 1.8. The chest x-ray showed perihilar fluid and no significant infiltrate. Obstructive series revealed no obstruction, no free air, just moderate bilateral loops. Urinalysis indicated no infection.

Hospital Course:
This patient received intravenous fluids to treat his dehydration, and received Lomotil, AZT, Rocephin, Peri-Colace, Reglan, Septra, Amitriptyline, and Tagamet. Erythromycin was tried but discontinued because the patient could not tolerate the side effect of an increase in vomiting. The diarrhea was not controlled because the *Cryptosporidium* infection has no specific treatment. After the patient was well hydrated, a central line was placed on the left side to allow intensive nursing care at his home, including intravenous fluid administration. The patient was discharged moderately dehydrated, but requested to go home since home health nursing care could provide enough intravenous fluids through his central line. The patient was then discharged with no further workup planned.

Discharge Medications:
AZT 100 mg five times a day; Tagamet 300 mg b.i.d.; Lomotil two tablets t.i.d.; Reglan 10 mg q.i.d.; Amitriptyline 25 mg t.i.d.; Potassium 40 mg p.o. b.i.d.; Septra DS one tablet p.o. q.d.

Discharge Diagnoses:
Acquire immunodeficiency syndrome.

Cryptosporidium infection of the intestine.

Dehydration, not well controlled.

Instructions for Care:
Regular diet plus a can of Ensure t.i.d. The patient is to have home health nursing care, especially for the administration of intravenous fluids and electrolytes.

Follow-Up:
The patient is to return to the infectious disease clinic in one week.

Codes: _____

5
CHAPTER

ICD Coding: Mental Disorders; Nervous System, Eye, and Ear Diseases and Operations

LEARNING OBJECTIVES

Upon completion of this chapter the learner should be able to:

1. Describe the clinical modifications of the ICD coding system in the sections for mental disorders.
2. Explain Appendix C and the glossary of mental disorders.
3. Describe the parameters for coding and reporting mental or behavioral disorders.
4. Describe the parameters for coding and reporting substance abuse.
5. Describe the parameters for coding and reporting cataract surgery.
6. Explain the table for coding legal blindness.
7. Describe the parameters for coding and reporting otitis.
8. Discuss the impact of comorbidities and complications on billing and reimbursement for mental or behavioral disorders.
9. Discuss the impact of comorbidities and complications on billing and reimbursement for diagnoses and procedures involving the nervous system and sense organs.
10. Apply knowledge of coding principles by assigning accurate and precise codes to report diagnoses of mental disorders.
11. Apply knowledge of coding principles by assigning accurate and precise codes to report diagnoses of chemical dependencies.
12. Apply knowledge of coding principles by assigning accurate and precise codes to report diagnoses and procedures pertaining to the nervous system.
13. Apply knowledge of coding principles by assigning accurate and precise codes to report diagnoses and procedures pertaining to the eye.
14. Apply knowledge of coding principles by assigning accurate and precise codes to report diagnoses and procedures pertaining to the ear.

ICD CODING OF MENTAL DISORDERS AND BEHAVIORAL DISORDERS

Chapter 5 of the ICD-9-CM diagnostic tabular volume is designated for listings of mental or behavioral disorders and closely corresponds with the tabular DSM-IV coding system. ICD-9-CM contains a glossary with definitions for the content of each category of mental or behavioral disorders. However, this glossary is not a part of the main text of the classification. The chapter on mental and behavioral disorders consists of three sections (Table 5–1).

The section on psychoses encompasses listings for psychotic organic brain syndrome, senile and presenile organic psychotic conditions, alcoholic psychoses, drug-induced psychoses, transient organic psychotic conditions, schizophrenic disorders, affective psychoses, paranoid states, psychoses with origin specific to childhood, and so forth. An additional E code should be used to report psychoses associated with the consumption of drugs. Additionally, a separate code may be used to identify any related drug dependence.

The second section of Chapter 5 contains listings for neurotic disorders and personality disorders. An additional code should also be reported with personality disorders to identify any associated neurosis or psychosis. This section also includes listings for sexual deviations, alcohol and drug dependence or abuse (maladaptive effect of substance taken on own initiative to detriment of personal functioning), psychogenic physical symptoms, stress reactions, adjustment reactions, depressive disorders, disturbances of conduct, disturbances of emotions, hyperkinetic syndrome, developmental delays, and psychic factors associated with diseases classified elsewhere. An additional code should be reported to indicate any other associated psychiatric condition or any associated physical condition.

The listings for mental retardation are contained in the third section of Chapter 5. An additional code should be utilized to report associated physical or psychological conditions.

ICD CODING OF DISEASES AND OPERATIONS OF THE NERVOUS SYSTEM AND SENSE ORGANS

Chapter 6 of the ICD-9-CM diagnostic tabular volume is designated for listings of diseases of the nervous system and sense organs, encompassing eye conditions and ear conditions. The chapter consists of six sections (Table 5–2).

The section for listings of inflammatory diseases of the central nervous system includes codes and narrative titles for meningitis, encephalitis, myelitis, encephalomyelitis, intracranial or intraspinal abscess, and intracranial phlebitis or thrombophlebitis. An additional code should be used to report any underlying disease.

Category *326 Late effects of intracranial abscess or pyogenic infection* should be used to indicate conditions that are primarily classified to a listing within categories 320–325 (with certain exclusions as indicated) as the cause of late effects, which are classifiable elsewhere.

TABLE 5–1

Sections and Subsections in Chapter 5, Volume 1 of ICD-9-CM

1. Psychoses (category range 290–299) with subsections Organic Psychotic Conditions (category range 290–294) and Other Psychoses (category range 295–299)
2. Neurotic Disorders, Personality Disorders, and Other Nonpsychotic Mental Disorders (category range 300–316)
3. Mental Retardation (category range 317–319)

The late effects include conditions specified as such, or specified as sequelae present after the onset of the causal condition.

Hereditary and degenerative diseases of the central nervous system in the second section of this chapter encompass cerebral degeneration, Parkinson's disease and other extrapyramidal diseases, spinocerebellar disease, anterior horn cell disease and other diseases of spinal cord, as well as disorders of the autonomic nervous system.

In the third section of Chapter 6, other disorders of the central nervous system include multiple sclerosis and other demyelinating diseases, hemiplegia, cerebral palsy and other paralytic syndromes, epilepsy, migraine, cataplexy, and narcolepsy.

Category 342 should be used when hemiplegia (complete) (incomplete) was documented without further specification, or when hemiplegia was stated to be old or longstanding, but of unspecified cause. This category should also be used for multiple coding to identify these types of hemiplegia resulting from any cause. Category 344 should be used when the listed conditions were documented without further specification or were stated to be old or longstanding, but of unspecified cause. This category should also be used in multiple coding to identify these conditions resulting from any cause. The listings include paralysis (complete) (incomplete) except as classifiable to category 342 or category 343.

Disorders of the peripheral nervous system in the fourth section of this chapter include trigeminal nerve disorders, facial nerve disorders, and other disorders of the cranial nerves. Other conditions included in this section are nerve root and plexus disorders, mononeuritis, hereditary and idiopathic peripheral neuropathy, inflammatory and toxic neuropathy, myoneural disorders, muscular dystrophies, and other related myopathies. The underlying disease should always be coded and reported with the documented manifestation.

Categories of listings in Chapter 1 of Volume 3 of ICD-9-CM are established for surgical procedures on the components of the nervous system. These include category range 01–05 for: incision, excision, and other operations on the skull, brain, and cerebral meninges; operations on the spinal cord and other spinal canal structures; operations on cranial and peripheral nerves; and operations on sympathetic nerves or ganglia.

Many varied disorders of the eye and adnexa are classified in the fifth section of Chapter 6 in Volume 1. These include disorders of the globe, retinal detachments, retinal defects and other retinal disorders, chorioretinal inflammations and other disorders of the choroid, disorders of the iris and ciliary body, glaucoma, cataracts, disorders of refraction and accommodation, visual disturbances, blindness, and low vision.

Visual impairment refers to a functional limitation of the eye, such as limited visual acuity, and is distinguished from a visual disability such as limited reading skills and from a visual handicap such as limited mobility. Definitions of blindness vary in different settings.

TABLE 5–2

Sections and Subsections in Chapter 6, Volume 1 of ICD-9-CM

1. Inflammatory Diseases of the Central Nervous System (category range 320–326)
2. Hereditary and Degenerative Diseases of the Central Nervous System (category range 330–337)
3. Other Disorders of the Central Nervous System (category range 340–349)
4. Disorders of the Peripheral Nervous System (category range 350–359)
5. Disorders of the Eye and Adnexa (category range 360–379)
6. Diseases of the Ear and Mastoid Process (category range 380–389)

In the United States, the definition of legal blindness as severe impairment is generally used. ICD-9-CM supplies a table for coding and reporting blindness according to World Health Organization definitions.

Other eye disorders encompass keratitis, corneal opacity and other disorders of the cornea, disorders of conjunctiva, inflammation and other disorders of eyelids, disorders of the lacrimal system, disorders of the orbit, disorders of the optic nerve and visual pathways, strabismus and other disorders of binocular eye movements.

Categories of listings in Chapter 3 of Volume 3 of ICD-9-CM are established for surgical procedures on the eye. These include category range 08–16 for: operations on eyelids; operations on the lacrimal system; operations on the conjunctiva; operations on the cornea; operations on the ciliary body, sclera, and anterior chamber; operations on the lens; operations on the retina, choroid, vitreous, and posterior chamber; operations on the extraocular muscles; and operations on the orbit.

Ear diseases are classified in the sixth section of Chapter 6 in Volume 1. These include disorders of the external ear, otitis media (suppurative and nonsuppurative), Eustachian tube disorders, mastoiditis and related conditions, disorders of the tympanic membrane, disorders of the middle ear, vertiginous syndromes and other disorders of the vestibular system, otosclerosis, and hearing loss.

Categories of listings in Chapter 4 of Volume 3 of ICD-9-CM are established for surgical procedures on the ear. These include category range 18–20 for: operations on the external ear; reconstructive operations on the middle ear; and other operations on the middle ear and on the inner ear.

MENTAL AND BEHAVIORAL HEALTHCARE REPORTING FOR BILLING

Submission of insurance claims to third-party payors involves the preparation and dissemination of diagnostic and procedural patient information. Psychiatric, mental health, and behavioral health inpatient admissions are usually much lengthier than typical medical or surgical admissions. Similarly, outpatient encounters for mental or behavioral disorders often extend throughout a series of care episodes. In most cases, the principal diagnosis determines the appropriate duration of care for psychiatric, mental health, or behavioral health services.

Generally, diagnostic data determines reimbursement and procedural data has relatively little impact on provider claims that are submitted for mental or behavioral healthcare. Exceptions occur, however, if procedures such as electroconvulsive therapy are rendered, or if medical or surgical procedures are rendered for disease conditions unrelated to the mental or behavioral disorder.

Because many patients receiving mental or behavioral health services may suffer from longstanding chronic conditions, a single diagnostic entity may provide the impetus for continuing admissions or encounters with healthcare providers. However, insurance carriers usually accept claims reporting only those diagnoses specifically assessed or treated during the admission or encounter. Inactive problems and minor untreated conditions should not be reported on the claims submitted.

Mental or behavioral disorders should be reported as specifically as possible, using fifth-digit subclassifications as appropriate. Codes from the residual subcategories should not be used if avoidable. Adequate documentation in the patient health record should ensure precise coding and reporting of diagnoses for mental and behavioral disorders.

Despite efforts to overcome barriers of misunderstanding among the populace, certain third-party payors and self-insured employers attach a stigma to mental and behavioral disorders, especially those involving psychotic conditions and chemical dependencies. Therefore, many healthcare facilities develop special policies for coding and reporting such problems. In fact, the release of patient information concerning psychiatric disorders as well as drug and alcohol abuse or dependency are governed by special legislation in most states.

All patient healthcare information should be considered as confidential data. But because of the repercussions that may surround patient information involving psychiatric care or substance abuse rehabilitation, specific policies for the processing of patient data in mental and behavioral health or chemical dependency rehabilitation are frequently maintained by providers and facilities.

In situations in which mental or behavioral disorders are documented in the patient health record as secondary diagnoses, an ethical dilemma may arise. For instance, a patient admitted to an acute care facility for injuries sustained in an accident may become depressed and receive psychiatric care (counseling and medications) concurrently with the treatment of other injuries. As a result, documentation in the medical record may indicate a diagnosis such as situational depression or anxiety depression. If the diagnosis of depression was coded and reported to the third-party payor, the patient may become stigmatized as a person with psychiatric problems.

An analogous situation might occur if a patient with a past history of schizophrenia, affective psychosis, or chemical dependency now in remission, was admitted for a surgical procedure. If the diagnostic data submitted to the third-party payor included the psychiatric or substance abuse diagnosis, notwithstanding appropriate coding with the fifth-digit to indicate remission of the disease, the patient might incur adverse stigmatization due to the inclusion of such diagnostic information.

Consequently, certain healthcare facilities denote secondary psychiatric or substance abuse diagnoses as unreportable, and certain practitioners omit these types of secondary conditions from their discharge summaries. However, another ethical dilemma is presented by the fact that particular carriers recognize specific ICD-9-CM codes for mental or behavioral disorders as comorbidities. And therefore, increased reimbursement might be obtained if the codes for these conditions are reported on the submitted claim. Thus, a conflict may evolve between protecting the confidentiality and the personal interests of the patient and optimizing the revenue received by the healthcare provider.

The Medicare prospective payment system recognizes specific comorbidities among the psychiatric, mental health, and behavioral health disorders. The following ICD-9-CM code numbers represent those comorbidities:

291.0	291.1	291.2
291.3	291.4	291.8
291.9	292.0	292.11
292.12	292.2	292.81
292.82	292.83	292.84
292.89	292.9	293.81
293.82	293.83	295.00
295.01	295.02	295.03
295.04	295.10	295.11
295.12	295.13	295.14
295.21	295.22	295.23
295.24	295.30	295.31
295.32	295.33	295.34
295.40	295.41	295.42
295.43	295.44	295.60

295.61	295.62	295.63
295.64	295.70	295.71
295.72	295.73	295.74
295.80	295.82	295.83
295.84	295.90	295.91
295.92	295.93	295.94
296.04	296.14	296.34
296.44	296.54	296.64
298.0	298.3	298.4
299.00	299.10	299.80
299.90	303.00	303.01
303.02	303.90	303.91
303.92	304.00	304.01
304.02	034.10	304.11
304.12	304.20	304.21
304.22	304.40	304.41
304.42	304.50	304.51
304.52	304.60	304.61
304.62	304.70	304.71
304.72	304.80	304.81
304.82	304.90	304.91
304.92	305.00	305.01
305.02	305.30	305.31
305.32	305.40	305.41
305.42	305.50	305.51
305.52	305.60	305.61
305.62	305.70	305.71
305.72	305.90	305.91
305.92	307.1	

Special federal reimbursement regulations apply to mental and behavioral healthcare and to substance abuse programs. Psychiatric units and mental or behavioral healthcare facilities are exempt from major provisions of the prospective payment system that is based upon diagnosis related groups (DRG's), determined by the reporting of ICD-9-CM code numbers.

Nevertheless, DRG's for psychiatric conditions and chemical dependencies are established. The DRG's relevant to psychiatric care are assigned to MDC 19, Mental Diseases and Disorders (Table 5–3). The DRG's pertinent to substance abuse treatment are assigned to MDC 20, Alcohol/Drug Use and Alcohol/Drug-Induced Organic Mental Disorders (Table 5–4).

NEUROLOGY AND NEUROSURGERY REPORTING FOR BILLING

The care and treatment of nervous system conditions sometimes involves complex diagnostics and intricate therapeutic operative procedures. Accurate and precise documentation in the patient record with the use of specific terminology is essential for the competent coding and reporting of neurological and neurosurgical diagnostic and procedural data.

The staff responsible for coding and billing should endeavor to fulfill the objective of submitting complete and adequate data to the third-party payors and to maintain data useful for

TABLE 5–3

Diagnosis Related Groups for Mental and Behavioral Disorders

DRG 424, Operating Room Procedures with Principal Diagnosis of Mental Illness
DRG 425, Acute Adjustment Reactions and Disturbances of Psychosocial Dysfunction
DRG 426, Depressive Neuroses
DRG 427, Neuroses Except Depressive
DRG 428, Disorders of Personality and Impulse Control
DRG 429, Organic Disturbances and Mental Retardation
DRG 430, Psychoses
DRG 431, Childhood Mental Disorders
DRG 432, Other Mental Disorder Diagnoses

statistical research. The reporting of ICD-9-CM code numbers for vague and nonspecific entities contradicts that objective.

Coding and billing personnel should comply with the basic guidelines for reporting principal and secondary diagnoses and procedures. With nervous system disorders, the suspected diagnosis at admission may be ruled out and superseded by a diagnosis established after diagnostic study to be responsible for the episode of care. If multiple problems are present concurrently, the condition presenting the most significant risk to the patient may be regarded as the principal diagnosis.

Patients afflicted with diseases and disorders of the nervous system may also suffer from other comorbid conditions. All conditions specifically evaluated or treated during the encounter or admission should be coded and reported on the claim submitted by the provider to the third-party payor.

Conversely, malignant neoplasms and endocrine diseases, such as diabetes and hypothyroidism may cause nervous system disorders that constitute secondary diagnoses. These secondary conditions should also be accurately and precisely coded and reported in descending order of clinical significance and resource intensity.

For inpatient admission, particular diseases of the nervous system are recognized as comorbidities by Medicare and certain other third-party payors. The reporting of such comorbid conditions may increase the amount of reimbursement received by the healthcare provider.

TABLE 5–4

Diagnosis Related Groups for Substance Abuse

DRG 433, Alcohol/Drug Abuse or Dependence, Left Against Medical Advice
DRG 434, Alcohol/Drug Abuse or Dependence, Detoxification, or Other Symptomatic Treatment with Comorbidity or Complication
DRG 435, Alcohol/Drug Abuse or Dependence, Detoxification, or Other Symptomatic Treatment without Comorbidity or Complication
DRG 436, Alcohol/Drug Dependence with Rehabilitation Therapy
DRG 437, Alcohol/Drug Dependence with Combined Rehabilitation and Detoxification Therapy

Comorbidities among nervous system diseases are represented by the following ICD-9-CM code numbers:

320.0	320.1	320.2
320.3	320.7	320.81
320.82	320.89	320.9
321.0	321.1	321.2
321.3	321.4	321.8
322.0	322.1	322.2
322.9	324.0	324.1
324.9	325	331.4
335.0	335.10	335.11
335.19	335.20	335.21
335.22	335.23	335.24
335.29	335.8	335.9
340	343.2	344.00
344.01	344.02	344.03
344.04	344.09	345.01
345.10	345.11	345.2
345.3	345.41	345.51
345.61	345.71	345.81
345.91	348.1	349.1
349.81	349.82	357.0
358.0	358.1	359.0
359.1		

Diagnosis related groups (DRG's), as a component of the Medicare prospective payment system, are determined by the ICD-9-CM code numbers reported on the claims submitted by providers to third-party payors. These DRG's are distributed into major diagnostic categories (MDC's). The DRG's associated with neurological and neurosurgical conditions are assigned to MDC 1, Diseases and Disorders of the Nervous System (Table 5–5).

OPHTHALMOLOGY REPORTING FOR BILLING

Eye disorders are predominantly treated in the office or outpatient setting. If an inpatient admission is necessitated for medical or surgical care of the eye, the length of stay is typically shorter than that required for care of conditions associated with other organs or body systems.

Reimbursement received for ophthalmological services is often based on the procedures rendered. One or more concurrent comorbid conditions may impact the revenue received by the provider of eye services to a patient. Similarly, a secondary diagnosis of certain eye disorders may increase the reimbursement obtained from third-party payors by the providers of medical or surgical care to that patient.

The Medicare prospective payment system recognizes specific comorbidities among eye diseases and disorders. Those comorbid conditions are represented by the following ICD-9-CM code numbers:

377.00	377.01	377.02

Diagnosis related groups (DRG's) are determined by the ICD-9-CM code numbers reported on claims submitted by providers to third-party payors. The DRG's associated with

TABLE 5-5

Diagnosis Related Groups for Nervous System Diseases and Disorders

DRG 1, Craniotomy, Age Greater than 17 except for Trauma
DRG 2, Craniotomy for Trauma, Age Greater than 17
DRG 3, Craniotomy, Age 0–17
DRG 4, Spinal Procedures
DRG 5, Extracranial Vascular Procedures
DRG 6, Carpal Tunnel Release
DRG 7, Peripheral and Cranial Nerve and Other Nervous System Procedures with Comorbidity or Complication
DRG 8, Peripheral and Cranial Nerve and Other Nervous System Procedures without Comorbidity or Complication
DRG 9, Spinal Disorders and Injuries
DRG 12, Degenerative Nervous System Disorders
DRG 13, Multiple Sclerosis and Cerebellar Ataxia
DRG 14, Specific Cerebrovascular Disorders except Transient Ischemic Attack
DRG 15, Transient Ischemic Attack and Precerebral Occlusions
DRG 16, Nonspecific Cerebrovascular Disorders with Comorbidity or Complication
DRG 17, Nonspecific Cerebrovascular Disorders without Comorbidity or Complication
DRG 18, Cranial and Peripheral Nerve Disorders with Comorbidity or Complication
DRG 19, Cranial and Peripheral Nerve Disorders without Comorbidity or Complication
DRG 20, Nervous System Infection except Viral Meningitis
DRG 21, Viral Meningitis
DRG 22, Hypertensive Encephalopathy
DRG 23, Nontraumatic Stupor and Coma
DRG 24, Seizure and Headache, Age Greater than 17 with Comorbidity or Complication
DRG 25, Seizure and Headache, Age Greater than 17 without Comorbidity or Complication
DRG 26, Seizure and Headache, Age 0–17
DRG 27, Traumatic Stupor and Coma, Coma Greater than One Hour
DRG 28, Traumatic Stupor and Coma, Coma Less than One Hour, Age Greater than 17 with Comorbidity or Complication
DRG 29, Traumatic Stupor and Coma, Coma Less than One Hour, Age Greater than 17 without Comorbidity or Complication
DRG 30, Traumatic Stupor and Coma, Coma Less than One Hour, Age 0–17
DRG 31, Concussion, Age Greater than 17 with Comorbidity or Complication
DRG 32, Concussion, Age Greater than 17 without Comorbidity or Complication
DRG 33, Concussion, Age 0–17
DRG 34, Other Disorders of Nervous System with Comorbidity or Complication
DRG 35, Other Disorders of Nervous System without Comorbidity or Complication

ophthalmological conditions are assigned to a specific major diagnostic category, MDC 2, Diseases and Disorders of the Eye (Table 5–6).

OTOLOGY REPORTING FOR BILLING

Comparable to services for the sense organ of the eye, ear disorders also are primarily treated in the office or outpatient setting. And likewise, if an inpatient admission is necessitated for medical or surgical care of the ear, the length of stay is typically shorter than that required for care of conditions associated with other body systems.

TABLE 5–6

Diagnosis Related Groups for Eye Diseases and Disorders

DRG 36, Retinal Procedures
DRG 37, Orbital Procedures
DRG 38, Primary Iris Procedures
DRG 39, Lens Procedures with or without Vitrectomy
DRG 40, Extraocular Procedures except Orbit, Age Greater than 17
DRG 41, Extraocular Procedures except Orbit, Age 0–17
DRG 42, Intraocular Procedures except Retina, Iris, and Lens
DRG 43, Hyphema
DRG 44, Acute Major Eye Infections
DRG 45, Neurological Eye Disorders
DRG 46, Other Disorders of the Eye, Age Greater than 17 with Comorbidity or Complication
DRG 47, Other Disorders of the Eye, Age Greater than 17 without Comorbidity or Complication
DRG 48, Other Disorders of the Eye, Age 0–17

Similarly, reimbursement received for otological services is usually predicated on the procedures rendered. One or more concurrent comorbid conditions diagnosed in a patient may impact the revenue received by the provider of care and treatment for an ear disorder in that patient. A secondary diagnosis of particular ear disorders may also increase the reimbursement obtained from third-party payors by the providers of medical or surgical care to that patient.

The Medicare prospective payment system recognizes specific comorbidities among ear diseases and disorders. Those comorbid conditions are represented by the following ICD-9-CM code numbers:

383.01   383.30   383.81

Not every code and narrative in the ICD-9-CM classification, however, represents an entity that may be reported as a principal diagnosis. Certain ICD-9-CM codes are commonly considered as an unacceptable principal diagnosis by a majority of third-party payors including Medicare and Medicaid. Code number *380.4 Impacted cerumen* is an ear condition designated as a questionable or unacceptable principal diagnosis for inpatient admission.

TABLE 5–7

Diagnosis Related Groups for Ear Diseases and Disorders

DRG 55, Miscellaneous Ear, Nose, Mouth, and Throat Procedures
DRG 61, Myringotomy with Tube Insertion, Age Greater than 1
DRG 62, Myringotomy with Tube Insertion, Age 0–17
DRG 63, Other Ear, Nose, Mouth, and Throat Operating Room Procedures
DRG 65, Dysequilibrium
DRG 68, Otitis Media and Upper Respiratory Infection, Age Greater than 17 with Comorbidity or Complication
DRG 69, Otitis Media and Upper Respiratory Infection, Age Greater than 17 without Comorbidity or Complication
DRG 70, Otitis Media and Upper Respiratory Infection, Age 0–17
DRG 73, Other Ear, Nose, Mouth, and Throat Diagnoses, Age Greater than 17
DRG 74, Other Ear, Nose, Mouth, and Throat Diagnoses, Age 0–17

Under the Medicare prospective payment system, the DRG's associated with ear conditions are assigned to a specific major diagnostic category, MDC 3, Diseases and Disorders of the Ear, Nose, Mouth, and Throat (Table 5–7).

KEY CONCEPTS

behavioral health _____

chemical dependency _____

clinical modification _____

comorbidity _____

complication _____

confidentiality _____

diagnosis related groups _____

DSM-IV coding system _____

glossary _____

late effect _____

lozenge _____

major diagnostic category _____

manifestation _____

mental health _____

principal diagnosis _____

principal procedure _____

prospective payment system _____

questionable diagnosis _____

rehabilitation _____

subclassification _____

substance abuse _____

underlying disease _____

REVIEW QUESTIONS

1. Compare and contrast the content of the DSM-IV coding system with that of the ICD-9-CM chapter on mental disorders. _____
_____
_____

2. Describe the purpose of the fifth digit subclassification for the coding of schizophrenia and major affective disorder. _____
_____
_____

3. Describe the purpose of the fifth-digit subclassification for the coding of substance abuse. ___
_____
_____

4. Prioritize (rank in order for reporting purposes) the following clusters of diagnoses:
   A. episodic cannabis abuse, acute exacerbation of chronic paranoid schizophrenia, mild mental retardation _____
   _____
   _____

   B. carpal tunnel syndrome, bacterial meningitis, eczema _____
   _____
   _____

   C. color blindness, astigmatism, partial retinal detachment _____
   _____
   _____

   D. toxic encephalitis, acne vulgaris, obsessive compulsive disorder _____
   _____
   _____

5. Identify at least ten codes and narrative titles that represent mental or behavioral conditions which are recognized by Medicare as complications or comorbidities.

6. Identify at least ten codes and narrative titles that represent nervous system conditions which are recognized by Medicare as complications or comorbidities.

7. Identify at least five codes and narrative titles that represent ear disorders or eye disorders which are recognized by Medicare as complications or comorbidities.

8. Assign precise, accurate code numbers from the ICD-9-CM volume for the following mental or behavioral disorders:

A. arteriosclerotic dementia _____

B. unspecified mental retardation _____

C. alcoholic jealousy _____

D. severe mental retardation _____

E. drug-induced delirium _____

F. mild mental retardation _____

G. subacute delirium _____

H. psychic factors associated with diseases classified elsewhere _____

I. Korsakoff's psychosis _____

J. alexia _____

K. schizophrenia simplex _____

L. attention deficit disorder, with hyperactivity _____

M. manic depressive psychosis, mixed circular type _____

N. sibling jealousy _____

O. simple paranoid state _____

P. pathological gambling _____

Q. acute hysterical psychosis _____

R. depressive disorder _____

S. Heller's syndrome _____

T. presbyophrenia _____

U. panic attack _____

V. separation anxiety disorder _____

W. narcissistic personality _____

X. mixed disorders as reaction to stress _____

Y. nymphomania _____

Z. stammering _____

AA. chronic alcoholism _____

BB. psychogenic paralysis _____

CC. cocaine dependence _____

DD. dependence on tobacco _____

EE. presenile dementia with delirium _____

FF. profound mental retardation _____

GG. pathological alcoholic intoxication _____

HH. mixed development disorder _____

II. hallucinatory state induced by drugs _____

JJ.   hyperkinetic conduct disorder _____

KK.   chronic delirium _____

LL.   identity disorder _____

MM. epileptic psychosis _____

NN.   aggressive outburst _____

OO.   residual schizophrenia _____

PP.   cardiovascular neurosis _____

QQ.   manic bipolar affective disorder _____

RR.   postconcussion syndrome _____

SS.   paranoia querulans _____

TT.   chronic posttraumatic stress disorder _____

UU.   psychogenic stupor _____

VV.   fugue as acute reaction to gross stress _____

WW. unspecified child psychosis _____

XX.   Gilles de la Tourette's disorder _____

9. Assign precise, accurate code numbers from the ICD-9-CM volume for the following diseases
   of the nervous system and sense organs:
   A.   nonpyogenic meningitis _____

   B.   acute perichondritis of pinna _____

   C.   Krabbe's disease _____

   D.   Thygeson's superficial punctate keratitis _____

   E.   encephalitis periaxialis _____

   F.   siderosis of the eye _____

   G.   atypical facial pain _____

   H.   encephalitis due to lead _____

I.   patulous Eustachian tube _____

_____

J.   carotid sinus syndrome _____

K.   macular corneal dystrophy _____

L.   headache after lumbar puncture _____

M.   primary retinal cyst _____

N.   unspecified myopathy _____

O.   meningitis due to trypanosomiasis _____

P.   acute necrotizing otitis media _____

Q.   Pick's disease of brain _____

R.   serous nonviral conjunctivitis _____

S.   spastic hemiplegia _____

T.   atrophic senile macular degeneration _____

U.   Bell's palsy _____

V.   intraspinal abscess _____

W.   mucosal cyst of postmastoidectomy cavity

_____

X.   drug-induced myelopathy _____

Y.   xeroderma of eyelid _____

Z.   brain calcification _____

AA.   central areolar choroidal dystrophy _____

BB.   myasthenia gravis _____

CC.   thrombophlebitis of intercranial venous sinus _____

DD.   perforation of eardrum _____

EE.   idiopathic Parkinson's disease _____

FF.   vascular anomalies of eyelid _____

GG. paralysis of both legs _____

HH. prolapse of iris _____

II. Collet-Sicard syndrome _____

JJ. meningitis in typhoid fever _____

KK. adhesive otitis _____

LL. Kugelberg-Welander disease _____

MM. lacrimal fistula _____

NN. narcolepsy _____

OO. hypersecretion glaucoma _____

PP. hereditary sensory neuropathy _____

QQ. late effect of streptococcal meningitis _____

RR. cholesteatoma of middle ear and mastoid _____

SS. idiopathic torsion dystonia _____

TT. intermittent monocular esotropia _____

UU. grand mal epilepsy _____

VV. pseudoexfoliation of lens capsule _____

WW. postinfectious polyneuritis neuritis _____

XX. suppurative meningitis _____

10. Assign precise, accurate code numbers from the ICD-9-CM volume for the following operations
    on the nervous system:
    A. cranial decompression _____

    B. strip craniectomy _____

    C. debridement of spinal cord _____

    D. peripheral nerve injection _____

    E. injection of neurolytic agent into sympathetic nerve _____

F. resection of cerebral meninges _____

G. implantation of electroencephalographic receiver _____

H. removal of foreign body from spinal canal _____

I. open biopsy of cranial nerve _____

J. division of sympathetic nerve _____

K. subdural tap through fontanel _____

L. ventriculopleural anastomosis _____

M. lysis of adhesions of spinal cord and nerve roots _____

N. nerve transplantation _____

O. presacral sympathectomy _____

P. chemothalamectomy _____

Q. simple suture of dura mater of brain _____

R. removal of spinal neurostimulator _____

S. neurectasis _____

T. repair of sympathetic nerve _____

U. open biopsy of cerebral meninges _____

V. replacement of ventricular shunt _____

W. spinal subarachnoid-peritoneal shunt _____

X. peripheral nerve graft _____

Y. biopsy of sympathetic nerve _____

11. Assign precise, accurate code numbers from the ICD-9-CM volume for the following operations on the eye:

A. repair of blepharoptosis by tarsal technique _____

B. repair of retinal tear by laser photocoagulation _____

C. incision of cornea for removal of foreign body _____

D. revision of enucleation socket with graft _____

E. insertion of stent into nasolacrimal duct _____

F. repair of laceration of conjunctiva _____

G. insertion of pseudophacos _____

H. shortening procedure on one extraocular muscle _____

I. removal of intraocular foreign body from anterior segment of eye with use of magnet ____

J. excision of lacrimal sac and passage _____

K. extracapsular extraction of lens by linear extraction _____

L. linear repair of laceration of eyelid _____

M. orbitotomy with insertion of orbital implant _____

N. thermokeratoplasty _____

O. mechanical vitrectomy by anterior approach _____

P. biopsy of conjunctiva _____

Q. revision of extraocular muscle surgery _____

R. cyclodialysis _____

S. excision of chalazion _____

T. biopsy of extraocular tendon _____

U. repair of scleral fistula _____

V. suture of corneal laceration _____

W. repair of symblepharon with free graft _____

X. retrobulbar injection of therapeutic agent _____

Y. total dacryoadenectomy _____

12. Assign precise, accurate code numbers from the ICD-9-CM volume for the following operations
    on the ear:
    A. otoscopy _____

    B. revision of mastoidectomy _____

C. type I tympanoplasty _____

D. surgical correction of prominent ear _____

E. closure of mastoid fistula _____

F. aspiration of middle ear _____

G. stapedectomy with incus homograft _____

H. removal of tympanostomy tube _____

I. piercing of ear lobe _____

J. otoplasty _____

K. remobilization of stapes _____

L. electrocochleography _____

M. endolymphatic shunt _____

N. radical excision of preauricular cyst _____

O. type III tympanoplasty _____

P. atticotomy _____

Q. ossiculectomy _____

R. reattachment of amputated ear _____

S. simple mastoidectomy _____

T. canaloplasty of external auditory meatus _____

U. stapediolysis _____

V. tympanectomy _____

W. revision of stapedectomy with incus replacement _____

X. radical excision of lesion of external ear _____

Y. revision of fenestration of inner ear _____

CODING OF CLINICAL DOCUMENTATION

Read the following clinical reports and assign precise, accurate diagnostic and procedural code numbers from the appropriate sections of the ICD-9-CM volumes.

PATIENT: Padberg, Herbert   **MR#:** 99-05-01

ADMITTING PHYSICIAN: Bates

History of Present Illness:

This 52-year-old white male with a history of alcohol abuse and tobacco use was brought to the ER after being picked up by police while he was wandering around in the streets, confused and hallucinating. The patient resides in an apartment above a bar. According to the bartender, he is a withdrawn person who rarely leaves the apartment. He drinks heavily, and stores trash in his apartment including the 39 cases of empty beer cans found today. Supposedly he was going door-to-door today searching for a friend and conversing with imaginary persons. He was also wandering through traffic smoking an imaginary cigarette. In the ER, the patient believes he is in the bar and cannot provide a reliable history. The patient had a phone conversation with the bartender who confirmed that the patient was confused and was not at his baseline.

Medications on Admission:

Supposedly on Haldol, Cogentin, and aspirin. No known drug allergies.

Past Medical History:

Peptic ulcer disease; status post appendectomy; status post T & A; patient stated that he has a disease of the nerves for which he takes little pills in a brown bag.

Family History:

Positive for leukemia and throat cancer.

Social History:

Smokes about one pack per day; drinks about twelve beers per day. He is divorced, has five children, and was recently arrested for failure to pay child support.

Physical Examination:

Cooperative white male. ***Pulse:*** 55; ***Resp:*** 28; ***Temp:*** 36.4; ***BP:*** 108/64.
HEENT: normocephalic and atraumatic; throat clear; sclerae anicteric.
Neck: supple without any abnormalities.
Chest: clear to auscultation.
Cardiovascular: regular rate and rhythm; S-1 normal; S-2 normal; no murmurs or gallops.
Abdomen: soft; non-tender; hepatomegaly, which was palpable and percussible 6 cm below the costal margin.
Extremities: without clubbing, cyanosis, or edema.
Rectal: normal tone with no masses; guaiac negative.
Neurological: alert, oriented to name but not to place or time, believes the bar was turned into a doctor's office to give physical examinations; normal psychomotor activity; flow of thought was sequential with occasionally illogical thought content; actively hallucinating and delusional regarding a cigarette in his hand but denied visual or auditory hallucinations; memory was 3/3 at 5 minutes; distant memory intact; serial 3's rapid and correct; calculations intact; named Presidents Clinton to Kennedy; pupils were 4 by 4 reacting down to 2 by 3; visual fields were full to confrontation; fundi benign; extraocular movements full; end point gaze nystagmus; face symmetric; bilaterally symmetric upgoing tongue; Barre without drift; good fine finger movements; diffuse muscle without fasciculations; strength

5/5 throughout; mildly tremulous, mostly postural tremor; relatively multifocal myoclonus; deep tendon reflexes were 2+ and toes downgoing bilaterally; sensation intact to light touch, pin prick, temperature, and joint position; mild decrease in vibration in toes; finger-nose-finger and heel-shin without dysmetria; gait mildly wide-based and unsteady with increased tremulousness.

Laboratory Data:
On admission, chest X ray was clear with slight cardiomegaly. The electrocardiogram showed sinus bradycardia with minimal left ventricular hypertrophy. SMA-12 revealed low albumin of 2.8, low total protein of 5.8, ALT of 51, AST of 70, calcium of 8.2, LDH of 254, BUN of 7, sodium of 139, potassium of 3.8, chloride of 109, CO2 of 24, glucose of 116, and creatinine of 0.7. Drug screen revealed the presence of acetone in the urine. B-12 was 320, folic acid was 12.6, and iron and total iron binding capacity were low with normal male ferritin levels. PT was 12.3, PTT was 25.7, and reticulocyte count was 0.5 with a retic index of 226. Sedimentation rate was 30, WBC was 6100, hemoglobin was 11.1, hematocrit was 32.9, platelet count was 372000, and MCV was 94.5. Thyroid function tests were within normal limits. Glucose was 69. Blood alcohol was less than .10. RPR was non-reactive. Urinalysis was clear. Cerebrospinal fluid protein was 24. Cerebrospinal fluid routine culture was negative for any growth.

Hospital Course:
The assessment on admission was alcoholic hallucinations. He was started on Librium, thiamine, and multivitamins. Clonidine was also added as part of the treatment for alcohol withdrawal. He did remarkably better with this regimen, and by the second day of admission, his sensorium was clear, and he was not hallucinating further. His discharge was delayed, however, because of placement problems. He was finally discharged to a VA shelter.

Discharge Diagnosis:
Alcoholic hallucinosis and withdrawal.

Discharge Medications:
Multivitamins one tablet p.o. q.d.

Thiamine 100 mg p.o. q.d.

Codes: _____

PATIENT: Mueller, Joan   **MR#:** 99-05-02

ADMITTING PHYSICIAN: Phillips

Chief Complaint:
This 37-year-old woman was admitted with increasing chronic anxiety and severe depressive symptoms.

Laboratory Studies:
Hemoglobin 12.8; hematocrit 38 with MCV of 101; WBC 6300; normal differential; platelets 324000; serum sodium 143; potassium 4.2; chloride 111; BUN 7; creatinine 0.9; glucose 62; cholesterol 196; SMA otherwise normal; total T4 6.8; TSH 0.6; urinalysis negative; B12 level 577; folic acid 6.4; MRI of the cervical spine negative.

Hospital Course:
The patient was given anti-anxiety medication. She was seen by Dr. Henderson, a neurosurgical consultant, whose impression was cervical strain. The consultant recommended treatment with physical therapy, heat, and ultrasound electric stimulation. She was also given

Voltaren 75 mg b.i.d. The patient was additionally seen by Dr. Fitzpatrick, a neurology consultant, whose impression also was cervical strain. The neurologist agreed with the recommendation of physical therapy as well as the use of Voltaren and muscle relaxants. The patient attended psychodrama. She was continued on treatment with lithium, although this medication was discontinued prior to discharge. The patient felt that she had improved and was discharged, to be followed in outpatient psychiatry. She also is to be followed up by Dr. Rubenstein, an orthopedic physician.

Discharge Diagnoses:

Major depression, recurrent.

Acute and chronic cervical strain.

Allergic rhinitis.

Chronic bronchitis.

Spastic colitis.

Duodenal ulcer by history.

Codes: _____

6

CHAPTER

ICD Coding: Circulatory System and Respiratory System Diseases and Operations

LEARNING OBJECTIVES

Upon completion of this chapter the learner should be able to:

1. Describe the parameters for coding and reporting hypertensive disease.
2. Explain the proper usage of the table for coding hypertension.
3. Explain the distinction between a condition diagnosed "with" another condition in contrast to a condition diagnosed "due to" another condition.
4. Describe the parameters for coding and reporting myocardial infarction.
5. Describe the parameters for coding and reporting cardiac catheterization, angioplasty, and coronary bypass surgery.
6. Describe the parameters for coding and reporting cardiac arrhythmias.
7. Describe the parameters for coding and reporting cerebrovascular disease.
8. Describe the parameters for coding and reporting endarterectomy.
9. Describe proper sequencing in reporting the late effects of cerebrovascular disease.
10. Describe the parameters for coding and reporting peripheral vascular disease.
11. Describe the parameters for coding and reporting pneumonia.
12. Describe the parameters for coding and reporting obstructive pulmonary disease.
13. Describe the parameters for coding and reporting bronchoscopy procedures.
14. Describe the parameters for coding and reporting respiratory distress.
15. Discuss the impact of comorbidities and complications on billing and reimbursement for diagnoses involving the cardiovascular system.
16. Discuss the impact of nonoperative procedures on billing and reimbursement involving the cardiovascular system.
17. Discuss the impact of comorbidities and complications on billing and reimbursement for diagnoses involving the respiratory system.
18. Discuss the impact of nonoperative procedures on billing and reimbursement involving the respiratory system.
19. Apply knowledge of coding principles by assigning accurate and precise codes to report diagnoses and procedures pertaining to the cardiovascular system.

20. Apply knowledge of coding principles by assigning accurate and precise codes to report diagnoses and procedures pertaining to the respiratory system.

ICD CODING OF CARDIOVASCULAR SYSTEM DISEASES AND OPERATIONS

Chapter 7 of the ICD-9-CM diagnostic tabular volume, designated for listings of diagnoses of the circulatory system, is one of the most frequently utilized chapters in that volume. This chapter consists of the nine sections listed in Table 6–1.

The first and second sections of Chapter 7 contain listings for acute rheumatic fever and chronic rheumatic heart disease. These listings encompass rheumatic fever with or without heart involvement, rheumatic chorea, chronic rheumatic pericarditis, diseases of the mitral valve, diseases of the aortic valve, diseases of other endocardial structures, and other rheumatic diseases.

The third section of this chapter is comprised of listings for hypertensive disease. These listings encompass essential hypertension including hyperpiesis, hypertensive vascular disease, hypertensive heart disease including hypertensive cardiomegaly, hypertensive cardiomyopathy, and hypertensive cardiovascular disease. These listings also encompass hypertensive renal disease including arteriolar nephritis, arteriosclerotic nephritis, hypertensive nephropathy, hypertensive renal failure, hypertensive uremia, nephrosclerosis, and renal sclerosis with hypertension, hypertensive heart and renal disease including cardiorenal disease and cardiovascular renal disease, as well as secondary hypertension.

Documentation of hypertension (arterial, essential, primary, systemic, or not otherwise specified) should be assigned to a code number within category 401, using the appropriate fourth digit to indicate malignant (.0), benign (.1), or unspecified (.9). An appropriate code from within category range 401 through 405 should be selected and assigned to report the documentation of controlled hypertension. This diagnostic statement usually refers to a preexisting condition of hypertension presently under control by therapy.

Uncontrolled hypertension may refer to untreated hypertension or to hypertension not responding to a current therapeutic regimen. In either case, an appropriate code from within category range 401 through 405 should be selected and assigned to designate the type of hypertension that was documented.

T A B L E   6–1

Sections in Chapter 7, Volume 1 of ICD-9-CM

1. Acute Rheumatic Fever (category range 390–392)
2. Chronic Rheumatic Heart Disease (category range 393–398)
3. Hypertensive Disease (category range 401–405)
4. Ischemic Heart Disease (category range 410–414)
5. Diseases of Pulmonary Circulation (category range 415–417)
6. Other Forms of Heart Disease (category range 420–429)
7. Cerebrovascular Disease (category range 430–438)
8. Diseases of Arteries, Arterioles, and Capillaries (category range 440–448)
9. Diseases of Veins and Lymphatics, and Other Diseases of Circulatory System (category range 451–459)

Code number *796.2, Elevated blood pressure reading without diagnosis of hypertension,* should be selected to report transient hypertension or elevated blood pressure documented without further specificity, unless an established diagnosis of hypertension was stated. A code number from within subcategory *642.3* should be selected to report transient hypertension of pregnancy.

Certain cardiovascular conditions, indicated by codes 428.0 through 428.9, 429.0 through 429.3, 429.8, and 429.9, should be coded and reported with a code number within category 402 if a causal relationship was stated as due to hypertension, or implied by the term "hypertensive." In such cases, only the code number from category 402 should be used.

These conditions, if documented in the patient record along with hypertension, but without a stated causal relationship, are coded and reported separately. Each diagnosis should be sequenced according to the circumstances of the admission or encounter.

Code numbers from category *403, Hypertensive renal disease,* should be selected and assigned if conditions classified to categories 585 through 587 were documented. Unlike the guideline for coding hypertension with heart disease, ICD-9-CM presumes a cause and effect relationship, and therefore renal failure with hypertension should be classified as hypertensive renal disease.

Code numbers from the combination category *404, Hypertensive heart and renal disease* should be assigned if both hypertensive renal disease and hypertensive heart disease were stated in the diagnosis. A causal relationship between the hypertension and the renal disease should be assumed for classification purposes, whether or not the conditions were documented as related.

Code numbers from categories 430 through 438, the section containing listings for cerebrovascular disease, should be selected and assigned using the appropriate code from category range 401 through 405 to represent the diagnosis of hypertension, if conditions listed in both sections were documented.

Two codes are necessary to identify the condition of hypertensive retinopathy. A code number from subcategory *362.11, Hypertensive retinopathy* should be reported with an appropriate code from within category range 401 through 405 to indicate the type of hypertension.

Two codes are also required to report secondary hypertension. One code is needed to identify the underlying condition, and another code from category 405 is needed to identify the diagnosis of hypertension. Sequencing of these codes should be determined by the reason for the admission or the encounter for care.

In the fourth section of Chapter 7, the listings for ischemic heart disease encompass acute myocardial infarction, coronary embolism, coronary occlusion, other acute and subacute forms of ischemic heart disease, old myocardial infarction, angina pectoris, and other forms of chronic ischemic heart disease.

The fifth section of Chapter 7 includes listings for diseases of pulmonary circulation. These listings encompass acute and chronic pulmonary heart disease such as pulmonary embolism and pulmonary hypertension.

The sixth section of this chapter is a varied section of listings for other forms of heart disease. The listings in this section include acute pericarditis, acute and subacute endocarditis, acute myocarditis, and other diseases of the pericardium and endocardium. This sixth section also contains listings for cardiomyopathy, conduction disorders, cardiac dysarrhythmias, heart failure, and other ill-defined descriptions and complications of heart disease. An additional code should be reported to identify the presence of arteriosclerosis, if that diagnosis was documented along with these other disorders.

The seventh section of Chapter 7 contains listings for cerebrovascular disease and encompasses subarachnoid hemorrhage, intracerebral hemorrhage, and other intracranial hemorrhage. This section also contains listings for occlusion of precerebral and cerebral arteries including arterial stenosis, embolism, and thrombosis, transient cerebral ischemia including cerebrovascular insufficiency and spasm, cerebrovascular accident, and other ill-defined cerebrovascular disease.

Category *438, Late effects of cerebrovascular disease,* should be used to indicate conditions classifiable to categories 430 through 437 as the causes of late effects (neurologic deficits), which are classified elsewhere. These late effects include neurologic deficits that persist after the initial onset of conditions classifiable to categories 430 through 437. Unlike other late effects, the neurologic deficits caused by cerebrovascular disease are generally present from the onset of the disorder, rather than arising months later.

The code for the specific neurologic deficit (for example, aphasia, dysphagia, hemiplegia, and/or paralysis) should be selected and assigned, followed by the selection and assignment of code 438. Code number 438 should not be assigned if a current diagnosis classifiable to categories 430 through 437 was documented, but rather should be assigned only if there was no documentation of any particular deficits. For instance, code number 438 may be properly assigned for a diagnosis stated as "old cerebrovascular accident" or "old CVA." Code V12.5 instead of code 438 should be selected and assigned as an additional code to report a patient history of cerebrovascular disease if no neurologic deficits were documented in the patient health record.

The eighth section of the circulatory system chapter of the diagnostic tabular is comprised of listings for diseases of the arteries, arterioles, and capillaries. These listings encompass atherosclerosis including arteriosclerosis, arteriolosclerosis, arteriosclerotic vascular disease or degeneration, endarteritis, aortic or other aneurysm and aneurysmal varix, and peripheral vascular disease. These listings also encompass arterial embolism and thrombosis including embolic or thrombotic infarction or occlusion, polyarteritis nodosa, and other allied conditions.

The ninth and final section of the circulatory system chapter of the diagnostic tabular is comprised of listings for diseases of the veins and lymphatics. These listings include phlebitis, thrombophlebitis, endophlebitis, periphlebitis, portal vein thrombosis, and other venous embolism and thrombosis. This section also includes listings for varicose veins of the lower extremities and other sites, hemorrhoids, noninfectious disorders of the lymphatic channels, hypotension, and certain other disorders of the circulatory system.

Categories of listings in Chapter 7 of Volume 3 of ICD-9 are established for surgical procedures on the components of the cardiovascular system. These include listings in category range 35–39 for: operations on the valves and septa of the heart; operations on the vessels of the heart; and incision, excision, or occlusion of blood vessels.

Open heart operation codes implicitly include the reporting of median sternotomy as an operative approach. Cardiopulmonary bypass, (extracorporeal circulation via heart-lung machine) should always be reported as an additional code, if applicable. For example, repair of atrial septal defect by open technique (code number *35.51*) should be reported with an additional code for extracorporeal circulation ancillary to open heart surgery (code number *39.61*).

Reporting the insertion of a cardiac pacemaker requires two ICD-9-CM codes. One code reports the insertion, revision, replacement, or removal of the pacemaker, and the other code reports the insertion, revision, replacement, or removal of the leads. For example, insertion of a single-chamber pacemaker with a transvenous lead into the atrium should be reported with code numbers *37.81* and *37.73*.

TABLE 6–2

Sections in Chapter 8, Volume 1, of ICD-9-CM

1. Acute Respiratory Infections (category range 460–466)
2. Other Diseases of the Upper Respiratory Tract (category range 470–478)
3. Pneumonia and Influenza (category range 480–487)
4. Chronic Obstructive Pulmonary Disease and Allied Conditions (category range 490–496)
5. Pneumoconioses and Other Lung Disease due to External Agents (category range 500–508)
6. Other Diseases of the Respiratory System (category range 510–519)

ICD CODING OF RESPIRATORY SYSTEM DISEASES AND OPERATIONS

Chapter 8 of the ICD-9-CM diagnostic tabular volume, designated for listings of diagnoses of the respiratory system, is another frequently utilized chapter of Volume 1. The chapter consists of the six sections listed in Table 6–2.

The initial section of Chapter 8 contains listings for acute respiratory infections. These listings encompass acute nasopharyngitis, acute sinusitis including abscess, empyema, infection, inflammation, or suppuration of sinus, acute pharyngitis, acute tonsillitis, acute laryngitis, acute tracheitis, acute bronchitis, acute bronchiolitis, and acute respiratory infection of multiple sites.

The second section of this chapter is comprised of listings for other diseases of the upper respiratory tract. This section encompasses listings for conditions such as deviated nasal septum, nasal polyps, chronic pharyngitis or nasopharyngitis, chronic sinusitis including abscess, empyema, infection or suppuration of sinus, chronic disease of the tonsils or adenoids, and peritonsillar abscess. This section also encompasses listings for chronic laryngitis or laryngotracheitis, allergic rhinitis including hay fever or spasmodic rhinorrhea, and certain other diseases of the upper respiratory tract.

The third section of the respiratory system chapter in the diagnostic tabular contains listings for pneumonia and influenza. These listings include viral pneumonia, pneumococcal and other bacterial pneumonia, pneumonia due to other organisms, pneumonia in infectious diseases classified elsewhere, and bronchopneumonia. Any underlying disease should be coded and reported along with the documented manifestation stated in the patient health record.

The fourth section of Chapter 8 is comprised of listings for chronic obstructive pulmonary disease and allied conditions that include chronic bronchitis, emphysema, asthma, bronchiectasis, extrinsic allergic alveolitis (including allergic alveolitis or pneumonitis due to inhaled particles), and chronic airway obstruction. An additional code should be reported to identify any acute exacerbation of a respiratory condition that was documented in the patient health record.

The fifth section of the respiratory system chapter in the diagnostic tabular volume is comprised of listings for pneumoconioses and other lung diseases due to external agents. These listings include coal workers' pneumoconiosis, asbestosis, pneumopathy due to inhalation of silica or other inorganic dust, respiratory conditions due to chemical fumes and vapors, pneumonitis due to solids and liquids, as well as respiratory conditions due to other external causes.

The sixth and final section of Chapter 8 contains listings for other diseases of the respiratory system. These listings encompass empyema, pleurisy, pneumothorax, abscess of lung and mediastinum, pulmonary congestion and hypostasis, postinflammatory pulmonary fibrosis, other alveolar and parietoalveolar pneumopathy, and lung involvement in diseases classified elsewhere.

Categories of listings in Volume 3 of ICD-9 are established for surgical procedures on the nose, mouth, pharynx, and components of the respiratory system. In Chapter 5 of Volume 3, these include categories 21 and 22 for listings of operations on the nose and nasal sinuses, and categories 28 and 29 for listings of operations on the tonsils, adenoids, and pharynx. In Chapter 6 of Volume 3, category range 30 through 34 contains listings for excision and other operations on the larynx and trachea, excision and other operations of the lung and bronchus, and operations on the chest wall, pleura, mediastinum, and diaphragm.

Thoracic cavity operation codes implicitly include the reporting of median sternotomy and/or rib resection as an operative approach. For example, incision of lung (code number *33.1*) includes any operative approach technique.

CARDIOLOGY AND CARDIOVASCULAR SURGERY REPORTING FOR BILLING

As a coding guideline for all clinical services, the principal diagnosis is defined as that condition responsible for the admission of the patient for the health service admission, encounter, or episode of care. Likewise, the principal procedure is defined as that procedure most closely associated with the patient's principal diagnosis for the specific admission, encounter, or episode of care.

Usually, the diagnosis or procedure that presents the greatest risk to the patient is also the most resource intensive diagnosis or procedure. And consequently, the provider is reimbursed at a relatively higher rate for rendering that entity to the patient.

Coding guidelines specify that the principal diagnosis should be sequenced first. To exemplify, a serious condition such as ventricular tachycardia should be sequenced before a lesser condition such as atrial flutter. Similarly, a significant procedure such as cardiac catheterization should be sequenced before a lesser procedure such as an echocardiogram.

However, under exceptional circumstances, especially those involving a hospitalized patient, the most resource intensive diagnosis or procedure or the diagnosis or procedure posing the greatest risk to the patient may be unrelated to that patient's principal diagnosis for the particular episode of inpatient service. Such a situation could occur if a patient was admitted for a relatively minor problem and major complications resulted unexpectedly. To exemplify, a patient might be admitted for evaluation of chronic myocarditis, and meanwhile during the hospitalization, the patient might sustain an acute inferior myocardial infarction.

Insurance claim policies ordinarily limit coding and reporting to only those diagnoses that are specifically assessed or treated during the admission, encounter, or episode of care. Additionally, these third-party payor criteria generally limit coding and reporting to those procedures actually rendered in entirety.

In all cases, the principal diagnosis or procedure should be sequenced and reported first, and followed by all relevant secondary diagnoses or procedures in descending order of clinical significance and resource intensity. Thus, a diagnosis of unstable angina should be sequenced before a diagnosis of essential hypertension.

Specific ICD-9-CM codes are recognized and designated as comorbidities by certain third-party payors, especially the carriers offering reimbursement under the Medicare prospective payment system. For inpatient admissions, these comorbid conditions may increase the amount of reimbursement received by the provider. Comorbidities among the listed circulatory system conditions are represented by the following ICD-9-CM code numbers:

394.0	394.1	394.2
394.9	395.0	395.1
395.2	395.9	396.0
396.1	396.2	396.3
396.8	396.9	397.0
397.1	397.9	398.0
398.91	401.0	402.00
402.01	402.11	402.91
403.00	403.01	403.11
403.91	404.00	404.01
404.02	404.03	404.11
404.12	404.13	404.91
404.92	404.93	405.01
405.09	410.01	410.11
410.21	410.31	410.41
410.51	410.91	411.0
411.81	411.89	413.0
413.1	413.9	415.0
415.1	416.0	420.0
420.90	420.91	420.99
421.0	421.1	421.9
422.0	422.90	422.91
422.92	422.93	422.99
423.0	423.1	423.2
424.0	424.1	424.2
424.3	424.90	424.91
424.99	425.0	425.1
425.2	425.3	425.4
425.5	425.7	425.8
425.9	426.0	426.12
426.13	426.53	426.54
426.6	426.7	427.0
427.1	427.2	427.31
427.32	427.41	427.42
427.5	428.0	428.1
428.9	429.4	429.5
429.6	429.71	429.79
429.81	429.82	430
431	432.0	432.1
433.01	433.11	433.21
433.31	433.81	433.91
434.01	434.11	434.91
436	437.2	437.4
437.5	437.6	440.24
441.00	441.01	441.02
441.03	441.1	441.3
441.5	441.6	444.0
444.1	444.21	444.22
444.81	444.89	444.9

446.0	446.20	446.21
446.29	446.3	446.4
446.5	446.6	446.7
451.0	451.11	451.19
451.2	451.81	452
453.0	453.1	453.2
453.3	453.8	453.9
456.0	456.2	459.0

However, not every code and narrative title in the ICD-9-CM classification represents an entity that may be accepted by the third-party payor as a principal or a primary diagnosis. Selected ICD-9-CM codes are commonly considered as an unacceptable principal or primary diagnosis by a majority of third-party payors including Medicare and Medicaid. Unacceptable principal or primary diagnoses codes for circulatory system conditions are as follows:

424.91	425.7	425.8

Additionally, several codes for circulatory system conditions are generally deemed as questionable, if these codes are reported as a principal or primary diagnosis. Diagnoses deemed as questionable if sequenced first are represented by codes:

401.1	426.2	426.3
426.4		

Certain non-operating room procedures listed among the operations on the cardiovascular system impact reimbursement under the prospective payment system. Codes from Chapter 7 of Volume 3 representing nonoperative procedures that affect DRG assignment are:

37.70	37.71	37.72
37.73	37.81	37.82
37.83		

Codes from Chapter 16 of Volume 3 for cardiovascular related procedures which are non-operative services that affect DRG assignment are:

85.52	85.53	85.54
88.55	85.56	85.57
85.58		

The reporting of code numbers for nonspecific or unspecified cardiovascular diagnoses or procedures should be avoided, if possible. Personnel responsible for coding and billing should attempt to ascertain the most specific code not only for reimbursement purposes but also to generate meaningful data for statistical and research purposes. Accurate, complete, and timely documentation in the patient health record may improve the quality of data obtained through the reporting of codes for cardiovascular diagnoses and procedures.

The DRG's associated with circulatory conditions are distributed into a specific major diagnostic category, MDC 5, Diseases and Disorders of the Circulatory System (Table 6–3).

TABLE 6-3

Diagnosis Related Groups for Diseases and Disorders of the Circulatory System

DRG 103, Heart Transplant
DRG 104, Cardiac Valve Procedures with Cardiac Catheterization
DRG 105, Cardiac Valve Procedures without Cardiac Catheterization
DRG 106, Coronary Bypass with Cardiac Catheterization
DRG 107, Coronary Bypass without Cardiac Catheterization
DRG 108, Other Cardiothoracic Procedures
DRG 110, Major Cardiovascular Procedures with Comorbidity or Complication
DRG 111, Major Cardiovascular Procedures without Comorbidity or Complication
DRG 112, Percutaneous Cardiovascular Procedures
DRG 113, Amputation for Circulatory System Disorders Except Upper Limb and Toe
DRG 114, Upper Limb and Toe Amputation for Circulatory System Disorders
DRG 115, Permanent Cardiac Pacemaker Implant with Acute Myocardial Infarction, Heart Failure, or Shock
DRG 116, Other Permanent Cardiac Pacemaker Implant or Generator Procedure
DRG 117, Cardiac Pacemaker Revision Except Device Replacement
DRG 118, Cardiac Pacemaker Device Replacement
DRG 119, Vein Ligation and Stripping
DRG 120, Other Circulatory System Operating Room Procedures
DRG 121, Circulatory Disorders with Acute Myocardial Infarction and Cardiovascular Complication, Discharged Alive
DRG 122, Circulatory Disorders with Acute Myocardial Infarction without Cardiovascular Complication, Discharged Alive
DRG 123, Circulatory Disorders with Acute Myocardial Infarction, Expired
DRG 124, Circulatory Disorders Except Acute Myocardial Infarction with Cardiac Catheterization and Complex Diagnosis
DRG 125, Circulatory Disorders except Acute Myocardial Infarction with Cardiac Catheterization without Complex Diagnosis
DRG 126, Acute and Subacute Endocarditis
DRG 127, Heart Failure and Shock
DRG 128, Deep Vein Thrombophlebitis
DRG 129, Cardiac Arrest, Unexplained
DRG 130, Peripheral Vascular Disorders with Comorbidity or Complication
DRG 131, Peripheral Vascular Disorders without Comorbidity or Complication
DRG 132, Atherosclerosis with Comorbidity or Complication
DRG 133, Atherosclerosis without Comorbidity or Complication
DRG 134, Hypertension
DRG 135, Cardiac Congenital and Valvular Disorders, Age Greater than 17 with Comorbidity or Complication
DRG 136, Cardiac Congenital and Valvular Disorders, Age Greater than 17 without Comorbidity or Complication
DRG 137, Cardiac Congenital and Valvular Disorders, Age 0-17
DRG 138, Cardiac Arrhythmia and Conduction Disorders with Comorbidity or Complication
DRG 139, Cardiac Arrhythmia and Conduction Disorders without Comorbidity or Complication
DRG 140, Angina Pectoris
DRG 141, Syncope and Collapse with Comorbidity or Complication
DRG 142, Syncope and Collapse without Comorbidity or Complication
DRG 143, Chest Pain
DRG 144, Other Circulatory System Diagnoses with Comorbidity or Complication
DRG 145, Other Circulatory System Diagnoses without Comorbidity or Complication
DRG 478, Other Vascular Procedures with Comorbidity or Complication
DRG 479, Other Vascular Procedures without Comorbidity or Complication

PULMONOLOGY AND THORACIC SURGERY REPORTING FOR BILLING

As previously discussed, a coding guideline for all clinical services defines the principal diagnosis as that condition responsible for the admission of the patient to the health service admission, encounter, or episode of care. Likewise, the principal procedure is that procedure most closely associated with the patient's principal diagnosis for that admission, encounter, or episode of care.

Coding guidelines specify that the principal diagnosis should be sequenced first. As examples, an acute condition such as a pulmonary embolism should be sequenced before a lesser condition such as chronic sinusitis. Moreover, a significant procedure such as a fiberoptic bronchoscopy should be sequenced before a lesser procedure such as a sinogram of the chest wall.

In all reported cases, the principal diagnosis or procedure should be sequenced first, and followed by all relevant secondary diagnoses or procedures in descending order of clinical significance and resource intensity. Thus, a diagnosis of pulmonary edema should be sequenced before secondary diagnoses of nasal polyps or chronic sinusitis.

Specific ICD-9-CM codes are designated and recognized as comorbidities by certain third-party payors, especially the carriers offering reimbursement under the Medicare prospective payment system. For inpatient admissions, these comorbid conditions may increase the amount of reimbursement received by the provider. Comorbidities among the listed respiratory system conditions are represented by the following ICD-9-CM code numbers:

464.11	464.21	464.31
475	478.21	478.22
478.24	478.30	478.31
478.32	478.33	478.34
481	482.0	482.1
482.2	482.30	482.31
482.32	482.39	482.4
482.81	482.82	482.83
482.89	482.9	483.0
483.8	484.1	484.3
484.5	484.6	484.7
484.8	485	486
487.0	491.1	491.20
491.21	491.8	491.9
492.8	493.01	493.11
493.20	493.21	493.91
494	495.0	495.1
495.2	495.3	495.4
495.5	495.6	495.7
495.8	495.9	496
506.0	506.1	507.0
507.1	507.8	508.0
508.1	510.0	510.9
511.1	511.8	511.9
512.0	512.1	512.8

513.0	513.1	515
516.0	516.1	516.2
516.3	516.8	516.9
517.1	517.2	517.8
518.0	518.1	518.4
518.5	518.81	518.82
519.0	519.2	

The DRG's associated with nose and throat conditions are assigned to a specific major diagnostic category, MDC 3, Diseases and Disorders of the Ear, Nose, Mouth, and Throat (Table 6–4). The DRG's associated with respiratory conditions are distributed into another major diagnostic category, MDC 4, Diseases and Disorders of the Respiratory System (Table 6–5).

TABLE 6-4

Diagnosis Related Groups for Diseases and Disorders of the Nose and Throat

DRG 49, Major Head and Neck Procedures

DRG 50, Sialoadenectomy

DRG 51, Salivary Gland Procedures except Sialoadenectomy

DRG 52, Cleft Lip and Palate Repair

DRG 53, Sinus and Mastoid Procedures, Age Greater than 17

DRG 54, Sinus and Mastoid Procedures, Age 0–17

DRG 55, Miscellaneous Ear, Nose, Mouth, and Throat Procedures

DRG 56, Rhinoplasty

DRG 57, Tonsillectomy and Adenoidectomy Procedures except Tonsillectomy and/or Adenoidectomy Only, Age Greater than 17

DRG 58, Tonsillectomy and Adenoidectomy Procedures except Tonsillectomy and/or Adenoidectomy Only, Age 0–17

DRG 59, Tonsillectomy and/or Adenoidectomy Only, Age Greater than 17

DRG 60, Tonsillectomy and/or Adenoidectomy Only, Age 0–17

DRG 63, Other Ear, Nose, Mouth, and Throat Operating Room Procedures

DRG 66, Epistaxis

DRG 67, Epiglottitis

DRG 68, Otitis Media and Upper Respiratory Infection, Age Greater than 17 with Comorbidity or Complication

DRG 69, Otitis Media and Upper Respiratory Infection, Age Greater than 17 without Comorbidity or Complication

DRG 70, Otitis Media and Upper Respiratory Infection, Age 0–17

DRG 71, Laryngotracheitis

DRG 72, Nasal Trauma and Deformity

DRG 73, Other Ear, Nose, Mouth, and Throat Diagnoses, Age Greater than 17

DRG 74, Other Ear, Nose, Mouth, and Throat Diagnoses, Age 0–17

DRG 168, Mouth Procedures with Comorbidity or Complication

DRG 169, Mouth Procedures without Comorbidity or Complication

DRG 482, Tracheostomy for Face, Mouth, and Neck Diagnoses

T A B L E 6–5

Diagnosis Related Groups for Diseases and Disorders of the Respiratory System

DRG 75, Major Chest Procedures
DRG 76, Other Respiratory System Operating Room Procedures with Comorbidity and Complication
DRG 77, Other Respiratory System Operating Room Procedures without Comorbidity or Complication
DRG 78, Pulmonary Embolism
DRG 79, Respiratory Infections and Inflammations, Age Greater than 17 with Comorbidity or Complication
DRG 80, Respiratory Infections and Inflammations, Age Greater than 17 without Comorbidity or Complication
DRG 81, Respiratory Infections and Inflammations, Age 0–17
DRG 83, Major Chest Trauma with Comorbidity or Complication
DRG 84, Major Chest Trauma without Comorbidity or Complication
DRG 85, Pleural Effusion with Comorbidity or Complication
DRG 86, Pleural Effusion without Comorbidity or Complication
DRG 87, Pulmonary Edema and Respiratory Failure
DRG 88, Chronic Obstructive Pulmonary Disease
DRG 89, Simple Pneumonia and Pleurisy, Age Greater than 17 with Comorbidity or Complication
DRG 90, Simple Pneumonia and Pleurisy, Age Greater than 17 without Comorbidity or Complication
DRG 91, Simple Pneumonia and Pleurisy, Age 0–17
DRG 92, Interstitial Lung Disease with Comorbidity or Complication
DRG 93, Interstitial Lung Disease without Comorbidity or Complication
DRG 94, Pneumothorax with Comorbidity or Complication
DRG 95, Pneumothorax without Comorbidity or Complication
DRG 96, Bronchitis and Asthma, Age Greater than 17 with Comorbidity or Complication
DRG 97, Bronchitis and Asthma, Age Greater than 17 without Comorbidity or Complication
DRG 98, Bronchitis and Asthma, Age 0–17
DRG 99, Respiratory Signs and Symptoms with Comorbidity or Complication
DRG 100, Respiratory Signs and Symptoms without Comorbidity or Complication
DRG 101, Other Respiratory System Diagnoses with Comorbidity or Complication
DRG 102, Other Respiratory System Diagnoses without Comorbidity or Complication
DRG 475, Respiratory System Diagnosis with Ventilator Support
DRG 483, Tracheostomy Except for Face, Mouth, and Neck Diagnoses
DRG 495, Lung Transplant

Certain non-operating room procedures listed among the operations on the respiratory system impact reimbursement under the prospective payment system. Codes from Chapter 6 of Volume 3 representing nonoperative procedures that affect DRG assignment are:

31.1	31.41	31.42
31.43	31.44	33.21
33.22	33.23	34.05

The reporting of code numbers for nonspecific or unspecified respiratory diagnoses or procedures should be avoided, if possible. Staff members responsible for coding and billing should attempt to determine the most specific code not only for reimbursement purposes but also to generate meaningful data for statistical and research purposes. Precise, complete, and timely documentation in the patient health record may improve the quality of data obtained through the reporting of codes for pulmonary diagnoses and procedures.

KEY CONCEPTS

category range _____

causal relationship _____

combination code _____

comorbidity _____

complication _____

diagnosis related groups _____

hypertension table _____

late effect _____

major diagnostic category _____

manifestation _____

nonoperative procedure _____

nonspecific diagnosis _____

principal diagnosis _____

principal procedure _____

questionable diagnosis _____

sequelae _____

unacceptable diagnosis _____

underlying disease _____

unspecified diagnosis _____

REVIEW QUESTIONS

1. Differentiate the causal relationship in disease etiology by explaining the contrast in conditions reported "with" another condition as opposed to conditions reported "due to" another condition. _____

_____

_____

2. Discuss the usage of each of the columns in the hypertension table in the alphabetic index. _____

_____

3. Describe the purpose of the fifth-digit subclassification for the coding of hypertensive heart disease. _____

_____

_____

4. Describe the purpose of the fifth-digit subclassification for the coding of acute myocardial infarction. _____

_____

_____

5. Explain the significance of the various modifiers essential in the coding of pneumonia. _____

_____

_____

6. Describe the purpose of the fifth-digit subclassification for the coding of asthma. _____

_____

_____

7. Prioritize (rank in order for reporting purposes) the following clusters of diagnoses.

   A. old myocardial infarction, ventricular tachycardia, atrial fibrillation _____

   B. unstable angina, arteriosclerotic heart disease, chronic obstructive pulmonary disease __

   C. cardiac pacemaker in situ, status post cerebrovascular accident, internal hemorrhoids, abdominal aortic aneurysm _____

    D. lumbar strain, chronic bronchitis, pulmonary embolism, degenerative joint disease _____

    E. transient tachycardia, accelerated hypertension, rheumatoid arthritis, Parkinson's disease

    _____

    F. intrinsic asthma, hypertension, ventricular tachycardia, angina pectoris _____

8. Identify at least ten codes and narrative titles that represent circulatory system conditions which are recognized by Medicare as complications or comorbidities.

    _____   _____

    _____   _____

    _____   _____

    _____   _____

    _____   _____

9. Identify at least five codes and narrative titles that represent nonoperative cardiovascular procedures which impact reimbursement under the Medicare prospective payment system.

    _____

    _____

    _____

    _____

    _____

10. Identify at least ten codes and narrative titles that represent respiratory system conditions which are recognized by Medicare as complications or comorbidities.

    _____   _____

    _____   _____

    _____   _____

    _____   _____

    _____   _____

11. Identify at least five codes and narrative titles that represent nonoperative respiratory procedures which impact reimbursement under the Medicare prospective payment system.

    _____

    _____

    _____

    _____

    _____

12. Assign precise, accurate code numbers from the ICD-9-CM volume for the following diseases of the circulatory system:

    A.   active rheumatic fever _____

    B.   congestive heart failure _____

    C.   acute myocardial infarction _____

    D.   aneurysm of coronary vessels _____

E. chronic endocarditis, valve unspecified _____

F. arterial hypotension _____

G. femoral arterial embolism _____

H. aneurysm of subclavian artery _____

I. Marable's syndrome _____

J. aneurysm of pulmonary artery _____

K. acute pericarditis _____

L. acute pneumococcal myocarditis _____

M. cerebral embolism _____

N. Moyamoya disease _____

O. impending cerebrovascular accident _____

P. atherosclerosis of aorta _____

Q. aneurysm of iliac artery _____

R. Goodpasture's syndrome _____

S. embolism of renal vein _____

T. varicose veins of lower extremities _____

U. spider veins _____

V. superficial phlebitis of the chest wall _____

W. portal thrombosis _____

X. ulcerated scrotum _____

Y. phlebofibrosis _____

Z. acute rheumatic carditis _____

AA. mitral stenosis with regurgitation _____

BB. malignant renovascular hypertension _____

CC. calcific aortitis _____

DD. hepatic vein thrombosis _____

EE. bleeding hemorrhoids _____

FF. chronic hypotension _____

GG. bleeding esophageal varices _____

HH. rheumatic left ventricle failure _____

II. apical-lateral myocardial infarction _____

JJ. Prinzmetal's angina _____

KK. acute infective endocarditis due to typhoid fever _____

LL. adherent pericarditis _____

MM. bilateral bundle branch block _____

NN. atrial fibrillation _____

OO. right heart failure _____

PP. myocardial degeneration of heart _____

QQ. rupture of papillary muscle _____

RR. ruptured subarachnoid hemorrhage _____

SS. cerebral embolism _____

TT. Mönckeberg's sclerosis _____

UU. ruptured abdominal aneurysm _____

VV. Raynaud's syndrome _____

WW. arterial embolism _____

XX. nonfilarial elephantiasis _____

13. Assign precise, accurate code numbers from the ICD-9-CM volume for the following operations on the cardiovascular system:

A. replacement of aortic valve with tissue graft _____

B. removal of coronary artery obstruction _____

C. combined right and left heart cardiac catheterization _____

D. percutaneous angioscopy _____

E. intra-abdominal venous shunt _____

F. suture of artery _____

G. ligation and stripping of lower limb varicose veins _____

H. pericardiocentesis _____

I. cardio-omentopexy _____

J. Blalock-Hanlon operation _____

K. repair of atrioventricular canal with tissue graft _____

L. repair of aneurysm of coronary vessel _____

M. insertion of heart pump _____

N. plication of vena cava _____

O. removal of arteriovenous shunt for renal dialysis _____

P. intraoperative cardiac pacemaker _____

Q. arterial catheterization _____

R. excision of aneurysm of heart _____

S. aortocoronary bypass of six coronary arteries _____

T. creation of shunt between right ventricle and distal pulmonary artery _____

U. closed heart valvotomy _____

V. indirect heart revascularization _____

W. repair of electrode by removal with reinsertion _____

X. excision of blood vessel _____

Y. replacement of vessel to vessel cannula _____

14. Assign precise, accurate code numbers from the ICD-9-CM volume for the following diseases of the respiratory system:

A.   acute frontal sinusitis _____

_____

B.   empyema with pleural fistula _____

C.   chronic maxillary sinusitis _____

D.   black lung disease _____

E.   pneumonia due to parainfluenza virus _____

F.   bronchitis _____

G.   acute viral tonsillitis _____

H.   pleurisy with effusion _____

I.   deviated nasal septum _____

J.   detergent asthma _____

K.   lobar pneumonia _____

L.   chronic tracheitis _____

M.   capillary pneumonia _____

N.   chronic pneumothorax _____

O.   sphenoidal polyp of sinus _____

P.   asbestosis _____

Q.   pneumonia due to staphylococcus _____

R.   Macleod's syndrome _____

S.   acute infective pharyngitis _____

T.   abscess of mediastinum _____

U.   chronic sore throat _____

V.   silicosis _____

W.   pneumonia due to Eaton's agent _____

X. intrinsic asthma _____

_____

Y. acute nasal catarrh _____

_____

Z. hypostatic bronchopneumonia _____

_____

AA. calculus of tonsil _____

_____

BB. bauxite fibrosis of lung _____

_____

CC. pneumonia in cytomegalic inclusion disease _____

_____

DD. bronchiectasis _____

_____

EE. viral epiglottitis with obstruction _____

_____

FF. fibrosis of lung _____

_____

GG. quinsy _____

_____

HH. fibrosis of lung following radiation _____

_____

II. lobular pneumonia _____

_____

JJ. farmer's lung _____

_____

KK. acute laryngopharyngitis _____

_____

LL. pulmonary alveolar microlithiasis _____

_____

MM. chronic laryngitis _____

_____

NN. pneumoconiosis _____

_____

OO. pneumonia _____

_____

PP. chronic lung disease _____

_____

QQ. acute tracheitis with acute laryngitis _____

_____

RR. middle lobe syndrome _____

_____

SS. allergic rhinitis due to pollen _____

_____

TT. acute chemical pulmonary edema _____

_____

UU. abdominal influenza _____

_____

VV. alveolitis due to *Cryptostroma corticale* _____

_____

WW. acute antritis _____

_____

XX. mediastinitis _____

_____

15. Assign precise, accurate code numbers from the ICD-9-CM volume for the following operations on the nose, mouth, and pharynx.

A. rhinoseptoplasty _____

_____

B. excision of lesion of tonsil and adenoid _____

_____

C. revision of cleft palate repair _____

_____

D. partial glossectomy _____

_____

E. puncture of nasal sinus for aspiration _____

_____

F. suture of laceration of gum _____

_____

G. incision of palate _____

_____

H. pharyngoscopy _____

_____

I. incision of salivary duct _____

_____

J. ethmoidotomy _____

_____

K. fascial sling of tongue _____

_____

L. tonsillectomy with adenoidectomy _____

_____

M. submucous resection of nasal septum _____

_____

N. labial frenectomy _____

_____

O. gingivoplasty _____

P. radical sialoadenectomy _____

_____

Q. correction of nasopharyngeal atresia _____

_____

R. ethmoidotomy _____

_____

S. control of epistaxis by anterior nasal packing _____

_____

T. division of glossopharyngeal nerve _____

_____

U. reconstruction of frontonasal duct _____

V. excision of lingual tonsil _____

W. tip rhinoplasty _____

X. pharyngeal diverticulotomy _____

Y. lysis of adhesions of tongue _____

16. Assign precise, accurate code numbers from the ICD-9-CM volume for the following operations on the respiratory system:

A. complete pneumonectomy _____

B. hemilaryngectomy _____

C. exploratory thoracotomy _____

D. mediastinal tracheostomy _____

E. bronchial dilation _____

F. pleural biopsy _____

G. fiberoptic bronchoscopy _____

H. resection of bronchus _____

I. laryngopharyngectomy _____

J. open biopsy of trachea _____

K. endoscopic excision of lesion of bronchus _____

L. decortication of lung _____

M. marsupialization of laryngeal cyst _____

N. incision of bronchus _____

O. suture of laceration of trachea _____

P. excision of vocal cords _____

Q. partial lobectomy _____

R. repair of chest wall _____

S. replacement of tracheal stent _____

_____

T. thoracoplasty _____

_____

U. radical laryngectomy _____

_____

V. repair of laryngeal fracture _____

_____

W. plication of emphysematous bleb _____

_____

X. lung transplant _____

_____

Y. implantation of diaphragmatic pacemaker _____

_____

CODING OF CLINICAL DOCUMENTATION

Read the following clinical reports and assign precise, accurate diagnostic and procedural code numbers from the appropriate sections of the ICD-9 volumes.

PATIENT: Burke, Norman   **MR#:** 99-06-01

SURGEON: Dvorak   **ASSISTANT:** Keller

Preoperative Diagnosis:
Intermittent atrial flutter and atrial fibrillation with severe ventricular bradycardia.

Postoperative Diagnosis:
Intermittent atrial flutter and atrial fibrillation with severe ventricular bradycardia.

Operation:
Implantation of permanent transvenous cardiac pacemaker (Medtronic model 5985).

Clinical History:
Patient was admitted with episodes of atrial flutter and atrial fibrillation with very slow ventricular response (in the low 40s). Patient was entirely uncooperative and combative during the course of the operation. Five staff members were needed to hold him on the cath table. In addition, his heart rate was between 140 and 180. He has very small veins in the region of the deltapectoral groove. All of these problems led to great difficulty in the insertion of this pacemaker. However, the electrode was finally positioned in the apex of the right ventricle, with an assumably satisfactory threshold. It appeared that the threshold was an MA of 0.8, voltage 0.5 with resistance of 610 ohms. R-wave sensitivity was 7.3.

Procedure:
With the patient in the supine position, the right pectoral region was prepped and draped in the usual fashion. As mentioned above, the patient was entirely combative and uncooperative with five people needed to hold him down. After satisfactory local anesthesia and regional anesthesia were induced, a transverse incision was made and the deltapectoral groove was dissected. One vein appeared to be slightly larger than the rest of the very small venules in this area and this vein was cannulated with a cardiac electrode, which with some difficulty was put into the apex of the right ventricle under fluoroscopic control. As mentioned above, the patient's threshold appeared to be satisfactory, though this was not entirely certain. Electrode was ligated in place with heavy silk, after which it was attached to the Medtronic pacemaker model 5985. The unit was implanted into the subcutaneous pocket. It should be noted that the patient has practically no subcutaneous fat, so that only a very, very thin layer of subcutaneous tissue and skin overlies the pacemaker. The wound was closed in two layers. Dressings were applied, and the patient was taken back to his room.

Codes: _____

PATIENT: Griffith, Delores   **MR#:** 99-06-02

ATTENDING PHYSICIAN: Johnston

Chest:
Consolidation of the left lower lobe has increased since the previous film. There is also involvement of the left upper lobe to a lesser degree. The decubitus view shows a small mobile left pleural effusion. There is linear atelectasis in the right base.

Impression:
Increasing consolidation of the left lung. Small left pleural effusion.

Obstructive Series:
Standard supine and upright views of the abdomen demonstrate no evidence of free air under the diaphragm. Scattered bowel gas is noted in the small and large bowel without significant distention or fluid levels, and there is no radiological evidence for bowel obstruction. The bowel gas pattern is considered to be nonspecific.

Codes: _____

PATIENT: Miller, Steven   **MR#:** 99-06-03

ATTENDING PHYSICIAN: Skaggs

Pulmonary Ventilation/Perfusion Scan:
Isotope: Tc-99m DTPA, 40 mCi; Tc-99m MAA, 5 mCi

Findings:
There is marked decrease in ventilation and perfusion of the left lung, corresponding to extensive consolidation on the chest X ray.

Impression:
Intermediate probability for pulmonary embolus.

Codes: _____

PATIENT: Sanders, Anthony   **MR#:** 99-06-04

ATTENDING PHYSICIAN: Hughes

Chest:
The cardiac size appears within normal limits. Interstitial pneumonic infiltrates involving the right upper and lower lung fields are consistent with pneumonia. No pleural effusion is identified.

Impression:
Infiltrates, right upper and lower lobes, rule out pneumonia.

Codes: _____

PATIENT: Hiashi, Takara   **MR#:** 99-06-05

ATTENDING PHYSICIAN: Barber

Portable Chest:
There is pulmonary vascular congestion. Questionable infiltrates are noted in the left upper lung. There are linear densities in the left midlung, which could result from linear atelectasis or fluid. Prominent left basal vascular markings are noted. There is a left chest tube. There is a left subcutaneous emphysema. There is dextroscoliosis of the thoracic spine.

Codes: _____

PATIENT: Abrams, George   **MR#:** 99-06-06

ATTENDING PHYSICIAN: Ott

History of Present Illness:

This 77-year-old male with a history of exertional dyspnea recently underwent exercise stress testing. There were ST-T changes suggestive of ischemia. The patient had a mild decrease of his systolic blood pressure as well as exercise-induced Wenckebach and ventricular ectopy. This was interpreted as a positive exercise stress test and he was referred for cardiac catheterization. Details of his cardiac catheterization are contained in the previously dictated cardiac catheterization note.

Physical Examination:

The patient is a pleasant white male with a resting blood pressure of 140/80. His skin is warm and dry. The head, eyes, ears, nose, and throat are unremarkable. The chest is somewhat barreled in configuration with decreased breath sounds and scattered wheezes. Cardiac exam reveals normal PMI, regular in rate, no evidence of S-2, S-3, or S-4. The carotid artery pulses are 2+ without bruits. The extremities are normal.

Hospital Course:

The patient was admitted and underwent left and right heart catheterization, ventriculography, and coronary arteriography. He was found to have normal systemic arterial hemodynamics and pulmonary arterial hypertension with pressures of 30–32/14. Cardiac output was normal. Ventricular function, systolic and diastolic, was normal; and coronary arteriography was normal. The patient experienced no difficulties from the cardiac catheterization, and by the following morning his groin was healing well without evidence of hematoma and with good distal pulse. On telemetry it was noted that he was bradycardic into the 40s and had a brief transitory period of Wenckebach type 20 A-V block. He was asymptomatic during this time. He was discharged with no ill effects from the cardiac catheterization, and is to follow up with Dr. Rivera in two weeks for pulmonary consultation and pulmonary function testing. The patient was informed that his heart is fine and that the likely reason for his dyspnea seems to be pulmonary in origin.

Discharge Diagnosis:

Dyspnea on exertion.

Pulmonary arterial hypertension.

Chronic obstructive lung disease by history.

Normal coronary arteriography.

Wenckebach A-V block, asymptomatic.

Procedures:

Left and right heart catheterization with ventriculography and coronary arteriography.

Discharge Medications:

Alupent 10 mg b.i.d.; Sloxin 400 mg b.i.d.; Dilatrate 40 mg b.i.d.

Codes: _____

PATIENT: Huebner, Percy   **MR#:** 99-06-07

ATTENDING PHYSICIAN: Mason

History of Present Illness:

This patient is a 49-year-old white male who was admitted to the intensive care unit as a result of chest pain. He complained of sudden chest pain that radiated to the medial aspect of the left arm. This pain lasted for about two hours, he then slept two hours, but awakened with the pain more intense. He denied shortness of breath, nausea, or back pain. The patient took Tagamet, but the pain was not relieved. Therefore, he came to the emergency room.

Past Medical History:

Hypertension, not treated; epigastric discomfort, treated by himself with Tagamet; chronic cough; and a history of alcohol abuse.

Family History

Father has hypertension; mother died of breast cancer.

Physical Examination:

Alert and in no acute distress; *BP:* 160/100; *Pulse:* 88; afebrile.
HEENT: essentially unremarkable.
Lungs: clear.
Heart: S-1, S-2, no gallop.
Abdomen: soft; mild epigastric tenderness.
Extremities: no edema.

Laboratory Data:

CBC was unremarkable. ASTRA-8 was unremarkable. CK on admission was 157, LD was 212, PT and PTT were within normal limits. Electrocardiogram showed normal sinus rhythm, Q-wave on leads 2 and 3, AVF and inversion in lead 1, AVL in V-3 and V-6, questionable ST elevation in V-1 and V-2.

Hospital Course:

The patient was admitted to the intensive care unit and was treated medically with myocardial infarction protocol. He proved to have non-Q-wave myocardial infarction with positive enzymes. The patient improved and underwent echocardiogram, which revealed left ventricular hypertrophy, posterior basilar and anterior basilar hypokinesia, and mild decrease in left ventricular systolic function. Stress test was negative for five minutes without chest pain, and upper GI series showed superficial ulcerations of the distal antrum, the pyloric channel, and the duodenal bulb. The patient was treated with Tagamet, Cardizem, Isordil, and enteric-coated aspirin, and was discharged in stable condition.

Discharge Medications:

Tagamet 400 mg p.o. b.i.d.; Enteric-coated aspirin b.i.d.; Compazine 60 mg b.i.d.; Isordil 10 mg p.o. t.i.d.; Nitroglycerin 0.4 mg p.r.n.

Discharge Diagnosis:

Non-Q-wave myocardial infarction.

History of alcohol abuse.

Instruction on Discharge:

Wait 5 to 6 weeks for full stress Thallium scan and follow-up in the office.

Codes: _____

PATIENT: Fletcher, Raymond   **MR#:** 99-06-08

ATTENDING PHYSICIAN: Jenkins

Admitting Diagnosis:
Supraglottitis.

Discharge Diagnosis:
Same.

History:
The patient is a 28-year-old male who experienced a gradual increase in throat soreness and difficulty swallowing on the morning of admission. The patient was eating chicken the previous evening, but the next morning he experienced a progressive increase in throat soreness with mild shortness of breath. The patient reported mild nausea during the prior two days and also had a bout of diarrhea.

Past Medical History:
Negative.

Past Surgical History:
None.

Medications on Admission:
None. No known drug allergies.

Physical Examination:
On admission, temperature was 99.5, and the other vital signs were normal. The patient was noted to have hoarseness; he had no stridor. On fiberoptic examination, he had moderate supraglottic edema with a 6-mm to 7-mm airway and erythema of the supraglottis. His vocal cords were mobile. His chest was clear, his abdomen was soft, his heart was regular, and his extremities were within normal limits. His neck was noted to have tenderness on palpation of the larynx.

Laboratory Data:
On admission, the WBC was 9700, the hematocrit was 41, and the platelet count was 227000. His SMA-6 revealed a sodium of 138, a potassium of 4.1, a chloride of 99, a bicarbonate of 27, a glucose of 109, and a creatinine of 1.2.

Hospital Course:
The patient was admitted and given IV antibiotics and three doses of Decadron. The patient was given IV Ceftazidine and remained afebrile during his hospitalization. The patient had mild gastric discomfort and was given Tagamet as well as Maalox with subsequent resolution of these symptoms. The patient improved dramatically. The patient was discharged on Clindamycin 300 mg p.o. q. 6 hours, Tagamet, and Maalox. The patient was instructed to eat soft foods and to continue oral rinses with salt water. If any swelling, fever, or difficulty breathing occurs, he was instructed to immediately return to the emergency room.

Discharge Diagnosis:
Supraglottitis.

Follow-up:
In ENT clinic.

Codes: _____

PATIENT: Wilkerson, Fred   **MR#:** 99-06-09

ATTENDING PHYSICIAN: Pagano   **ASSISTANT:** Albright

Preoperative Diagnosis:
Chronic diarrhea secondary to Cryptosporidium infection.

Postoperative Diagnosis:
Same.

Operation:
Raaf catheter placement in left subclavian vein.

Brief Clinical History:
The patient is a white male with a several month history of chronic diarrhea, nausea, and vomiting secondary to Cryptosporidium gastrointestinal infection. He presents now for intravenous access for hydration.

Description of Procedure:
The patient was brought to the OR and placed in the supine position on the operating table with a shoulder roll under his scapula. He was then prepped in the usual sterile manner. Anesthesia was by 1% Lidocaine used to infuse inferiorly to the left clavicle. Then a seeker needle was used without difficulty to find the left subclavian vein. A guide wire was passed through the seeker needle and the seeker needle was removed. Then an X ray was obtained that showed that the wire was clearly in the left subclavian vein down to the superior vena cava. After this was completed, a second incision was made just lateral to the sternum, about level with the breast, and a #15 blade was used to make the incision down through the subcutaneous tissue. Lidocaine was used to infuse the skin between the second incision and the guide wire. The guide wire incision was made at the site where the guide wire entered the skin. Both incisions were approximately 1 cm in length. A tunneler was used to enter through the first incision down to the second and the Raaf catheter was brought under the skin. After this was completed, the dilator sheath and the introducer were both placed over the wire into the vein, and the dilator and wire were removed. Subsequently, the catheter was brought down into the guide sheath in the vein and the guide sheath was peeled away and removed. After the catheter was placed in the subclavian vein, it was then aspirated per the Raaf catheter, and the Raaf catheter was found to be functioning well. The catheter was in proper position and was infused with Heparin flush. The first incision site was closed with a 3-0 subcutaneous suture times one and then the skin was closed with a 4-0 running subcuticular. At the second incision site, one stitch was thrown with 2-0 Nylon and tied, and then a locking stitch was tied around the catheter. Sterile dressings were then applied and the patient was transferred to the post-anesthesia recovery area in stable condition. A postoperative X ray was ordered to again check the catheter placement.

Codes: _____

7 CHAPTER

ICD Coding: Digestive System and Genitourinary System Diseases and Operations

LEARNING OBJECTIVES

Upon completion of this chapter the learner should be able to:

1. Describe the parameters for coding and reporting peptic ulcer disease.
2. Describe the parameters for coding and reporting hernias.
3. Describe the parameters for coding and reporting gastrointestinal hemorrhage.
4. Describe the parameters for coding and reporting renal failure.
5. Describe the parameters for coding and reporting urinary tract infection.
6. Discuss the impact of comorbidities and complications on billing and reimbursement for diagnoses involving the digestive system.
7. Discuss the impact of nonoperative procedures on billing and reimbursement involving the digestive system.
8. Discuss the impact of comorbidities and complications on billing and reimbursement for diagnoses and procedures involving the genitourinary system.
9. Discuss the impact of nonoperative procedures on billing and reimbursement involving the genitourinary system.
10. Apply knowledge of coding principles by assigning accurate and precise codes to report diagnoses and procedures pertaining to the digestive system.
11. Apply knowledge of coding principles by assigning accurate and precise codes to report dental diagnoses and dental procedures.
12. Apply knowledge of coding principles by assigning accurate and precise codes to report diagnoses and procedures pertaining to the urinary system.
13. Apply knowledge of coding principles by assigning accurate and precise codes to report procedures performed on the male genital system.
14. Apply knowledge of coding principles by assigning accurate and precise codes to report procedures performed on the female genital system.

ICD CODING OF DIGESTIVE SYSTEM DISEASES AND OPERATIONS

Chapter 9 of the ICD-9-CM diagnostic tabular volume is designated for listings of digestive system diagnoses and includes dental diagnoses and oral diagnoses. The digestive system disease chapter consists of seven sections (Table 7–1).

The section of Chapter 9 is comprised of listings for diseases of the oral cavity, salivary glands, and jaws. This section includes listings for disorders of tooth development and eruption, diseases of the hard tissues of teeth, diseases of the pulp and periapical tissues, gingival and periodontal diseases, dentofacial anomalies and malocclusion, as well as other diseases and conditions of the teeth and supporting oral structures. This section also includes listings for diseases of the oral soft tissues, and for diseases and other conditions of the tongue.

The second section of this chapter encompasses listings for diseases of the esophagus, the stomach, and the duodenum. These listings include gastric ulcer and erosion, duodenal ulcer and erosion, peptic ulcer, gastrojejunal ulcer, gastritis, duodenitis, and functional or other disorders of the stomach and the duodenum. The relatively brief third section of Chapter 9 contains listings for appendicitis including acute or other appendicitis, as well as other diseases of the appendix.

The fourth section of the digestive system chapter in the diagnostic tabular encompasses listings for hernia of the abdominal cavity including inguinal hernia and bubonocele (with or without obstruction or gangrene), as well as other hernias such as diaphragmatic hernia or hiatal hernia. The fifth section of Chapter 9 is comprised of listings for noninfectious enteritis and colitis including regional enteritis, idiopathic proctocolitis, vascular insufficiency of intestine, and noninfectious gastroenteritis.

The sixth section of this chapter contains listings for other diseases of the intestines and the peritoneum. These listings include intestinal obstruction without mention of hernia, diverticula of intestine, functional digestive disorders, anal fissure or fistula, abscess of anal and rectal regions, and peritonitis. An additional code should be reported to identify any associated hemorrhage or peritonitis that was documented with other conditions in the patient health record.

The seventh and final section of the digestive system chapter in the diagnostic tabular is comprised of listings for other diseases of the digestive system, particularly those involving the hepatobiliary system. These listings include conditions of acute and subacute necrosis of liver, chronic liver disease and cirrhosis, liver abscess and sequelae of chronic liver disease, as well as other disorders of the liver. This section of Chapter 9 also includes listings for cholelithiasis, certain other disorders of the gallbladder and biliary tract, diseases of the pancreas, gastrointestinal hemorrhage, and intestinal malabsorption.

TABLE 7–1

Sections in Chapter 9, Volume 1 of ICD-9-CM

1. Diseases of the Oral Cavity, Salivary Glands, and Jaws (category range 520–529)
2. Diseases of the Esophagus, Stomach, and Duodenum (category range 530–537)
3. Appendicitis (category range 540–543)
4. Hernia of Abdominal Cavity (category range 550–553)
5. Noninfectious Enteritis and Colitis (category range 555–558)
6. Other Diseases of Intestines and Peritoneum (category range 560–569)
7. Other Diseases of Digestive System (category range 570–579)

Categories of listings in Chapter 9 of Volume 3 of ICD-9-CM are established for surgical procedures on the components of the digestive system. These listings are included in category range 42–54 for: operations on the esophagus; incision, excision, and other operations of the stomach; incision, excision, anastomosis, and other operations of the intestine; operations on the appendix and appendiceal stump; operations on the rectum, rectosigmoid, and perirectal tissue; and operations on the anus. These procedural categories also include listings for: operations on the liver; operations on the gallbladder and biliary tract (encompassing common bile duct, cystic duct, hepatic duct, intrahepatic bile duct, and sphincter of Oddi); operations on the pancreas and pancreatic duct; repair and reduction of hernia; as well as certain other operations of the abdominal region encompassing epigastric region, flank, groin region, hypochondrium, inguinal region, loin region, male pelvic cavity, mesentery, omentum, peritoneum, and retroperitoneal tissue space.

Other procedures related to the digestive system are contained among the listings of categories 23–27 in Chapter 5 of Volume 3 of ICD-9-CM. These listings include: removal and restoration of teeth; other operations on the teeth, gums, and alveoli; operations on the tongue; operations on the salivary glands; and other operations on the soft tissue of the mouth.

ICD CODING OF GENITOURINARY SYSTEM DISEASES AND OPERATIONS

Chapter 10 of the ICD-9-CM diagnostic tabular volume is designated for listings of genitourinary system diagnoses. This chapter includes diagnoses relating to both the male genital system and the female genital system. This chapter consists of six sections (Table 7–2).

The first section of Chapter 10 contains listings for nephritis, nephrotic syndrome, and nephrosis. These listings include acute nephritis and glomerulonephritis, nephrotic syndrome and chronic nephritis, as well as other nephropathy. This section also includes listings for acute renal failure, chronic renal failure, renal sclerosis, disorders resulting from impaired renal function, and small kidney of unknown cause.

The second section in the genitourinary chapter of the diagnostic tabular contains listings for other diseases of the urinary system. These listings encompass infections of the kidney; hydronephrosis; calculus of the kidney, the ureter, or the lower urinary tract; cystitis; urethritis; urethral syndrome; urethral stricture; and certain other disorders of the kidney, ureter, bladder, or urethra. An additional code should be reported to identify any infectious organism that was the cause of a condition that was documented in the patient health record.

Categories of listings in Chapter 10 of Volume 3 of ICD-9-CM are established for surgical procedures on the components of the urinary system. These listings are included in category range 55–59 for: operations on the kidney and renal pelvis; operations on the ureter; operations on the urinary bladder; operations on the urethra and periurethral tissue; as well as other operations on the urinary tract.

TABLE 7–2

Sections in Chapter 10, Volume 1 of ICD-9-CM

1. Nephritis, Nephrotic Syndrome, and Nephrosis (category range 580–589)
2. Other Diseases of Urinary System (category range 590–599)
3. Diseases of Male Genital Organs (category range 600–608)
4. Disorders of Breast (category range 610–611)
5. Inflammatory Disease of Female Pelvic Organs (category range 614–616)
6. Other Disorders of Female Genital Tract (category range 617–629)

The third section of Chapter 10 in the diagnostic tabular volume is comprised of listings for diseases of the male genital organs. These listings include: hyperplasia, inflammatory diseases, and other disorders of the prostate; hydrocele; orchitis; epididymitis; redundant prepuce; phimosis; male infertility; and other disorders of the penis and male genital organs. An additional code should be reported to identify any infectious organism that was the cause of a condition that was documented in the patient health record.

Categories of listings in Chapter 11 of Volume 3 of ICD-9-CM are established for surgical procedures on the components of the male genital organs. These include the listings in category range 60–64 for: operations on the prostate, seminal vesicles, and periprostatic tissue; operations on the scrotum and tunica vaginalis; operations on the testes; operations on the spermatic cord, epididymis, and vas deferens; as well as operations on the penis and prepuce.

The fourth section of Chapter 10 in Volume 1 contains listings for disorders of the breast including benign mammary dysplasias. An additional code should be reported to identify any infectious organism that was documented in the patient health record as the cause of a stated condition.

The fifth section of Chapter 10 in the diagnostic tabular is comprised of listings for inflammatory disease of the female pelvic organs. These listings include inflammatory disease of the ovary, the fallopian tubes, pelvic cellular tissue, the peritoneum, the uterus, the cervix, the vagina, and the vulva.

The sixth and final section of Chapter 10 in Volume 1 is comprised of listings for other disorders of the female genital tract. These listings include: endometriosis; genital prolapse; fistula involving the female genital tract; noninflammatory disorders of the cervix, the vagina, the vulva, and the perineum; as well as pain and other symptoms associated with the female genital organs. This section also includes listings for: disorders of menstruation and other abnormal bleeding from the female genital tract; menopausal and postmenopausal disorders; female infertility; and certain other disorders of the female genital organs.

Categories of listings in Chapter 12 of Volume 3 of ICD-9-CM are established for surgical procedures on the components of the female genital organs. These include the listings within category range 65–71 for: operations on the ovary; operations on the fallopian tubes; operations on the cervix; other incision and excision of the uterus; certain other operations on the uterus and supporting structures; operations on the vagina and the cul-de-sac; and operations on the vulva and the perineum.

ORAL SURGERY REPORTING FOR BILLING

Surgical procedures on the mouth and oral cavity are sometimes rendered in an inpatient setting, and therefore the established coding guidelines for sequencing and reporting of ICD-9-CM codes are applicable. Reimbursement policies under the prospective payment system are impacted by the assignment of the patient admission into one of several diagnostic related groups.

The DRG's associated with dental and oral conditions are distributed into the major diagnostic category primarily associated with otorhinolaryngology, namely MDC 3, Diseases and Disorders of the Ear, Nose, Mouth, and Throat (Table 7–3).

GASTROENTEROLOGY AND ABDOMINAL SURGERY REPORTING FOR BILLING

Coding and sequencing guidelines for principal diagnosis and principal procedure are comparable to those established for all other clinical services. The principal diagnosis is the condition responsible for the admission of the patient for the health service admission, encounter,

TABLE 7-3

Diagnosis Related Groups for Dental and Oral Diseases

DRG 185, Dental and Oral Diseases except Extractions and Restorations, Age Greater than 17
DRG 186, Dental and Oral Diseases except Extractions and Restorations, Age 0–17
DRG 187, Dental Extractions and Restorations

or episode of care; and the principal procedure is the procedure most closely associated with the patient's principal diagnosis for that specific admission, encounter, or episode of care.

Generally, the diagnosis or procedure having the greatest potential for risk to the patient is also the most resource intensive diagnosis or procedure. Nevertheless, under exceptional circumstances, especially those involving a patient in an acute care facility, the diagnosis or procedure having the most risk or the most resource intensive diagnosis or procedure may not be the principal diagnosis for that episode of inpatient service. Such a situation could occur if a patient was admitted for a relatively minor problem and major complications occurred unexpectedly. For example, a patient could be admitted for evaluation of irritable bowel syndrome, and subsequently this patient could sustain a ruptured appendix, necessitating an emergency appendectomy.

Insurance claim regulations ordinarily limit coding and reporting only to diagnoses specifically assessed or treated during the admission, encounter, or episode of care. Similarly, these regulations limit coding and reporting to procedures actually rendered during the interval of that particular admission, encounter, or episode of care. An inactive chronic condition such as an incisional hernia should not be coded or reported with the submitted claim.

The code number for the principal diagnosis or procedure should be sequenced first followed by secondary diagnoses or procedures, sequenced in descending order of clinical significance and resource intensity. For instance, an acute condition such as hemorrhagic peptic ulcer should receive sequencing priority before a lesser condition such as dyspepsia.

Certain ICD-9-CM codes are recognized as comorbidities by specific third-party payors such as Medicare. For inpatient admissions, these comorbid conditions may increase the amount of reimbursement received by the provider. Comorbidities among the digestive system and hepatobiliary system conditions are represented by the following ICD-9-CM code numbers:

527.3	527.4	528.3
530.4	530.7	530.82
530.84	531.00	531.01
531.10	531.11	531.20
531.21	531.31	531.40
531.41	531.50	531.51
531.60	531.61	531.71
531.91	532.00	532.01
532.10	532.11	532.20
532.21	532.31	532.40
532.41	532.50	532.51
532.60	532.61	532.71
532.91	533.00	533.01
533.10	533.11	533.20

533.21	533.31	533.40
533.41	533.50	533.51
533.60	533.61	533.71
533.91	534.00	534.01
534.10	534.11	534.20
534.21	534.31	534.40
534.41	534.50	534.51
534.60	534.61	534.71
534.91	535.01	535.11
535.21	535.31	535.41
535.51	535.61	536.1
537.0	537.3	537.4
537.83	540.0	540.1
540.9	550.00	550.01
550.02	550.03	550.10
550.11	550.12	550.13
551.00	551.01	551.02
551.03	551.1	551.20
551.21	551.29	551.3
551.8	551.9	552.00
552.01	552.02	552.03
552.1	552.20	552.21
552.29	552.3	552.8
552.9	557.0	558.1
558.2	560.0	560.1
560.2	560.30	560.31
560.39	560.81	560.89
560.9	562.02	562.03
562.12	562.13	566
567.0	567.1	567.2
567.8	567.9	568.81
569.3	569.5	569.6
569.83	569.85	570
571.2	571.49	571.5
571.6	572.0	572.1
572.2	572.4	573.1
573.2	573.3	573.4
574.00	574.01	574.10
574.11	574.21	574.30
574.31	574.40	574.41
574.50	574.51	575.0
575.2	575.3	575.4
575.5	576.1	576.3
576.4	577.0	577.2
578.0	578.1	578.9
579.3		

Reporting code numbers for unspecified or nonspecific gastrointestinal diagnoses or procedures should be avoided, if possible. The personnel responsible for coding and billing should attempt to obtain the most specific code not only for reimbursement purposes, but also to generate meaningful data for statistical and research purposes. Accurate, precise, complete, and timely documentation in the patient medical record may upgrade the quality of reported codes for gastrointestinal diagnoses and procedures.

The DRG's associated with digestive system conditions are assigned to a specific major diagnostic category, MDC 6, Diseases and Disorders of the Digestive System (Table 7–4). The DRG's associated with hepatobiliary and pancreatic conditions are distributed into a separate major diagnostic category, MDC 7, Diseases and Disorders of the Hepatobiliary System and Pancreas (Table 7–5).

TABLE 7–4

Diagnosis Related Groups for Diseases and Disorders of the Digestive System

DRG 146, Rectal Resection with Comorbidity or Complication

DRG 147, Rectal Resection without Comorbidity or Complication

DRG 148, Major Small and Large Bowel Procedures with Comorbidity or Complication

DRG 149, Major Small and Large Bowel Procedures without Comorbidity or Complication

DRG 150, Peritoneal Adhesiolysis with Comorbidity or Complication

DRG 151, Peritoneal Adhesiolysis without Cormorbidity or Complication

DRG 152, Minor Small and Large Bowel Procedures with Comorbidity or Complication

DRG 153, Minor Small and Large Bowel Procedures without Comorbidity or Complication

DRG 154, Stomach, Esophageal, and Duodenal Procedures, Age Greater than 17 with Comorbidity or Complication

DRG 155, Stomach, Esophageal, and Duodenal Procedures, Age Greater than 17 without Comorbidity or Complication

DRG 156, Stomach, Esophageal and Duodenal Procedures, Age 0–17

DRG 157, Anal and Stomal Procedures with Comorbidity or Complication

DRG 158, Anal and Stomal Procedures without Comorbidity or Complication

DRG 159, Hernia Procedures except Inguinal and Femoral, Age Greater than 17 with Comorbidity or Complication

DRG 160, Hernia Procedures except Inguinal and Femoral, Age Greater than 17 without Comorbidity or Complication

DRG 161, Inguinal and Femoral Hernia Procedures, Age Greater than 17 with Comorbidity or Complication

DRG 162, Inguinal and Femoral Hernia Procedures, Age Greater than 17 without Comorbidity or Complication

DRG 163, Hernia Procedures, Age 0–17

DRG 164, Appendectomy with Complicated Principal Diagnosis with Comorbidity or Complication

DRG 165, Appendectomy with Complicated Principal Diagnosis without Comorbidity or Complication

DRG 166, Appendectomy without Complicated Principal Diagnosis with Comorbidity or Complication

DRG 167, Appendectomy without Complicated Principal Diagnosis without Comorbidity or Complication

DRG 170, Other Digestive System Operating Room Procedures with Comorbidity or Complication

DRG 171, Other Digestive System Operating Room Procedures without Comorbidity or Complication

DRG 174, Gastrointestinal Hemorrhage with Comorbidity or Complication

DRG 175, Gastrointestinal Hemorrhage without Comorbidity or Complication

DRG 176, Complicated Peptic Ulcer

DRG 177, Uncomplicated Peptic Ulcer with Comorbidity or Complication

DRG 178, Uncomplicated Peptic Ulcer without Comorbidity or Complication

DRG 179, Inflammatory Bowel Disease

T A B L E 7–4

Diagnosis Related Groups for Diseases and Disorders of the Digestive System—cont'd

DRG 180, Gastrointestinal Obstruction with Comorbidity or Complication

DRG 181, Gastrointestinal Obstruction without Comorbidity or Complication

DRG 182, Esophagitis, Gastroenteritis, and Miscellaneous Digestive Disorders, Age Greater than 17 with Comorbidity or Complication

DRG 183, Esophagitis, Gastroenteritis, and Miscellaneous Digestive Disorders, Age Greater than 17 without Comorbidity or Complication

DRG 184, Esophagitis, Gastroenteritis, and Miscellaneous Digestive Disorders, Age 0–17

DRG 188, Other Digestive System Diagnoses, Age Greater than 17 with Comorbidity or Complication

DRG 189, Other Digestive System Diagnoses, Age Greater than 17 without Comorbidity or Complication

DRG 190, Other Digestive System Diagnoses, Age 0–17

Certain non-operating room procedures listed among the operations on the digestive system and the hepatobiliary system impact reimbursement under the prospective payment system. Codes from Chapter 9 of Volume 3 representing nonoperative procedures that affect DRG assignment are:

42.22	42.23	42.24
42.39	43.41	45.12
45.13	45.14	45.16
45.22	45.23	45.24
45.25	45.30	45.42
45.43	48.22	48.23
48.24	48.36	49.31
51.10	51.11	51.14
51.64	51.84	51.85
51.86	51.87	52.13
52.14	52.21	52.93
52.97	52.98	

UROLOGY AND GYNECOLOGY REPORTING FOR BILLING

As previously discussed, the principal diagnosis is defined as the condition responsible for the admission of the patient for the health service admission, encounter, or episode of care; and the principal procedure is the procedure most closely associated with the patient's principal diagnosis. Occasionally, exceptional circumstances result in a deviation from this guideline. For example, prostatic surgery may be performed on a patient admitted for an unrelated medical diagnosis, and thus the principal procedure and principal diagnosis are not clinically associated.

Insurance claim rules and regulations ordinarily restrict coding and reporting to diagnoses specifically assessed or treated during the admission, encounter, or episode of care, and to procedures actually rendered during that particular service. The principal diagnosis or procedure normally should be sequenced first, and should be followed by secondary diagnoses or procedures in descending order of clinical significance and resource intensity. For example, chronic renal failure should be reported before chronic cystitis.

TABLE 7–5

Diagnosis Related Groups for Hepatobiliary and Pancreatic Diseases and Disorders

DRG 191, Pancreas, Liver, and Shunt Procedures with Comorbidity or Complication

DRG 192, Pancreas, Liver, and Shunt Procedures without Comorbidity or Complication

DRG 193, Biliary Tract Procedures except Only Cholecystectomy with or without Common Duct Exploration with Comorbidity or Complication

DRG 194, Biliary Tract Procedures except Only Cholecystectomy with or without Common Duct Exploration without Comorbidity or Complication

DRG 195, Cholecystectomy with Common Duct Exploration with Comorbidity or Complication

DRG 196, Cholecystectomy with Common Duct Exploration without Comorbidity or Complication

DRG 197, Cholecystectomy except by Laparoscope without Common Duct Exploration with Comorbidity or Complication

DRG 198, Cholecystectomy except by Laparoscope without Common Duct Exploration without Comorbidity or Complication

DRG 200, Hepatobiliary Diagnostic Procedure for Nonmalignancy

DRG 201, Other Hepatobiliary or Pancreas Operating Room Procedures

DRG 202, Cirrhosis and Alcoholic Hepatitis

DRG 204, Disorders of Pancreas except Malignancy

DRG 205, Disorders of Liver except Malignancy, Cirrhosis, and Alcoholic Hepatitis with Comorbidity or Complication

DRG 206, Disorders of Liver except Malignancy, Cirrhosis, and Alcoholic Hepatitis without Comorbidity or Complication

DRG 207, Disorders of the Biliary Tract with Comorbidity or Complication

DRG 208, Disorders of the Biliary Tract without Comorbidity or Complication

DRG 480, Liver Transplant

DRG 493, Laparoscopic Cholecystectomy without Common Duct Exploration with Comorbidity or Complication

DRG 494, Laparoscopic Cholecystectomy without Common Duct Exploration without Comorbidity or Complication

Particular ICD-9-CM codes are recognized and designated as comorbidities by certain third-party payors, such as Medicare, under the prospective payment system. For inpatient admissions, these comorbid conditions may increase the amount of reimbursement received by the provider. Comorbidities among the urinary system conditions are represented by the following ICD-9-CM code numbers:

580.0	580.4	580.81
580.89	580.9	581.0
581.1	581.2	581.3
581.81	581.89	581.9
583.4	584.5	584.6
584.7	584.8	584.9
585	590.10	590.11
590.2	590.3	590.80
590.81	590.9	591
592.1	593.5	595.0
595.1	595.2	595.4
595.81	595.82	595.89
595.9	596.0	596.1

TABLE 7–6

Diagnosis Related Groups for Diseases and Disorders of the Kidney and Urinary Tract

---

DRG 302, Kidney Transplant

DRG 304, Kidney, Ureter, and Major Bladder Procedures for Nonneoplasms with Comorbidity or Complication

DRG 305, Kidney, Ureter, and Major Bladder Procedures for Nonneoplasms without Comorbidity or Complication

DRG 306, Prostatectomy with Comorbidity or Complication

DRG 307, Prostatectomy without Comorbidity or Complication

DRG 308, Minor Bladder Procedures with Comorbidity or Complication

DRG 309, Minor Bladder Procedures without Comorbidity or Complication

DRG 310, Transurethral Procedures with Comorbidity or Complication

DRG 311, Transurethral Procedures without Comorbidity or Complication

DRG 312, Urethral Procedures, Age Greater than 17 with Comorbidity or Complication

DRG 313, Urethral Procedures, Age Greater than 17 without Comorbidity or Complication

DRG 314, Urethral Procedures, Age 0–17

DRG 315, Other Kidney and Urinary Tract Operating Room Procedures

DRG 316, Renal Failure

DRG 317, Admission for Renal Dialysis

DRG 320, Kidney and Urinary Tract Infections, Age Greater than 17 with Comorbidity or Complication

DRG 321, Kidney and Urinary Tract Infections, Age Greater than 17 without Comorbidity or Complication

DRG 322, Kidney and Urinary Tract Infections, Age 0–17

DRG 323, Urinary Stones with Comorbidity or Complication and/or Extracorporeal Shockwave Lithotripsy

DRG 324, Urinary Stones without Comorbidity or Complication

DRG 325, Kidney and Urinary Tract Signs and Symptoms, Age Greater than 17 with Comorbidity or Complication

DRG 326, Kidney and Urinary Tract Signs and Symptoms, Age Greater than 17 without Comorbidity or Complication

DRG 327, Kidney and Urinary Tract Signs and Symptoms, Age 0–17

DRG 328, Urethral Stricture, Age Greater than 17 with Comorbidity or Complication

DRG 329, Urethral Stricture, Age Greater than 17 without Comorbidity or Complication

DRG 330, Urethral Stricture, Age 0–17

DRG 331, Other Kidney and Urinary Tract Diagnoses, Age Greater than 17 with Comorbidity or Complication

DRG 332, Other Kidney and Urinary Tract Diagnoses, Age Greater than 17 without Comorbidity or Complication

DRG 333, Other Kidney and Urinary Tract Diagnoses, Age 0–17

596.2	596.4	596.6
596.7	597.0	598.1
598.2	599.0	599.4
599.7		

Comorbidities among the male genital system conditions are represented by the following ICD-9-CM code numbers:

| 601.0 | 601.2 | 601.3 |
| 602.1 | 603.1 | 604.0 |

Comorbidities among the female genital system conditions are represented by the following ICD-9-CM code numbers:

TABLE 7-7

Diagnosis Related Groups for Diseases and Disorders of the Male Reproductive System

DRG 334, Major Male Pelvic Procedures with Comorbidity or Complication
DRG 335, Major Male Pelvic Procedures without Comorbidity or Complication
DRG 336, Transurethral Prostatectomy with Comorbidity or Complication
DRG 337, Transurethral Prostatectomy without Comorbidity or Complication
DRG 339, Testes Procedures for Nonmalignancy, Age Greater than 17
DRG 340, Testes Procedures for Nonmalignancy, Age 0–17
DRG 341, Penis Procedures
DRG 342, Circumcision, Age Greater than 17
DRG 343, Circumcision, Age 0–17
DRG 345, Other Male Reproductive System Operating Room Procedures Except for Malignancy
DRG 348, Benign Prostatic Hypertrophy with Comorbidity or Complication
DRG 349, Benign Prostatic Hypertrophy without Comorbidity or Complication
DRG 350, Inflammation of the Male Reproductive System
DRG 351, Sterilization, Male
DRG 352, Other Male Reproductive System Diagnoses
DRG 476, Prostatic Operating Room Procedure Unrelated to Principal Diagnosis

611.72	614.0	614.3
614.5	615.0	616.3
616.4	620.7	

The DRG's associated with kidney and urinary tract conditions are distributed into a specific major diagnostic category, MDC 11, Diseases and Disorders of the Kidney and Urinary Tract (Table 7–6).

Specific non-operating room procedures listed among the operations on the digestive system and the hepatobiliary system impact reimbursement under the prospective payment system. Codes from Chapter 10 of Volume 3 representing nonoperative procedures that affect DRG assignment are:

55.21	55.22	56.31
57.31	57.32	

One code from Chapter 16 of Volume 3 represents a nonoperative urinary system related procedure that affects DRG assignment. Code number listing *98.51, Extracorporeal shockwave lithotripsy of the kidney, ureter, and/or bladder* may impact reimbursement if reported.

The DRG's associated with male genital conditions are assigned to MDC 12, Diseases and Disorders of the Male Reproductive System (Table 7–7).

The DRG's associated with female genital conditions are assigned to MDC 13, Diseases and Disorders of the Female Reproductive System (Table 7–8).

Several non-operating room procedures listed among the operations on the female genital system impact reimbursement under the prospective payment system. Codes from Chapter 12 of Volume 3 representing nonoperative procedures that affect DRG assignment are:

68.22	70.21	70.22

T A B L E 7–8

Diagnosis Related Groups for Diseases and Disorders of the Female Reproductive System

DRG 353, Pelvic Evisceration, Radical Hysterectomy, and Radical Vulvectomy
DRG 356, Female Reproductive System Reconstructive Procedures
DRG 358, Uterine and Adnexa Procedures for Nonmalignancy with Comorbidity or Complication
DRG 359, Uterine and Adnexa Procedures for Nonmalignancy without Comorbidity or Complication
DRG 360, Vagina, Cervix, and Vulva Procedures
DRG 361, Laparoscopy and Incisional Tubal Interruption
DRG 362, Endoscopic Tubal Interruption
DRG 364, Dilatation and Curettage, Conization except for Malignancy
DRG 365, Other Female Reproductive System Operating Room Procedures
DRG 368, Infections of Female Reproductive System
DRG 369, Menstrual and Other Female Reproductive System Disorders

Reporting code numbers for nonspecific or unspecified genitourinary diagnoses or procedures should be avoided, if possible. The staff responsible for coding and billing should attempt to obtain the most specific code not only for reimbursement purposes but also to facilitate meaningful data for statistical and research purposes. Precise, accurate, complete, and timely documentation in the patient medical record may upgrade the quality of patient healthcare data and thereby alleviate the necessity of reporting codes for unspecified genitourinary diagnoses and procedures.

KEY CONCEPTS

category range _____   nonspecific diagnosis _____
combination code _____   nonspecific procedure _____
comorbidity _____   principal diagnosis _____
complication _____   principal procedure _____
diagnosis related groups _____ prospective payment system _____
major diagnostic category _____ subclassification _____
manifestation _____   underlying disease _____
nonoperative procedure _____   unspecified diagnosis _____

REVIEW QUESTIONS

1. Describe the purpose of the fifth-digit subclassification for the coding of peptic ulcer disease.

   _____

   _____

2. Describe the purpose of the fifth-digit subclassification for the coding of specific hernias.

   _____

   _____

3. Prioritize (rank in order for reporting purposes) the following clusters of diagnoses:

   A. Crohn's disease, aphthous stomatitis, chronic duodenal ulcer, irritable bowel syndrome

   _____

B. bacteriuria, acute renal failure, impotence, male infertility _____

C. cervical polyp, menomenorrhagia, grand multiparity, seborrhea _____

D. hematuria, carcinoma of prostate, urethral calculus, chronic gastritis _____

4. Identify at least ten codes and narrative titles that represent digestive system or hepatobiliary system conditions which are recognized by Medicare as comorbidities or complications.

_____   _____
_____   _____
_____   _____
_____   _____
_____   _____
_____   _____

5. Identify at least five codes and narrative titles that represent nonoperative procedures involving the digestive system or hepatobiliary system, and which impact reimbursement under the prospective payment system.

_____   _____
_____   _____
_____   _____
_____   _____
_____   _____
_____   _____

6. Identify at least ten codes and narrative titles that represent urinary system conditions which are recognized by Medicare as comorbidities or complications.

_____   _____
_____   _____
_____   _____
_____   _____
_____   _____
_____   _____

7. Identify at least five codes and narrative titles that represent nonoperative procedures involving the urinary system or female genital system, and which impact reimbursement under the prospective payment system.

_____   _____
_____   _____
_____   _____
_____   _____
_____   _____
_____   _____

8. Assign precise, accurate code numbers from the ICD-9-CM volume for the following diseases of the digestive system:

A. allergic parotitis _____

B. postoperative blind loop syndrome _____

C.   lymphoepithelial cyst of mouth _____

D.   blood in stool _____

E.   rupture of esophagus _____

F.   senile atrophy of pancreas _____

G.   acute gastritis _____

H.   recurrent cholangitis _____

I.   hyperplasia of appendix _____

J.   nonfunctioning gallbladder _____

K.   cirrhosis of pancreas _____

L.   chronic cholecystitis with choledocholithiasis _____

M.   nasopalatine cyst _____

N.   hepatic infarction _____

O.   sialodocholithiasis _____

P.   portal hypertension _____

Q.   gangrenous stomatitis _____

R.   florid cirrhosis of liver _____

S.   glossopyrosis _____

T.   acute necrosis of liver _____

U.   abscess of esophagus _____

V.   solitary ulcer of anus _____

W.   acute gastric ulcer _____

X.   nontraumatic hemoperitoneum _____

Y.   acute erosion of duodenum with hemorrhage and obstruction _____

Z.   pneumococcal peritonitis _____

AA. peptic ulcer _____

BB. anal cellulitis _____

CC. chronic jejunal ulcer with perforation _____

DD. rectal fistula _____

EE. acute alcoholic gastritis _____

FF. anal spasm _____

GG. hourglass contraction of stomach _____

HH. diverticulitis of colon _____

II. chronic duodenal ileus _____

JJ. impaction of intestine _____

KK. cascade stomach _____

LL. radiation enterocolitis _____

MM. acute distention of stomach _____

NN. abdominal angina _____

OO. abscess of appendix _____

PP. chronic ulcerative colitis _____

QQ. appendicitis _____

RR. granulomatous colitis _____

SS. relapsing appendicitis _____

TT. bilateral femoral hernia _____

UU. hyperplasia of appendix _____

VV. hiatal hernia with obstruction _____

WW. unspecified inguinal hernia with gangrene _____

XX. ventral hernia with gangrene _____

9. Assign precise, accurate code numbers from the ICD-9-CM volume for the following operations on the digestive system:

A. anastomosis of esophagus to intestinal segment _____

_____

B. exploratory laparotomy _____

_____

C. pyloromyotomy _____

_____

D. repair of diaphragmatic hernia by abdominal approach _____

_____

E. suture of duodenal ulcer site _____

_____

F. total pancreatectomy _____

_____

G. flexible fiberoptic colonoscopy _____

_____

H. choledochectomy _____

_____

I. temporary ileostomy _____

_____

J. localized perfusion of liver _____

_____

K. appendectomy _____

_____

L. reduction of hemorrhoids _____

_____

M. proctostomy _____

_____

N. reduction of anal prolapse _____

_____

O. closure of esophagostomy _____

_____

P. anastomosis of appendix _____

_____

Q. peritoneal dialysis _____

_____

R. Stromeyer-Little operation _____

_____

S. total gastrectomy with internal interposition _____

_____

T. ileopexy _____

_____

U. unilateral repair of femoral hernia with graft _____

_____

V. hepatocholedochostomy _____

_____

W. dilation of pylorus by incision _____

_____

    X. total intra-abdominal colectomy _____

    Y. pancreatic transplant _____

10. Assign precise, accurate code numbers from the ICD-9-CM volume for the following dental conditions:

    A. dilaceration of tooth _____

    B. cementation hyperplasia _____

    C. periapical granuloma _____

    D. chronic desquamative gingivitis _____

    E. excessive overbite _____

    F. irregular alveolar process _____

    G. dentinal dysplasia _____

    H. irradiated enamel _____

    I. subgingival dental calculus _____

    J. derangement of temporomandibular joint _____

    K. tooth development disorder _____

    L. discoloration of teeth due to copper _____

    M. pulp gangrene _____

    N. gingival cysts _____

    O. maxillary asymmetry _____

    P. aveolar mandibular hypoplasia _____

    Q. paradontal abscess _____

    R. irregular dentin _____

    S. habitual abrasion of teeth _____

    T. impacted wisdom teeth _____

11. Assign precise, accurate code numbers from the ICD-9-CM volume for the following dental services:

   A. restoration of tooth by filling _____
   _____

   B. repair of dental arch _____
   _____

   C. implantation of tooth _____
   _____

   D. biopsy of gum _____
   _____

   E. extraction of deciduous tooth _____
   _____

   F. excision of odontogenic lesion _____
   _____

   G. root canal therapy with apicoectomy _____
   _____

   H. sutures of laceration of gum _____
   _____

   I. removal of impacted teeth _____
   _____

   J. fitting of orthodontic obturator _____
   _____

   K. restoration of tooth by inlay _____
   _____

   L. apical alveolotomy _____
   _____

   M. insertion of fixed bridge _____
   _____

   N. gingivoplasty with bone graft _____
   _____

   O. endosseous dental implant _____
   _____

   P. simple alveolectomy _____
   _____

   Q. extraction of tooth _____
   _____

   R. exposure of tooth _____
   _____

   S. root canal therapy _____
   _____

   T. extension of lingual sulcus _____
   _____

12. Assign precise, accurate code numbers from the ICD-9-CM volume for the following diseases of the genitourinary system:

   A. acute necrotizing glomerulitis _____
   _____

   B. senile involution of ovary _____
   _____

C. foot process disease _____

D. hyperplastic endometritis _____

E. lobular glomerulonephritis _____

F. leukoplakia of cervix _____

G. nephritis with necrotizing glomerulitis _____

H. vaginal polyps _____

I. acute renal failure _____

J. hypertrophy of labia _____

K. chronic uremia _____

L. Taylor's syndrome _____

M. uremia _____

N. amenorrhea _____

O. renal failure _____

P. postmenopausal bleeding _____

Q. hypokalemic nephropathy _____

R. infertility associated with dysmucorrhea _____

S. bilateral small kidneys _____

T. canal of Nuck cyst _____

U. ureteritis cystica _____

V. fibroma of prostate _____

W. hydronephrosis _____

X. prostatic stone _____

Y. ureteric stones _____

Z. encysted hydrocele _____

AA. hypertrophy of kidney _____

BB. testicular abscess _____

CC. urinary bladder stone _____

DD. tight foreskin _____

EE. follicular cystitis _____

FF. infertility due to radiation _____

GG. diverticulitis of bladder _____

HH. painful erection _____

II.   abscess of Cowper's gland _____

JJ. hematoma of vas deferens _____

KK. postobstetric stricture of urethra _____

LL. periductal mastitis _____

MM. prolapse of urethra _____

NN. gynecomastia _____

OO. prostatocystitis _____

PP. oophoritis _____

QQ. rectovulval fistula _____

RR. chronic endometritis _____

SS. decensus uteri _____

TT. Bartholin's gland cyst _____

UU. adenomyosis _____

VV. acute glomerulonephritis with exudative nephritis _____

WW. female hematocele _____

XX. absolute infertility _____

13. Assign precise, accurate code numbers from the ICD-9-CM volume for the following operations on the urinary system:

A. pyelostomy _____

B. revision of ureterointestinal anastomosis _____

C. percutaneous aspiration of bladder _____

D. urethral meatoplasty _____

E. insertion of ureteral stent _____

F. closed endoscopic biopsy of ureter _____

G. perineal urethroscopy _____

H. insertion of indwelling urinary catheter _____

I. Kelly-Stoeckel urethral plication _____

J. marsupialization of kidney lesion _____

K. cystourethopexy with levator muscle sling _____

L. perineal urethrostomy _____

M. transurethral lysis of intraluminal adhesions _____

N. ureteral meatotomy _____

O. nephropexy _____

P. trigonectomy _____

Q. transureteroureterostomy _____

R. fulguration of urethral lesion _____

S. nephrotomy _____

T. Marshall-Marchetti-Krantz operation _____

U. correction of ureteropelvic junction _____

V. dilation of ureteral meatus _____

W. cystoscopy through artificial stoma _____

X. internal urethral meatotomy _____
_____

Y. incision of perirenal abscess _____
_____

14. Assign precise, accurate code numbers from the ICD-9-CM volume for the following operations on the male genital organs:

A. open biopsy of prostate _____

B. removal of internal prosthesis of penis _____

C. percutaneous aspiration of tunica vaginalis _____

D. high ligation of spermatic vein _____

E. mobilization and replacement of testis in scrotum _____

F. circumcision _____

G. ligation of spermatic cord _____

H. excision of appendix testis _____

I. repair of scrotal fistula _____

J. percutaneous aspiration of prostate _____

K. retropubic prostatectomy _____

L. biopsy of penis _____

M. reduction of elephantiasis of scrotum _____

N. removal of valve from vas deferens _____

O. suture of laceration of testis _____

P. suture of laceration of penis _____

Q. epididymotomy _____

R. bilateral orchidectomy _____

S. incision and drainage of scrotum and tunica vaginalis _____

T. spermatocystectomy _____

U. amputation of penis _____
_____

V. transvesical prostatectomy _____

W. spermatocelectomy _____

X. excision of hydrocele of tunica vaginalis _____

Y. open biopsy of testis _____

15. Assign precise, accurate code numbers from the ICD-9-CM volume for the following operations on the female genital organs:

A. aspiration biopsy of ovary _____

B. bilateral endoscopic ligation and division of fallopian tubes _____

C. electroconization of cervix _____

D. digital examination of uterus _____

E. aspiration curettage following delivery _____

F. hymenectomy _____

G. female circumcision _____

H. modified radical hysterectomy _____

I. artificial insemination _____

J. repair of old obstetric laceration of cervix _____

K. culdocentesis _____

L. removal of prosthesis of fallopian tube _____

M. repair of fistula of perineum _____

N. unilateral salpingo-oophorectomy _____

O. division of Skene's gland _____

P. vaginal reconstruction _____

Q. removal of intraligamentous ectopic pregnancy _____

R. lysis of intraluminal uterine adhesions _____

S. conization of cervix _____

T. salpingoureterostomy _____

_____

U. simple suture of ovary _____

_____

V. vaginal repair of chronic inversion of uterus _____

_____

W. manual rupture of ovarian cyst _____

_____

X. radical vulvectomy _____

_____

Y. endocervical biopsy _____

_____

CODING OF CLINICAL DOCUMENTATION

Read the following clinical reports and assign precise, accurate diagnostic and procedural code numbers from the appropriate sections of the ICD-9-CM volumes.

PATIENT: Weber, Jane   **MR#:** 99-07-01

SURGEON: Shaw   **ASSISTANT:** Ferrara

Preoperative Diagnosis:
Vulvovaginal condyloma.

Postoperative Diagnosis:
Vulvar, perirectal, and periclitoral condyloma.

Procedure:
Laser surgery to perineum.

Brief Clinical History:
The patient is a 20-year-old white female, gravida 0, who has several month history of condyloma refractory to both Podophyllin and TCA.

Description of Procedure:
The patient was brought to the OR where she was administered a general anesthesia and then placed in the dorsal lithotomy position. The physical examination rendered at that time revealed no lesions of the cervix or the vagina. However, lesions were noted in the periclitoral area, along the right and left labia, and in the perirectal region. She was prepped and then draped with wet towels and the CO_2 laser was set on 10 continuous beam. Starting superiorly, the lesions were cauterized with the laser down to the reticular layer just beneath the epidermis. This was carried out all the way down to the perirectal area covering all lesions. No hemorrhoids were noted. Several small bleeders were noted during the procedure. The beam was simply defocused and these were easily coagulated. After they were burned, these lesions were wiped with acetic acid. All were found to be treated and beneath skin level by the end of the procedure. She was awakened from general anesthesia without difficulty.

Codes: _____

PATIENT: Shelton, Louise   **MR#:** 99-07-02

SURGEON: Winters   **ASSISTANT:** Holmes

Preoperative Diagnosis:
Peritonitis, possible free air.

Postoperative Diagnosis:
Volvulus of mid-small intestine with total proximal obstruction and perforation, gross peritoneal sepsis, hemorrhage from liver surface secondary to disruption of adhesions.

Operation:
Resection of small bowel and extensive adhesiolysis

Relevant Clinical History:

The patient is a 33-year-old black female who was 17 weeks pregnant and presented to the hospital with increasing abdominal distention. She was seen initially by the OB/GYN service on the day of admission with vague lower abdominal pain that was paraumbilical in nature and radiated down to both lower quadrants. The examination at that time was unremarkable for a WBC of 7600. The patient was admitted to the OB/GYN service for observation and re-hydration. A surgery consultation was obtained. The patient was afebrile with a temperature of 37.5. The abdominal examination revealed a distended tympanic abdomen without bowel sounds. There was bilateral minimal lower quadrant tenderness without rebound. The rectal examination revealed heme negative stool and no tenderness. Bimanual examination revealed no masses. During the following two days, the patient continued to complain of diffuse abdominal pain. The patient was prepared for surgery because of continued severe pain and a WBC elevation to 30000. A repeat WBC just prior to surgery revealed that the WBC had decreased to 14000. The patient's examination remained equivocal and the plans to take the patient to the OR for appendectomy were deferred.

The next day, the patient was feeling better. Her abdominal pain, nausea, and vomiting appeared to resolve with nasogastric suctioning. The patient continued to be followed by the Surgery service. A left upper quadrant and a right upper quadrant ultrasound were obtained in order to investigate the possibility of a pseudocyst that may have developed due to prior abdominal trauma that she has experienced. The ultrasounds were negative, however, the patient continued to complain of abdominal pain. The evening of that day she had a spontaneous breech delivery of a nonviable infant. The next morning, the patient became hypotensive with a blood pressure of 60/40. Her WBC was 13700, and an obstructive series was obtained, which revealed the presence of free air. Given the patient's marked change in clinical status to one of diffuse pain with distention, leukocytosis, and possible free air, the patient was taken to the OR for emergency exploration.

Operative Procedure:

The patient was brought to the OR and placed on the operating table in the supine position. General endotracheal anesthesia was induced. The patient's abdomen was prepped and draped in the usual sterile fashion. The abdomen was entered through a midline incision. Immediately upon entering the abdomen, gross, foul-smelling pus was detected. Aerobic and anaerobic cultures were sent. The abdomen was thoroughly explored. There were dense adhesions between loops of small bowel. In the distal jejunum and proximal ileum, a segment of small bowel was detected with a volvulus and a perforation. This twisted loop of small bowel was totally necrotic and gelatinous. The proximal bowel was massively distended. The distal bowel was collapsed. The uterus was moderately enlarged. The tubes and ovaries appeared edematous and had a gray discoloration to them. There was also a gray discoloration on the surface of the mesentery of the right colon and on the right colon itself. The descending colon similarly had grayish discoloration on the exposed surface. The transverse colon appeared grossly normal. The right and left colons were thoroughly mobilized. The retroperitoneal surfaces of each were noted to be pink and clearly viable. Removal of the peritoneum, which was affected by this gray discoloration, revealed underlying viable large bowel on both the right and left sides. The appendix was normal.

After an extensive adhesiolysis of the small bowel, the area of the small bowel volvulus was totally resected and submitted to pathology. A side-to-side functional end-to-end stapled anastomosis was performed between the remaining ends after the sulcus entericus of the proximal bowel had been removed by suction. The bowel was then irrigated until clear with copious amounts of sterile Saline and then with an antibiotic containing normal Saline. The abdomen was reexamined. Dense adhesions were noted between the surface of the liver and the anterior abdominal wall, and these were taken down bluntly. Hemorrhage started and was difficult to control. The blood loss at this point in the operation had been 800 cc's. Bleeding was subsequently controlled using compression packs soaked with thrombin. Before adequate hemostasis was obtained, an additional 1200 cc's of blood was lost. During the period of hemorrhage, the patient's blood pressure, which had been very stable at about 120 mm of Mercury, dropped momentarily to 98 mm Mercury. The BP was quickly restored with blood transfusion, as well as with low dose Dopamine. When hemostasis appeared to be adequate, the abdomen was closed with towel clips and covered with a sterile towel and a large iodine impregnated bio-drape. The patient will be brought back to the OR in two days for reexamination of her abdomen. The hematocrit at the end of the case, after transfusion of a total of eight units of blood, was 42%. The patient was subsequently taken from the OR, still intubated, with a BP of 110. The sponge and instrument count at the end of the procedure was incorrect, with the presence of three laparotomy sponges remaining in the abdomen.

Codes: _____

PATIENT: Russell, Paul **MR#:** 99-07-03

SURGEON: Milton **ASSISTANT:** Kirsch

Preoperative Diagnosis:
Left hemiscrotal mass.

Postoperative Diagnosis:
Left hemiscrotal mass.

Operation:
Excision of left hemiscrotal mass.

Brief Clinical History:
The patient is a 42-year-old white male with a hard palpable left hemiscrotal mass that he noticed increasing over the past year or so. The lesion is painless. The patient had the tumor markers alpha fetoprotein and Beta HCG measured, and these are within normal limits. The patient's testicular sonogram shows the mass to be completely separate from the testicle and his physical examination indicates the same.

Procedure:
The patient was brought to the OR and had general anesthesia induced. He was prepped and draped in the usual sterile fashion for scrotal surgery.

An incision was made in the scrotum approximately 2 cm in length. The incision was carried down through dartos layer and on down into the tunica vaginalis. The incision cut down right to the scrotal mass. The mass and testicle were both delivered out of the scrotal wound. The mass was noted to be adherent to the tail of the epididymis. The mass was removed from the epididymis using sharp and blunt dissection, and the Bovie cautery was used to control any small bleeding blood vessels. The mass was handed off the field once it was removed from the epididymis and pathology bisected it. Satisfied that there were no more bleeders along the epididymis where the dissection took place, the scrotum was closed, closing the dartos layer with a running 3-0 chromic stitch. The scrotal skin was closed with a running 3-0 chromic stitch. The scrotum was then wrapped with a turban type dressing and a scrotal support was applied.

The mass was opened by pathology in the OR and was a very well-circumscribed lesion that appeared to have a capsule around it. The inside of the mass was a fleshy white color with a hard texture that appeared to have concentric rings. The sponge and needle counts were correct at the end of the case. The patient tolerated the procedure very well. The patient was awakened and taken to the recovery room.

Codes: _____

PATIENT: Zimmer, Margaret   **MR#:** 99-07-04

SURGEON: Bachmann   **ASSISTANT:** Novak

Preoperative Diagnosis:
Submucosal lesion, left cheek.

Postoperative Diagnosis:
Submucosal lesion, left cheek.

Operation:
Transoral excision of submucosal lesion, left cheek.

Indications:
This is a 35-year-old female who has noticed a mass in the right cheek for several months. On physical examination, the patient was found to have a 1.5-cm firm mass in the submucosal area of the left anterior buccal gingival sulcus, just distal and inferior to the left oral commissure. This mass was completely mobile and free from the mandible and the mucosa overlying the mass appeared to be normal. The skin on the outside also appeared to be normal. The patient had no other intraoral lesions. There was no adenopathy noted anywhere in the neck or the parotid gland.

Procedure:
With the patient in the supine position, the head slightly elevated, the area of the mass was injected using 1% Lidocaine and 1:100000 Epinephrine circumferentially through the transoral route. Under satisfactory anesthesia, the mucosa overlying the mass was incised. Using sharp and blunt dissection, the mass was easily excised, leaving a cuff or buccal sac overlying it. It was removed in its entirety and handed off to pathology. The area was then inspected and hemostasis obtained. While still on the table, the patient was asked to animate the mouth, both in the smiling and frowning modes, and nerve function appeared completely intact. The mucosa was then closed using locking running sutures with 4-0 chromic material. The patient was then asked to rinse her mouth out with Listerine. The patient tolerated the procedure without any incident.

Codes: _____

PATIENT: Riggins, Dale   **MR#:** 99-07-05

SURGEON: Watkins   **ASSISTANT:** Graham

Preoperative Diagnosis:
Left testicular torsion.

Postoperative Diagnosis:
Same with viable testes.

Operation:
Scrotal exploration, detorsion of left testes, and bilateral orchiopexy.

Description of Procedure:
The patient was brought to the OR and general endotracheal anesthesia was induced. The patient was prepped and draped in the usual sterile fashion. A midline scrotal incision was then made. The left testes was delivered through the dartos tissue after sharp dissection, and a single torsion of the testes was noted with the typical bell clapper deformity. This was detorsed. The testes was noted to be quite viable and therefore without further delay it was pexed into place with two 2-0 silk sutures to the dartos fibers. Exploration of the contralateral testes revealed a normal testes again with bell clapper deformity. This was similarly pexed with two 2-0 sutures. They were dropped back into the cavity. The dartos was loosely approximated with 3-0 chromic sutures. The skin was approximated with 4-0 chromic sutures. Scrotal suspensory and fluff dressing were applied. The patient was taken to the floor in stable condition without apparent intraoperative complications. The final needle and sponge counts were correct. There were no drains.

Codes: _____

PATIENT: Fuller, Jerry   **MR#:** 99-07-06

SURGEON: Pierce   **ASSISTANT:** Shah

Preoperative Diagnosis:
Supraumbilical ventral hernia.

Postoperative Diagnosis:
Supraumbilical ventral hernia.

Operation:
Supraumbilical ventral hernia repair.

Brief Clinical History:
The patient is a 41-year-old black male with a history of alcoholic liver disease, who presented with complaint of a protruding mass above his umbilicus. He reports that the mass is especially prominent after meals. It is only slightly tender and it is always reducible. The patient also has a history of right inguinal hernia repair and still has a left inguinal hernia that will be repaired at a later date.

Description of Procedure:
The patient was brought to the OR, and after the induction of spinal anesthesia, was placed in the supine position. His abdomen was prepped and draped. An approximately 4-cm midline incision was made just superior to the umbilicus overlying a quarter-sized midline palpable defect with a slight bulge. Once beyond the dermis, the hernia sac was evident. Bovie cautery was used to continue to complete the opening of the dermal layer. Then blunt dissection combined with Bovie cautery was used to free up the hernia sac from the surrounding fascia. With this complete, the hernia sac was incised. There were no fixed contents within the sac. A small amount of free peritoneal fluid was seen within the abdomen, but there was no free-flowing fluid exiting the opened hernia sac. The sac was put on tension and amputated. Hemostasis was achieved with Bovie cautery. The skin flaps were elevated in all directions above the fascial layer. The fascial layer was closed with four interrupted 3-0 Vicryl sutures. The wound was then irrigated and the skin was closed with vertical mattress 3-0 Nylon sutures. Betadine

ointment was then applied and the wound was covered with a dry sterile dressing. The patient was taken to the recovery room in satisfactory condition.

Codes: _____

PATIENT: Chen, Lucy   **MR#:** 99-07-07

SURGEON: Vaughn   **ASSISTANT:** O'Reilly

Preoperative Diagnosis:
Status post colostomy secondary to gunshot wound.

Postoperative Diagnosis:
Same.

Operation:
Take down of loop colostomy.

Description of Procedure:
The patient was brought to the OR and placed in the supine position. The abdomen was prepped with Betadine and draped in a sterile fashion. Ostomy was taken down with blunt and sharp dissection. Once the colon was mobilized, a GIA stapler was used to connect the ostomy and the mucous fistula assuring that the mesentery was not in the anastomosis site. The end of the mucous fistula and ostomy were then closed with a GIA stapler. The distal ostomy was sent to pathology. Hemostasis was assured with electrocautery and Lembert sutures inverted the anastomosis. There was no significant bleeding. The fascial opening was extended medially and laterally in order to easily pass the bowel back into the peritoneum. Hemostasis was then assured with electrocautery and the posterior fascia was reapproximated with two figure-eight 1-0 Prolene sutures. The anterior fascia was then also reapproximated with two figure-eight 1-0 Prolene sutures. The wound was then packed with Saline-soaked fine mesh gauze. The patient tolerated the procedure well and was discharged to the floor.

Codes: _____

PATIENT: Knight, Catherine   **MR#:** 99-07-08

SURGEON: Hodges   **ASSISTANT:** Newman

Preoperative Diagnosis:
Gallstone pancreatitis.

Peripancreatic fluid collections.

Postoperative Diagnosis:
Gallstone pancreatitis.

Peritoneal adhesions.

Omental fat necrosis.

Operation:
Cholecystectomy.

Intraoperative cholangiogram.

Anesthesia:
General endotracheal.

Indications for Operation:

The patient is a 38-year-old white female with a history of intravenous drug abuse and depression, who presented six weeks ago to the medical service, febrile and with abdominal pain. Ultrasound demonstrated gallstones with a normal common bile duct. The patient began to develop a fulminant pancreatitis with an extensive pancreatic phlegmon. She was treated with intravenous antibiotics and total parenteral nutrition. She remained persistently febrile with white blood counts in the 200.0 range. Repeat CT scan demonstrated the formation of several large fluid collections. Percutaneous aspiration of this fluid remained sterile. The patient failed to improve and was therefore admitted for drainage of these fluid collections. The bilirubin was 3 and alkaline phosphatase was 250. These elevations were attributed to the presence of pancreatitis.

Description of Operative Procedure:

The patient was sterilely prepped and draped in the supine position after induction of satisfactory general endotracheal anesthesia. The abdomen was entered through an upper midline incision. There were multiple filmy adhesions between the small bowel and the anterior peritoneum, which were manually broken to develop the peritoneal cavity. In the superior aspect of the incision, anterior to the liver and stomach, there was a large fluid collection palpable. Besides the presence of the previously mentioned fresh and moist adhesions, there was also fat necrosis in the omentum and in the region of the pancreatic head.

Codes: _____

PATIENT: Pittman, Richard   **MR#:** 99-07-09

SURGEON: Collins   **ASSISTANT:** Freeman

Preoperative Diagnosis:
Gynecomastia.

Postoperative Diagnosis:
Gynecomastia.

Operation:
Bilateral simple mastectomy.

Brief Clinical History:
The patient is a 20-year-old black male with an approximate six-year history of bilateral breast enlargement, who presents now requesting simple bilateral mastectomy for removal of gynecomastia.

Description of Procedure:
The patient was brought into the OR and placed supine on the operating table. Then he was prepped and draped in the usual sterile fashion. Anesthesia was by general endotracheal.

Then an inferior circumareolar incision was made on the left side down to the subcutaneous tissue. A pair of hooks were placed on the skin inferiorly and heavy Mayos were used to dissect down to the subcutaneous tissue around the enlarged breast tissue. Allis clamps were then used to grasp the breast tissue. The upper flap was then dissected free with sharp dissection with curved heavy Mayos. After this was completed, the inferior aspect of the breast tissue over the pectoralis fascia was freed up. Once it was felt that the tissue had been adequately removed, the sample was completely dissected and sent to pathology. The wound was then irrigated with copious amounts of normal saline. Electrocautery was used for hemostasis. Then the wound was irrigated again and checked for bleeding. Once it was adequately stopped, the wound was closed with 4-0 Vicryl subcutaneous sutures, used simple, times seven, and then a running subcuticular 4-0 Vicryl.

The other side was completed with an inferior circumareolar incision. Skin hooks were then used to hold the inferior flap back as heavy Mayos were used to dissect the breast tissue free down to the superficial pectoral fascia. Then the superior flap was freed and incised down to the pectoral fascia. Once this was completed, the tissue overlying the fascia was dissected out and the sample was removed and sent to pathology. The wound was then irrigated copiously with normal saline. Electrocautery was used for hemostasis. Then the wound was probed and all the breast tissue was felt to be removed, ensuring that equal amounts of tissue were removed on both sides. After this was completed, the wound was then irrigated once more and checked for hemostasis. Once adequate hemostasis was maintained, the wound was closed with 4-0 Vicryl subcutaneous stitch, used simple, times eight, and then a running subcuticular 4-0 Vicryl. Steri-strips were then applied on both wounds. A bulky pressure dressing was applied bilaterally. The patient tolerated the procedure without complications and was transferred back to the post-anesthesia recovery area in stable condition.

Estimated Blood Loss:
About 50 cc's.

Intravenous Fluids:
Approximately one liter of crystalloid was administered.

Codes: _____

PATIENT: Kohler, Ernest   **MR#:** 99-07-10

SURGEON: Reese   **ASSISTANT:** Wynn

Preoperative Diagnosis:
Balanitis.

Postoperative Diagnosis:
Balanitis.

Operation:
Circumcision.

Procedure:
The patient was brought into the OR and placed on the operating table in the supine position. He was prepped and draped in the usual sterile fashion for circumcision. A penile nerve block was injected at the level of the pubic bone. Next the base of the penis was circumferentially anesthetized with 1% Lidocaine without Epinephrine. After testing to ascertain that the entire penis was well anesthetized, the procedure was begun.

First, the desired line of incision was indicated with the marking pen on the outer skin and on the inner prepuce skin. Next, the knife was used to incise the foreskin on its inner portion, taking care at the ventral side not to cut too deep and damage the urethra. After completely incising circumferentially on the inner prepuce, the outer foreskin was incised in the same manner. Next the foreskin, which was cut in a double sleeve fashion, was incised across its dorsal edge to completely free it from the penis. The foreskin was then completely removed from the shaft of the penis using sharp and blunt dissection with the Mayo scissors, taking care to cut as close as possible to the foreskin being removed. Great care was exercised on the ventral side of the penis to insure that there was no injury to the urethra. After the foreskin was removed, hemostasis was obtained with Bovie electrocautery. The skin edges were reapproximated with a 3-0 chromic stitch. Stay stitches were placed at the 12, 3, 6 and 9 o'clock positions to be used as traction. Once this was completed, a running stitch of 3-0 chromic was placed between these stitches. The penis was wiped clean and a bandage consisting of a wrap of Vaseline gauze and a wrap of Kerlix gauze was placed. This completed the procedure and the patient was taken back to the outpatient surgery area for discharge.

The patient was instructed to remove the dressing tomorrow and to return in a few weeks to the Genitourinary Clinic. He was instructed not to engage in any sexual activity. He was given a prescription for Keflex and a prescription for pain pills. He was also given a prescription for Amyl Nitrate to take if he should get an erection.

Codes: _____

PATIENT: Summers, Donald   **MR#:** 99-07-11

SURGEON: Gardner   **ASSISTANT:** Morgan

Preoperative Diagnosis:
Chronic constipation.

Irritable bowel syndrome.

Postoperative Diagnosis:
Chronic constipation.

Irritable bowel syndrome.

Colonoscopy:
Instrument: Olympus CF1TL flexible colonoscope.

Procedure:
The patient was premedicated with Demerol 50 mg and Valium 20 mg and an additional 10 mg of Valium IV was given during the procedure. The colonoscope was passed to the cecum with mild difficulty.

Findings:
The patient was poorly prepped and there was some spasm in the sigmoid colon, but otherwise, there were no mucosal lesions, mass lesions, friability, or ulcerations seen throughout the colon.

Impression:
Normal examination except for some spasm in the sigmoid colon.

Recommendations:
Antispasmodics.

High-fiber diet.

Codes: _____

PATIENT: Eisenberg, Marie   **MR#:** 99-07-12

SURGEON: James   **ASSISTANT:** Nollman

Preoperative Diagnosis:
Status post excision of volvuli of small intestine with perforation and towel clip closure

Operation:
Reexploration of abdomen, secondary towel clip closure, and removal of four laparotomy packs from right upper quadrant of abdomen

Brief Clinical History:
The patient is a thirty-two year-old white female who was surgically explored for peritonitis, septicemic shock, and free air four days prior to this surgery. Findings at the time of surgery included a volvulus of the mid-intestine with necrosis of the volvulized segment and free perforation into the peritoneal cavity. The small bowel was resected and functional end-to-end stapled anastomosis was performed. During exploration of the abdomen slight hemorrhage resulted from adhesions taken down from the liver and abdominal wall. Therefore, four laparotomy packs were placed during that surgery. The patient was closed with towel clips and admitted to the intensive care unit. Her postoperative course was initially characterized by hemodynamic instability with blood pressures between 90 and 110. However, with treatment by antibiotics, Neosynephrine, and Dopamine, the patient's hemodynamic parameters stabilized. She was successfully diuresed and brought back to the operating room for reexploration of the abdomen and removal of the laparotomy packs.

Operative Procedure:
The patient was brought to the operating room and placed on the operating table in supine position. General endotracheal anesthesia was induced. The towel clips closing the abdomen were removed under sterile conditions. The abdomen was prepped and draped in sterile fashion. The abdomen was reopened and 500 cc of serous fluid were removed from the abdominal cavity. Four packs were removed from the right upper quadrant, two subhepatic and two suprahepatic. A foul odor was associated with the removal of these packs. Cultures, aerobic and anaerobic, were sent to microbiology. The right upper quadrant was irrigated until clear with two liters of saline. The small bowel anastomosis was inspected and the anastomosis was patent with no evidence of perforation. However, an area of serosal denuding was noted on a portion of the anastomosed small intestine. The anastomosis was placed in the left lower quadrant, adjacent to the inferior aspect of the wound, by reason that the contents would be immediately accessible to drainage from the inferior portion of the wound, in the event of perforation of this segment. The abdomen was closed again with towel clips. A sterile iodinized biodressing was then placed over the entire abdomen. The patient was then transferred from the operating room to the surgical intensive care unit, intubated, in stable condition. The sponge and instrument counts were correct with no remaining packs left in the abdomen. Blood loss was minimal.

Codes: _____

PATIENT: Taber, Betty   **MR#:** 99-07-13

SURGEON: Oldenhaus   **ASSISTANT:** Sutphin

Operation:
Exploratory laparotomy with incision and drainage of the abdomen and irrigation of the abdomen with antibiotic solution

Indications:
The patient is status post exploratory laparotomy in which the wound was unable to be closed. The patient was brought to the operating room for attempted closure of the wound and debridement of the known wound infection.

Procedure:
The patient was prepped and draped in sterile manner and placed in supine position and inducted with general anesthesia. After Betadine scrub, retention clamps were removed from the abdomen of the patient. The abdominal wall was opened with blunt dissection to expose the abdominal cavity, and purulent discharge was encountered. Anaerobic and aerobic bacterial cultures were taken from the purulent material. The abdomen was irrigated copiously with five liters of antibiotic solution. The omentum and bowel were freed from the peritoneal lining and the peritoneal gutters were freely irrigated. No abscess cavities were discovered. The liver appeared clean. The entire area was thoroughly irrigated, and following this irrigation, attempt was made at closing the wound. The fascia was still too far apart to be approximated, but the skin however, was able to be approximated. Therefore, abdominal skin closure was obtained with a running 1-0 Prolene suture. Two peritoneal Jackson-Pratt drains were placed for continuous drainage of the retroperitoneal fluid, until return to the operating room in several days to complete the fascial closure. The patient tolerated the procedure well without complications. The patient remained on the ventilator and was returned to the surgical intensive care unit in good condition. Vital signs remained stable and she remained afebrile.

Codes: _____

PATIENT: Quartz, Leona   **MR#:** 99-07-14

SURGEON: Webb   **ASSISTANT:** Farmer

Preoperative Diagnosis:
Small bowel fistula

Postoperative Diagnosis:
Small bowel fistula

Operation:
Exploratory laparotomy and Foley catheter decompression of small bowel through fistula tract

Procedure:
The patient was brought to the operating room and placed supine on the operating table. After successful induction of general endotracheal anesthesia, the wound was prepped and draped in the usual fashion. Previously placed nylon sutures were removed and the incision was allowed to open spontaneously. The fascia was not previously closed and accordingly matted small bowel loops were encountered immediately under the skin incision. There was a fair amount of enteric small bowel contents within the wound, and this area was vigorously irrigated. The wound was then carefully explored and a small hole of approximately 2 mm in a small bowel loop was noted. Surrounding this area were small silk sutures, possibly from prior repair of a serosal tear. It appeared obvious that any attempt to dissect these inflamed matted loops of bowel and to directly repair this fistula would be impossible, and would likely create greater damage. Instead, this uncontrolled leak was converted to a controlled enterocutaneous fistula by placing a #16 French Foley catheter through the opening in the small bowel and inflating the balloon with 2 cc of saline. The balloon was pulled up to tent it against the small bowel wall and immediately the leak stopped. The catheter was gently suctioned and free flow of enteric contents was obtained through the catheter. The skin edges were reapproximated, leaving the fascia open over the length of the wound and at the point at which the catheter came through the skin, the skin edges were simply approximated around the

catheter. The catheter exited the small bowel opening at an approximately 90 degree angle. There was no leak around the catheter and it drained freely, attached to a Foley bag for dependent drainage. The wound was dressed and the patient was returned to the intensive care unit in serious condition after tolerating the procedure without incident. All counts were correct times two.

Codes: _____

PATIENT: Yates, Geneva   **MR#:** 99-07-15

SURGEON: Monroe   **ASSISTANT:** Tasma

Preoperative Diagnosis:
Presumptive colonic perforation

Postoperative Diagnosis:
Right colon perforation

Operation:
Exploratory laparotomy with placement of a cecostomy tube and bilateral gutter drains

Procedure:
The patient was brought to the operating room and placed supine on the operating table. Following successful induction of general endotracheal anesthesia, the patient was prepped and draped in routine manner. The patient's abdomen was entered by removal of the skin sutures, which were placed several days prior during previous surgery. Immediately upon removal of the skin sutures, copious amounts of purulent bloody fluid and frank stool were liberated. The mass of matted small bowel was then carefully freed from the anterior abdominal wall using blunt dissection from gutter to gutter and from xiphoid to pubis. No holes were created during this dissection, and after completed mobilization of the bowel, the findings consisted of one persistent small bowel leak around the previously placed Foley catheter and a 5-mm distal cecal perforation. The gutters and mass of bowel were copiously irrigated with antibiotic saline solution. A #24 Malecot catheter with the tip cut off was inserted through the perforation into the right colon and subsequently brought out through the lateral abdominal wall as a cecostomy tube. A 3-0 silk pursestring suture was placed around the entry site of the cecostomy tube and gently snugged. Three 3-0 silk sutures were then used to tack the cecum to the lateral abdominal wall around the cecostomy tube. A 3-0 silk suture was placed in pursestring fashion around the Foley catheter and gently snugged up to stop the leak. The abdominal cavity was again irrigated with plain saline solution, antibiotic Ancef solution, and Amphotericin solution. The site of the cecostomy was again inspected and no leak around the tube was noted. Two #14 irrigating gastric tubes were placed in each gutter for adequate drainage and these two-way tubes allowed the installation of saline into the gutters. Two 10-mm Jackson-Pratt drains were placed next to these tubes and all of these tubes and drains were then brought out through the lower aspect of the incision. Their placement allowed continuous irrigation and suction of the peritoneal gutters to prevent the collection of any purulent material or drainage fluid. The skin was closed using interrupted 2-0 nylon sutures. The patient was returned to the intensive care unit in stable condition.

Codes: _____

PATIENT: Cook, Tina   **MR#:** 99-07-16

SURGEON: McKinney   **ASSISTANT:** Urbaniak

Preoperative Diagnosis:
Possible colon perforation

Postoperative Diagnosis:
Perforation of the right colon

Operation:
Exploratory laparotomy; Cecostomy tube placement; Incision and drainage of intra-abdominal fecal contents

Indications:
The patient is a thirty-three year-old black female, status post small bowel resection for small bowel fistula, who was noted last evening to have fecal contents leaking from a Jackson-Pratt drain. The patient was suspected of having a perforated right colon and after evaluation, it was decided that the patient needed exploratory laparotomy to exclude colon perforation or to repair the colon in the event of perforation.

Procedure:
At midnight, the patient was brought to the operating room on an emergency basis and placed in the supine position. An endotracheal tube was inserted and the patient was induced with a satisfactory general anesthetic. Her abdominal wall was prepped and draped in the usual sterile manner. Nylon sutures over the abdominal wall were removed and the abdominal cavity was explored. The Foley catheter remained in place in the small bowel fistula. There was minimal enteric content leaking around the Foley catheter. Further examination noted old blood mixed with fecal content in the lower abdomen and under the right gutter. A small perforation of the right colon was noted and a cecostomy tube was inserted with a pursestring suture placed around it. The cecostomy tube was brought out through the abdominal wall and it was tagged to the abdominal wall with 3-0 silk sutures inside the abdomen and secured on the outside skin with 2-0 nylon sutures. The Foley catheter in the small bowel fistula was also secured with pursestring sutures. The wound was copiously irrigated with saline as well as with antibiotic solution containing Amphotericin. Two irrigation tubes were placed into both gutters and Jackson-Pratt drains were also placed into each gutter. The tubes were brought out through the lower part of the incision and the incision was closed with 2-0 interrupted vertical mattress nylon stitches. The patient tolerated the procedure well with minimal blood loss estimated at about 50 cc. The patient was returned to the intensive care unit, intubated, and in stable condition.

Codes: _____

PATIENT: Nevens, Ingrid   **MR#:** 99-07-17

SURGEON: LaBianca   **ASSISTANT:** O'Malley

Preoperative Diagnosis:
Small bowel and right colon perforation

Postoperative Diagnosis:
Small bowel and right colon perforation

Operation:
Extensive small bowel resection and right colectomy with jejunostomy

Procedure:
The patient was brought to the operating room and placed supine on the operating room table. Following induction of general endotracheal anesthesia, the patient was prepped and draped in a routine fashion. The previously placed Jackson-Pratt drains, the previously placed Foley catheter, and the previously placed cecostomy tube were removed. The existing midline sutures were removed and the entire mass of matted small bowel and large bowel were mobilized off the abdominal wall. Persistent right colonic perforation as well as an adjacent smaller perforation and an additional persistent perforation noted in the mid-jejunum were ascertained. The ligament of Treitz was identified and the small bowel was mobilized from that point for approximately 70 cm to 80 cm, at which point a densely matted segment of small bowel was encountered. Further mobilization became impossible. Using heavy Kelly clamps, the distal small bowel was resected from a point 75 cm from the ligament of Treitz to the right ileocolic junction. Each of the Kelly clamps placed across the mesenteric pedicle were oversewn with running 2-0 chromic sutures. The small bowel specimen was removed from the field and the right colon was mobilized to the hepatic flexure. The mesentery supplying the colon was divided between heavy Kelly clamps and each of these Kelly clamps across the vascular pedicle of the mesentery was oversewn using 2-0 chromic sutures. The right colonic specimen was then removed from the field. The abdominal cavity was copiously irrigated with sterile saline. Several points of persistent mesenteric bleeding were further oversewn with 2-0 Vicryl sutures. The remainder of the colon was inspected and in mobilizing the sigmoid to inspect it, a large anterior tear in the rectosigmoid was created. This tear, approximately 7 cm long, was repaired with an inverting Connell stitch of 2-0 chromic and was further oversewn with interrupted 3-0 silk sutures. The abdominal cavity was again copiously irrigated with sterile saline. Jackson-Pratt drains were placed in the gutters and a 10-mm Jackson-Pratt drain was placed in the pelvis. These were brought out through stab wounds in the flanks. The fascia would not close, so the anterior rectus fascia was mobilized over the length of the muscle, and flaps were rotated medially to effectively close the gap between the two edges of fascia. Subsequently, the fascia was closed using 0 Vicryl intermittent sutures above and 0 Vicryl running sutures below. At approximately the midpoint of the closure, a gap was left to pull through the stapled end of the jejunum. A 2-cm tear in the jejunum was noted approximately 1 cm proximal to the staple line. The anterior abdominal fascia was copiously irrigated and closure was reassessed a final time. Jackson-Pratt drains were placed on top of each of the large fascial flaps and the skin was then closed using interrupted 2-0 nylon mattress sutures. After closing the skin, an enterostomy bag was placed around the jejunostomy and the wound was dressed. The patient tolerated the procedure reasonably well, however, there was a significant amount of bleeding for which the patient was transfused. The patient was taken to the recovery room, intubated, and in serious, but stable, condition.

Codes: _____

PATIENT: Vitt, Ethel   **MR#:** 99-07-18

SURGEON: Uchiama   **ASSISTANT:** Diener

Preoperative Diagnosis:
Status post jejunostomy and resection of small bowel and right colon

Postoperative Diagnosis:
Status post jejunostomy and resection of small bowel and right colon

Operation:
Jejunostomy takedown

Procedure:
The patient was brought to the operating room and placed supine on the operating table. After successful induction of general endotracheal anesthesia, the abdomen was prepped and draped in routine fashion. The skin around the jejunostomy was incised with a knife and the incision was carried down through very thick and very tough scar tissue until the cavity was entered. Several small points of bleeding were Bovie electrocauterized. The jejunum was successfully mobilized and the proximal limb of large bowel was identified. The midline incision inadvertently entered the large bowel and this laceration was oversewn using 3-0 chromic sutures followed by imbricating 2-0 silk sutures. A stab wound was made in the left lower quadrant and a Burlisher was inserted by palpation through the anterior abdominal wall into this segment of the colon. The tip of the Burlisher was visualized within the lumen. An umbilical tape was pulled through the stab wound and the external end of the umbilical tape was tied to a Foley catheter, which was pulled through the stab wound and into the lumen of the large bowel. The catheter was inflated with saline and secured in place at the skin. The defunctionalized closed loop of large bowel was decompressed via the Foley catheter following oversewing of the open end. A jejunocolic anastomosis was created in the immediate subfascial space using a two-layer anastomosis, the first layer consisting of running 3-0 chromic sutures and the second layer consisting of seromuscular 3-0 silk Lembert sutures. By virtue of the tethering effects of both the proximal jejunum and the distal colon, the anastomosis could not be completely reduced below the fascial level. Thus, flaps of subcutaneous tissue and scar tissue were developed to adequately close over the anastomosis. The area was thoroughly irrigated with antibiotic saline solution and a 7-mm Jackson-Pratt drain was placed adjacent to the anastomosis. The skin over the anastomosis was closed with interrupted 2-0 nylon horizontal mattress sutures. The Jackson-Pratt drain was connected to bulb suction and the wound was covered with a sterile dressing. The patient tolerated the procedure well and was transferred to the recovery room in stable condition.

Codes: _____

PATIENT: Streppler, Louella   **MR#:** 99-07-19

SURGEON: Martske

Clinical Diagnosis:
Status post perforation of small bowel with enteric fistula

Operative Procedures:
Exploratory laparotomy; Small bowel resection; Right colectomy; Ileostomy

Specimens:
Right colon segment, Posterior segment of small bowel

Gross:
The specimen consists of multiple loops of small intestine matted together by dense fibrous adhesions. The serosa is diffusely covered by shaggy reddish-brown fibrinous and hemorrhagic

exudate. Focal areas of yellow-tan discoloration measuring approximately 7 cm in greatest diameter are consistent with deposits of fibrin and areas of adhesions. The small bowel mucosa is grossly unremarkable. The wall of the bowel appears somewhat edematous and thickened but otherwise is grossly within normal limits. The segment of right colon measures approximately 8 cm in length and notably exhibits red discoloration on the serosa. The colon mucosa is grossly unremarkable. Multiple representative sections are submitted in Block A through Block F.

Microscopic:
The sections of small intestine display moderate acute and chronic inflammatory cell infiltrates in the serosa and subserosa. Fairly large areas of fibrosis containing dilated capillaries are noted in the subserosa. A fistula tract containing numerous acute inflammatory cell infiltrates in its wall is also noted. The sections of large bowel similarly display marked edema and interstitial hemorrhage with acute and chronic inflammatory cell infiltrates primarily on the serosa and foci of multinucleated foreign body type giant cells containing foreign body material.

Diagnosis:
Acute and chronic inflammation with focal foreign body granuloma

Codes: _____

PATIENT: Amberg, Linus   **MR#:** 99-07-20

SURGEON: Sunil

Clinical Diagnosis:
Status post bowel resection

Operative Procedure:
Jejunostomy takedown

Specimen:
Portion of small bowel

Gross:
The specimen consists of two irregular fragments of soft tissue with the larger fragment measuring 5 cm by 4 cm by 2 cm and the smaller fragment measuring 3 cm by 2 cm by 1 cm. The larger fragment represents a bowel segment that is partially distorted and focal areas of yellowish discoloration as well as firm tissue suggestive of fibrosis are noted. Representative sections are submitted as Block A and Block B.

Microscopic:
Sections of the jejunum reveal marked chronic inflammation with foreign body reaction. The inflammatory cells consist of lymphocytes and histiocytes with numerous multinucleated giant cells. Inflammation accompanied by reactive fibrosis is noted mostly on the external aspect of the bowel. Block A consists mainly of fibroadipose tissue revealing chronic inflammation, reactive fibrosis, and foreign body reaction.

Diagnosis:
Chronic inflammation and reactive fibrosis with foreign body reaction

Codes: _____

PATIENT: Wallace, Barbara   **MR#:** 99-07-21

ATTENDING PHYSICIAN: Mills

Sonogram Abdomen:
Shows gallstone. There is thickening of the gallbladder wall due to edema. Common bile duct is 4.5 mm and is normal. Pancreas is normal. There is fluid density around both kidneys. No mass or abscess of kidneys is seen. Liver is normal.

Impression:
Gallstone. Edema of gallbladder wall. Perinephric fluid in both kidneys, questionable perinephritis. Recommend CT scan.

Codes: _____

PATIENT: Carpenter, Mark   **MR#:** 99-07-22

ATTENDING PHYSICIAN: Stephens

IVP:
The scout film shows a large calcification in the left pelvis measuring about 4 cm × 6 cm. There is also a calcification overlying the right kidney region. There is good excretion of contrast material bilaterally. The size and shape of both kidneys are normal. There is a small dromedary hump on the left side. There is minimal dilation of the collecting system on the left, and there is moderate dilation of the left ureter. The calyceal system on the right shows partial duplication but is otherwise normal. The right ureter is normal. The bladder is also within normal limits. The distal left ureter does point right towards the stone seen on the scout film.

Impression:
Large left ureteral stone in the distal left ureter, which is causing only minimal obstructive symptoms.

Codes: _____

PATIENT: Vickers, Peter   **MR#:** 99-07-23

SURGEON: Delaney

Clinical Diagnosis:
Ventral hernia.

Postoperative Diagnosis:
Ventral hernia.

Operative Procedure:
Ventral hernia repair.

Specimen:
Ventral hernia sac.

Gross:
The specimen labeled "ventral hernia sac" consists of a piece of soft tissue showing focal areas of fibrous thickening with membranous appearance measuring approximately 3.7 cm in length. A representative section is submitted in Block A.

Microscopic:

The sections of hernia sac show diffuse areas of fibrosis. Foci of mild chronic inflammatory cell infiltrates are also seen.

Diagnosis:

Soft tissue, abdominal wall, excision and repair of ventral hernia. Hernia sac with fibrosis and chronic inflammation.

Codes: _____

PATIENT: Schmitt, Laura   **MR#:** 99-07-24

SURGEON: Haynes

Clinical Diagnosis:
Status Post Colostomy.

Postoperative Diagnosis:
Same.

Operative Procedure:
Colostomy takedown.

Specimen:
Distal anastomotic site of colostomy takedown.

Gross:
The specimen is labeled as "colostomy takedown" and consists of a linear piece of tissue that is 6.0 cm × 0.3 cm in greatest dimensions and is reddish brown in appearance. The specimen is totally submitted and labeled as Block A.

Microscopic:
The section of the colostomy stump shows a portion of the colonic wall, which shows chronic inflammation with fibrosis. In focal areas, foreign body giant cell reaction to suture material is also noted. No evidence of malignancy is noted.

Diagnosis:
Chronic inflammation with fibrosis of colonic wall.

Foreign body giant cell reaction to suture material.

Codes: _____

PATIENT: Baldwin, Sandra   **MR#:** 99-07-25

SURGEON: Jackson

Specimen:
Gallbladder.

Gross:
There is a single calculus that is yellow to brown 0.7 cm diameter mulberry type. The previously opened gallbladder consists of two portions, one measuring 6.0 cm × 3.5 cm × 1.2 cm showing abundant fat and multiple staples, the other portion measuring 6.0 cm × 3.0 cm × 1.5 cm is the portion of fundus that was previously opened.

Microscopic Diagnoses:
1. Chronic cholecystitis.
2. Cholelithiasis.

Codes: _____

PATIENT: Tucker, Gary   **MR#:** 99-07-26

SURGEON: Mayfield

Clinical Diagnosis:
Left scrotal mass.

Postoperative Diagnosis:
Left scrotal mass.

Operative Procedure:
Excision left scrotal mass.

Specimen:
Left scrotal mass.

Gross:
The specimen labeled "rectal scrotal mass" consists of a piece of grayish tan soft tissue that is roughly ovoid in shape, measuring approximately 2.3 cm in length and 2.0 cm in greatest diameter. In cut section it is moderately firm in consistency, grayish tan in color, and slightly trabeculated. A representative section is submitted in Block A.

Microscopic:
The sections show a mass made up of groups and nests of cells with moderate amount of pink cytoplasm, round or oval-shaped nuclei with inconspicuous nucleoli arranged in chords or glandular fashion around empty spaces that are somewhat variable in size and shape, separated from each other by strands of fibrocollagenous soft tissue. The histological features are characteristic of adenomatoid tumor.

Diagnosis:
Adenomatoid tumor.

Codes: _____

PATIENT: Ewing, Carol   **MR#:** 99-07-27

SURGEON: Hudson

Clinical Diagnosis:
Partial small bowel obstruction.

Perforated viscus.

Intrauterine pregnancy of 17 weeks gestation.

Postoperative Diagnosis:
Partial small bowel obstruction.

Perforated viscus.

Complete second trimester miscarriage.

Operative Procedure:
Exploratory laparotomy and small bowel resection.

Specimens:
Small bowel, non-viable fetus, membranes, cord, placenta.

Gross:
The specimen is received in two parts.

The first part of the specimen is labeled "small bowel" and consists of a segment of bowel measuring approximately 22 cm in length and 4 cm in greatest diameter. Located approximately in the middle of the specimen there appears to be constriction of the lumen due to the specimen being twisted. In this constricted area, there is a marked softening and necrosis of the intestine, which has a grayish discoloration and is fragmented. The discoloration also extends into half of the bowel on one side. In this discolored area, the mucosal surface shows focal areas of congestion and hemorrhage with marked edema, however, the entire mucosal wall does not appear to be necrotic, except in the area of obstruction. The external surface in the other half shows yellowish white exudate. The mucosal surface is unremarkable except for edema. Also included in the same container is an irregular fragment of grayish soft tissue, which appears necrotic and measures approximately 9 cm × 6 cm × 1 cm in greatest dimension. Representative sections are submitted as Block A. Sections from the discolored half of the bowel area are submitted as Block B and Block C. Sections from the relatively normal appearing bowel are submitted as Block D. A section of the separate necrotic fetus is submitted as Block E. The head is normocephalic, and no external deformities are identified. All four extremities include the usual five digits. A segment of umbilical cord measuring approximately 24 cm in length is attached to the fetus; the umbilical cord measures approximately 8 mm in greatest diameter and appears to contain three umbilical vessels. Representative sections of the fetal liver and umbilical cord are submitted as Block F. The placenta weighs approximately 57 grams and the umbilical cord is completely separated from the placenta. The membranes are translucent. The placenta measures approximately 9.5 cm by 8.5 cm by 0.5 cm in greatest dimensions. On the maternal surface, the cotyledons appear intact. Representative sections of the placenta and membranes are submitted as Block G and Block H.

Microscopic:
In Block A, sections of the small bowel exhibit complete necrosis and hemorrhage at the site of the obstruction. These necrotic changes extend to and involve the adjacent mesentery. In Block B and in Block C there is marked congestion with focal hemorrhage in the mucosa. The submucosa is edematous and with acute inflammatory reaction on the serosal surface. Block D also exhibits edema with acute inflammatory reaction on the serosal surface that is consistent with peritonitis. Block E consists of adipose tissue with marked congestion and focal areas of hemorrhage with acute inflammation. Sections of fetal tissue exhibit partially autolyzed hepatic tissue with prominent extramedullary hematopoiesis. Sections of the placenta exhibit immature chorionic villi and decidua. The villi appear hypercellular and several blood vessels are identified. The umbilical cord contains three blood vessels.

Diagnosis:
Necrosis with a history of obstruction; Edema with acute peritonitis; Fetal demise at approximately 17 to 18 weeks of gestational age

Codes: _____

PATIENT: Foster, Linda   **MR#:** 99-07-28

SURGEON: Rodgers

Clinical Diagnosis:
Cholelithiasis.

Postoperative Diagnosis:
Cholelithiasis.

Pancreatic pseudocyst.

Operative Procedure:
Exploratory laparotomy, cholecystectomy, biopsy.

Specimen:
Gallbladder.

Biopsy of cyst wall.

Gross:
The specimen is received in two parts.

The first part of the specimen is labeled "gallbladder" and consists of a gallbladder that is 9.5 cm × 3.5 cm in greatest dimensions. The serosal surface of the gallbladder is discolored green. On opening the gallbladder, it contains a large amount of bile and a few small mulberry-shaped stones are also noted. These stones range from 3 cm to 4 mm in greatest dimension. The wall of the gallbladder is thickened and the mucosa is granular and slightly speckled in appearance. Representative sections are submitted and labeled as Block A.

The second part of the specimen is labeled as "biopsy, cyst wall" and consists of an elliptical piece of tissue that is 3.0 cm × 1.0 cm × 1.0 cm in greatest dimensions. One surface of this cyst wall is hemorrhagic in appearance. Representative sections are submitted and labeled as Block B.

Microscopic:
The sections of the gallbladder show fibromuscular thickening of the wall and the interstitium is infiltrated by chronic inflammatory cells. The overlying epithelium is secretory and no evidence of malignancy is noted.

The sections of the biopsy of the cyst wall show fibroconnective tissue in which no definite epithelial lining is noted. The wall is infiltrated by acute and chronic inflammatory cells. The inner surface of the cyst is lined by granulation tissue and a large number of acute inflammatory cells are also noted with proliferation of the fibroblasts. No evidence of malignancy is noted.

Diagnosis:
Chronic cholecystitis.

Cholelithiasis.

Pancreatic pseudocyst.

Acute and chronic inflammation of pancreatic pseudocyst wall.

Codes: _____

PATIENT: Smoot, Donna   **MR#:** 99-07-29

SURGEON: Li

Clinical Diagnosis:
Mammary hyperplasia.

Postoperative Diagnosis:
Mammary hyperplasia.

Operative Procedure:
Bilateral mastectomy.

Specimen:
Left breast tissue.
Right breast tissue.

Gross:
The specimen is received in two parts.

Specimen 1, labeled "left breast tissue" consists of two irregular fragments of yellowish tan soft tissue measuring approximately 5.0 cm × 4.5 cm × 3.0 cm and 3.5 cm × 3.2 cm × 2.6 cm in greatest dimensions, respectively. The external surface is irregular. On sectioning, part of the specimen appears to be white in color and indurated. The area of induration is irregular, measuring approximately 2.2 cm × 3.5 cm. Representative sections are submitted as Block A, Block B, and Block C.

Specimen 2, labeled "right breast tissue" consists of two irregular fragments of soft tissue partly covered by fat. The fragments measure 5.5 cm × 4.5 cm × 2.7 cm and 5.5 cm × 4.4 cm × 2.8 cm in greatest dimensions, respectively. Sectioning shows focal areas of whitish induration. The bulk of the tissue consists of yellow lobulated fat. Representative sections are submitted as Block D, Block E, and Block F.

Microscopic:
Sections of the left and right breast tissue show extensive stromal fibrosis and hyalinization. Few mammary ducts are identified and some of these show slight hyperplasia. No definite periductal edema or inflammation is seen. The histologic changes, other than the stromal fibrosis, are very slight, but consistent with mammary hyperplasia.

Diagnosis:
Intraductal hyperplasia, mild, focal with stromal fibrosis.

Codes: _____

PATIENT: Goldstein, Rose   **MR#:** 99-07-30

ADMITTING PHYSICIAN: Yaeger

Chief Complaint and History of Present Illness:
This 78-year-old white female was admitted for evaluation of abdominal pain, nausea, and vomiting with reports of coffee-ground emesis. Several weeks ago she was evaluated as an out-patient for similar symptoms and was told she has several ulcers in her distal esophagus. She was subsequently started on medications and did fairly well after the initiation of medications, but over the course of the past three days prior to admission, she had increasing left upper quadrant discomfort along with nausea, vomiting, and hematemesis. She also states a

history of a 35-pound weight loss over the last 18 months. She underwent another evaluation and was found to have erosive gastritis with duodenitis as well as reflux esophagitis. She also has left upper quadrant pain that is attributed to post herpes zoster neuritis. The patient previously had a colecystectomy and an appendectomy.

Physical Examination on Admission:
Multiple well-healed abdominal scars are present. No masses are palpable. There is mild discomfort in the left upper quadrant on palpation. Bowel sounds are normal.

Laboratory Data on Admission:
Hemoglobin was 13.8 and WBC was 8000. Urinalysis showed 3+ protein with 1 to 3 RBC's/HPF. SMAC was normal except for a slight elevation of BUN at 38.

Hospital Course:
The patient underwent esophagogastroduodenoscopy by Dr. Mattingly with findings of some mild erythema in the prepyloric area. Otherwise the exam was unremarkable. CT scan of the abdomen was normal. Serum gastrin was slightly elevated at 256, and gastric analysis showed a quite low basal rate of 0.3 mEq/hr, and also a low maximal acid output of 7.1, and a peak acid output of 10 mEq/hr. Zantac was discontinued about 24 hours prior to the gastric analysis. Barium enema was performed, and was grossly normal. The patient has atrophic gastritis. She was started on Reglan and displayed marked improvement with regard to her nausea and abdominal discomfort. The patient has irritable bowel syndrome. A high-fiber diet was instituted with the continuation of Reglan and Zantac. She was instructed to continue a bland diet and to add additional foods gradually. She is to return to the office in three weeks for follow-up.

Diagnoses:
Atrophic gastritis.

Irritable bowel syndrome.

Procedures:
Esophagogastroduodenoscopy.

Discharge Medications:
Zantac 150 mg p.o. b.i.d.; Reglan 10 mg p.o. a.c and h.s.; Restoril 30 mg h.s. p.r.n. for sleep; Darvocet-N 100 1 q. 4 hours p.r.n for pain.

Codes: _____

PATIENT: Atkinson, Dana   **MR#:** 99-07-31

ADMITTING PHYSICIAN: Townsend

Chief Complaint and History of Present Illness:
The patient is a 51-year-old black male with a history of hypertension, end stage renal disease on peritoneal dialysis, and adult onset diabetes, who was in his usual state of health until four days prior to admission when on the way to a family reunion he began having abdominal cramping and sharp abdominal pain without radiation around his peritoneal dialysis catheter site. He also forgot his medications and was unable to take them as scheduled. The patient began to feel diffuse weakness and lightheadedness. In addition, he noticed that his Dialysate had been draining out as cloudy yellow fluid. Over the next three days prior to admission, he had continued weakness and abdominal pain with occasional vomiting. He denies fever, night

sweats, headaches, blurred vision, or chest pain. He had chills and a slight increase in baseline dyspnea on exertion.

Past Medical History:

As above. No surgeries except peritoneal dialysis catheter placement. Admission for peritonitis three months ago. Adult onset diabetes and hypertension for ten years. No known drug allergies.

Admission Medications:

Calcium carbonate 1 gm p.o. b.i.d.; Procardia XL 90 mg p.o. q. a.m.; Lobetalol 600 mg p.o. b.i.d.; Clonidine 0.2 mg p.o. b.i.d.

Family History:

Mother with hypertension and diabetes mellitus. Father with hypertension and gout. Sister with hypertension.

Social History:

The patient is divorced, has four children. He does not drink alcohol. His last alcoholic drink was fifteen years ago. He does not smoke. His last cigarette was fifteen years ago. He smoked one pack per day for twenty years. He denies IV drug abuse and takes no medications without a prescription.

Admission Physical Examination:

His temperature was 36.8, pulse 64, respirations 20, and blood pressure was 140/80 (after receiving four liters of fluid). In general, he is a well-developed, well-nourished, cooperative black male in mild acute distress.

HEENT examination: nonicteric sclerae; pupils equal and reactive to light and accommodation; extraocular movements intact; oral nasal mucosa slightly dry; oropharynx without exudate or erythema; neck supple without lymphadenopathy or masses; no thyromegaly.

Fundoscopic examination: AV nicking bilaterally; with no hemorrhages or exudates.

Chest examination: lungs clear to auscultation bilaterally; no CVA tenderness.

Cardiovascular examination: regular rate and rhythm with a grade II/IV systolic ejection murmur along the left sternal border radiating to the apex and axillae; no S-3, but S-4 present.

Abdominal examination: abdomen slightly distended with mild diffuse tenderness, greatest by the peritoneal dialysis catheter site with plus-minus rebound and positive guarding; trace bowel sounds; no masses; no hepatosplenomegaly; shifting dullness.

Neurological examination: sensory intact to light touch; 5/5 motor strength throughout; cranial nerves II/XII grossly intact.

Extremity examination: no clubbing or cyanosis; 1+ pitting edema. Chest X ray: no infiltrate or acute disease seen.

Obstructive series: unremarkable.

Admission Laboratory Data:

White count of 5.9; hemoglobin of 9.0; hematocrit of 27.0 with 282000 platelets; differential on CBC was 68 segs, 6 bands, 19 lymphs, and 7 monos; sodium of 137; potassium of 4.2; chloride of 102; bicarb of 27; BUN of 64; creatinine of 14; and glucose of 172.

Hospital Course:

The patient was orthostatic on admission and subsequently rehydrated. Peritoneal dialysis was continued with Vancomycin in his Dialysate. Culture of his Dialysate indicated *Pseudomonas aeruginosa* and subsequently he was given Gentamicin in his Dialysate, four exchanges per day. Over his hospital stay, his abdominal pain resolved. The patient remained afebrile throughout his hospital course.

Discharge Diagnoses:
1. Peritonitis.
2. End stage renal disease.
3. Chronic ambulatory peritoneal dialysis.
4. Hypertension.
5. Adult onset diabetes mellitus.

Discharge Medications:
Procardia XL 90 mg p.o. q. a.m.; Lobetalol 600 mg p.o. b.i.d.; Clonidine 0.3 mg p.o. b.i.d.; Gentamicin 6 mg in each bag of Dialysate.

Codes: _____

PATIENT: Andrews, Elizabeth   **MR#:** 99-07-32

ADMITTING PHYSICIAN: Weiss

History of Present Illness:
The patient is a 27-year-old female admitted to the hospital with severe abdominal pain and fever. She has a significant past history of an abdominal hysterectomy with a bout of acute urinary retention approximately three months ago. The patient had a history of chronic neurogenic bladder so the acute urinary retention was not really that unexpected with the trauma of the pelvic surgery. She was advised to learn intermittent catheterization but decided that she could not handle the procedure. Therefore, as an outpatient, she had a suprapubic tube placed to allow her to open and close the tube on her own and thus to void spontaneously. The patient developed progressive abdominal discomfort last night. She was seen in the emergency room and had a WBC count of 19600 and a sed rate of 56 with severe abdominal pain that appeared to be quite acute in nature. It was decided that the patient possibly had pelvic cellulitis or sepsis causing her pain.

Laboratory Data upon Admission:
The initial admission SMA-6 was essentially normal. Creatinine was 2.3, BUN was 18, and glucose was 24. The next day, creatinine was 1.0 and BUN was 8 and basically remained at those levels through the entire hospital course. The initial admission SMA-12 revealed a calcium of 10.6, a phosphorus of 1.6, an SGOT of 13, a total bilirubin of 1.2, with the rest of the SMA-12 essentially normal. The patient had a urinalysis upon admission showing large amount of blood (consistent with recent suprapubic tube placement), negative nitrates, moderate leukocytes, 25–30 WBC's, and 8–10 RBC's. PT and PTT were essentially normal. The patient had blood cultures that showed no growth. A urine culture showed greater than 100000 *Klebsiella oxytoca* and less than 10000 Beta hemolytic strep group B. Culture after treatment showed no growth. The patient's initial hemoglobin was 13.1, subsequently dropped down to 10, and remained at approximately that level throughout the rest of the hospital course. The admission white count was 196.0 and the discharge white count was 92.0.

Hospital Course:
The patient was started on broad-spectrum antibiotics, Ampicillin and Gentamicin. Pending the culture results, a consultation was obtained from Dr. Ross. A CT scan of the abdomen revealed evidence of a soft tissue density in the pelvis consistent with the possibility of hematoma, possibly inflammation secondary to either the vaginal hysterectomy or the suprapubic

tube placement, all consistent with pelvic cellulitis. The patient continued to have abdominal discomfort with nausea and vomiting, and was seen by Dr. Alvarez in GI consultation. He concluded that the patient's known Crohn's disease would not cause the acute exacerbation of the patient's pain. Her fever may have been related to the diarrhea, which may have been related to the patient's Crohn's disease. She has been tried on multiple medications in the past, as documented in her chart. Contrast was injected into the suprapubic tube, revealing it intact and in good position with no extravasation. The patient continued to have abdominal pain, and was seen in infectious disease consultation by Dr. Price. The patient's antibiotics were changed by adding Flagyl, continuing Gentamicin, discontinuing Unasyn, and adding Piperacillin. The patient also was seen in the gynecologic consultation by Dr. Krueger who concluded that the patient had a stable pelvis, and that she had pelvic cellulitis post abdominal hysterectomy. During the next week, the patient slowly deffervesced, her white count improved, and her pain and discomfort also improved somewhat. She appeared to be having probable bladder spasms, perhaps related to the suprapubic tube in place. Repeat CT scan continued to reveal some cellulitis. The patient's suprapubic tube was removed and a Foley catheter was placed to attempt to alleviate the patient's pain. She continued with pain although the pain was not quite as severe. The patient's Foley catheter was discontinued and she voided spontaneously without problems except for some spasms during micturition. The patient's diet was advanced, her nausea improved, and she remained afebrile.

Discharge Medications:
Zantac 100 mg b.i.d.; Voltaren 75 mg b.i.d.; Soma with codeine q. 8 hours p.r.n.; Ativan 1 mg t.i.d. p.r.n.; Butabel 1 q.i.d. p.r.n.

Codes: _____

PATIENT: Schwartz, Martha   **MR#:** 99-07-33

ADMITTING PHYSICIAN: Bennett

History of Present Illness:
The patient is a 42-year-old white female who was admitted for vomiting blood. She vomited dark blood the night before admission and in the morning of the day of admission she vomited dark blood again. She also had diarrhea with dark contents that morning. She was nauseated but had neither abdominal pain nor chest pain. She did have mild shortness of breath and did feel light-headed.

Past Medical History:
The patient has a history of manic depression for three years. She was involved in a motor vehicle accident last year. She drinks alcohol occasionally but not to excess. She has no known drug allergies.

Medications on Admission:
Thioridazine 25 mg p.o. q. h.s.; Pamelor 75 mg p.o. q. h.s.; Lithonate 300 mg p.o. t.i.d.

Physical Examination:
Temp: 95.2; *BP:* 100/70 lying down, 90/70 sitting up; *Pulse:* 100; *Resp:* 16.
General: appearance of distress from nausea and vomiting; nasogastric tube suctioning bright red blood; sweating during the examination.
HEENT: slightly pale; neck supple; no nodes.
Heart: tachycardia; normal sounds.

Lungs: clear on both sides.

Abdomen: soft; no tenderness.

Extremities: no lesions; no edema.

Neurological: alert and oriented times three; moves all extremities.

Laboratory Data:

CBC: WBC 11470; hemoglobin 10.8; hematocrit 33.4; MCV 98.0; platelet count 195000.

ASTRA-8: sodium 139; potassium 4.8; chloride 106; bicarbonate 22; BUN 24; creatinine 1.0; total bilirubin 0.8; amylase 199.

ABG: pH 7.36; PO2 127; PCO2 38; bicarbonate 21; oxygen saturation 98.4%.

Electrocardiogram:

Normal sinus rhythm; Q-wave in lead number 3; no ST change.

Initial Impression:

Acute upper gastrointestinal bleeding.

Manic depressive disorder.

Hospital Course:

She was admitted to the hospital and received intravenous fluid resuscitation with D5 and normal Saline 150 cc's per hour. She was typed and crossed with six units of packed red blood cells and transfused with two units packed red blood cells. She received triple lumen insertion in her right groin and a Foley catheter. Reglan 10 mg IV push q. 8 hours was given, as well as Tagamet infusion 900 mg in 24 hours, and Compazine 10 mg IM p.r.n. for nausea and vomiting. CBC check was done every six hours while she was on bed rest. She received an upper GI endoscopy, which revealed a Mallory-Weiss tear at the distal end of her esophagus. She received Vasopressin 20 units IV bolus in 20 minutes. This was followed by 0.4 units per minute IV drip. She also received Tridil drip 10 micrograms to keep systolic blood pressure higher than 130, and she received a total of 11 units of packed red blood cells and 10 units of platelets. The bleeding ceased and the hemoglobin and hematocrit remained stable. Her last CBC showed a WBC of 8200; a hemoglobin of 9.3; a hematocrit of 26.2; and a platelet count of 105000. The patient was discharged in stable condition with no restrictions on activity.

Discharge Medications:

Lithonate 300 mg p.o. t.i.d.; Pamelor 75 mg p.o. q. h.s.; Thioridazine 25 mg p.o. q. h.s.; Cimetidine 800 mg p.o. q. h.s.; Reglan 10 mg p.o. t.i.d. one hour a.c.; Ferrous Sulfate 325 mg p.o. t.i.d.; Folic Acid 1 mg p.o. q. a.m.; Multivitamin one tablet p.o. q. a.m.; Neutra-phos 250 mg 2 tablets p.o. b.i.d. for five days.

Discharge Diagnoses:

Mallory-Weiss tear at the lower end of the esophagus, which caused the upper GI bleeding.

Manic depressive disorder.

Procedures:

Upper GI endoscopy.

Operations.

None.

Codes: _____

ICD Coding: Complications of Pregnancy, Obstetrical Procedures, and Congenital Conditions

LEARNING OBJECTIVES

Upon completion of this chapter the learner should be able to:

1. Describe the fifth-digit subclassification with regard to coding and reporting antepartum conditions.
2. Describe the fifth-digit subclassification with regard to coding and reporting complications of labor and delivery.
3. Describe the fifth-digit subclassification with regard to coding and reporting postpartum conditions.
4. Discuss the impact of comorbidities and complications on billing and reimbursement for obstetric diagnoses and procedures.
5. Discuss the impact of comorbidities and complications on billing and reimbursement for neonatal or perinatal diagnoses and procedures.
6. Apply knowledge of coding principles by assigning accurate and precise codes to report obstetric diagnoses and obstetric procedures.
7. Apply knowledge of coding principles by assigning accurate and precise codes to report neonatal and perinatal conditions.
8. Apply knowledge of coding principles by assigning accurate and precise codes to report congenital anomalies.
9. Apply knowledge of coding principles by assigning accurate and precise codes to report maternal conditions affecting the newborn.

ICD CODING OF OBSTETRIC CONDITIONS AND PROCEDURES

Chapter 11 of the ICD-9-CM diagnostic tabular volume is designated for listings of obstetrical diagnoses. The code numbers in this chapter predominantly consist of five digits. This chapter

TABLE 8-1

Sections in Chapter 11, Volume 1 of ICD-9-CM

1. Ectopic and Molar Pregnancy (category range 630–633)
2. Other Pregnancy with Abortive Outcome (category range 634–639)
3. Complications Mainly Related to Pregnancy (category range 640–648)
4. Normal Delivery and Other Indications for Care in Pregnancy, Labor, and Delivery (category range 650–659)
5. Complications Occurring Mainly in the Course of Labor and Delivery (category range 660–669)
6. Complications of the Puerperium (category range 670–677)

contains listings for conditions and complications of pregnancy, childbirth, and the puerperium and encompasses six sections (Table 8–1).

The first section of Chapter 11 is comprised of listings for ectopic and molar pregnancy. These listings include hydatidiform mole, other abnormal product of conception, and ectopic pregnancy. The second section of this chapter contains listings for pregnancy with an abortive outcome.

Category 639 is provided for use if deemed necessary to classify separately the complications classifiable to the fourth-digit level in category range 634–638. This category could be utilized if an obstetric complication was responsible for an episode of medical care, if the ectopic or molar pregnancy was treated in a previous episode of care, or if the conditions documented were immediate complications of ectopic or molar pregnancy that are classifiable to category range 630–633 which lacks specificity for classification at the fourth-digit level.

The third section of Chapter 11, comprised of category range 640–648, primarily classifies antepartum complications of pregnancy. Nevertheless, this section includes the listed conditions even if these diagnoses were present or became activated during labor, delivery, or the puerperium.

This section includes listings for: antepartum hemorrhage, abruptio placentae, and placenta previa; hypertension complicating pregnancy, childbirth, or the puerperium; hyperemesis gravidarum; and early or threatened labor. This section also includes listings for: prolonged or post term pregnancy; infectious and parasitic conditions complicating pregnancy, childbirth, or the puerperium; and encompasses other current medical conditions prompting a primary reason for obstetric care.

If an obstetric patient was admitted either due to a condition that was a complication of pregnancy per se or due to a medical disorder that was complicating the pregnancy, the code for the obstetric complication should be reported as the principal diagnosis. An additional code may also be selected and assigned as needed to provide specificity in reporting.

Category 650 should be used only to report delivery in a completely normal case, a case without abnormality or complication classifiable elsewhere in the chapter. A normal delivery implies spontaneous cephalic delivery without mention of fetal manipulation.

The fourth section of Chapter 11 contains listings for other indications for care in pregnancy, labor, or delivery. These listings encompass: multiple gestation; malposition and malpresentation of fetus; maternal fetal disproportion; and abnormality of organs and soft tissues of the pelvis. These listings also encompass: known or suspected fetal abnormality affecting the management of the mother; other fetal and placental problems affecting the management of the mother; polyhydramnios; and certain problems associated with the amniotic cavity and membranes.

Codes from category *655, Known or suspected fetal abnormality affecting management of mother,* and codes from category *656, Other fetal and placental problems affecting management of mother,* should be assigned only if the fetal condition was actually responsible for modifying the management of the mother by requiring diagnostic studies, additional observation, special care, or termination of pregnancy. The fact that the fetal condition existed and was documented in the patient health record does not justify the selection and assignment of a code from these categories to report the diagnostic entities in the maternal health record.

The fifth section of this chapter is comprised of listings for complications occurring mainly in the course of labor and delivery. These listings include: obstructed labor; abnormality of the forces of labor; long labor; and umbilical cord complications. These listings also include: trauma and damage from instruments to the perineum and vulva during delivery; postpartum hemorrhage; retained placenta or membranes; and complications of anesthetic administration or other sedation in labor and delivery.

The sixth and final section of Chapter 11 contains listings for complications of the puerperium. These listings of postpartum conditions encompass: major puerperal infection; venous complications in pregnancy and the puerperium, pyrexia of unknown origin during the puerperium; obstetrical pulmonary embolism; infections of the breast and nipple associated with childbirth; and disorders of lactation. All of the categories in this section, with the exceptions of 670 and 672, include the listed conditions even if the disorder occurred during pregnancy or childbirth.

The following categories within Chapter 11 require coding and reporting with the fifth-digit subclassification:

634	635	636
637	638	640
641	642	643
644	645	646
647	648	651
652	653	654
655	656	657
658	659	660
661	662	663
664	665	666
667	668	669
670	671	672
673	674	675
676		

The outcome of delivery (stillborn or liveborn and single birth or multiple birth) should be reported on the maternal health record. Codes for reporting the outcome of delivery are listed in category V27 of a supplementary classification in the diagnostic tabular volume.

Categories of listings in Chapter 13 of Volume 3 of ICD-9-CM are established for obstetrical procedures. These listings include category range 72–75 for: forceps, vacuum, and breech delivery; other procedures inducing or assisting delivery; cesarean section and removal of fetus; and other obstetric conditions. Other synchronous procedures that were performed during labor and delivery should also be coded and reported secondarily.

ICD CODING OF NEONATAL AND PERINATAL CONDITIONS

Two chapters of the ICD-9-CM diagnostic tabular volume are designated for listings of neonatal and perinatal conditions and complications. These chapters for listings of diagnoses pertaining to the newborn are:

Chapter 14—Congenital Anomalies (category range 740–759)

Chapter 15—Certain Conditions Originating in the Perinatal Period (category range 760–779)

Chapter 15 is divided into the following two sections:

1. Maternal Causes of Perinatal Morbidity and Mortality (category range 760–763)
2. Other Conditions Originating in the Perinatal Period (category range 764–779)

Chapter 14 includes listings for congenital anomalies. Among these listings are: anencephalus and similar anomalies; spina bifida and other congenital anomalies of the nervous system; congenital anomalies of the eye, ear, face, and neck; bulbus cordis anomalies and anomalies of cardiac septal closure; as well as other congenital anomalies of the heart and the circulatory system. The listings in this chapter also include: congenital anomalies of the respiratory system; cleft palate and cleft lip; other congenital anomalies of the upper alimentary tract and the digestive system; congenital anomalies of the genital organs and the urinary system; certain congenital musculoskeletal deformities and congenital anomalies of the limbs; congenital anomalies of the integument (skin, subcutaneous tissue, hair, nails, and breast); and finally, chromosomal anomalies.

Codes from category range 760–763, Maternal Causes of Perinatal Morbidity, should be selected and assigned only if the documented maternal condition actually affected the fetus or the newborn. The fact that the mother was diagnosed with an associated medical condition or that she experienced a complication of pregnancy, labor, or delivery does not justify the selection and assignment of codes from these categories to report on the newborn healthcare record.

The first section of Chapter 15 containing listings of maternal causes of perinatal morbidity and mortality includes: complications involving placenta, cord, or membranes that affected the newborn as well as other complications of labor and delivery that affected the fetus or the newborn. However, these listings exclude the reporting of maternal endocrine or metabolic disorders that affected the fetus or the newborn.

This section of listings in Chapter 15 includes conditions originating in the perinatal period, even though morbidity or mortality occurred much later. For example, during the post-World War II era, many pregnant women were prescribed with diethylstilbestrol (DES), a pharmaceutical substance later determined to be carcinogenic in their offspring. An adult diagnosed with cancer due to maternal use of DES occurring decades earlier would still be regarded as affected by a maternal cause of the disorder.

The second section of Chapter 15 includes listings of other conditions originating in the perinatal period. These listings encompass: slow fetal growth and fetal malnutrition; disorders relating to short gestation and low birthweight; disorders relating to long gestation and high birthweight; birth trauma; intrauterine hypoxia, birth asphyxia, or anoxia during labor; respiratory distress syndrome; and other respiratory conditions of the fetus or the newborn. The listings in this chapter also encompass: infections specific to the perinatal period acquired before or during birth or via the umbilicus; fetal and neonatal hemorrhage; hemolytic disease of the fetus or the newborn due to isoimmunization; perinatal jaundice; transient endocrine and metabolic disturbances specific to the fetus or the newborn; hematological disorders of the fetus or the newborn; perinatal disorders of the digestive system; and conditions involving the integument and temperature regulation of the fetus or the newborn.

OBSTETRICS REPORTING FOR BILLING

The principal diagnosis is defined as the condition responsible for the admission of the patient for the health service admission, encounter, or episode of care. In obstetric cases, the primary reason for admission to the hospital involves labor and delivery. Therefore, codes from the fourth and fifth section of Chapter 11 generally receive precedence in sequencing and reporting.

In reporting inpatient obstetric care, the more generic codes should be sequenced before the more specific codes. For example, multiple gestation or breech presentation represent diagnostic entities that direct the overall care and treatment of the obstetric patient. Perineal laceration or retained placenta represent diagnostic entities of lesser significance in this episode of care, and consequently should receive a lower sequencing priority. Medical antepartum complications such as diabetes or anemia should be coded, but reported with less priority than current active conditions affecting labor and delivery. An exception would occur if life-threatening complications such as renal failure were diagnosed.

The principal procedure reported in obstetric cases should be the procedure most closely associated with the delivery. Procedures ancillary to delivery should be coded and reported secondarily. The clinical significance of the procedures rendered should determine their sequencing for reporting purposes.

Insurance claim regulations ordinarily mandate the coding and reporting of only diagnoses specifically assessed or treated during the admission, encounter, or episode of care. Physicians rendering care and treatment throughout the antepartum, intrapartum, and postpartum periods should code and report all diagnoses and procedures managed during that interval. Healthcare facilities, however, should code and report only those diagnoses or procedures managed during the period of confinement.

Although most obstetric cases are not affected by the prospective payment system, designated ICD-9-CM codes are recognized as comorbidities by certain third-party payors, especially Medicare. For inpatient admissions, these comorbid conditions may increase the amount of reimbursement received by the provider. Comorbidities among the listed obstetric conditions are represented by the following ICD-9-CM code numbers:

634.00	634.01	634.02
634.10	634.11	634.12
634.20	634.21	634.22
634.30	634.31	634.32
634.40	634.41	634.42
634.50	634.51	634.52
634.60	634.61	634.62
634.70	634.71	634.72
634.80	634.81	634.82
634.90	634.91	634.92
639.0	639.1	639.2
639.3	639.4	639.5
639.6	639.8	639.9
640.00	640.01	640.03

640.80	640.81	640.83
640.90	640.91	640.93
641.00	641.01	641.03
641.10	641.11	641.13
641.30	641.31	641.33
641.80	641.81	641.83
641.90	641.91	641.93
642.40	642.41	642.42
642.43	642.44	642.50
642.51	642.52	642.53
642.54	642.60	642.61
642.62	642.63	642.64
642.70	642.71	642.72
642.73	642.74	644.00
644.03	644.10	644.13
646.60	646.61	646.62
646.63	646.64	646.70
646.71	646.73	647.30
647.31	647.32	647.33
647.34	647.40	647.41
647.42	647.43	647.44
648.00	648.01	648.02
648.03	648.04	648.20
648.21	648.22	648.23
648.24	648.30	648.31
648.32	648.33	648.34
648.50	648.51	648.52
648.53	648.54	648.60
648.61	648.62	648.63
648.64	659.30	659.31
659.33	665.00	665.01
665.03	665.10	665.11
666.32	666.34	668.00
668.01	668.02	668.03
668.04	668.10	668.11
668.12	668.13	668.14
668.20	668.21	668.22
668.23	668.24	668.80
668.81	668.82	668.83
668.84	668.90	668.91
668.92	668.93	668.94
669.10	669.11	669.12
669.13	669.14	669.30
669.32	669.34	670.00
670.00	670.02	670.04
671.20	671.21	671.22
671.23	671.24	671.30
671.31	671.33	671.40

671.42	671.44	673.00
673.01	673.02	673.03
673.04	673.10	673.11
673.12	673.13	673.14
673.20	673.21	673.22
673.23	673.24	673.30
673.31	673.32	673.33
673.34	673.80	673.81
673.82	673.83	673.84
674.00	674.01	674.02
674.03	674.04	674.10
674.12	674.20	674.22
674.24	675.10	675.11
675.12		

Most procedures involving delivery are performed in the labor room or in a birthing center. However, certain obstetrical procedures are designated under the prospective payment system as valid operating room procedures. The following ICD-9-CM code numbers represent obstetrical procedures that may be reported with operating room charges:

73.94	73.99	74.0
74.1	74.2	74.3
74.4	74.91	74.99
75.36	75.50	75.51
75.52	75.61	75.93
75.99		

TABLE 8–2

Diagnosis Related Groups for Pregnancy, Childbirth, and the Puerperium

DRG 370, Cesarean Section with Comorbidity or Complication

DRG 371, Cesarean Section without Comorbidity or Complication

DRG 372, Vaginal Delivery with Complicating Diagnoses

DRG 373, Vaginal Delivery without Complicating Diagnoses

DRG 374, Vaginal Delivery with Sterilization and/or Dilatation and Curettage

DRG 375, Vaginal Delivery with Operating Room Procedure except Sterilization and/or Dilatation and Curettage

DRG 376, Postpartum and Postabortion Diagnoses without Operating Room Procedure

DRG 377, Postpartum and Postabortion Diagnoses with Operating Room Procedure

DRG 378, Ectopic Pregnancy

DRG 379, Threatened Abortion

DRG 380, Abortion with Dilatation and Curettage

DRG 381, Abortion with Dilatation and Curettage, Aspiration Curettage, or Hysterotomy

DRG 382, False Labor

DRG 383, Other Antepartum Diagnoses with Medical Complications

DRG 384, Other Antepartum Diagnoses without Medical Complications

Reporting code numbers for nonspecific or unspecified obstetrical diagnoses or procedures indicates deficient documentation and should be avoided. The personnel responsible for coding and billing should attempt to determine the most specific code not only for reimbursement purposes but also to facilitate useful data for statistical and research purposes. Accurate, precise, complete, and timely documentation in the obstetric patient record may alleviate the necessity of reporting codes for nonspecific or unspecified obstetrical diagnoses and procedures.

Although infrequently utilized, obstetric conditions are classified into a major diagnostic category under the prospective payment system. The DRG's associated with pregnancy and delivery are distributed into MDC 14, Pregnancy, Childbirth, and the Puerperium (Table 8–2).

NEONATOLOGY AND PERINATOLOGY REPORTING FOR BILLING

As discussed in the preceding section, the principal diagnosis is defined as the condition responsible for the admission of the patient to the health service admission, encounter, or episode of care. Similarly, the principal procedure is the procedure most closely associated with the principal diagnosis for that specific admission, encounter, or episode of care.

Often newborns in intensive care units may be diagnosed with several concurrent congenital conditions and may endure more than one surgical procedure. Usually, the diagnosis or procedure presenting the greatest health risk to the newborn is sequenced as the principal diagnosis or as the principal procedure.

If the risk posed by two or more simultaneously existing conditions or operations is clinically equivalent, for reporting purposes, the most resource intensive diagnosis or procedure may be sequenced as the principal. Exceptions to this guideline for the sequencing of a principal procedure may occur if complications developed during the neonatal or perinatal period, and these complications necessitated surgical operations that were not expressly stated in the original care and treatment plan. All secondary diagnoses and additional procedures should be sequenced in descending order of clinical significance and resource intensity.

Notwithstanding that most neonatal and perinatal care is not subject to the regulations of the prospective payment system, specific ICD-9-CM codes are designated as comorbidities by particular third-party payors, especially Medicare. For inpatient admissions, these comorbid conditions may increase the amount of reimbursement received by the provider. Comorbidities among the listed perinatal conditions are represented by the following ICD-9-CM code numbers:

741.00	741.02	741.03
741.90	741.92	741.93
745.0	745.10	745.11
745.12	745.19	745.2
745.3	745.4	745.60
745.69	745.7	746.01
746.02	746.1	746.2
746.3	746.4	746.5
746.6	746.7	746.81
746.82	746.83	746.84
746.86	747.11	747.22
748.4	748.5	748.61
765.01	765.02	765.03
765.04	765.05	765.06
765.07	765.08	767.0

T A B L E   8–3

Diagnosis Related Groups for Neonatal and Perinatal Conditions

DRG 385, Neonates, Died or Transferred to Another Acute Care Facility

DRG 386, Extreme Immaturity or Respiratory Distress Syndrome of Neonate

DRG 387, Prematurity with Major Problems

DRG 388, Prematurity without Major Problems

DRG 389, Full Term Neonate with Major Problems

DRG 390, Neonate with Other Significant Problems

DRG 391, Normal Newborn

768.5	769	770.0
770.1	770.2	770.3
770.4	770.5	770.7
771.0	771.1	771.3
771.8	772.1	772.2
772.4	772.5	773.0
773.1	773.2	773.3
773.4	774.0	774.1
774.2	774.30	774.31
774.39	774.4	774.5
774.7	775.1	775.2
775.3	775.4	775.5
775.6	775.7	776.0
776.1	776.2	776.3
777.1	777.2	777.5
777.6	778.0	779.0
779.1	779.3	779.4

The reporting of code numbers for unspecified or nonspecific neonatal or perinatal diagnoses or procedures should be avoided, if possible. Staff members responsible for coding and billing should attempt to report the most specific code, not only for reimbursement purposes, but also to generate meaningful data for statistical and research purposes. Adequate and timely documentation in the newborn patient record may preclude the need to report codes for unspecified or nonspecific neonatal or perinatal diagnoses and procedures.

Certain neonatal and perinatal conditions are grouped into a specific major diagnostic category under the prospective payment system. The DRG's associated with neonatal or perinatal conditions are distributed into MDC 15, Newborns and Other Neonates with Conditions Originating in the Perinatal Period (Table 8–3).

KEY CONCEPTS

acquired condition _____	congenital condition _____
anomaly _____	diagnosis related groups _____
antepartum period _____	labor and delivery _____
comorbidity _____	major diagnostic category _____
complication _____	neonatal period _____

nonspecific diagnosis _____

perinatal period _____

postpartum period _____

principal diagnosis _____

principal procedure _____

prospective payment system _____

puerperium _____

subclassification _____

unspecified diagnosis _____

REVIEW QUESTIONS

1. Describe the purpose of the fifth-digit subclassification for the coding of obstetric conditions.

   _____

   _____

2. Explain the purpose of the outcome of delivery codes. _____

   _____

   _____

3. Describe the purpose of the fourth-digit subclassification for the newborn codes. _____

   _____

   _____

4. Explain the distinction provided in the ICD-9-CM classification system between the coding of congenital conditions and the coding of acquired conditions. _____

   _____

   _____

5. Assign precise, accurate code numbers from the ICD-9-CM volume for the following complications of pregnancy, childbirth, and the puerperium:

   A. vesticular mole _____

   _____

   B. blighted ovum _____

   C. antepartum icterus gravis _____

   _____

   D. ovarian pregnancy _____

   E. miscarriage complicated by shock _____

   _____

   F. antepartum condition of mentum presentation _____

   _____

   G. antepartum toxemia with convulsions _____

   _____

   H. post term pregnancy delivered _____

   _____

   I. mild antepartum hyperemesis gravidarum _____

   _____

   J. blood clot embolism following miscarriage _____

   _____

   K. antepartum cephalopelvic disproportion _____

   _____

   L. ablatio placentae _____

   _____

M.   mild preeclampsia with preexisting hypertension _____

N.   unstable lie malposition at delivery _____

O.   false labor _____

P.   prolonged pregnancy _____

Q.   asymptomatic postpartum bacteriuria in pregnancy _____

R.   rubeola during pregnancy _____

S.   anemia during pregnancy _____

T.   normal spontaneous delivery _____

U.   triplet pregnancy delivered _____

V.   breech delivery _____

W.   conjoined twins causing disproportion _____

X.   rigid cervix _____

Y.   suspected damage to fetus from maternal rubella _____

Z.   fetal acidemia _____

AA. hydramnios _____

BB. amnionitis _____

CC. delivery by elderly primigravida _____

DD. failed trial of labor _____

EE. arrested active phase of labor _____

FF. prolonged second stage of labor _____

GG. know in umbilical cord _____

HH. first degree perineal laceration involving the labia _____

II. inversion of the uterus _____

JJ. postpartum afibrinogenemia _____

KK. retained portion of placenta without hemorrhage _____

LL. Mendelson's syndrome following sedation in delivery _____

MM. obstetric shock following delivery _____

NN. puerperal pyemia following delivery _____

OO. varicose veins of legs during pregnancy _____

PP. puerperal pyrexia _____

QQ. obstetrical blood clot embolism _____

RR. placental polyp _____

SS. lymphangitis of breast _____

TT. agalactia _____

UU. intraperitoneal pregnancy _____

VV. antepartum fetal disproportion _____

WW. bruising of umbilical cord _____

XX. amniotic fluid embolism _____

6. Indicate which of the diagnostic entities in the preceding exercise are subject to the guidelines for the fifth-digit subclassification, and indicate which of the available fifth-digits are not applicable to the diagnostic entities that require expansion to the five-digit rubric.

	Fifth-Digit Required **Yes** or **No**	Applicable Fifth-Digits If Required
A.	_____	_____
B.	_____	_____
C.	_____	_____
D.	_____	_____
E.	_____	_____
F.	_____	_____
G.	_____	_____
H.	_____	_____
I.	_____	_____
J.	_____	_____
K.	_____	_____
L.	_____	_____
M.	_____	_____
N.	_____	_____

O.   _____   _____
P.   _____   _____
Q.   _____   _____
R.   _____   _____
S.   _____   _____
T.   _____   _____
U.   _____   _____
V.   _____   _____
W.   _____   _____
X.   _____   _____
Y.   _____   _____
Z.   _____   _____
AA.   _____   _____
BB.   _____   _____
CC.   _____   _____
DD.   _____   _____
EE.   _____   _____
FF.   _____   _____
GG.   _____   _____
HH.   _____   _____
II.   _____   _____
JJ.   _____   _____
KK.   _____   _____
LL.   _____   _____
MM.   _____   _____
NN.   _____   _____
OO.   _____   _____
PP.   _____   _____
QQ.   _____   _____
RR.   _____   _____
SS.   _____   _____
TT.   _____   _____
UU.   _____   _____
VV.   _____   _____
WW.   _____   _____
XX.   _____   _____

7. Assign precise, accurate code numbers from the ICD-9-CM volume for the following obstetrical procedures:

A. repair of current obstetric laceration of cervix _____
_____

B. classical cesarean section _____
_____

C. application of forceps without delivery _____
_____

D. forceps rotation of fetal head _____
_____

E. induction by cervical dilation _____
_____

F. vaginal cesarean section _____

_____

G. Piper forceps operation _____

_____

H. obstetrical hysterotomy _____

_____

I. low forceps operation with episiotomy _____

_____

J. episioproctotomy _____

_____

K. low cervical cesarean section _____

_____

L. repair of current obstetric laceration of bladder and urethra _____

_____

M. obstetric tamponade of vagina _____

_____

N. supravesical cesarean section _____

_____

O. clavicotomy on fetus _____

_____

P. total breech extraction with forceps to after coming head _____

_____

Q. mid forceps operation with episiotomy _____

_____

R. replacement of prolapsed umbilical cord _____

_____

S. lower uterine segment cesarean section _____

_____

T. fetal blood sampling and biopsy _____

_____

U. medical induction of labor _____

_____

V. removal of ectopic abdominal pregnancy _____

_____

W. unspecified instrumental delivery _____

_____

X. manual removal of retained placenta _____

_____

Y. induction by cervical dilation _____

_____

8. Assign precise, accurate code numbers from the ICD-9-CM volume for the following congenital anomalies:

A. craniorachischisis _____

_____

B. Arnold-Chiari syndrome type II _____

_____

C. congenital cerebral cyst _____

_____

D. congenital glaucoma _____

E. cervical auricle _____

F. congenital aortic stenosis _____

G. endocardial cushion defect _____

H. interruption of aortic arch _____

I. congenital bronchiectasis _____

J. cleft palate with cleft lip _____

K. absence of salivary gland _____

L. ectopic anus _____

M. imperforate hymen _____

N. congenital displaced kidney _____

O. talipes varus _____

P. congenital deformity of clavicle _____

Q. osteopoikilosis _____

R. congenital ectodermal dysplasia _____

S. Klinefelter's syndrome _____

T. absent parathyroid gland _____

U. inencephaly _____

V. hydromyelocele _____

W. jaw-winking syndrome _____

X. aniridia _____

Y. microcheilia _____

9. Assign precise, accurate code numbers from the ICD-9-CM volume for the following conditions originating in the neonatal or perinatal period:

A. fetus affected by surgical operation on mother _____

B. triplet gestation _____

C. vasa previa of umbilical cord _____

D. breech delivery affecting newborn _____

E. fetal growth retardation _____

F. extreme immaturity _____

G. exceptionally large baby _____

H. caput succedaneum _____

I. fetal death from anoxia during labor _____

J. pulmonary hypoperfusion syndrome _____

K. Wilson-Mikity syndrome _____

L. ophthalmia neonatorum _____

M. superficial hematoma in newborn _____

N. hydrops fetalis due to isoimmunization _____

O. bilirubin encephalopathy _____

P. neonatal myasthenia gravis _____

Q. isoimmune neutropenia _____

R. meconium peritonitis _____

S. edema neonatorum _____

T. regurgitation of food in newborn _____

U. fetal alcohol syndrome _____

V. abruptio placentae affecting fetus _____

W. newborn affected by precipitate delivery _____

X. congenital rubella _____

Y. neonatal jaundice due to delayed conjunction _____

9

ICD Coding: Integumentary System and Musculoskeletal System Diseases and Operations

LEARNING OBJECTIVES

Upon completion of this chapter the learner should be able to:

1. Describe the parameters for coding and reporting degenerative joint disease.
2. Explain the distinction between a congenital condition and an acquired condition.
3. Explain the distinction between an old injury and a current injury.
4. Describe the parameters for coding and reporting the internal derangement of a joint.
5. Discuss the impact of comorbidities and complications on billing and reimbursement for diagnoses involving the integumentary system.
6. Discuss the impact of comorbidities and complications on billing and reimbursement for diagnoses involving the musculoskeletal system.
7. Apply knowledge of coding principles by assigning accurate and precise codes to report diagnoses and procedures pertaining to the integumentary system.
8. Apply knowledge of coding principles by assigning accurate and precise codes to report diagnoses and procedures pertaining to the musculoskeletal system.

ICD CODING OF INTEGUMENTARY SYSTEM DISEASES AND OPERATIONS

Chapter 12 of the ICD-9-CM diagnostic tabular volume is designated for listings of integumentary system diagnoses, and largely consists of non-traumatic conditions affecting this body system. The skin and subcutaneous tissue disease chapter consists of three sections (Table 9–1).

The first section of Chapter 12 contains listings for infections of the skin and subcutaneous tissue. This section excludes the reporting of skin infections classified in Chapter 1 of the diagnostic tabular. Among the listings encompassed in this section are: carbuncle and furuncle; cellulitis and abscess of the skin and subcutaneous tissue; acute lymphadenitis; impetigo; and pilonidal cyst or pilonidal fistula. An additional code should be reported to identify any infectious organism associated with a skin condition.

TABLE 9–1

Sections in Chapter 12, Volume 1 of ICD-9-CM

1. Infections of Skin and Subcutaneous Tissue (category range 680–686)
2. Other Inflammatory Conditions of Skin and Subcutaneous Tissue (category range 690–698)
3. Other Diseases of Skin and Subcutaneous Tissue (category range 700–709)

The second section of this chapter includes listings for other inflammatory conditions of the skin and subcutaneous tissue. The listings in this section encompass: erythematosquamous dermatosis; atopic dermatitis and related conditions; contact dermatitis and other eczema; dermatitis due to substances taken internally; bullous dermatoses; erythematous conditions; psoriasis and similar disorders; lichen; pruritus; and related conditions.

The third section of Chapter 12 is comprised of listings for other diseases of the skin and subcutaneous tissue. This section excludes both the reporting of congenital conditions as well as conditions confined to the eyelids, but encompasses varied other entities. These listings include: corns and callosities; hypertrophic and atrophic conditions of the skin and other dermatoses; diseases of the nail; diseases of the hair and hair follicles; disorders of the sweat glands; diseases of the sebaceous glands; chronic ulcer of the skin (excluding gangrene and infections); and urticaria.

Categories of listings in Chapter 15 of Volume 3 of ICD-9-CM are established for integumentary system procedures. These include the listings in categories 85 and 86 for: operations on the breast (including procedures on the male breast or previous mastectomy site), and operations on the skin and subcutaneous tissue (encompassing procedures on hair, nails, sweat glands, and so forth). These listings exclude the reporting of procedures on the skin of the anus, breast, ear, eyebrow, eyelids, lips, nose, penis, scrotum, or vulva. Many of these procedures, however, are rendered as a consequence of traumatic injuries to the integumentary system. The coding and reporting of traumatic injuries is explained in Chapter 11.

ICD CODING OF MUSCULOSKELETAL SYSTEM DISEASES AND OPERATIONS

Chapter 13 of the ICD-9-CM diagnostic tabular volume, designated for listings of musculoskeletal system diagnoses, also consists mostly of non-traumatic conditions affecting the bones, joints, and associated structures. The musculoskeletal system and connective tissue disease chapter consists of four sections (Table 9–2).

The first section of Chapter 13 is comprised of listings for arthropathies and related disorders. This section excludes the reporting of disorders of the spine. Among the listings encompassed in this section are: diffuse diseases of connective tissue such as collagen diseases;

TABLE 9–2

Sections in Chapter 13, Volume 1 of ICD-9-CM

1. Arthropathies and Related Disorders (category range 710–719)
2. Dorsopathies (category range 720–724)
3. Rheumatism, Excluding the Back (category range 725–729)
4. Osteopathies, Chondropathies, and Acquired Musculoskeletal Deformities (category range 730–739)

arthropathy associated with infections; crystal arthopathies; arthropathy associated with disorders classified elsewhere; and rheumatoid arthritis as well as other inflammatory arthropathies. The underlying disease or manifestation should be coded and reported with all arthropathies as applicable.

This section of listings for arthropathies and allied disorders also includes: osteoarthrosis and related disorders such as hypertrophic arthritis, polyarthritis, degenerative joint disease, and osteoarthritis; internal derangement of the knee; and other derangement of a joint. In general, bilateral joint involvement of the same anatomic site should be coded and reported with a single diagnostic code, but bilateral joint procedures on the same anatomic structures should be coded and reported with two codes (by repeating the same appropriate code).

The second section of the musculoskeletal system chapter in the diagnostic tabular contains listings for dorsopathies, but excludes the reporting of curvature of the spine. The listings in this section include: ankylosing spondylitis and other inflammatory spondylopathies; spondylosis and related disorders; intervertebral disc disorders; and certain other disorders of the cervical region and the back.

The third section of Chapter 13 is comprised of listings for rheumatism. These listings include disorders of muscles and tendons and their attachments such as polymyalgia rheumatica, as well as peripheral enthesopathies and allied syndromes, and disorders of peripheral ligamentous attachments. This section also includes listings for other disorders of the synovium, tendon, bursa, muscle, ligament, fascia, and soft tissues.

The fourth section of the musculoskeletal system chapter in the diagnostic tabular includes listings for osteopathies, chondropathies, and acquired musculoskeletal deformities. Among the listings of this section are: osteomyelitis, periostitis, and other infections involving bone; osteitis deformans and osteopathies associated with disorders classified elsewhere; osteochrondropathies and other disorders of bone and cartilage; flat foot and acquired deformities of the toe and limbs; curvature of spine and other deformities; as well as nonallopathic lesions encompassing segmental dysfunction and somatic dysfunction.

The listings of this final section of Chapter 13 exclude the reporting of congenital deformities and curvatures. Congenital conditions should be coded and reported with the listings contained within Chapter 14 of Volume 1. If applicable, an additional code should be reported to identify any infectious organism or any underlying disease associated with the documented osteopathy, chrondropathy, or musculoskeletal deformity.

Categories of listings in Chapter 14 of Volume 3 of ICD-9-CM are established for musculoskeletal system and connective tissue procedures. These include category range 76–84 for: operations on skull bones, facial bones, and related joints; incision, excision, and division of other bones; reduction of fracture and reduction of dislocation with or without cast or splint application and with or without internal fixation; incision and excision of joint structures; repair and plastic operations on joint structures; operations on muscle, fascia, tendon, or bursa; as well as certain other procedures on the musculoskeletal system and connective tissue. Many of these procedures, however, are rendered as a consequence of traumatic injuries to the musculoskeletal system. The coding and reporting of traumatic injuries is explained in Chapter 11.

DERMATOLOGY REPORTING FOR BILLING

As a general guideline, the principal diagnosis is that condition responsible for the admission of the patient for the health service admission, encounter, or episode of care. And similarly, the principal procedure is the procedure most closely associated with the patient's principal diagnosis for that specific admission, encounter, or episode of care.

Usually, the diagnosis or procedure posing the greatest risk to the patient is the most resource intensive diagnosis or procedure, and thus receives sequencing priority. For example, care and treatment rendered for a diagnosis of cellulitis would surpass the care and treatment rendered for a concurrent diagnosis of dermatitis. Therefore, if both conditions were documented as active problems in the patient health record, the code for the cellulitis should have sequencing priority over the code for the dermatitis.

However, under exceptional circumstances, especially those involving a hospitalized patient, the most resource intensive diagnosis or procedure or the diagnosis or procedure presenting the greatest risk to the patient may be unrelated to that patient's principal diagnosis for that episode of inpatient service. Such a situation could occur if a patient was admitted for a relatively minor problem and major complications occurred unexpectedly. For instance, a patient who was admitted for treatment of a skin ulcer might suddenly develop a serious infection or gangrene. Although complications and even life-threatening comorbidities might emerge, the principal diagnosis is that condition which originally necessitated the patient admission.

Insurance claim regulations ordinarily direct the reporting of only those diagnoses that are specifically assessed or treated during the admission, encounter, or episode of care. Secondary diagnoses should be reported in descending order of clinical significance and resource intensity. Likewise, secondary procedures should be reported in the same manner. For example, the code for a full-thickness skin graft should be sequenced before the code for suturing.

Designated ICD-9-CM codes are recognized as comorbidities by certain third-party payors such as Medicare. For inpatient admissions, these comorbid conditions may increase the amount of reimbursement received by the healthcare provider. Comorbidities among the integumentary system conditions are represented by the following ICD-9-CM code numbers:

680.0	680.1	680.2
680.3	680.4	680.5
680.6	680.7	680.8
680.9	682.0	682.1
682.2	682.3	682.5
682.6	682.7	682.8
682.9	684	685.0
694.4	694.5	695.0
696.0	707.0	707.1

The reporting of code numbers for nonspecific and unspecified integumentary system diagnoses and dermatological procedures should be avoided, if possible. Personnel responsible for coding and billing should attempt to determine the most specific code not only for reimbursement purposes but also to generate meaningful data for statistical research purposes. Accurate, precise, complete, and timely documentation in the patient health record may alleviate the necessity of reporting codes for such nonspecific or unspecified diagnoses and procedures.

The DRG's associated with integumentary system diseases and disorders are assigned to MDC 9, Diseases and Disorders of the Skin, Subcutaneous Tissue, and Breast (Table 9–3). Although the diagnostic tabular of ICD-9-CM classifies breast disorders within the diseases of the female genitourinary system, the procedural tabular of ICD-9-CM classifies breast operations with those of the skin and subcutaneous tissue. The prospective payment system

T A B L E   9–3

Diagnosis Related Groups for Diseases and Disorders of the Skin, Subcutaneous Tissue, and Breast

DRG 261, Breast Procedure for Nonmalignancy except Biopsy and Local Excision

DRG 262, Breast Biopsy and Local Excision for Nonmalignancy

DRG 263, Skin Graft and/or Debridement for Skin Ulcer or Cellulitis with Comorbidity or Complication

DRG 264, Skin Graft and/or Debridement for Skin Ulcer or Cellulitis without Comorbidity or Complication

DRG 265, Skin Graft and/or Debridement except for Skin Ulcer or Cellulitis with Comorbidity or Complication

DRG 266, Skin Graft and/or Debridement except for Skin Ulcer or Cellulitis without Comorbidity or Complication

DRG 267, Perianal and Pilonidal Procedures

DRG 268, Skin, Subcutaneous Tissue, and Breast Plastic Procedures

DRG 269, Other Skin, Subcutaneous Tissue, and Breast Procedures with Comorbidity or Complication

DRG 270, Other Skin, Subcutaneous Tissue, and Breast Procedures without Comorbidity or Complication

DRG 271, Skin Ulcers

DRG 272, Major Skin Disorders with Comorbidity or Complication

DRG 273, Major Skin Disorders without Comorbidity or Complication

DRG 276, Nonmalignant Breast Disorders

DRG 277, Cellulitis, Age Greater than 17 with Comorbidity or Complication

DRG 278, Cellulitis, Age Greater than 17 without Comorbidity or Complication

DRG 279, Cellulitis, Age 0–17

DRG 280, Trauma to Skin, Subcutaneous Tissue, and Breast, Age Greater than 17 with Comorbidity or Complication

DRG 281, Trauma to Skin, Subcutaneous Tissue, and Breast, Age Greater than 17 without Comorbidity or Complication

DRG 282, Trauma to Skin, Subcutaneous Tissue, and Breast, Age 0–17

DRG 283, Minor Skin Disorders with Comorbidity or Complication

DRG 284, Minor Skin Disorders without Comorbidity or Complication

also distributes breast disorders and operations into a major category along with disorders and operations of the integumentary system.

RHEUMATOLOGY REPORTING FOR BILLING

As guidelines for all clinical services, the principal diagnosis is the condition responsible for the admission of the patient for the health service encounter or episode of care; and the principal procedure is the procedure most closely associated with the patient's principal diagnosis for that specific encounter or episode of care.

In the case of two or more concurrent diagnoses, the diagnosis that involves the most resource intensive care and treatment may be sequenced as the principal diagnosis. For instance, the code for a diagnosis of acute osteomyelitis should precede the code for a concurrent diagnosis of degenerative arthritis.

Under exceptional circumstances, especially those involving a hospitalized patient, the most resource intensive diagnosis or the diagnosis presenting the greatest risk to the patient may be unrelated to that patient's principal diagnosis for the reported episode of inpatient care. Such a situation could occur if a patient was admitted for a treatment of chronic problem (such as a bunionectomy for hallux valgus) and major complications occurred unexpectedly (such as a herniated lumbar disk treated with intervertebral chemonucleolysis).

Insurance claim regulations ordinarily mandate the coding and reporting of only diagnoses that are specifically assessed or treated during the admission, encounter, or episode of care. Secondary diagnoses should be sequenced in descending order of clinical significance and resource intensity. Thus, the code for an acute bursitis condition should be sequenced before the code for a chronic synovitis condition.

Specific ICD-9-CM codes are recognized and designated as comorbidities by certain third-party payors, especially Medicare under the prospective payment system. For inpatient admissions, these comorbid conditions may increase the amount of reimbursement received by the healthcare provider. Comorbidities among the musculoskeletal system conditions are represented by the following ICD-9-CM code numbers:

710.0	710.3	710.4
710.5	710.8	711.00
711.01	711.02	711.03
711.04	711.05	711.06
711.07	711.08	711.09
711.60	711.61	711.62
711.63	711.64	711.65
711.66	711.67	711.68
711.69	714.1	714.2
714.30	714.31	714.32
714.33	722.80	722.81
722.82	722.83	723.4
723.5	728.0	730.00
730.01	730.02	730.03
730.04	730.05	730.06
730.07	730.08	730.09
730.80	730.83	730.84
730.85	730.86	730.87
730.88	730.89	730.90
730.91	730.92	730.93
730.94	730.95	730.96
730.97	730.98	730.99
733.10	733.11	733.12
733.13	733.14	733.15
733.16	733.19	733.81
733.82		

Reporting code numbers for unspecified or nonspecific musculoskeletal system diagnoses or rheumatological procedures should be avoided, if possible. Staff members responsible for coding and billing should attempt to ascertain the most specific code, not only for reimbursement purposes, but also to generate meaningful data for statistical and research purposes. Accurate, complete, adequate, and timely documentation in the patient health record may alleviate the necessity of reporting codes for unspecified or nonspecific diagnoses and procedures.

Several nonoperating room procedures listed among the operations on the integumentary system impact reimbursement under the prospective payment system. The following codes from Chapter 14 of Volume 3 of ICD-9-CM represent nonoperative procedures that affect DRG assignment:

86.07   86.09   86.3

The DRG's associated with musculoskeletal system diseases and disorders are assigned to a specific major diagnostic category, MDC 8, Diseases and Disorders of the Musculoskeletal System and Connective Tissue (Table 9–4).

T A B L E 9–4

Diagnosis Related Groups for Diseases and Disorders of the Musculoskeletal System and Connective Tissue

DRG 209, Major Joint and Limb Reattachment Procedures of Lower Extremity

DRG 210, Hip and Femur Procedures except Major Joint Procedures, Age Greater than 17 with Comorbidity or Complication

DRG 211, Hip and Femur Procedures except Major Joint Procedures, Age Greater than 17 without Comorbidity or Complication

DRG 212, Hip and Femur Procedures except Major Joint Procedures, Age 0–17

DRG 213, Amputation for Musculoskeletal System and Connective Tissue Disorders

DRG 214, Back and Neck Procedures with Comorbidity or Complication

DRG 215, Back and Neck Procedures without Comorbidity or Complication

DRG 216, Biopsies of Musculoskeletal System and Connective Tissue

DRG 217, Wound Debridement and Skin Graft except Hand for Musculoskeletal and Connective Tissue Disorders

DRG 218, Lower Extremity and Humerus Procedures except Hip, Foot, and Femur, Age Greater than 17 with Comorbidity or Complication

DRG 219, Lower Extremity and Humerus Procedures except Hip, Foot, and Femur, Age Greater than 17 without Comorbidity or Complication

DRG 220, Lower Extremity and Humerus Procedures except Hip, Foot, and Femur, Age 0–17

DRG 221, Knee Procedures with Comorbidity or Complication

DRG 222, Knee Procedures without Comorbidity or Complication

DRG 223, Major Shoulder/Elbow Procedures or Other Upper Extremity Procedures with Comorbidity or Complication

DRG 224, Shoulder, Elbow, or Forearm Procedures except Major Joint Procedures without Comorbidity or Complication

DRG 225, Foot Procedures

DRG 226, Soft Tissue Procedures with Comorbidity or Complication

DRG 227, Soft Tissue Procedures without Comorbidity or Complication

DRG 228, Major Thumb or Joint Procedures or Other Hand or Wrist Procedures with Comorbidity or Complication

DRG 229, Hand or Wrist Procedures except Major Joint Procedures without Comorbidity or Complication

DRG 230, Local Excision and Removal of Internal Fixation Devices of Hip and Femur

DRG 231, Local Excision and Removal of Internal Fixation Devices except Hip and Femur

DRG 232, Arthroscopy

DRG 233, Other Musculoskeletal System and Connective Tissue Operating Room Procedures with Comorbidity or Complication

DRG 234, Other Musculoskeletal System and Connective Tissue Operating Room Procedures without Comorbidity or Complication

DRG 235, Fractures of Femur

DRG 236, Fractures of Hip and Pelvis

T A B L E   9–4

Diagnosis Related Groups for Diseases and Disorders of the Muscuoloskeletal System and Connective Tissue—cont'd

DRG 237, Sprains, Strains, and Dislocations of Hip, Pelvis, and Thigh

DRG 238, Osteomyelitis

DRG 240, Connective Tissue Disorders with Comorbidity or Complication

DRG 241, Connective Tissue Disorders without Comorbidity or Complication

DRG 242, Septic Arthritis

DRG 243, Medical Back Problems

DRG 244, Bone Diseases and Specific Arthropathies with Comorbidity or Complication

DRG 245, Bone Diseases and Specific Arthropathies without Comorbidity or Complication

DRG 246, Nonspecific Arthropathies

DRG 247, Signs and Symptoms of Musculoskeletal System and Connective Tissue

DRG 248, Tendonitis, Myositis, and Bursitis

DRG 249, Aftercare, Musculoskeletal System and Connective Tissue

DRG 250, Fractures, Sprains, Strains, and Dislocations of Forearm, Hand, and Foot, Age Greater than 17 with Comorbidity or Complication

DRG 251, Fractures, Sprains, Strains, and Dislocations of Forearm, Hand, and Foot, Age Greater than 17 without Comorbidity or Complication

DRG 252, Fractures, Sprains, Strains, and Dislocations of Forearm, Hand, and Foot, Age 0–17

DRG 253, Fractures, Sprains, Strains, and Dislocations of Upper Arm and Lower Leg except Foot, Age Greater than 17 with Comorbidity or Complication

DRG 254, Fractures, Sprains, Strains, and Dislocations of Upper Arm and Lower Leg except Foot, Age Greater than 17 without Comorbidity or Complication

DRG 255, Fractures, Sprains, Strains, and Dislocations of Upper Arm and Lower Leg except Foot, Age 0–17

DRG 256, Other Musculoskeletal System and Connective Tissue Diagnoses

DRG 471, Bilateral or Multiple Major Joint Procedures of Lower Extremity

DRG 491, Major Joint and Limb Reattachment Procedures of Upper Extremity

K E Y   C O N C E P T S

acquired condition _____

comorbidity _____

complication _____

congenital condition _____

current injury _____

diagnosis related groups _____

major diagnostic category _____

manifestation _____

nonoperative procedure _____

nonspecific diagnosis _____

nontraumatic condition _____

old injury _____

principal diagnosis _____

principal procedure _____

traumatic condition _____

underlying disease _____

unspecified diagnosis _____

R E V I E W   Q U E S T I O N S

1. Differentiate traumatic conditions of the integumentary system and the musculoskeletal system from non-traumatic conditions of the same body systems. _____

_____

_____

2. Explain the distinction provided in the ICD-9-CM classification system between the coding of current orthopedic injuries and the coding of old orthopedic injuries. _____

_____

_____

3. Describe the purpose of the fifth-digit subclassification for the coding of degenerative joint disease. _____

_____

_____

4. Identify at least five codes and narrative titles that represent integumentary system conditions which are recognized by Medicare as complications or comorbidities.

_____   _____

_____   _____

_____   _____

_____   _____

_____   _____

_____   _____

5. Identify at least five codes and narrative titles that represent musculoskeletal system conditions which are recognized by Medicare as complications or comorbidities.

_____   _____

_____   _____

_____   _____

_____   _____

_____   _____

6. Assign precise, accurate code numbers from the ICD-9-CM volume for the following diseases of the skin and subcutaneous tissue:

A.   carbuncle of the ankle _____

_____

B.   panaritium of toe _____

_____

C.   acute lymphangitis _____

_____

D.   acute adenitis _____

_____

E.   bullous impetigo of the eyelid _____

_____

F.   pilonidal cyst with abscess _____

_____

G.   purulent dermatitis _____

_____

H.   dandruff _____

_____

I.   diaper rash _____

_____

J.   contact dermatitis due to detergents _____

_____

K.   dermatitis due to milk _____

_____

L. Sneddon-Wilkinson syndrome _____

M. Ritter's disease _____

N. acrodermatitis continua _____

O. ruber planus lichen _____

P. Hyde's disease _____

Q. callus _____

R. keratosis nigricans _____

S. senile keratoma _____

T. onycholysis _____

U. polytrichia _____

V. granulosis rubra nasi _____

W. xerosis cutis _____

X. chronic ulcer of skin _____

Y. idiopathic urticaria _____

Z. vesicular eruption _____

AA. furuncle of the shoulder _____

BB. abscess of the axilla _____

CC. cellulitis of the ankle _____

DD. Besnier's prurigo _____

EE. allergic dermatitis due to phenols _____

FF. dermatitis due to eating unspecified substance _____

GG. juvenile pemphigoid _____

HH. Lyell's syndrome _____

II. Devergie's disease _____

JJ. lichen _____

KK. winter itch _____

LL. cutis laxa senilis _____

MM. unguis incarnatus _____

NN. seborrhea capitis _____

OO. prickly heat _____

PP. blackhead _____

QQ. bed sore _____

RR. vibratory urticaria _____

SS. angioma serpiginosum _____

TT. pulp abscess of finger _____

UU. dermatitis vegetans _____

VV. dermatitis due to poison ivy _____

WW. ocular pemphigus _____

XX. hypertrophic scar _____

7. Assign precise, accurate code numbers from the ICD-9-CM volume for the following operations on the integumentary system:

A. mammotomy _____

B. excision of pilonidal cyst _____

C. revision of breast implant _____

D. excision of skin for graft _____

E. excision of ectopic breast tissue _____

F. unilateral breast implant _____

G. suture of laceration of breast _____

H. insertion of totally implantable infusion pump _____

I. open biopsy of breast _____

J. size reduction of buttock _____

K. amputative mammoplasty _____

L. reimplantation of scalp _____

M. subcutaneous mammectomy _____

N. biopsy of skin and subcutaneous tissue _____

O. bilateral breast implants _____

P. destruction of skin by cryosurgery _____

Q. bilateral extended simple mastectomy _____

R. full-thickness skin graft to hand _____

S. extended radical mastectomy _____

T. radical excision of skin lesion _____

U. augmentation mammoplasty _____

V. cutting and preparation of pedicle graft _____

W. mastopexy _____

X. advancement of pedicle graft to hand _____

Y. total reconstruction of breast _____

8. Assign precise, accurate code numbers from the ICD-9-CM volume for the following diseases of the musculoskeletal system and connective tissue:

A. keratoconjunctivitis sicca _____

B. acute infective arthritis _____

C. unspecified chondrocalcinosis _____

D. Charcot's arthropathy _____

E. Felty's syndrome _____

F. Otto's pelvis _____

G. Kaschin-Beck disease of the ankle _____

H.   joint mice of knee _____

I.   protrusio acetabuli _____

J.   intermittent hydarthrosis _____

K.   Romanus lesion _____

L.   thoracic osteoarthritis _____

M.   Schmorl's nodes of thoracic region _____

N.   cervical radiculitis _____

O.   low back pain _____

P.   polymyalgia rheumatica _____

Q.   rotator cuff syndrome _____

R.   ganglion of tendon sheath _____

S.   amyotrophia _____

T.   pain in limb _____

U.   osteopathy resulting from poliomyelitis _____

V.   Bamberger-Marie disease _____

W.   osteochondritis dissecans _____

X.   postmenopausal osteoporosis _____

Y.   acquired talipes planus _____

Z.   acquired claw toe _____

AA. mallet finger _____

BB. adolescent postural kyphosis _____

CC. degenerative spondylolisthesis _____

DD. nonallopathic lesions of the sacral region _____

EE. nonallopathic lesions of the lower extremities _____

FF. cauliflower ear _____

GG. acquired lordosis _____

HH. acquired cavus deformity of foot _____

II. acquired hallux valgus _____

JJ. Sudeck's atrophy _____

KK. juvenile osteochrondrosis of clavicle _____

LL. Paget's disease of bone _____

MM. abscess of periosteum _____

NN. rheumatism _____

OO. interstitial myositis _____

PP. short Achilles tendon _____

QQ. patellar tendonitis _____

RR. hypermobility of coccyx _____

SS. Klippel's disease _____

TT. degenerative disc disease _____

UU. ankylosing vertebral hyperostosis _____

VV. rheumatoid arthritis of spine _____

WW. snapping hip _____

XX. recurrent dislocation of hip _____

9. Assign precise, accurate code numbers from the ICD-9-CM volume for the following operations on the musculoskeletal system:

A. temporomandibular arthroplasty _____

B. partial phalangectomy of hammer toe _____

C. epiphyseal stapling of humerus _____

D. closed reduction of dislocation of hip _____

E. biopsy of ankle joint _____

_____

F. spinal fusion _____

_____

G. reconstruction for opponensplasty _____

_____

H. tenosynovectomy_____

_____

I. disarticulation of ankle _____

_____

J. diskectomy _____

_____

K. open reduction of fracture of radius without internal fixation _____

_____

L. total wrist replacement _____

_____

M. removal of internal fixation device from femur _____

_____

N. suture of tendon sheath of hand _____

_____

O. local excision of lesion of bone _____

_____

P. bursotomy_____

_____

Q. closed reduction of maxillary fracture _____

_____

R. fitting of prosthesis above knee _____

_____

S. reattachment of thumb _____

_____

T. tendon graft _____

_____

U. bursotomy of hand _____

_____

V. bipolar endoprosthesis _____

_____

W. excision of meniscus of knee _____

_____

X. debridement of compound fracture of fibula _____

_____

Y. lengthening of patella with bone graft _____

_____

CODING OF CLINICAL DOCUMENTATION

Read the following clinical reports and assign precise, accurate diagnostic and procedural code numbers from the appropriate sections of the ICD-9-CM volumes.

PATIENT: Harding, Aaron   **MR#:** 99-09-01

SURGEON: Bailey   **ASSISTANT:** Duvall

Preoperative Diagnosis:
Posttraumatic arthritis, right knee.

Postoperative Diagnosis:
Posttraumatic arthritis, right knee with partial thickness cartilaginous loss of the patella.

Operation:
Arthroscopy with patellar debridement.

Brief Clinical History:
This is a 31-year-old white male status post right femur fracture, which subsequently healed in the shortened position. The patient underwent femoral lengthening procedure and has been doing well except for complaints of leg length inequality and knee pain. Radiographs revealed that there is not a significant leg length discrepancy, however, the patient's knee pain persisted. Therefore, a decision was made to perform arthroscopy on the patient.

Operative Procedure:
Following satisfactory induction of general endotracheal anesthesia, the patient was placed in the supine position on the operating table and his right lower extremity was prepped and draped in the usual sterile fashion.

The usual portals were made for arthroscopy including medial inflow portal, superior and medial to the patella, and the lateral scope portal, just lateral to the patellar tendon at the joint line. The patellofemoral joint was then observed and the patient was noted to have partial thickness cartilage loss on the undersurface of the patella. The medial gutter was then scoped and the medial joint entered in this fashion. The medial meniscus was noted to be intact. A second medial portal was made after an initial attempt was too close to the patellar tendon. This second portal was just medial to the first. The medial meniscus was once again probed and noted to be intact. The cartilage of the medial compartment was noted to be in good shape. The lateral compartment was also scoped and the meniscus was noted to be intact and the cartilage was noted to be in fairly good condition. Attention was once again turned to the patellofemoral joint. A fourth portal was made lateral and superior to the patellar tendon for introduction of the shaver. The cartilaginous lesion was then shaved and debrided. The cartilage was noted to be quite soft. Following this, the knee was irrigated with several hundred cc's of irrigant. The knee was then injected with 80 mg of Kenalog and 10 cc of Marcaine.

Following this, the C-arm was brought in and a screw was placed in the intercondylar region to reattach the lateral collateral ligament, identified and located using biplanar fluoroscopy. A 3 cm incision was made on the lateral aspect of the knee and carried down sharply through the subcutaneous tissue and fascia lata down to the bone. The screw was localized and removed along with its washer. The wound was irrigated and closed with nylon in the skin. Sterile dressing was then applied to the knee and the patient was awakened, extubated, and taken to the recovery room in good condition.

Codes: _____

PATIENT: Massey, Joseph　　**MR#:** 99-09-02

SURGEON: Payne　　**ASSISTANT:** Garrett

Preoperative Diagnosis:
Right medial meniscus tear.

Postoperative Diagnosis:
Healed medial meniscus repair with no new tear.

Operation:
Arthroscopy, right knee.

Indications:
This patient is a young male who is status post medial meniscus repair about three months ago. He has been doing well but began having recurrent pain. He has clicking and popping in his knee and pain that was similar to his original pain before the meniscal repair. A tentative diagnosis of failed meniscus repair was made and the patient was brought to the OR for exploration and treatment.

Description of Procedure:
The patient was brought to the OR and placed on the operating table in the supine position. After the satisfactory induction of general endotracheal anesthesia, a right thigh tourniquet was placed, and the extremity was placed in the arthroscopy leg holder. His knee, leg, and foot were prepped and draped in the usual sterile fashion.

The old arthroscopy portal was used, making a superior medial inflow portal and then an inferior anterolateral arthroscopy portal. The patellofemoral joint was visualized and there was no fraying. The cartilage looked good. Next the medial gutter was exposed and there was no evidence of any foreign body or any abnormalities of the medial gutter. Next the medial joint and the area where the meniscal repair was made were examined. The anterior cruciate ligament and notch were examined and there were no abnormalities. The lateral meniscus also had no abnormalities upon exploration of the lateral joint compartment. A medial portal was made with an 18-gauge needle under direct visualization. The medial meniscus was probed. The meniscus could not be displaced into the joint and did not show any evidence of tear. A grabber was used to pull the meniscus into the joint and to dislodge it and bring it into the joint. There was no evidence of any tear. The lateral meniscus was similarly probed and there was no tear. The joint was irrigated. The arthroscope was removed. The cannula for the inflow was used to extract the water out of the knee. A single 4-0 nylon stitch was made in each portal. Then 15 cc's of Marcaine and 40 mg of Kenalog were injected into the knee joint. Dry sterile dressings were applied and he was taken to the recovery room in stable condition. The sponge, needle, and instrument counts were correct.

Codes: _____

PATIENT: Ludwig, Harvey　　**MR#:** 99-09-03

ATTENDING PHYSICIAN: Shea

This gentleman was admitted for an elective cervical microdiskectomy. He underwent the procedure at the C6–7 level, with removal of a large, free fragment. Postoperatively, he did well and was discharged on the first postoperative day to be followed by Dr. Scott.

Discharge Diagnoses:

Cervical disk disease, degenerative.

Status post cervical microdiskectomy.

Operation:

As indicated.

Codes: _____

PATIENT: Ghani, Anastasia   **MR#:** 99-09-04

SURGEON: Doherty   **ASSISTANT:** Jordan

Preoperative Diagnosis:

Medial meniscus tear and grade II chondromalacia of medial patellar facet and lateral tibial plateau

Postoperative Diagnosis:

Medial meniscus tear and grade II chondromalacia of medial patellar facet and lateral tibial plateau

Operation:

Arthroscopic partial medial meniscectomy with shaving of lateral tibial defect and shaving of patellar defect

Procedure:

The patient was prepped and draped in the usual fashion and induced with general anesthesia. Ancef was administered in dosage of 1 gm. The skin was prepped by scrubbing with Iodophor solution. A mechanical leg holder was used to stabilize the extremity. An arthroscope approximately 3.5 mm in diameter with a lens angle of approximately 30 degrees was inserted into the knee through a superolateral portal, a medial patellar lateral portal, and a mid patellar medial portal. Thorough examination of the menisci revealed a vertical longitudinal tear in the medial meniscus. The articular surfaces were examined and articular cartilage was noted to be split or fractured. The articular surface of the patella displayed deep fissures and fragmentation. The articular surface of the lateral tibial plateau also displayed deep fissures and fragmentation. The knee was examined for ligament instability. The anterior cruciate ligament appeared completely normal and the posterior cruciate ligament appeared completely normal. The medial gutter was inspected with valgus stress applied to the knee. The medial collateral ligament was normal. The lateral gutter was inspected with varus stress applied to the knee. The lateral capsular ligaments were normal. The medial meniscus was partially excised, removing the unstable torn fragments and any adjacent degenerative tissue, leaving the free margin smoothly contoured. This procedure was accomplished entirely with arthroscopically controlled techniques. The hyaline cartilage on the lateral tibial plateau and on the patella was thoroughly washed to remove proteolytic enzymes and any small chips of cartilage debris. The articular surface of the lateral tibial plateau and patella was shaved to reduce the profile of degenerative tags of cartilage. All arthroscopic instruments were withdrawn after aspirating the remaining irrigation fluid. Passive range-of-knee-motion postoperatively was from 0 degrees to at least 120 degrees. A nonabsorbable suture skin closure was performed. A sterile compressive bandage was applied to the knee. The patient was transferred to the recovery room in good condition.

Codes: _____

ICD Coding: Symptoms and Signs; Factors Influencing Health Status; and Contact with Health Services

LEARNING OBJECTIVES

Upon completion of this chapter the learner should be able to:

1. Differentiate the coding and reporting of unconfirmed diagnoses rendered in inpatient care and treatment from that rendered in outpatient or office care and treatment.
2. Explain the use and function of the V codes.
3. Differentiate status codes from service codes.
4. Explain the purpose of codes to report the personal history of conditions.
5. Explain the purpose of codes to report the family history of conditions.
6. Apply knowledge of coding principles by assigning accurate and precise codes to report symptoms, nonspecific abnormal findings, and ill-defined and unknown causes of morbidity and mortality.
7. Apply knowledge of coding principles by assigning accurate and precise codes to report miscellaneous diagnostic and therapeutic procedures.
8. Apply knowledge of coding principles by assigning accurate and precise codes to report factors influencing health status.
9. Apply knowledge of coding principles by assigning accurate and precise codes to report contact with health services.

ICD CODING OF SYMPTOMS, SIGNS, AND ILL-DEFINED CONDITIONS

Chapter 16 of the ICD-9-CM diagnostic tabular volume, designated for listings of signs, symptoms, and ill-defined conditions, is utilized considerably in ambulatory care, outpatient clinics, and office practices. This chapter consists of three sections, one for symptoms, one for nonspecific abnormal findings, and one for ill-defined and unknown causes of morbidity and mortality (Table 10–1).

Chapter 16 includes listings of symptoms, signs, abnormal results of laboratory and other diagnostic procedures, as well as vaguely documented conditions that cannot be classified elsewhere. Signs and symptoms that indicate or signify a definitive diagnosis should be

TABLE 10-1

Sections in Chapter 16, Volume 1 of ICD-9-CM

1. Symptoms (category range 780–789)
2. Nonspecific Abnormal Findings (category range 790–796)
3. Ill-defined and Unknown Causes of Morbidity and Mortality (category range 797–799)

assigned with a code number and title listed in the preceding fifteen chapters of the ICD-9-CM diagnostic classification.

In general, category range 780 through 786 is comprised of symptomatic conditions that indicate or signify perhaps equal likelihood of two or more diseases, or equal likehood of disorders affecting two or more systems of the body. In most of these cases, the necessary investigative study was not completed to ascertain a final diagnosis. Practically all of the categories in this section could be designated as "not otherwise specified," or as "of unknown etiology."

The alphabetic index in Volume 2 of ICD-9-CM should be consulted to determine which symptoms and signs should be reported with the listings in Chapter 16 of Volume 1, and which should be reported with more specific listings among the other chapters of this diagnostic classification. The residual subcategories (numbered .9) throughout these other chapters are provided for relevant symptoms associated with the disorders classified in that chapter, and that are not listed elsewhere in the classification.

The conditions and signs or symptoms included in category range 780 through 796 consist of listings applicable to report:

1. Entities for which a specific diagnosis cannot be made even after all the diagnostic facts bearing on the case were investigated.

2. Signs or symptoms existing at the time of the initial patient encounter that proved to be transient and whose etiology could not be determined.

3. Provisional diagnoses established for a patient who failed to return for further testing or treatment.

4. Conditions referred elsewhere for diagnosis or therapy before a final diagnosis was made.

5. Entities for which a more precise diagnosis was not available for any other reason.

6. Certain symptoms that represent important problems in medical care that are significant to classify in addition to a known causative factor.

The first section of Chapter 16 contains listings for the reporting of: general bodily symptoms; symptoms involving the nervous system; symptoms involving the musculoskeletal system; symptoms involving the skin and other integumentary tissue with the exception of breast symptoms; symptoms concerning nutrition, metabolism, and development; and symptoms involving the head and neck with the exception of specific neck symptoms classifiable to category 723. This section also contains listings for the reporting of symptoms involving the cardiovascular system; symptoms involving the respiratory system and other chest symptoms; symptoms involving the digestive system with the exception of constipation and diarrhea; symptoms involving the urinary system with the exception of hematuria and uremia; and other symptoms involving the abdomen and pelvis with the exception of symptoms referable to the genital organs.

The second section of Chapter 16 comprises listings for the reporting of: nonspecific findings on examination of blood, urine, or other body substances, with the exception of those found in chromosomal analysis; and nonspecific abnormal findings on radiological, thermo-graphic, ultrasonographic, or other imaging of body structures. This section also comprises listings for the reporting of: nonspecific abnormal results of function studies including ra-dioisotope scans, uptake studies, and scintiphotography; as well as nonspecific abnormal his-tological or immunological findings.

The relatively brief third section of Chapter 16 includes listings for the reporting of ill-defined and unknown causes of morbidity and mortality. Among these listings are codes to re-port entities such as senility without mention of psychosis and unknown cause of sudden death.

The following subcategories within Chapter 16 require coding and reporting with the fifth-digit subclassification:

780.0	780.5	782.6
784.4	784.6	785.5
786.0	786.5	787.0
787.9	788.2	788.3
788.4	788.6	789.0
789.3	789.4	789.6
790.9	794.0	794.1
794.3	795.7	

Categories of listings in Chapter 16 of Volume 3 of ICD-9-CM are established for miscel-laneous diagnostic and therapeutic procedures, services often rendered to patients presenting with symptoms or signs of unknown etiology. These include category range 87 through 99 for: diagnostic radiology and related techniques; interview, evaluation, consultation, and exami-nation; microscopic examination; nuclear medicine; physical therapy, respiratory therapy, re-habilitation, and related procedures; procedures related to the psyche; ophthalmologic and oto-logic diagnosis and treatment; nonoperative intubation and irrigation, replacement and removal of therapeutic appliances; and nonoperative removal of foreign body or calculus.

The vast majority of the miscellaneous diagnostic and therapeutic procedures listed in Chapter 16 of Volume 3 of ICD-9-CM are not performed in an operating room or in an out-patient surgery center. However, several of these procedures are designated by certain insur-ance carriers (especially Medicare) as valid for reporting as operating room procedures. The ICD-9-CM listing *92.27, Implantation or insertion of radioactive elements,* represents miscel-laneous procedures that may be reported with operating room charges.

Designated ICD-9-CM codes are recognized as comorbidities by Medicare and certain other third-party payors. These comorbid conditions may increase the amount of reimburse-ment received by the provider. Several signs and symptoms are regarded by Medicare as co-morbidities. Those entities are represented by the following ICD-9-CM code numbers:

780.01	780.03	780.1
780.3	781.7	785.4
785.50	785.51	785.59
786.3	788.20	788.29
789.5	790.7	791.1
791.3	799.1	799.4

Not every code and narrative in the ICD-9-CM classification represents an entity that may be reported as a principal or primary diagnosis. Designated ICD-9-CM codes are commonly considered as an unacceptable principal or primary diagnosis by a majority of third-party payors including Medicare and Medicaid. Unacceptable principal or primary diagnoses using signs or symptoms are as follows:

798.1	798.2	798.9

ICD CODING OF HEALTH STATUS AND CONTACT WITH HEALTH SERVICES

The classification known as the Supplementary Classification of Factors Influencing Health Status and Contact with Health Services, category range V01 through V82, is provided to deal with encounters in which circumstances other than a disease or injury classifiable to categories 001 through 999 (the main bulk of ICD-9-CM), are documented as "diagnoses" or "problems." This type of documentation may occur in two general situations.

The first situation could occur if a person who was not sick encountered health services for a specific purpose, such as to receive prophylactic immunization or to be counseled for a problem that was per se not a disease or an injury. This situation would constitute a rare occurrence among hospital inpatients, but appears quite frequently among hospital outpatients and patients of family practice physicians or ambulatory care health clinics.

In these circumstances, it is permissible for the V code to be reported in primary cause tabulations, or in other words, to be reported as the principal diagnosis for that encounter or episode of care. If V codes are used in this manner, they are essentially codes that report a patient service.

The second situation could occur if an established diagnosis or problem influenced the patient's health status but was not per se a current illness or injury. Such health factors might be elicited during population screenings or might be a documented supplementary consideration that impacts the care and treatment rendered for a current illness or injury. A prosthetic orthopedic device, an artificial heart valve in situ, and a personal history of a malignant neoplasm are examples of entities that could comprise complicating factors in the rendering of patient care and treatment for a diagnostic problem categorized in the main classification of ICD-9-CM.

If V codes are used in this manner, they are essentially codes that report a patient status. In these circumstances, the V code should be utilized only as a supplementary code, and should not be sequenced in primary cause tabulations or reported as a principal diagnosis or a primary diagnosis.

Sections of this supplementary classification encompassing the V codes include nine groupings of listings that generally are either status codes reflecting the patient's past health history, or service codes reflecting procedures performed or services rendered during the current episode of care. The sections of the Supplementary Classification of Factors Influencing Health Status and Contact with Health Services are summarized in Table 10–2.

The group of categories with listings of potential health hazards related to communicable diseases excludes the reporting of family or personal history of infectious or parasitic diseases. Nonetheless, this section does contain listings of codes and titles to report: personal contact with or exposure to communicable diseases; status as a carrier or a suspected carrier of infectious disease; and the need for prophylactic vaccination and inoculation against bacterial, viral, or other diseases or combinations of diseases.

The group of categories with listings to report potential health hazards related to personal and family history includes codes and titles for reporting the personal history of: malignant neoplasm; mental disorder; allergy to medicinal agents; and other hazards to health. This

T A B L E 10–2

Sections in the V Code Supplement of ICD-9-CM

---

1. Persons with Potential Health Hazards Related to Communicable Diseases (category range V01–V06)
2. Persons with Need For Isolation, Other Potential Health Hazards and Prophylactic Measures (category range V07–V09)
3. Persons with Potential Health Hazards Related to Personal and Family History (category range V10–V19)
4. Persons Encountering Health Services in Circumstances Related to Reproduction and Development (category range V20–V28)
5. Liveborn Infants According to Type of Birth (category range V30–V39)
6. Persons with a Condition Influencing Their Health Status (category range V40–V49)
7. Persons Encountering Health Services for Specific Procedures and Aftercare (category range V50–V59)
8. Persons Encountering Health Services in Other Circumstances (category range V60–V68)
9. Persons without Reported Diagnosis Encountered During Examination and Investigation of Individuals and Populations (category range V70–V82)

---

grouping also includes categories with listings of codes and titles for reporting a family history of: malignant neoplasm; certain chronic disabling diseases; and other specific conditions.

The group of categories with listings to report persons encountering health services in circumstances related to reproduction and development excludes the reporting of obstetric aftercare or obstetric care in which fetal investigation was the reason for observation or management. This group of categories contains listings of codes and titles for the reporting of: health supervision of the infant or child; assessment or evaluation of constitutional states in development; care during normal pregnancy; supervision of high-risk pregnancy; postpartum care and examination; contraceptive management; procreative management; antenatal screening, and the outcome of delivery.

Category 27 provides listings intended for coding and reporting the outcome of delivery on the maternal health record, and not for tabulation on the health record of the newborn. Category range V30 through V39 provides listings intended for coding and reporting the healthcare services provided to liveborn infants throughout the duration of crib or bassinet occupancy in a designated healthcare facility. The section classifying liveborn infants according to type of birth includes listings of codes and titles to report: a single liveborn; a twin with a mate liveborn; a twin with a mate stillborn; multiple mates, all liveborn; multiple mates, all stillborn; and multiple mates, liveborn and stillborn.

The group of categories with listings to report persons who have a condition influencing personal health status contains codes and titles for: existing mental and behavioral problems; concurrent problems with special senses and other special functions; status post organ or tissue replaced by transplant or by other means; artificial opening status; postsurgical status; physiological dependence on machines; existing problems with internal organs; and concurrent problems with the head, neck, trunk or limbs.

Category range V51 through V58 provides listings intended for use to indicate a reason for the encounter or episode of care in patients who were previously treated for a disease or injury that was not present at the time of the reported encounter or episode of care. Usually such patients received care to consolidate the treatment, to assess or evaluate the residual effects of the disease or injury, or to prevent recurrence of the condition. The listings in these categories exclude the reporting of a follow-up examination for medical surveillance following treatment.

The group of categories with listings to report persons encountering health services for specific procedures and aftercare services includes codes and titles for: elective surgery rendered for purposes other than remedying disease or injury (mostly cosmetic surgical procedures); aftercare involving the use of plastic surgery; fitting and adjustment of prosthetic device or other device (excluding the reporting of that provided for malfunction or complication of the device); orthopedic aftercare; attention to artificial openings (excluding the reporting of complications of external stoma); aftercare involving intermittent dialysis (including the reporting of dialysis preparation and treatment); care involving use of rehabilitation procedures; and patient status as an organ or tissue donor.

The group of categories with listings to report persons encountering health services in other circumstances contains codes and titles for: problems entailing housing, household, and economic circumstances; problems involving family circumstances; problems concerning psychosocial circumstances; unavailability of other medical facilities for care; admission for specific procedures or services that were not performed or rendered; consultation offered without present complaint or illness; convalescence care; follow-up examination for surveillance following treatment; as well as encounters for administrative purposes.

Category V71 is provided to report cases in which a patient presented with symptoms or with evidence of an abnormal condition that appeared to require further assessment or evaluation, but which after study and observation revealed no need for further treatment or care. Nonspecific abnormal findings may be established at the time of such investigations that are classified in category range V70 through V82. These findings, however, are classified in category range 790 through 796 in Chapter 16, and should be reported with codes and titles from within those listings.

The group of categories with listings to report persons without reported diagnosis encountered during examination and investigation of individuals and populations includes codes and titles for general medical examination, for observation and evaluation for suspected conditions, and for special investigations and examinations including the routine examination of a specific body system. This grouping of categories also contains listings of codes and titles to report special screening for: viral, bacterial, spirochetal, and other infectious diseases; malignant neoplasms; endocrine, nutritional, metabolic, and immunity disorders; disorders of blood and blood-forming organs; mental disorders and developmental handicaps; neurological, eye, and ear diseases; and cardiovascular, respiratory, and genitourinary diseases. Category range V73 through V82 should not be used to report examinations of individual patients; these categories are designated solely for the reporting of screenings administered to specifically defined populations.

A common misconception surrounds the reporting of V codes to represent a principal or primary diagnosis. Certain personnel among billers and insurance claim specialists mistakenly conclude that all V codes are unacceptable for such designation. Many V codes represent entities that comprise a completely valid reason for necessitating the admission or encounter. However, many V codes are inherently unacceptable for reporting as a principal or primary diagnosis. The following list is comprised of V codes from the ICD-9-CM supplementary classification that are unacceptable for sequencing as a primary or principal diagnosis:

V01.0	V01.1	V01.2
V01.3	V01.4	V01.5
V01.6	V01.7	V01.8
V01.9	V02.0	V02.1
V02.2	V02.3	V02.4

V02.5	V02.6	V02.7
V02.8	V02.9	V03.0
V03.1	V03.2	V03.3
V03.4	V03.5	V03.6
V03.7	V03.81	V03.82
V03.89	V03.9	V04.0
V04.1	V04.2	V04.3
V04.4	V04.5	V04.6
V04.7	V04.8	V05.0
V05.1	V05.2	V05.3
V05.4	V05.8	V05.9
V06.0	V06.1	V06.2
V06.3	V06.4	V06.5
V06.6	V06.8	V06.9
V07.1	V07.2	V07.31
V07.39	V07.4	V09.0
V09.1	V09.2	V09.3
V09.4	V09.50	V09.51
V09.6	V09.70	V09.71
V09.80	V09.81	V09.90
V09.91	V10.00	V10.01
V10.02	V10.03	V10.04
V10.05	V10.06	V10.07
V10.09	V10.11	V10.12
V10.20	V10.21	V10.22
V10.29	V10.3	V10.40
V10.41	V10.42	V10.43
V10.44	V10.45	V10.46
V10.47	V10.49	V10.50
V10.51	V10.52	V10.59
V10.60	V10.61	V10.62
V10.63	V10.69	V10.71
V10.72	V10.79	V10.80
V10.81	V10.82	V10.83
V10.84	V10.85	V10.86
V10.9	V11.0	V11.1
V11.2	V11.3	V11.8
V11.9	V12.00	V12.01
V12.02	V12.03	V12.4
V12.50	V12.51	V12.52
V12.59	V12.6	V12.70
V12.71	V12.72	V12.79
V13.00	V13.01	V13.09
V13.1	V13.2	V13.3
V13.4	V13.5	V13.6
V13.7	V13.8	V13.9
V14.0	V14.1	V14.2
V14.3	V14.4	V14.5
V14.6	V14.7	V14.8

V14.9	V15.0	V15.1
V15.2	V15.3	V15.41
V15.42	V15.49	V15.5
V15.6	V15.7	V15.81
V15.82	V15.84	V15.85
V15.86	V15.89	V15.9
V16.0	V16.1	V16.2
V16.3	V16.4	V16.5
V16.6	V16.7	V16.8
V16.9	V17.0	V17.1
V17.2	V17.3	V17.4
V17.5	V17.6	V17.7
V17.8	V18.0	V18.1
V18.2	V18.3	V18.4
V18.5	V18.6	V18.7
V18.8	V19.0	V19.1
V19.2	V19.3	V19.4
V19.5	V19.6	V19.7
V19.8	V20.1	V20.2
V21.0	V21.1	V21.2
V21.8	V21.9	V22.0
V22.1	V22.2	V23.0
V23.1	V23.2	V23.3
V23.4	V23.5	V23.7
V23.8	V23.9	V24.1
V24.2	V25.01	V25.02
V25.09	V25.1	V25.40
V25.41	V25.42	V25.43
V25.49	V25.5	V25.8
V25.9	V26.1	V26.2
V26.3	V26.4	V26.8
V26.9	V27.0	V27.1
V27.2	V27.3	V27.4
V27.5	V27.6	V27.7
V27.9	V28.0	V28.1
V28.2	V28.3	V28.4
V28.5	V28.8	V28.9
V29.9	V40.0	V40.1
V40.2	V40.3	V40.9
V41.0	V41.1	V41.2
V41.3	V41.4	V41.5
V41.6	V41.7	V41.8
V41.9	V42.0	V42.1
V42.2	V42.3	V42.4
V42.5	V42.6	V42.7
V42.8	V42.9	V43.0
V43.1	V43.2	V43.4
V43.5	V43.60	V43.61
V43.62	V43.63	V43.64

V43.65	V43.66	V43.69
V43.7	V43.81	V43.82
V43.89	V44.0	V44.1
V44.2	V44.3	V44.4
V44.5	V44.6	V44.7
V44.8	V44.9	V45.00
V45.01	V45.02	V45.09
V45.1	V45.2	V45.3
V45.4	V45.51	V45.52
V45.59	V45.81	V45.82
V45.83	V45.89	V46.0
V46.1	V46.9	V47.0
V47.1	V47.2	V47.3
V47.4	V47.5	V47.9
V48.0	V48.1	V48.2
V48.3	V48.4	V48.5
V48.6	V48.7	V48.8
V48.9	V49.0	V49.1
V49.2	V49.3	V49.4
V49.5	V49.60	V49.61
V49.62	V49.63	V49.64
V49.65	V49.66	V49.67
V49.70	V49.71	V49.72
V49.73	V49.74	V49.75
V49.76	V49.77	V49.8
V49.9	V50.3	V50.8
V50.9	V52.9	V53.1
V53.2	V53.4	V53.5
V53.6	V53.7	V53.8
V53.9	V54.8	V54.9
V55.9	V57.0	V57.1
V57.21	V57.22	V57.3
V57.4	V57.81	V57.89
V58.2	V58.3	V58.5
V58.9	V59.01	V59.02
V59.09	V59.9	V60.0
V60.1	V60.2	V60.3
V60.4	V60.5	V60.6
V60.8	V60.9	V61.0
V61.1	V61.10	V61.11
V61.12	V61.20	V61.22
V61.29	V61.3	V61.41
V61.49	V61.5	V61.6
V61.7	V61.8	V61.9
V62.0	V62.2	V62.3
V62.4	V62.5	V62.6
V62.81	V62.82	V62.83
V62.89	V62.9	V63.0
V63.1	V63.2	V63.8

V63.9	V64.0	V64.1
V64.2	V64.3	V65.1
V65.3	V65.40	V65.41
V65.42	V65.43	V65.44
V65.45	V65.49	V65.5
V65.8	V65.9	V66.0
V66.1	V66.2	V66.3
V66.4	V66.5	V66.6
V66.7	V66.9	V67.9
V68.0	V68.1	V68.2
V68.81	V68.89	V68.9
V69.0	V69.1	V69.2
V69.3	V69.8	V69.9
V70.0	V70.1	V70.2
V70.3	V70.4	V70.5
V70.6	V70.7	V70.8
V70.9	V71.9	V72.0
V72.1	V72.2	V72.3
V72.4	V72.5	V72.6
V72.7	V72.81	V72.82
V72.83	V72.84	V72.85
V72.9	V73.0	V73.1
V73.2	V73.3	V73.4
V73.5	V73.6	V73.88
V73.89	V73.98	V73.99
V74.0	V74.1	V74.2
V74.3	V74.4	V74.5
V74.6	V74.8	V74.9
V75.0	V75.1	V75.2
V75.3	V75.4	V75.5
V75.6	V75.7	V75.8
V75.9	V76.0	V76.1
V76.2	V76.3	V76.41
V76.42	V76.43	V76.49
V76.8	V76.9	V77.0
V77.1	V77.2	V77.3
V77.4	V77.5	V77.6
V77.7	V77.8	V77.9
V78.0	V78.1	V78.2
V78.3	V78.8	V78.9
V79.0	V79.1	V79.2
V79.3	V79.8	V79.9
V80.0	V80.1	V80.2
V80.3	V81.0	V81.1
V81.2	V81.3	V81.4
V81.5	V81.6	V82.0
V82.1	V82.2	V82.3
V82.4	V82.5	V82.6
V82.8	V82.9	

Additionally, several codes for signs and symptoms and several V codes are generally deemed as questionable if reported as a principal or primary diagnosis. These codes are:

790.93	795.71	795.79
796.2	V53.31	V53.32
V53.39		

The Medicare prospective payment system distributes diagnosis related groups into major diagnostic categories. The DRG's associated with the entities among the V codes are distributed into MDC 23, Factors Influencing Health Status and Other Contacts with Health Services (Table 10–3).

The supplementary classification comprised of V codes includes listings of healthcare services that are administrative rather than clinical in orientation. The prospective payment system, similarly, incorporates diagnosis related groups that account for circumstances devoid of clinical significance. The following DRG's report such situations:

DRG 468, Extensive Operating Room Procedure Unrelated to Principal Diagnosis

DRG 469, Principal Diagnosis Invalid as Discharge Diagnosis

DRG 470, Ungroupable

DRG 477, Nonextensive Operating Room Procedure Unrelated to Principal Diagnosis

ICD CODING OF OUTPATIENT SERVICES

Coding guidelines for outpatient diagnoses were established primarily for use by healthcare facilities in coding and reporting outpatient services. The terms "encounter" and "visit" are often used interchangeably in describing outpatient service contacts and, therefore these two terms frequently appear together within coding guidelines, without distinguishing one term from the other. Nonetheless, usage of the term "encounter" is more prevalent, and usage of the term "visit" is somewhat outdated.

Coding guidelines for reporting diagnoses documented for outpatients vary in several instances from those guidelines to report diagnoses documented for inpatients. The generally recognized Uniform Hospital Discharge Data Set definition of principal diagnosis applies essentially to inpatients in acute, short-term, comprehensive healthcare facilities.

Moreover, coding guidelines for inconclusive diagnoses documented for inpatients, utilizing such qualifying words as "probable," "suspected," "possible," "likely," or "rule out," direct

---

T A B L E   10–3

Diagnosis Related Groups for Factors of Health Status and Contacts with Health Services

DRG 461, Operating Room Procedures with Diagnoses of Other Contact with Health Services
DRG 462, Rehabilitation
DRG 463, Signs and Symptoms with Comorbidity or Complication
DRG 464, Signs and Symptoms without Comorbidity or Complication
DRG 465, Aftercare with History of Malignancy as Secondary Diagnosis
DRG 466, Aftercare without History of Malignancy as Secondary Diagnosis
DRG 467, Other Factors Influencing Health Status

that these entities be coded and reported as confirmed diagnoses. Exceptions to this principle are upheld for the reporting of malignant neoplasms and significant infectious diseases such as septicemia, tuberculosis, and especially human immunodeficiency virus. In these types of cases, unconfirmed diagnoses should be reported only to the highest degree of certainty.

These guidelines pertaining to unconfirmed diagnoses, developed for inpatient reporting, are in most respects contrary to, and altogether not applicable for the reporting of outpatient services. By reason that clinical diagnoses often are not established at the time of the initial outpatient encounter, two or more encounters may elapse before a diagnosis can be confirmed.

Therefore, after a single encounter in a series of outpatient diagnostic or therapeutic sessions, a diagnosis documented with a qualifying term indicating its probability or likelihood, should be coded and reported according to the presenting symptoms or signs, acknowledging that the actual diagnostic condition is not yet established. Abnormal findings noted on physical examination or diagnostic test results should also be coded only to the highest degree of certainty in the reporting of outpatient services.

To exemplify, the coding and reporting of a diagnosis documented in the health record of an inpatient with "persistent polyuria, possible urinary tract infection," and that documented in the record of an outpatient ascribed with the same condition would differ.

> **Inpatient Diagnosis:** persistent polyuria, possible urinary tract infection, should be reported as if the condition was confirmed using code number 599.0
>
> **Outpatient Diagnosis:** persistent polyuria, possible urinary tract infection, should be reported according to the presenting symptom using code number 788.42.

If abnormal casts or cells were noted upon urinalysis, code number 791.7, should also be reported for the outpatient case, but not for the inpatient case.

Any of the codes from categories 001 through V82 in ICD-9-CM may be used to report the reason for the outpatient encounter or visit. A three-digit code should be reported only if the category is not further subdivided (for example, code number 600). If fourth-digit or fifth-digit classifications are provided, these digits must be assigned as applicable.

In reporting outpatient services, the ICD-9-CM code for the diagnosis, condition, problem, or other reason for the encounter should be documented in the patient medical record. This entity, which is chiefly responsible for occasioning the outpatient services provided, should be sequenced as the primary diagnosis. Additional codes may be reported to indicate secondary diagnoses representing coexisting active (not latent or inactive) conditions noted during the episode of care.

In certain instances, the physician or other healthcare practitioner may document the chief complaint of the patient as the reason for encounter. Vague descriptions such as "weakness" or "nervousness" may be documented as the diagnostic entity. With these cases, the coder should survey the patient health record to ascertain the laboratory or other tests performed to determine if any codable or reportable abnormal findings were noted.

However, coders should avoid reporting these encounters with generic (and virtually meaningless) V codes such as V72.6 Laboratory examination, or V72.5 Radiological examination, not elsewhere classified. In the preceding example, weakness should be sequenced as the primary diagnosis, appropriately reported with code number 780.7.

For reporting patients receiving specific ancillary diagnostic services during an encounter, the appropriate V code for the service should be sequenced first, and if documented, the problem for which these services were performed should be sequenced secondarily. For instance, the diagnostic service of mental health evaluation (code V70.2) should be sequenced and reported as the primary reason for the encounter, and the precipitating problem of paranoid tendency (code 301.0) should be sequenced secondarily.

For reporting patients receiving specific ancillary therapeutic services during an encounter, the appropriate V code for the service should also be sequenced first, and if documented, the problem for which the services were performed should be sequenced secondarily. For instance, the therapeutic service of fitting of contact lenses (code V53.1) should be sequenced and reported as the primary reason for the encounter, and the underlying problem of myopia (code 367.1) should be sequenced secondarily.

For reporting patients receiving outpatient surgical procedures, the diagnosis for which the surgery was performed should be coded as the primary diagnosis. If the postoperative diagnosis was different from that of the preoperative diagnosis, the postoperative diagnosis should be selected for coding and reporting.

Conditions or reasons for encounters classifiable to the supplementary classification comprised of category range V01 through V82, should also be used if appropriate to designate the diagnostic entity. To exemplify, if a patient was admitted for replacement of a peritoneal dialysis catheter, code V56.1 should be reported as the primary diagnosis.

Chronic diseases, such as emphysema or arthritis, treated in a continual series of outpatient encounters should be coded and reported as the primary diagnosis each time the patient received services for that condition. All other documented conditions that coexisted at the time of each encounter may also be coded and reported as secondary diagnoses, if these conditions required or affected patient care, treatment, or management. For instance, if a patient routinely encountered for management of diabetes also is maintained on medications to control hypertension, and if blood pressure of this patient is also monitored during each encounter, the hypertensive condition should be coded and reported as a secondary diagnosis.

Inactive problems should not be coded or reported. Certain physicians were trained to document significant diagnoses as a reference for further care, without indication of temporality. These practitioners document present conditions along with past conditions to formulate an ongoing recapitulation of the patient problem list that chronicles the health history of that person. For example, a diagnosis of "myocardial infarction" may be entered in the health record in each episode of care to indicate that the patient has a past history of myocardial infarction.

Particular practicing physicians additionally document physical observations such as "obesity" or "alopecia" among the listed diagnoses. If no care or treatment was rendered for these entities, they should not be coded or reported, even though technically they represent an existing condition.

Those physicians who document conditions previously treated and no longer existing, for instance, might list a diagnosis of hepatitis in the health record, without denoting that the condition is no longer an active problem. If the dates of occurrences are provided for the listed conditions, the coder may be able to ascertain the timeliness of these stated conditions.

A practicing physician, most frequently a generalist rather than a specialist, may document minor health problems or past operations with the prefix "status post," such as "status post tonsilectomy." Such documentation practices impede accurate and precise statistical tabulation for clinical or research purposes, although certain healthcare facilities maintain policies mandating the coding of every diagnostic entity documented by the physician, imputing only to him or her the clinical acumen to formulate a problem list or an account of relevant diagnostic and procedural entities.

Although specific and nonspecific V codes are extant to report essentially any problem documented in the patient health history, such codes should be reported secondarily only if the historical problem is directly related to the outpatient service rendered in that encounter.

Applicable V codes should be reported for related historical conditions, however, notwithstanding that the relationship may be indirect. For example, code V45.81 signifying aortocoronary bypass status is pertinent to all cardiovascular conditions, and code V45.1 signifying renal dialysis status is pertinent to all urological conditions, even if treated simply on an out-patient basis.

Coders must be competent in distinguishing between the documentation of conditions presently existing and the documentation of conditions existing in the past. Certain conditions such as a stroke are often marked by residuals or late effects that persist long after the original disease. The alphabetic index and diagnostic tabular should be surveyed to ascertain if such sequalae are distinctly codable and reportable.

The variability of physician documentation impacts the reliability and validity of statistical patient care data. Each physician is accountable for the documentation of diagnostic and procedural entities reportable for the patients whom he or she evaluated and treated. Due to the lack of uniformity in documentation protocol, the tabulated incidence of secondary conditions (and sometimes even primary conditions) often is merely an approximation of the actual incidence.

ICD CODING OF PHYSICIAN OFFICE SERVICES

The coding and reporting guidelines applicable to services rendered by physician office practices are very similar to those guidelines applicable to patient services rendered in outpatient clinics. Physician practices must use the appropriate ICD-9-CM diagnostic code or codes from categories 001 through V82 to identify diagnoses, symptoms, conditions, problems, complaints, or other reason for the patient encounter or visit.

The primary diagnosis reportable is that represented by the ICD-9-CM code for the condition, problem, or other reason for the episode of care that was documented in the medical record as chiefly responsible for the services provided. Reportable secondary diagnoses represent any coexisting conditions or problems noted in the duration of the encounter.

Physician office practices must report codes at their highest level of specificity, in accordance with the coding and reporting guidelines established and maintained for other healthcare providers. Three-digit codes should be selected and assigned only if there are no four-digit codes provided within that category of the classification. Four-digit codes should be selected and assigned only if there is no fifth-digit subclassification provided for that subcategory. Codes from the fifth-digit subclassification should be selected and assigned in those subcategories in which that option exists.

Conditions or problems documented in the patient health record as probable, suspected, questionable, or to be ruled out, should not be coded or reported as if they were established. Instead, these entities should be coded and reported to the highest degree of certainty for that encounter, utilizing the codes and titles for symptoms, signs, abnormal findings, or other reason for the episode of care.

Chronic diseases evaluated and treated on an ongoing basis may be coded and reported as many times as the patient received services for the condition. For reporting patients who received ancillary diagnostic services in the physician office during an encounter, the appropriate V code for the diagnostic examination should be sequenced first, and the diagnosis of the problem for which the services were performed should be sequenced secondarily. For reporting patients who received ancillary therapeutic services in the physician office during an encounter, the appropriate V code for the therapeutic session should be sequenced first, and the diagnosis of the problem for which the services were performed should be sequenced secondarily.

For reporting surgical procedures rendered in the physician office setting, the diagnosis necessitating the surgery that was performed should be sequenced as the primary diagnosis for that episode of care. If the postoperative diagnosis was determined to differ from the preoperative diagnosis, only the postoperative diagnosis should be reported for reimbursement purposes or for statistical tabulation.

All documented conditions that coexisted at the time of each patient encounter or visit in the physician office, and all documented conditions which required or affected patient care, treatment, or management should be coded and reported. Conditions previously treated, or conditions untreated but no longer existing, should not be coded or reported.

AMBULATORY CARE REPORTING FOR BILLING

The reporting of ambulatory care services is enhanced through a cooperative effort between the physician provider and the healthcare facility. A collaborative effort is essential to facilitate adequate, complete, and timely documentation; code selection and assignment; and reporting of diagnoses and procedures. Specific coding guidelines assist both the physician and the facility in identifying those primary and secondary diagnoses and procedures that should be reported.

The Uniform Hospital Discharge Data Set established definitions to report patient care data elements in a standardized manner. These data elements and corresponding definitions are periodically disseminated in the publication Coding Clinic. Secondary diagnoses, for instance, are defined as all conditions that coexisted at the time of the patient encounter, or that developed during the encounter, or that affected the treatment rendered and/or the duration of care. Secondary diagnoses that related to an earlier episode of care, and that have no effect on the current encounter should be excluded from the coding and reporting process. Likewise, for reporting purposes, the definition established for "other diagnoses" is interpreted as additional conditions that affect patient care in terms of clinical evaluation; diagnostic assessment, therapeutic treatment; as well as duration or intensity of care and/or monitoring.

Substantial variability exists in the documentation of ambulatory care services, and this variability impedes the tabulation necessary to index or classify data useful for research study purposes. Not only do documentation practices differ between the staffs of separate ambulatory healthcare facilities, but even among staff members at a specific healthcare facility, uniformity in the patient health record documentation protocol is an unfulfilled objective.

As a commonly noted example, many physicians who practice in the surgical specialties do not document diagnoses concerning problems outside of their clinical domain, although their notes indirectly indicate that such conditions are indeed active problems. For example, an orthopedic surgeon may record in the chart that a patient treated for a fractured femoral neck was maintained on medications for intrinsic asthma. Yet, the asthma diagnosis may not be stated on the list of diagnoses. Thus, the asthma condition most likely would not be coded or reported in ambulatory care billing.

Inconsistency in ambulatory care reporting often surrounds the coding of diagnostic entities. Conditions that are integral to an overall disease process should not be reported with additional codes. For instance, alcoholic cirrhosis of the liver implies an alcohol addiction (either current or past). Generally, in such cases, coding and reporting the alcohol problem is unnecessary, if the care and treatment was medical and not rehabilitative or psychiatric.

Conditions that are not an integral part of a disease process and conditions not routinely associated with a disease process should be coded and reported if these conditions are present at the time of the encounter. To exemplify, a bowel impaction produced by gallstones should necessitate the coding and reporting of both the primary problem (the impaction) and also the coexisting problem (the gallstones).

In ambulatory care reporting for billing, abnormal findings from laboratory reports, radiological reports, and other diagnostic results should not be coded and reported unless the physician specifically indicates their clinical significance in that episode of care. For instance, a chest X-ray record might denote an opacification or a slight atelectasis. If the physician did not remark upon such findings in his or her documentation in the progress notes, these incidental observations stated within the diagnostic reports fundamentally should be disregarded for purposes of ambulatory care coding and reporting.

If these observed findings were outside the normal range of results, and if based on this factor, the physician ordered subsequent procedures to assess or evaluate the condition or to prescribe treatment, then such abnormal findings may be appropriately coded and reported for ambulatory care billing. For example, if a patient's hematocrit and hemoglobin results indicated significant anemia, and if additional blood tests were consequently ordered, these abnormal findings may be coded and reported.

The primary diagnosis, the condition responsible for the admission of the patient to the health service encounter or episode of service, should always be sequenced first in reporting for ambulatory care billing. If several procedures are rendered, the principal procedure is the procedure most closely associated with the patient's primary diagnosis that was documented for the specific encounter. Secondary diagnoses and secondary procedures should be sequenced and reported in descending order of clinical significance. Insurance claim reimbursement policies ordinarily mandate the coding and reporting of only diagnoses specifically assessed or treated during the particular encounter or episode of service reported.

The reporting of code numbers for nonspecific diagnoses or procedures rendered in ambulatory care should be avoided, if possible. Personnel responsible for coding and billing should attempt to determine the most specific code both for reimbursement purposes and to generate meaningful data for statistical research purposes. Accurate, complete, and timely clinical documentation could alleviate the necessity of reporting codes for unspecified ambulatory care diagnoses and procedures.

KEY CONCEPTS

aftercare _____	primary tabulation _____
ambulatory care _____	principal diagnosis _____
comorbidity _____	principal procedure _____
complication _____	problem list _____
confirmed diagnosis _____	prospective payment system _____
diagnosis related group _____	questionable diagnosis _____
diagnostic condition _____	reimbursement _____
elective procedure _____	residual subcategory _____
encounter _____	screening _____
episode of care _____	secondary diagnosis _____
ill-defined condition _____	secondary procedure _____
major diagnostic category _____	service code _____
nonspecific abnormal finding _____	signs _____
nonspecific diagnosis _____	status code _____
observation _____	status post _____
outcome of delivery _____	subclassification _____
outpatient service _____	supplementary classification _____
physician billing _____	symptoms _____

unacceptable diagnosis _____   unspecified diagnosis _____
unconfirmed diagnosis _____   visit _____
unrelated procedure _____

REVIEW QUESTIONS

1. Explain the similarities and differences in coding unconfirmed diagnoses in an inpatient setting of care as opposed to coding unconfirmed diagnoses in an outpatient or office setting of care. _____
   _____
   _____

2. Discuss the similarities and differences between the residual subcategories throughout the main body of the disease classification and the categories and subcategories of the chapter with listings of symptoms and signs. _____
   _____
   _____

3. Explain the intent of the status codes and titles. _____
   _____
   _____

4. List the V code categories comprised of patient status listings. _____
   _____
   _____

5. Explain the intent of the service codes and titles. _____
   _____
   _____

6. List the V code categories comprised of patient service listings. _____
   _____
   _____

7. Discuss the differences and similarities between the observation codes and the screening codes. _____
   _____
   _____

8. Describe several idiosyncracies of physician clinical documentation between practitioners of various specialties. How do such practices impact the coding and reporting of diagnoses? ___
   _____
   _____

9. Discuss the impact of physician documentation of inactive problems in the patient health record upon coding and reporting. _____
   _____
   _____

10. Explain the consequences of variability in physician documentation practices upon the statistical tabulation of diagnostic and procedural data for research and study purposes. _____
    _____
    _____

11. Identify at least five codes and narrative titles that represent symptoms which are recognized by Medicare as complications or comorbidities.

_____   _____
_____   _____
_____   _____
_____   _____
_____   _____

12. Identify at least ten codes and narrative titles that represent V codes which are regarded by Medicare as unacceptable for reporting as primary diagnoses.

_____   _____
_____   _____
_____   _____
_____   _____
_____   _____

13. Assign precise, accurate code numbers from the ICD-9-CM volume for the following symptoms, signs, and ill-defined conditions:

A. auditory hallucinations _____

B. Dupré's syndrome _____

C. dropsy _____

D. anorexia _____

E. aphasia _____

F. lymphadenopathy _____

G. chest pain _____

H. pyrosis _____

I. extravasation of urine _____

J. hepatomegaly _____

K. cobalt abnormality of blood _____

L. glycosuria _____

M. abnormal cerebrospinal fluid _____

N. abnormal mammogram _____

O. abnormal echoencephalogram _____

P.   dyskaryotic cervical smear _____

_____

Q.   abnormal reflex _____

_____

R.   senility _____

_____

S.   sudden infant death syndrome _____

_____

T.   nervousness _____

_____

U.   unattended death _____

_____

V.   abnormal blood pressure reading _____

_____

W.   abnormal result of Mantoux test _____

_____

X.   abnormal electrocardiogram _____

_____

Y.   abnormal echocardiogram _____

_____

Z.   abnormal spermatozoa _____

_____

AA. hemoglobinuria _____

_____

BB. viremia _____

_____

CC. umbilical bleeding _____

_____

DD. painful urination _____

_____

EE. tenesmus _____

_____

FF. rales _____

_____

GG. heart palpitations _____

_____

HH. hemorrhage from throat _____

_____

II.   hyperalimentation _____

_____

JJ. thickening of skin _____

_____

KK. muscular incoordination _____

_____

LL. insomnia with sleep apnea _____

_____

MM. cachexia _____

_____

NN parageusia _____

OO. cholemia _____

PP. failure to thrive _____

QQ. aphonia _____

RR. bruit _____

SS. orthopnea _____

TT. hyperperistalsis _____

UU. nocturia _____

VV. umbilical swelling _____

WW. poikilocytosis _____

XX. chyluria _____

14. Assign precise, accurate code numbers from the ICD-9-CM volume for the following miscellaneous diagnostic or therapeutic procedures or services:

A. contrast dacryocystogram _____

B. acupuncture for anesthesia _____

C. magnetic resonance imaging of brain and brain stem _____

D. removal of intraluminal foreign body from larynx without incision _____

E. cardiovascular stress test using bicycle ergometer _____

F. removal of urethral stent _____

G. microscopic examination of blood _____

H. irrigation of nasal passages _____

I. microscopic examination of bursa _____

J. fitting of hearing aid _____

K. placental radioisotope scan _____

L. group therapy for psychosexual dysfunction _____

M. spinal traction using halo device _____

_____

N. barium swallow _____

_____

O. vaccination against yellow fever _____

_____

P. aortography _____

_____

Q. removal of foreign body from foot without incision _____

_____

R. general physical examination _____

_____

S. removal of tracheostomy tube _____

_____

T. microscopic examination of specimen from eye _____

_____

U. manual reduction of rectal prolapse _____

_____

V. microscopic examination of specimen from amnionic sac _____

_____

W. fluorescein angiography of eye _____

_____

X. liver scan and radioisotope function scan _____

_____

Y. psychiatric commitment evaluation _____

_____

15. Assign precise, accurate code numbers from the ICD-9-CM volume for the following uncon-firmed diagnoses presuming an inpatient setting of care:

A.   possible eastern equine encephalitis _____

B.   probable malignant neoplasm of ileum _____

C.   suspected hypopotassemia _____

D.   suspected hypertensive retinopathy _____

E.   possible protein deficiency anemia _____

F.   probable paranoid senile dementia _____

G.   probable rheumatic myocarditis _____

H.   possible viral epiglottitis _____

I.   suspected gastrojejunal ulcer _____

J.   suspected stricture of ureter _____

_____

K.   probable hyperemesis gravidarum _____

L.   possible contact dermatitis due to detergents _____

M.   possible bucket handle tear of lateral meniscus _____

N.   suspected displacement of brachial plexus _____

O.   probable cow's milk hypocalcemia _____

P.   possible abnormal spermatozoa _____

Q.   suspected injury to trigeminal nerve _____

R.   possible whooping cough due to *Bordetella parapertussis* _____

S.   suspected malignant neoplasm of the hippocampus _____

T.   probable pineal gland dysfunction _____

U.   probable bacterial meningitis _____

V.   suspected aplastic anemia due to drugs _____

W.   possible hysterical amnesia _____

X.   possible cerebral embolism _____

Y.   probable pneumonia due to streptococcus _____

Z.   probable acute appendicitis _____

AA. possible prostatic stone _____

BB. suspected major abnormality of bony pelvis _____

CC. possible Fox-Fordyce disease _____

DD. suspected spinal stenosis in cervical region _____

EE. possible fusion of ear ossicles _____

FF. probable neonatal infective mastitis _____

GG. suspected hypersomnia with sleep apnea _____

HH. possible poisoning by penicillin _____

II.   suspected hepatitis due to toxoplasmosis _____

JJ.   possible benign neoplasm of the cheek _____

KK.   possible iodine hypothyroidism _____

LL.   possible acoustic neuritis _____

MM.   probable thrombocytasthenia _____

NN.   suspected cannabis dependence _____

OO.   probable chronic hypotension _____

PP.   suspected acute pulmonary edema _____

QQ.   possible perforation of gallbladder _____

RR.   probable premenstrual tension _____

SS.   probable puerperal pulmonary embolism _____

TT.   suspected dermatitis due to medicine _____

UU.   suspected arrest of bone development _____

VV.   probable congenital preluxation of hip _____

WW.   suspected thrombosis of umbilical cord _____

XX.   possible symbolic dysfunction _____

YY.   probable heat exhaustion _____

16. Assign precise, accurate V codes for the following conditions documented in an episode of care.

A.   child with exposure to tuberculosis _____

B.   male admitted with exposure to venereal disease _____

C.   ninety-year-old man infected with microorganism resistant to tetracyclines _____

D.   patient infected with aminoglycoside microorganism _____

E.   elderly man infected with microorganism resistant to multiple drugs _____

F.   female with personal history of malignant neoplasm of the gastrointestinal tract _____

G. seventy-five-year-old patient with personal history of malignant neoplasm of the kidney _____

H. man admitted with an unspecified type of leukemia in remission _____

I. patient with history of Hodgkin's disease _____

J. woman with personal history of thyroid malignancy _____

K. personal history of alcoholism noted in patient's history and physical examination report _____

L. physician's history and physical notes reveal patient's personal history of blood diseases _____

M. personal history of chronic obstructive pulmonary disease _____

N. family history of diabetes mellitus documented in patient's record _____

O. patient with family history of endocrine and metabolic diseases _____

P. patient with personal history of allergy to Penicillin _____

Q. personal history of allergic reaction to tranquilizing narcotic agent _____

R. personal history of allergy to serum vaccine _____

S. man with history of allergy to unspecified medicinal agents _____

T. family reported that patient has personal history of non-compliance with medical treatment _____

U. patient with personal history of psychological trauma due to rape _____

V. patient with history of stroke following coronary artery bypass surgery _____

W. patient whose mother died of cerebral vascular accident five years ago _____

X. female with family history of ischemic heart disease _____

Y. man whose mother suffers from osteoarthritis _____

Z. woman whose father died in a mental institution _____

AA. male with family history of diabetes mellitus _____

BB. patient whose brother and sister each received kidney transplants _____

CC. patient whose aunt died of complications from a parasitic disease _____

DD. twenty-one-year-old with normal pregnancy _____

EE.   elderly patient with family history of blindness _____

FF.   adolescent with speech problems _____

GG.   person on waiting list undergoing social agency investigation _____

HH.   fifty-two-year-old male with kidney transplant _____

II.   patient who decided not to have surgery on knee _____

JJ.   triplets (two female, one male) born in hospital _____

KK.   woman who lost her sense of smell and taste _____

LL.   three-year-old girl showing signs of neglect _____

MM.   thirty-year-old male who refused treatment due to his religion _____

NN.   contraindication ruled out DPT shot in three month-old female child _____

OO.   thirty-five-year-old woman with a tracheostomy _____

PP.   sixty-six-year-old male with a carotid sinus pacemaker in situ _____

QQ.   teenage girl with a family history of asthma _____

RR.   young male with a history of noncompliance with treatment couple undergoing general counseling and advice on procreative management _____

SS.   male patient with a heart valve replacement _____

TT.   family with lack of heating in home _____

UU.   teenage girl with illegitimate pregnancy _____

VV.   medical services in home not available _____

WW.   forty-year-old male with cardiovascular exercise intolerance while performing ordinary activity _____

17. Assign precise, accurate V codes for the following services documented in an episode of care.

A.   infant who had contact with brother infected with diphtheria _____

B.   man with need for prophylactic tetanus toxin vaccination _____

C.   elderly woman given prophylactic vaccination for the common cold _____

D. patient who had contact with family member with mumps _____

E. patient given prophylactic influenza vaccination before discharge _____

F. thirty-year-old woman given rhogam as prophylactic immunotherapy _____

G. sixty-nine-year-old woman treated with post menopausal hormone replacement therapy

H. ten-year-old counseled after experiencing fondling by neighborhood friend _____

I. routine childhood health check _____

J. supervision of high risk pregnancy _____

K. pregnant woman with history of infertility _____

L. patient visit for postpartum care and examination _____

M. supervision of lactating mother _____

N. patient admitted for insertion of intrauterine contraceptive device _____

O. husband and wife seen for genetic counseling _____

P. pregnant teenager screened for chromosomal anomalies by amniocentesis _____

Q. pregnant thirty-five-year-old admitted with history of trophoblastic disease _____

R. patient encounter for contraceptive management _____

S. patient admitted for special screening for cardiovascular disease _____

T. screening of male smoker for emphysema _____

U. army recruit administered with health examination _____

V. screening patient for cataract _____

W. examination of victim of alleged rape _____

X. screening of child for mental retardation _____

Y. patient receiving a routine chest X-ray _____

Z. screening of patient for radiation exposure _____

AA. screening of patient for sickle-cell anemia _____

BB. rubella screening for child _____

CC. patient undergoing screening for mucoviscidosis _____

DD. teenager screened for venereal disease _____

EE. screening of patient for malaria _____

FF. screening for malignant neoplasm in mouth of user of chewing tobacco _____

GG. forty-eight-year-old woman undergoing face lift _____

HH. bone marrow donor _____

II. plastic surgery following healed injury due to auto accident _____

JJ. patient undergoing chemotherapy _____

KK. fitting of breast prosthesis following surgery _____

LL. patient undergoing renal dialysis _____

MM. fitting of orthopedic brace on child _____

NN. closure of tracheostomy _____

OO. changing of plaster cast on patient _____

PP. routine health check on six-month-old boy _____

QQ. supervision of pregnancy in woman with history of stillbirths _____

RR. screening for chromosomal anomalies by amniocentesis _____

SS. male undergoing vasoplasty after previous sterilization _____

TT. supervision of lactating mother _____

UU. checking of contraceptive device _____

VV. male needing vaccination for diphtheria _____

WW. vaccination for viral hepatitis _____

XX. postmenopausal hormone replacement therapy _____

CODING OF CLINICAL DOCUMENTATION

Read the following clinical reports, determine the reason for the encounter or visit, and assign precise, accurate diagnostic and procedural code numbers from the appropriate sections of the ICD-9-CM volumes.

PATIENT: Taylor, Lillian   **MR#:** 99-10-01

PHYSICIAN: Edwards

Chief Complaint:
"Fell and cut my chin"

History of Present Illness:
Patient experienced dizziness and fell, striking chin on coffee table, resulting in small laceration; no associated loss of consciousness, nausea, vomiting, headache, or angina; no previous history of loss of consciousness, seizures, cerebrovascular accident, or transient ischemic attack; status post mitral valve replacement, on Coumadin; adult type diabetes mellitus on insulin; chronic obstructive pulmonary disease for twenty years requiring nasal O_2.

Past Medical History:
Positive for measles; mumps; and rheumatic fever with three months in the hospital at age 14; total right hip replacement in 1989, after a fall on the ice; gravida 3, para 3, vaginal delivery × 3; no known allergies.

Medications:
Coumadin 10 mg q.d. p.o.; NPH insulin 80 units subq. q.d. at breakfast; nasal O_2 at 2L/min; ASA 500 mg t.i.d. p.r.n. for arthritis pain; vitamin pill q.d. p.o.

Review of Systems:
Multiple age spots on hands; crepitus both hands; decreased hearing both sides; sleeps better on three pillows.

Family Medical History:
Father died of heart attack at age 67; mother died of old age; sister died in childbirth; three children alive and well.

Social History:
Lives in nursing home with few visitors; husband died two years ago; smoked three packs per day for 30 years.

Reason for encounter: _____

_____

Codes: _____

PATIENT: Whitfield, Hunter   **MR#:** 99-10-02

PHYSICIAN: Sparks

Chief Complaint:
"Pain in my stomach and just feeling sick"

History of Present Illness:
Patient came to the hospital this morning with a three-day history of intermittent episodes of "crampy" pain in the right upper quadrant; this pain is diffuse without radiation and is related to eating of meals; this morning after the patient's breakfast, the pain worsened and became associ-

ated with nausea and vomiting; he is a sickle cell trait heterozygote diagnosed in 1970 after a prolonged ill feeling; he is hypertensive, well controlled on diuretic Furosemide 80 mg twice daily.

History of Past Illness:
Measles without complications, 1959; mumps with unilateral right-sided orchitis, 1964; prolonged ill feeling diagnosed as anemia with etiology of sickle cell trait, 1970; hypertension diagnosed on routine physical for work, 1976; right-sided wrist fracture from a racquetball accident, 1985.

Review of Systems:
No history of weight loss; no change of diet or appetite; no changes in sleep patterns; no changes in skin, nails, or hair; no enlarged lymph nodes; no pain in joints; no recent bleeding; no recent dizziness; no changes in bowel or bladder function or habits.

Family Medical History:
Mother and father still living; mother had gallbladder removed three years ago; father has high blood pressure and chronic anemia, and had a stroke in 1983; one older brother and a sister alive and well; children, three boys, alive and well; no family history of diabetes or cardiovascular disease.

Social History:
Patient is a full-time salesman, which involves travel across the country, but not into foreign countries; eats regular meals, low salt, and balanced three times per day; exercises regularly four times per week, running five miles in approximately 35–40 minutes; he is a non-smoker, and drinks socially approximately three beers per week.

Reason for encounter: _____

_____

Codes: _____

PATIENT: Mullins, Todd   **MR#:** 99-10-03

PHYSICIAN: Koenig

Chief Complaint:
Motor Vehicle Accident

History of Present Illness:
Patient was passenger (without seat belt on) in automobile that crossed median and struck another car head on; patient was brought in by ambulance comatose, with neck collar, intubated, and bagged; field vitals pulse 140, blood pressure 80/40.

Past Medical History:
No known allergies; no medications.

Review of Systems:
Non-contributory.

Family Medical History:
Mother has diabetes mellitus.

Social History:
Lives with mother, father, and one sister; freshman in high school.

Reason for encounter: _____

_____

Codes: _____

PATIENT: Cooper, Paula   **MR#:** 99-10-04

PHYSICIAN: Young

Chief Complaint:
"Pain in my stomach, then vomiting blood"

History of Present Illness:
Patient first noted pain in her stomach three days ago and attributed it to spicy foods, she took antacids and the pain dissipated; this morning before breakfast she felt similar pain more severely so she again took antacids and ate her breakfast; after breakfast she became nauseous and vomited approximately one cup of bright red blood with food; about one hour later she again vomited approximately one cup of blood; no history of dizziness, shortness of breath, diarrhea, previous hematemesis, or melena.

History of Past Illness:
No major injuries or illnesses; no hospitalizations other than normal vaginal deliveries; gravida 4, para 4; no known allergies.

Medications:
Antacid tablets, p.o. p.r.n. for stomach pain; ASA occasionally for headache.

Review of Systems:
Wears glasses; deviated septum; initial insomnia without daytime sleepiness.

Family Medical History:
Negative for ulcers, coagulopathies, diabetes, or cardiovascular disease; father has colon Ca with polyposis.

Social History:
Homemaker with children 12, 10, 8, and 5 years old; does not smoke; rarely drinks alcohol.

Reason for encounter: _____

_____

Codes: _____

PATIENT: Higgins, Thomas   **MR#:** 99-10-05

PHYSICIAN: Caldwell

Physical Examination:
Age: 47; *Sex:* male; *Weight:* 138 lbs; *Temp:* 100.2; *Pulse:* 62; *Resp:* 14; *BP:* 138/88.
General: well-developed, well-nourished white male appearing younger than stated age; supine in pain with legs drawn up.
Skin: without erythema or edema; normal male hair distribution.
Eyes: pupils equal, round, responsive to light and accommodation; no hypertensive changes; extraocular movements intact.
Ears: air conduction greater than bone conduction; both tympanic; both membranes clear; normal wax.
Nose: without inflammation, swelling, or blood.
Mouth: upper dentures; no inflammation or masses.
Neck: range of motion is intact; no lymph nodes palpable; thyroid not palpable.
Chest: lungs clear to auscultation and percussion; symmetrical diaphragm movement by percussion.
Heart: regular rate and rhythm; first and second heart sounds present; normal physiological splitting of second heart sound without murmur, gallop, or rub.

Pulses: (Scale 1+ to 4+) carotid++, radial++, ulnar+, brachial++, femoral++, popliteal+, dorsalis pedis++, posterior tibial+, symmetrically; no bruits carotid or femoral.

Abdomen: bowel sounds normoactive; tenderness to deep palpation in right upper quadrant without rebound; no palpable masses; liver 12 cm by percussion with a smooth edge; spleen not felt.

Extremities: range of motion intact; no femoral or axillary lymph nodes noted; without cyanosis, clubbing, or edema.

Genitourinary: normal male uncircumcised; bladder not distended; right testicle smaller than normal.

Rectal: prostate not enlarged; uniform density without local areas of hardness; no masses felt; stool present in anal vault; occult and gross blood not present.

Neurological: awake, alert, oriented to time, person, and place; good muscular strength; cranial nerves II through XII intact; normal sensory perception to pain and vibration; finger-to-nose test and heel-to-shin test intact; superficial long tract reflex responds in a plantar direction.

Diagnosis:
Pain due to cholangitis, probably associated with cholecystitis and cholelithiasis.

Reason for encounter: _____

_____

Codes: _____

PATIENT: Koch, Ella   **MR#:** 99-10-06

PHYSICIAN: Hauser

Physical Examination:
Age: 70; *Sex:* female; *Weight:* 98 lbs; *Temp:* 96.8; *Pulse:* 96; *Resp:* 8; *BP:* 164/104.

General: frail, elderly lady in no acute distress, laying supine and relaxed.

Skin: pink, warm, without edema; laceration 2 cm right chin, 1 cm from midline.

Eyes: pupils equal and reactive to light and accommodation; extraocular movements intact.

Ears: decreased hearing both sides; air conduction greater than bone conduction both sides; tympanic membranes clear.

Nose: without inflammation; dry mucosa; deviation to left.

Mouth: edentulous with dentures; no inflammation.

Neck: limited range of motion with crepitus; no nodes; thyroid firm.

Chest: bibasalar rales 1+; very resonant to percussion.

Heart: regular rate and rhythm; S-1 clicks (mechanical); S-2 normal; slight systolic flow; murmur II/IV.

Pulses: carotid+, radial+, ulnar−, brachial+, femoral+, popliteal−, dorsalis pedis+, posterior tibial− both sides; no bruits carotid or femoral.

Abdomen: protuberant with normoactive bowel sounds; transmitted heart sounds; liver palpable, 10 cm by percussion; spleen not felt.

Extremities: limited range of motion left with crepitus; right without crepitus but painful; no ulcers.

Genitourinary: normal female; dry mucosa; no masses.

Rectal: no masses; no stool; heme+.

Neurological: awake, but at times distant; oriented × 2; good strength but motion limited on left; cranial nerves II through XII intact; decreased sensory on left; finger-to-nose and heel-to-shin tremorous but grossly intact; speech at times slurred.

Diagnosis:
Transient ischemic attack secondary to emboli formed on mitral valve.

Reason for encounter: _____

_____

Codes: _____

PATIENT: Aubuchon, Lynn   **MR#:** 99-10-07

PHYSICIAN: Perez

Physical Examination:
Age: 32; *Sex:* female; *Weight:* 124 lbs; *Temp:* 101.2; *Pulse:* 86; *Resp:* 18; *BP:* 132/82.
General: well-developed, well-nourished white female looking tired and older than her stated age.
Skin: pale but warm; normal female hair.
Eyes: pupils equal and reactive to light and accommodation; extraocular movements intact; fundi orange.
Ears: excessive wax occluding both tympanic membranes; air conduction greater than bone conduction both sides.
Nose: without hemorrhage; without inflammation.
Mouth: without inflammation; teeth in good repair.
Neck: range of motion intact; submandibular nodes 2 cm diameter.
Chest: diaphragm symmetrical; right dull to percussion.
Heart: regular rate and rhythm; S-1 and S-2 normal.
Pulses: carotid++, brachial++, radial++, ulnar+, femoral++, popliteal++, dorsalis pedis++, posterior tibial+, symmetrical; no bruits carotid or femoral.
Abdomen: bowel sounds hyperactive; pain sub xiphoid.
Extremities: range of motion intact; warm hands; cold feet.
Rectal: good sphincter tone; occult blood+.
Neurological: awake, alert, oriented × 3; good speech; strength good; gait good; cranial nerves II through XII intact; normal sensory; plantar response.

Diagnosis:
Gastric ulcer, rule out ETOH gastritis; Pneumonia secondary to aspiration.

Reason for encounter: _____

_____

Codes: _____

PATIENT: Porter, Larry   **MR#:** 99-10-08

PHYSICIAN: Vogel

Physical Examination:
Age: 12; *Sex:* male; *Weight:* 135 lbs; *Temp:* 95.6; *Pulse:* 120; thready; *Resp:* 20; bagged; *BP:* 90/50.
General: well-developed, well-nourished white male adolescent of adult proportion; multiple lacerations on face; displaced right shoulder; right rib fractures with indentation; head covered with blood.
Skin: pale; shrunken with bleeding from multiple sites.

Eyes: right pupil fixed and dilated; left pinpoint pupil; no extraocular movement; positive for corneal reflex both sides.
Ears: blood in external canal.
Nose: displaced to left grossly with blood in vestibule.
Mouth: jaw displaced to left without fracture of mandible.
Throat: endotracheal tube in place.
Neck: cervical collar; no deviation of trachea; no deformity; jugular vein distention.
Chest: lungs clear to auscultation.
Heart: weak beat; S-1 and S-2 muffled.
Abdomen: absent bowel sounds; no masses.
Pulses: carotid+, femoral+, radial−, ulnar−, dorsalis pedis−, posterior tibial−.
Extremities: right humeral head displaced.
Rectal: heme negative; no masses.
Neurological: comatose; not responsive to pain; decorticate posture; Babinski left; plantar response right.

Diagnosis:
Hemorrhage with hypovolemic hypotension; Cranial damage, possibly epidural or subdural; Pericardiac tamponade.

Reason for encounter: _____

_____

Codes: _____

PATIENT: Pappas, Ellen   **MR#:** 99-10-09

ATTENDING PHYSICIAN: Hakeem

Chest:
Anteroposterior and Lateral
   Extensive consolidation of the left lung is unchanged. No significant pleural fluid layers on the decubitus view. There is linear atelectasis at the right base.

Impression:
Extensive left lung consolidation.

Codes: _____

PATIENT: Maxwell, Frank   **MR#:** 99-10-10

ATTENDING PHYSICIAN: Simmons

Chest:
There is a calcified nodule in the right upper lobe. There is no active cardiopulmonary disease or pleural effusion.

Impression:
No active disease.

Upper GI Series:
There is a superficial ulceration of the distal antrum, pyloric channel, and duodenal bulb.

Obstructive Series:
There is no free air under the diaphragm. No obstruction to the small or large bowel.

Impression:
Grossly negative abdomen.

Codes: _____

PATIENT: Eastmann, Leonard   **MR#:** 99-10-11

ATTENDING PHYSICIAN: Reynolds

Reason for Admission:
Colostomy takedown.
    The patient is a young male, status post gunshot wound and subsequent colostomy. He was admitted for colostomy takedown.

Past Surgical History:
Exploratory laparotomy.

Past Medical History:
Not significant.

No drug allergies known.

Medications on Admission:
None.

Physical Examination:
Benign on admission. The patient was brought to the operating room for a colostomy takedown, status post gunshot wound. He tolerated the procedure well without complications. The patient returned to the floor postoperatively. Vital signs remained stable and he was afebrile. The patient began to have bowel sounds on postoperative day three. His wound was noted to be clean, dry, and intact. The patient began to have bowel movements and tolerated clear liquid diet well. He was advanced to a regular diet and was discharged in good condition.

Discharge Medications:
Colace 100 mg p.o. b.i.d.; Tylenol p.r.n.

Discharge Instructions:
No heavy lifting or driving for six weeks.

Follow-up:
In office in one week.

Codes: _____

11

ICD Coding: Injury and Poisoning and External Causes of Injury and Poisoning

LEARNING OBJECTIVES

Upon completion of this chapter the learner should be able to:

1. Describe the parameters for coding and reporting fractures and dislocations.
2. Describe the parameters for coding and reporting head injuries.
3. Describe the parameters for coding and reporting internal injuries.
4. Describe the parameters for coding and reporting open wounds.
5. Describe the parameters for coding and reporting late effects of injury.
6. Describe the parameters for coding and reporting superficial injury.
7. Describe the parameters for coding and reporting burns.
8. Describe the parameters for coding and reporting poisoning.
9. Explain the proper usage of the table of poisoning.
10. Describe the parameters for coding and reporting complications of medical or surgical care.
11. Explain the use and function of the E codes.
12. Discuss the impact of comorbidities and complications on billing and reimbursement for diagnoses and procedures involving traumatic injury.
13. Apply knowledge of coding principles by assigning accurate and precise codes to report injury and poisoning.
14. Apply knowledge of coding principles by assigning accurate and precise codes to report complications of medical and surgical care.
15. Apply knowledge of coding principles by assigning accurate and precise codes to report external causes of injuries.

ICD CODING OF TRAUMA

Chapter 17 of the ICD-9-CM diagnostic tabular volume is designated for listings of injuries and poisoning, but also includes listings of other traumatic conditions and complications. This chapter consists of nineteen sections and seven subsections (Table 11–1).

TABLE 11-1

Sections and Subsections in Chapter 17, Volume 1 of ICD-9-CM

1. Fractures (category range 800–829)
   Fracture of Skull (category range 800–804)
   Fracture of Neck and Trunk (category range 805–809)
   Fracture of Upper Limb (category range 810–819)
   Fracture of Lower Limb (category range 820–829)
2. Dislocation (category range 830–839)
3. Sprains and Strains of Joints and Adjacent Muscles (category range 840–848)
4. Intracranial Injury, Excluding Those with Skull Fracture (category range 850–854)
5. Internal Injury of Thorax, Abdomen, and Pelvis (category range 860–869)
6. Open Wound (category range 870–897)
   Open Wound of Head, Neck, and Trunk (category range 870–879)
   Open Wound of Upper Limb (category range 880–887)
   Open Wound of Lower Limb (category range 890–897)
7. Injury to Blood Vessels (category range 900–904)
8. Late Effects of Injuries, Poisonings, Toxic Effects, Other External Causes (category range 905–909)
9. Superficial Injury (category range 910–919)
10. Contusion with Intact Skin Surface (category range 920–924)
11. Crushing Injury (category range 925–929)
12. Effects of Foreign Body Entering through Orifice (category range 930–939)
13. Burns (category range 940–949)
14. Injury to Nerves and Spinal Cord (category range 950–957)
15. Certain Traumatic Complications and Unspecified Injuries (category range 958–959)
16. Poisoning by Drugs, Medicinal, and Biological Substances (category range 960–979)
17. Toxic Effects of Substances Chiefly Nonmedicinal as to Source (category range 980–989)
18. Other and Unspecified Effects of External Causes (category range 990–995)
19. Complications of Surgical and Medical Care, Not Elsewhere Classified (category range 996–999)

The coding guidelines for reporting trauma adhere to the principle that multiple coding of injuries should be accomplished to the greatest extent possible. The combination categories for multiple injuries are provided for use only if insufficient detail was documented concerning the traumatic conditions (such as transitory care of cases that were transferred elsewhere), or for specific primary tabulation purposes in designated research projects.

As a general coding guideline, component injuries should be reported with separate and distinct code numbers. If multiple sites of injury are specified in the code titles within the tabular classification, the word "with" indicates involvement of both sites, and the word "and" indicates involvement of either or both sites.

In the event of reporting injuries such as multiple fractures, separate codes should be assigned for each fracture unless a combination code is specifically provided. For example, a concurrent closed fracture of the shaft of tibia and the fibula should be reported with code number *823.22*.

With the reporting of multiple injuries, the code for the most serious injury, as determined by the physician, should be sequenced first. To exemplify, a cerebral concussion with brief loss of consciousness (code number *850.1*) is a more serious injury than a laceration of the scalp (code number *873.0*) or a second degree burn of the thigh (code number *945.26*), and thus the concussion diagnosis should be sequenced first among the three conditions.

Superficial injuries such as abrasions or contusions should not be coded if these conditions are associated with more severe injuries of the same anatomic site. Therefore, an abrasion on a finger that was fractured would not be coded and reported, by reason that the fracture was the reportable diagnosis and the abrasion was incidental to the fracture.

If a major traumatic injury resulted in minor damage to peripheral nerves or blood vessels, the primary injury that must be sequenced first may be reported along with additional codes from category range *950* through *957, Injury to nerves and spinal cord,* and/or from category range *900* through *904, Injury to blood vessels.* These additional codes represent the secondary injuries to the nerves or blood vessels. However, if the nerve or blood vessel injury was documented in the patient health record as the reason for the admission or encounter, that condition should then be sequenced as the principal or primary diagnosis.

ICD CODING OF FRACTURES AND DISLOCATIONS

The first section of Chapter 17 in the diagnostic tabular of ICD-9-CM contains listings for fractures. The reporting of malunion, nonunion, as well as pathological or spontaneous fracture are excluded from the listings of this section.

In this section, the terms condyle, coronoid process, ramus, and symphysis predominantly indicate the portion of the bone that was fractured, and not the name of the bone involved. A fracture not documented as either closed or open should be coded and reported as a closed fracture. The descriptions, closed and open, used in the fourth-digit subcategories of this section inherently include specific synonyms.

Synonyms for closed fracture encompass: comminuted; depressed; elevated; fissured; greenstick; impacted; linear; march; simple; slipped epiphysis; and spiral.

Synonyms for open fracture encompass: compound; infected; missile; puncture; and with foreign body.

The section of Chapter 17 containing listings for fractures includes categorization for: fracture of the skull, fracture of the face bones; fracture of the vertebral column with or without spinal cord injury (paralysis, paraplegia, quadriplegia, and spinal concussion); fracture of the ribs, the sternum, the larynx, and the trachea; as well as fracture of the pelvis. This section also contains listings for: fracture of the clavicle; fracture of the scapula; fracture of the humerus; fracture of the radius, fracture of the ulna; fracture of the carpal bone; fracture of the metacarpal bone; fracture of one or more phalanges of the hand; fracture of the femur; fracture of the patella; fracture of the tibia, fracture of the fibula; fracture of the ankle; fracture of one or more tarsal or metatarsal bone; and fracture of one or more phalanges of the foot.

Multiple fractures of the same extremity that are classifiable to the same four-digit subcategory should be coded and reported with only one code. Multiple unilateral or bilateral fractures of same bones that may be classified to different fourth-digit subcategories within the same three-digit category should be reported with each individual code that is applicable.

Multiple fractures should be sequenced for reporting in accordance with the severity of the fracture as documented in the patient medical record. If doubt exists, the physician should be contacted to determine the order of severity among the fracture diagnoses.

The second section of Chapter 17 is comprised of listings to report dislocations. These listings in this section include the reporting of displacement and subluxation, although they exclude the reporting of congenital, pathological, or recurrent dislocation.

A dislocation not documented as either closed or open should be coded and reported as a closed dislocation. The descriptions, closed and open, used in the fourth-digit subcategories of this section inherently include specific synonyms.

Synonyms for closed dislocations encompass: complete; partial; simple; and uncomplicated.

Synonyms for open dislocations encompass: compound; infected; and with foreign body.

The section of Chapter 17 containing listings of dislocations includes categorization for: dislocation of the jaw; dislocation of the shoulder; dislocation of the elbow; dislocation of the wrist; dislocation of the finger; dislocation of the hip; dislocation of the knee; dislocation of the ankle; and dislocation of the foot.

The third section of Chapter 17 of the diagnostic tabular volume of ICD-9-CM is comprised of listings to report sprains and strains including avulsion, hemartrosis, laceration, rupture, or tear of capsule, ligament, muscle, or tendon. These listings in this section exclude the reporting of a laceration of a tendon in open wounds.

The section of Chapter 17 containing listings of sprains and strains encompasses categorization for: sprains and strains of the shoulder and the upper arm; sprains and strains of the elbow and the forearm; sprains and strains of the wrist and the hand; sprains and strains of the hip and the thigh; sprains and strains of the knee and the leg; sprains and strains of the ankle and the foot; sprains and strains of the sacroiliac region; and sprains and strains of other parts of the back.

ICD CODING OF INTERNAL INJURIES AND OPEN WOUNDS

The fourth section of Chapter 17, comprised of category range 850 through 854, includes listings for the reporting of intracranial injury. The description "with open intracranial wound" used in the fourth-digit subcategories of this section incorporates diagnoses specifying an open wound with documentation of an infection or a foreign body.

This section containing listings to report intracranial injury includes categorization for: concussion; subarachnoid, subdural, extradural, and other intracranial hemorrhage following trauma; cerebral laceration and contusion; as well as brain injury and head injury not otherwise specified.

The fifth section of Chapter 17, comprised of category range 860 through 869, contains listings to report blast injuries, blunt trauma, concussion injuries, crushing, hematoma, laceration, puncture, tear, or traumatic rupture of internal organs. The listings in these categories exclude the reporting of a foreign body entering through an orifice and exclude injury to blood vessels. The description "with open wound" used in the fourth-digit subcategories of this section incorporates diagnoses specifying the documentation of an infection or a foreign body.

This section comprised of listings to report an internal injury of the chest, the abdomen, or the pelvis includes categorization for: traumatic pneumothorax and hemothorax; injury to the heart or the lung; injury to other intrathoracic organs; injury to the gastrointestinal tract; injury to the liver; injury to the spleen; injury to the kidney; injury to the pelvic organs; and injury to other intra-abdominal organs.

The sixth section of Chapter 17 is comprised of listings to report open wounds. These listings throughout category range 870 through 897 may be utilized to report wounds involving animal bite, avulsion, cut, laceration, puncture, and traumatic amputation. However, these listings exclude the reporting of wounds resulting from burn, crushing, or superficial injury, as well as those wounds resulting from incidental dislocation, fracture, or internal injury. The term "complicated" used in the fourth-digit subcategories incorporates diagnoses specifying documentation of delayed healing, delayed treatment, foreign body, or major infection.

The section containing listings for categorization of open wound include: open wound of ocular adnexa; open wound of the eyeball; open wound of the ear; open wound of the head; open wound of the neck; open wound of the chest; open wound of the back; open wound of the buttock; and open wound of the genital organs. This section also contains listings for reporting: open wound of the shoulder and the upper arm; open wound of the elbow, the forearm, and the wrist; open wound of the hand and the finger; complete or partial traumatic amputation of the thumb, the finger, the hand, or the arm; open wound of the hip and the thigh; open wound of the knee and the ankle; open wound of the foot and the toe; and complete or partial traumatic amputation of the toe, the foot, or the leg.

The seventh section of Chapter 17 encompasses listings to report the injury of a blood vessel. These listings within category range 900 through 904 include diagnoses involving arterial hematoma, avulsion, cut, laceration, rupture, traumatic aneurysm, or traumatic fistula. These listings in these categories exclude the reporting of accidental puncture or laceration during a medical or surgical procedure.

This section comprised of listings to report injury to blood vessels includes categoration for: injury to blood vessels of the head and the neck; injury to blood vessels of the thorax; injury to blood vessels of the abdomen and the pelvis; and injury to blood vessels of the upper extremity and lower extremity.

The fourteenth section of Chapter 17 is comprised of listings to report injury to the nerves and the spinal cord. These listings within category range 950 through 957 incorporate diagnoses involving division of nerve, lesion in continuity, traumatic neuroma, or traumatic transient paralysis with or without an open wound. However, these listings exclude the reporting of accidental puncture or laceration during a medical, surgical, or other clinical procedure.

The section encompassing listings for reporting injury to nerves and spinal cord includes categorization for: injury to the optic nerve and pathways; injury to other cranial nerves; spinal cord injury without evidence of spinal bone injury; injury to nerve roots, spinal plexus or other nerves of the trunk; injury to peripheral nerves of the shoulder girdle and the upper limb; and injury to peripheral nerves of the pelvic girdle and the lower limb.

The brief fifteenth section of Chapter 17 is comprised of listings to report certain traumatic complications and unspecified injuries. This section provides two residual categories for reporting miscellaneous listings of early complications of trauma and for reporting injuries not otherwise specified.

The eighth section of Chapter 17 encompasses listings to report late effects. These listings among category range 905 through 909 should be used to report conditions classifiable to category range 800 through 999 as the cause of late effects that are classified elsewhere.

These "late effects" include conditions documented as such as well as sequelae resulting from the acute injury. This section containing listings to report late effects includes categorization for: late effects of musculoskeletal and connective tissue injuries; late effects of injuries to the skin and subcutaneous tissues; late effects of injuries to the nervous system; late effects of poisoning and toxic effects; and late effects of other external causes.

ICD CODING OF SUPERFICIAL INJURIES

The ninth section of Chapter 17 comprises listings to report superficial injury. These listings within category range 910 through 919, however, exclude the reporting of diagnoses involving a burn, a contusion, a foreign body, an insect bite, or an open wound with incidental foreign body.

This section encompassing listings for reporting superficial injury includes categorization for: superficial injury of the face, the neck, and the scalp; superficial injury of the trunk and the groin; superficial injury of the shoulder and the upper arm; superficial injury of the elbow, the forearm, and the wrist; superficial injury of the hand and the finger; superficial injury of the hip, the thigh, the leg, and the ankle; superficial injury of the foot and the toe; and superficial injury of the eye and adnexa.

The tenth section of Chapter 17 is comprised of category range 920 through 924 and contains listings to report diagnoses involving contusion with intact skin surface, such as those involving a bruise or hematoma without fracture or open wound. These listings exclude the reporting of a contusion incidental to crushing injury, dislocation, fracture, internal injury, intracranial injury, nerve injury, or open wound.

The section encompassing listings to report contusion with intact skin surface includes categorization for: contusion of the face, the scalp, and the neck; contusion of the eye and adnexa; contusion of the trunk; contusion of the upper limb; and contusion of the lower limb.

The eleventh section of Chapter 17 contains listings to report crushing injury. These listings within category range 925 through 929 exclude the reporting of diagnoses involving concussion or those involving crushing injury incidental to internal injury or intracranial injury.

The section encompassing listings for reporting crushing injury includes categorization for: crushing injury of the face, the scalp, and the neck; crushing injury of the trunk, and crushing injury of the upper limb or the lower limb.

The twelfth section of Chapter 17 is comprised of listings to report effects of foreign body entering through a bodily orifice. These listings within category range 930 through 939 exclude the reporting of diagnoses involving a foreign body in an open wound or with a superficial injury without a major open wound.

The section containing listings to report a foreign body includes categorization for: a foreign body on the external eye; a foreign body in the ear; a foreign body in the nose; a foreign body in the pharynx or the larynx; a foreign body in the trachea, the bronchus, or the lung; a foreign body in the mouth, the esophagus, or the stomach; a foreign body in the intestine or the colon; a foreign body in the anus or the rectum; as well as a foreign body in the genitourinary tract.

ICD CODING OF BURNS

The thirteenth section of Chapter 17 of the diagnostic tabular volume of ICD-9-CM is comprised of listings to report burn injuries. These listings with category range 940 through 949 incorporate diagnoses of burns sustained from heating appliances, electricity, flames, hot objects, lightning, radiation, chemicals, and scalds. However, these listings exclude the reporting of diagnoses involving friction burns and sunburn.

This section encompassing listings to report burns includes categorization for: burns confined to eye and adnexa; burns of the face, the head, and the neck; burns of the trunk; burns of the upper limb, burns of the wrist and the hand; burns of the lower limb; and burns of internal organs.

Burns may be classified and reported by depth, extent, and by causative agent with the utilization of supplementary E codes. E codes are explained in another section of this chapter. By depth, burns should be classified as first-degree (erythema), second-degree (blistering), or third-degree (full-thickness involvement).

In coding and reporting burns, the highest degree of burn should be sequenced as the primary burn. If first-degree and second-degree burns of different sites were documented, the principal burn diagnosis reported should ordinarily be the second-degree burn, unless a vital organ such as the eye was affected by a first-degree burn and the second-degree burn affected only flesh. In that instance, the eye injury should take precedence in sequencing.

Burns of the same local site (within the same three-digit category), but of different degrees, should be coded with the listings in the subcategory identifying the highest degree burn that was documented in the patient's medical record. For instance, with documentation of second-degree and third-degree burns of the wrist, only the third-degree burns should be coded and reported. Code number *958.3, Posttraumatic wound infection, not elsewhere classified,* should be selected and assigned as an additional code to report any documentation of an infected burn site.

Category *948, Burns classified according to extent of body surface involved,* is generally regarded as an optional category. This category may be used as an adjunct to category range 940 through 947 to indicate the percent of body surface that sustained a third-degree burn. The fourth-digit classification is used to denote the percentage of body surface involved in a burn of any degree, and the fifth-digit subclassification is used to denote the percentage of the body surface that was inflicted with a third-degree burn. The valid fifth-digits that may be selected and assigned are placed in brackets under each code in this category. This category should be utilized only if this additional data is needed for a designated purpose, such as the compilation of burn mortality by burn units in an acute care facility.

Treatment of severe burns usually entails extensive skin debridement. For coding and reporting purposes, code *86.22* for the reporting of excisional debridement should be assigned only if the procedure was performed by a physician. Nonexcisional debridement performed by the physician or nonphysician healthcare practitioner should be reported with code *86.28.* Any other excisional type of procedure rendered by a nonphysician should also be reported with code *86.28.*

ICD CODING OF POISONING

The sixteenth section of Chapter 17 of Volume 1 of ICD-9-CM encompasses listings to report poisoning by drugs, medicinals, and biological substances. These listings within category range 960 through 979 incorporate diagnoses of overdose of these substances listed, as well as diagnoses of a wrong substance given or taken in error.

The listings within these categories exclude the reporting of adverse effects of a pharmaceutical or medicinal substance that was properly administered. Such adverse effects should be coded and reported according to the nature of the adverse effect. Furthermore, the drug or biological substance precipitating the adverse effect should be identified by use of a supplementary code contained within category range E930 through E939 of the classification for external causes of injuries and poisonings.

This section containing listings to report poisoning by drugs, medicinals, and biological substances also excludes the reporting of diagnoses involving drug dependencies, drug reactions affecting the newborn, nondependent abuses of drugs, and pathological drug intoxications. However, any confirmed concurrent diagnosis of substance abuse or drug dependence should be coded and reported secondarily. The listings for reporting poisoning are applicable if an error (such as a dosage error) was made by the physician prescribing the drug or by the practitioner, patient, or other person administering the drug.

These poisoning cases should be reported with an appropriate diagnostic code from within the category range 960 through 979. If an overdose of a drug was intentionally taken or administered and therefore resulted in drug toxicity, this incident should also be reported as a poisoning by using an appropriate code from the category range 960 through 979. In addition, if a nonprescribed drug or medicinal agent was taken in combination with a correctly prescribed and properly administered drug, any drug toxicity or other reaction resulting from the interaction of the two drugs should likewise be coded and reported as a poisoning.

In coding and reporting a poisoning or a reaction to the improper usage of a medication (such as the wrong dosage, the wrong substance, or the wrong route of administration), the code representing the poisoning should be sequenced first, and a code representing the manifestation should be sequenced secondarily.

The section containing listings for reporting poisoning includes categorization for: poisoning by antibiotics and other anti-infectives; poisoning by hormones and synthetic substances; poisoning by primarily systemic drugs; poisoning by drugs primarily affecting blood constituents; poisoning by analgesics, antipyretics, and antirheumatics; poisoning by anticonvulsants and anti-Parkinsonism drugs; poisoning by sedatives and hypnotics; poisoning by central nervous system depressants and anesthetics; poisoning by psychotropic drugs; and poisoning by central nervous system stimulants.

This section with listings for reporting poisoning also includes categorization for: poisoning by drugs primarily affecting the autonomic nervous system; poisoning by drugs primarily affecting the cardiovascular system; poisoning by drugs primarily affecting the gastrointestinal system; poisoning by water, mineral, and uric acid metabolism drugs; poisoning by drugs primarily acting on the smooth and skeletal muscles or the respiratory system; poisoning by drugs primarily affecting the skin and mucous membranes, as well as poisoning by ophthalmological, otorhinolaryngological, and dental drugs; and poisoning by bacterial and other vaccines or biological substances.

The seventeenth section of Chapter 17 of the diagnostic tabular of ICD-9-CM is comprised of listings to report toxic effects of substances chiefly nonmedicinal as to source. These listings in category range 980 through 989 exclude the reporting of diagnoses involving burns from chemical agents, respiratory conditions due to external agents, and localized effects indexed elsewhere in the diagnostic classification.

The section containing listings for reporting toxic effects of nonmedicinal substances includes categorization for: the toxic effects of alcohol; the toxic effects of petroleum products and other solvents; the toxic effects of corrosive aromatics, acids, and caustic alkalis; the toxic effects of lead and other metals and their compounds; the toxic effects of carbon monoxide and other gases, fumes, or vapors; and the toxic effects of noxious substances eaten as food, although the reporting of an allergic reaction to food or food poisoning is excluded from reporting with these listings.

Codes for the reporting of poisoning or toxic effect of a substance should be supplemented with another code to report the causative factor involved. These codes are contained within the Supplementary Classification of External Causes of Injury and Poisoning and are accessed through a special index encompassed in Volume 1 of ICD-9-CM. The supplementary codes, entitled E codes, are explained in more detail in a subsequent section of this chapter.

Within the supplementary classification for external causes, category range E850 through E858 is comprised of listings for supplementing the reporting of: an accidental overdose of a drug; effects of an incorrect drug given or taken in error; and effects of a drug taken inadvertently. This section also encompasses listings for supplementing the reporting of accidents that occurred in the use of drugs and biologicals in medical, surgical, or other clinical procedures.

These listings of codes and titles in category range E850 through E858, however, are excluded from supplementing the reporting of substance administration with suicidal or homicidal intent or with any intent to harm, or for supplementing the reporting in circumstances in which the motivation for the drug administration was unknown or undetermined. The listings in this category range supplement the reporting of a poisoning and therefore are inherently excluded from supplementing the reporting of an adverse effect of a correct drug properly administered in therapeutic or prophylactic dosage.

The listings of codes and titles in category range E850 through E858 are designated to supplement the reporting of accidental poisoning by drugs, medicinal substances, and biologicals. Included among these listings are categorization for accidental poisoning by: analgesics, antipyretics, and antirheumatics; barbiturates, sedatives, hypnotics, tranquilizers, psychotropics, antibiotics, and anti-infectives.

The table of drugs and chemicals in the alphabetic index should be consulted for the categorization of specific drugs classified under the four-digit subcategory titles. The American Hospital Formulary Service list numbers can be used to classify new pharmaceuticals for which there are no index entries.

Category range E960 through E968 is designated for supplementing the reporting of the external cause of poisoning with primary tabulation classifiable to category range 980 through 989 in Volume 17. E codes with listings in the category range E960 through E969 may also be utilized to indicate the external causes of localized effects classified throughout the main portion of the diagnostic tabular classification (categories 001 through 799).

The supplementary classification of external causes also encompasses a section of code and title listings to supplement the reporting of accidental poisoning by solid and liquid substances or by gases and vapors, and contains listings for accidental poisoning by: alcohol; cleansers, polishes, disinfectants, paints, varnishes; corrosives, caustics, petroleum products, and other solvents and their vapors. Also encompassed in this section are code and title listings to supplement the reporting of accidental poisoning by agricultural or horticultural preparations of chemicals or pharmaceuticals; toxic effects of foodstuffs and poisonous plants (with the exception of food poisoning); toxic effects of utility gas or other gas distributed by pipeline; toxic effects of carbon monoxide and other gases or vapors (with the exception of anesthetics or smoke emanating from a conflagration or an explosion).

ICD CODING OF ADVERSE EFFECTS

The eighteenth section of Chapter 17 of Volume 1 of ICD-9-CM encompasses listings to report adverse effects of nature or the environment that affected the health status of an individual patient. These listings contained within category range 990 through 995 include categorization for: the adverse effects of radiation; the adverse effects of reduced or increased atmospheric temperature; the adverse effects of heat and light; the adverse effects of air pressure or other phenomenon such as lightning, electric current, motion, or gravity.

Category *990, Effects of radiation, unspecified,* excludes the reporting of diagnoses in which the adverse effects of radiation were specifically documented. In such cases, each condition documented in the health record should be coded and reported according to the nature of the adverse effect, and the type of radiation responsible for the adverse effect should be identified and reported with the utilization of E codes.

Category *995, Certain adverse effects not elsewhere classified,* is designated to identify and report adverse effects of unknown, undetermined, or ill-defined causes, essentially effects that are not classifiable elsewhere in the ICD-9-CM diagnostic tabular. These listings within this category should also be utilized to provide an additional code to identify and report adverse effects associated with conditions that are classified elsewhere in the tabular.

Codes for the reporting an adverse effect of a pharmaceutical or medicinal substance should be supplemented with another code to report the causative factor involved. These codes are contained within the Supplementary Classification of External Causes of Injury and Poisoning. These codes are accessed through a special index encompassed in Volume 1 of ICD-9-CM. The supplementary codes, entitled E codes, are explained in more detail in a subsequent section of this chapter.

The properties of certain drugs, medicinals, and biologicals, or combinations of such substances, may cause adverse effects known as toxic reactions. The occurrence of drug toxicity is classified in ICD-9-CM as an adverse effect if the drug was correctly prescribed and properly administered. In such circumstances, the code indicating the reaction should be reported in addition to the appropriate code from the E930 through E949 category range.

An adverse effect (such as a toxicity, a synergistic reaction, a side effect, or an idiosyncratic reaction) of a therapeutic substance correctly prescribed and properly administered may be due to inherent differences among patients, such as age, sex, coexisting disease, and genetic factors, or may be due to drug-related factors, such as the chemical components of the drug, the dosage, the route of administration, the duration of drug therapy, and its bioavailability.

Supplementary codes from the E930 through E949 category range should be reported to identify the causative factor of an adverse effect of a pharmaceutical, a medicinal, or a biological substance. The physiological adverse effect, such as delirium, tachycardia, respiratory failure, gastrointestinal hemorrhage, vomiting, hypokalemia, renal failure, or hepatitis should always be coded and reported with sequencing priority over the appropriate supplementary code from category range E930 through E949 that denotes the substance causing the adverse effect.

To reiterate, the listings within category range E930 through E949 are primarily intended to supplement the reporting of adverse effects resulting from a correct drug properly administered in therapeutic or prophylactic dosage. Otherwise, if an incorrect drug was administered, or if a correct drug was improperly administered, the incident should be regarded as a poisoning instead of an adverse effect.

Moreover, the listings of codes and titles in categories E930 through E949 are explicitly excluded from the supplementary reporting of: any adverse effects resulting from an accidental overdose of a drug or a drug given or taken in error; as well as any adverse effects resulting from the technique of administration of a pharmaceutical or a medicinal substance.

Listings comprised within category range E930 through E949 are excluded from the supplementary reporting of adverse effects as a consequence of: accidental puncture during an injection; contamination of a drug; or the administration of a drug with suicidal or homicidal intent or any documented intent to harm the victim.

The section of the supplementary classification of external causes of injuries and poisonings comprised of listings for drugs, medicinals, and biological substances causing adverse effects in therapeutic usage consists of categorization for: antibiotics; anti-infectives; hormones; synthetic hormonal substitutes; drugs affecting blood constituents; primary systemic drugs; analgesics; antipyretics; antirheumatics; anticonvulsants; sedatives; hypnotics; central nervous system depressants; central nervous system stimulants; anesthetics; and psychotropic drugs. This section also consists of categorization for: drugs primarily affecting the autonomic nervous system; drugs primarily affecting the cardiovascular system; drugs primarily affecting the gastrointestinal system; water, mineral, and uric acid metabolism drugs; drugs primarily affecting the smooth and skeletal muscles; drugs primarily affecting the respiratory system, drugs primarily affecting the skin and mucous membranes; ophthalmological, otorhinolaryngological, and dental drugs; as well as bacterial or other vaccines and biological substances.

The alphabetic index in Volume 2 of ICD-9-CM should be consulted for a more complete list of specific drugs that are classified under the fourth-digit subdivisions. The American Hospital Formulary Service list numbers can be used to categorize new drugs that are not yet indexed in Volume 2.

ICD CODING OF IATROGENIC COMPLICATIONS

Iatrogenic complications are problems that developed as a consequence of medical, surgical, or other clinical care. The nineteenth and final section of Chapter 17 in Volume 1 is comprised of listings to report medical and surgical complications of care and treatment. These listings in category range 996 through 999, include codes for reporting complications resulting from the use of artificial substitutes or natural sources involving anastomosis, graft, implant, internal device, reimplant, or transplant.

This section also contains codes for reporting: complications that resulted in shock; complications resulting from the administration of anesthesia; complications due to an artificial or synthetic implanted device or graft; complications associated with a reattached extremity or a transplanted organ; complications of dialysis or extracorporeal circulation; and complications of therapy involving hyperalimentation, immunization, infusion, inhalation, injection, inoculation, perfusion, transfusion, vaccination, or ventilation.

However, the listings contained within this section exclude the reporting of diagnoses involving: adverse effects of medicinal agents; complications of poisoning and toxic effects of drugs and chemicals; burns from local applications and irradiation; complications of clinical conditions for which the procedure was performed; and complications of surgical procedures rendered during labor and delivery. These listings also exclude the reporting of specific complications classified elsewhere, including those indexed as due to or resulting from a particular procedure.

If a patient admission was necessitated for the treatment of a complication resulting from surgical or other medical care, the code (from category range 996 through 999) representing the complication should be sequenced as the principal diagnosis. An additional code should be selected and assigned to report the specific complication.

Codes for the reporting of complications stemming from surgical or medical care may be supplemented with another code to report the factors entailed. These codes are contained within the Supplementary Classification of External Causes of Injury and Poisoning and are accessed through a special index encompassed in Volume 1 of ICD-9-CM. The supplementary codes, entitled E codes are explained in more detail in a subsequent section of this chapter.

Within the supplementary classification for external causes, category range E870 through E876 is comprised of listings of codes and titles for supplementing the reporting of misadventures to patients during surgical or medical care. This section contains listings for reporting a variety of iatrogenic injuries including: an accidental cut, puncture, perforation, or hemorrhage that occurred during medical or surgical care; a foreign object left in the body during a procedure; the failure of sterile precautions during a procedure; the failure to prepare the proper dosage of a medication or therapeutic substance; the mechanical failure of an instrument or apparatus during a procedure; the administration of contaminated or infected blood, fluid, drug, or biological substance; and many other misadventures that could occur during clinical patient care and treatment.

The listings in category range E870 through E876, however, are excluded from supplementing the reporting of an accidental overdose of a drug or a wrong drug given or taken in error. The listings in this category range also are excluded from supplementing the reporting of surgical, medical, or other clinical procedures as the causative factor of an abnormal reaction by the patient without documented iatrogenic misadventure at the time of the procedure or service. Such abnormal reaction should be augmented for reporting with codes and titles from category range E878 through E879 in the supplementary classification for external causes.

The listings in category range E878 and E879 are designated to supplement the reporting of abnormal reactions or subsequent complications arising from clinical patient care. These listings include codes and titles for reporting abnormal reactions such as: the displacement or malfunction of prosthetic device, postoperative hepatorenal failure, the malfunction of external stoma, postoperative intestinal obstruction, and the rejection of a transplanted organ. These listings are excluded from supplementing the reporting of an adverse effect from anesthetic management properly rendered, or the reporting of an adverse effect from infusion and transfusion without stated misadventure in the technique of the procedural service.

ORTHOPEDIC SURGERY REPORTING FOR BILLING

As a general principle maintained in all clinical services, the principal diagnosis is defined as that condition responsible for the admission of the patient to the health service encounter or episode of care. The principal procedure is defined as the procedure most closely associated with the patient's principal diagnosis for that specific admission.

The diagnosis or procedure that presents the greatest risk to the patient is not necessarily the most resource intensive diagnosis or procedure. A fracture of the skull, even if the fracture required no procedural intervention, might pose greater risk to the patient than a fracture of the ankle. Yet the ankle fracture might entail the utilization of operating room procedures that were relatively higher in terms of resource intensity. Similarly, a patient admitted for a diagnostic arthroscopy might slip and fall and sustain a fractured humerus requiring an operative procedure for reduction and fixation.

Insurance claim regulations ordinarily restrict coding and reporting to diagnoses specifically assessed or treated during the admission, encounter, or episode of care. The principal diagnosis (and principal procedure) should always be sequenced first, and followed by secondary or additional diagnoses (and secondary or additional procedures) in descending order of clinical significance and resource intensity. Thus, a fractured clavicle should ordinarily be sequenced before a fractured metacarpal, if both conditions were documented concurrently.

Designated ICD-9-CM codes are recognized as comorbidities by certain third-party payors, especially Medicare. For inpatient admissions, these comorbid conditions may increase the amount of reimbursement received by the provider. Comorbidities among orthopedic conditions are represented by the following ICD-9-CM codes:

820.00	820.01	820.02
820.03	820.09	820.10
820.11	820.12	820.13
820.19	820.20	820.21
820.22	820.30	820.31
820.32	820.8	820.9
821.00	821.01	821.10
821.11	838.19	839.00
839.01	839.02	839.03
839.04	839.05	839.06
839.07	839.08	839.10
839.11	839.12	839.13
839.14	839.15	839.16
839.17	839.18	

The Medicare prospective payment system comprises major diagnostic categories (MDC's) containing various diagnosis related groups (DRG's). The DRG's associated with orthopedic diagnoses and procedures are distributed into MDC 8, Diseases and Disorders of the Musculoskeletal System and Connective Tissue. Those DRG's relevant to orthopedics are enumerated in the following list (Table 11–2).

T A B L E 11–2

Diagnosis Related Groups for Diseases and Disorders of the Musculoskeletal System and Connective Tissue

DRG 209, Major Joint and Limb Reattachment Procedures of Lower Extremity

DRG 210, Hip and Femur Procedures except Major Joint Procedures, Age Greater than 17 with Comorbidity or Complication

DRG 211, Hip and Femur Procedures except Major Joint Procedures, Age Greater than 17 without Comorbidity or Complication

DRG 212, Hip and Femur Procedures except Major Joint Procedures, Age 0–17

DRG 213, Amputation for Musculoskeletal System and Connective Tissue Disorders

DRG 214, Back and Neck Procedures with Comorbidity or Complication

DRG 215, Back and Neck Procedures without Comorbidity or Complication

DRG 217, Wound Debridement and Skin Graft except Hand for Musculoskeletal and Connective Tissue Disorders

DRG 218, Lower Extremity and Humerus Procedures except Hip, Foot, and Femur, Age Greater than 17 with Comorbidity or Complication

DRG 219, Lower Extremity and Humerus Procedures except Hip, Foot, and Femur, Age Greater than 17 without Comorbidity or Complication

DRG 220, Lower Extremity and Humerus Procedures except Hip, Foot, and Femur, Age 0–17

DRG 221, Knee Procedures with Comorbidity or Complication

DRG 222, Knee Procedures without Comorbidity or Complication

DRG 223, Major Shoulder/Elbow Procedures or Other Upper Extremity Procedures with Comorbidity or Complication

DRG 224, Shoulder, Elbow, or Forearm Procedures except Major Joint Procedures without Comorbidity or Complication

DRG 225, Foot Procedures

DRG 228, Major Thumb or Joint Procedures or Other Hand or Wrist Procedures with Comorbidity or Complication

DRG 229, Hand or Wrist Procedures except Major Joint Procedures without Comorbidity or Complication

DRG 230, Local Excision and Removal of Internal Fixation Devices of Hip and Femur

DRG 231, Local Excision and Removal of Internal Fixation Devices except Hip and Femur

DRG 232, Arthroscopy

DRG 233, Other Musculoskeletal System and Connective Tissue Operating Room Procedures with Comorbidity or Complication

DRG 234, Other Musculoskeletal System and Connective Tissue Operating Room Procedures without Comorbidity or Complication

DRG 235, Fractures of Femur

DRG 236, Fractures of Hip and Pelvis

DRG 237, Sprains, Strains, and Dislocations of Hip, Pelvis, and Thigh

DRG 249, Aftercare, Musculoskeletal System and Connective Tissue

DRG 250, Fractures, Sprains, Strains, and Dislocations of Forearms, Hand, and Foot, Age Greater than 17 with Comorbidity or Complication

DRG 251, Fractures, Sprains, Strains, and Dislocations of Forearm, Hand, and Foot, Age Greater than 17 without Comorbidity or Complication

DRG 252, Fractures, Sprains, Strains, and Dislocations of Forearm, Hand, and Foot, Age 0–17

DRG 253, Fractures, Sprains, Strains, and Dislocations of Upper Arm and Lower Leg except Foot, Age Greater than 17 with Comorbidity or Complication

DRG 254, Fractures, Sprains, Strains, and Dislocations of Upper Arm and Lower Leg except Foot, Age Greater than 17 without Comorbidity or Complication

DRG 255, Fractures, Sprains, Strains, and Dislocations of Upper Arm and Lower Leg except Foot, Age 0–17

DRG 256, Other Musculoskeletal System and Connective Tissue Diagnoses

DRG 471, Bilateral or Multiple Major Joint Procedures of Lower Extremity

DRG 491, Major Joint and Limb Reattachment Procedures of Upper Extremity

The reporting of code numbers for nonspecific or unspecified orthopedic diagnoses or procedures should be avoided, if possible. The staff members responsible for coding and billing should attempt to determine the most specific code to report for reimbursement purposes and to generate meaningful data for statistical and research uses. Accurate, complete, and timely documentation in the patient medical record may alleviate the necessity of selecting and assigning codes for nonspecific or unspecified orthopedic diagnoses and procedures.

TRAUMA SURGERY REPORTING FOR BILLING

The general principle applicable to all clinical specialties defines the principal diagnosis as the condition responsible for the admission of the patient, and defines the principal procedure as the procedure most closely associated with the diagnosis for that specific admission. Trauma cases most likely involve multiple diagnoses of varying clinical significance and resource intensity. Life-threatening conditions, of course, should always be sequenced with priority over less significant ones. For instance, the coding and reporting of a laceration of the liver should precede in sequence the simultaneous coding and reporting of a laceration of the tongue.

However, in certain situations involving a patient in an acute care facility, major complications of greater resource intensity might unexpectedly result during the course of an admission for a less severe condition. For example, a patient admitted in stable status for repair of a gunshot wound might develop a serious postoperative infection requiring intensive therapeutic endeavors.

Insurance claim regulations ordinarily mandate that only those diagnoses specifically assessed or treated during the admission or encounter may be reported on a claim for that episode of care. The principal diagnosis and procedure should always be sequenced first, and followed by all pertinent secondary diagnoses and procedures reported in descending order of clinical significance and resource intensity. As examples, reporting of internal injuries should precede that of superficial injuries; and the reporting of open injuries should be sequenced to precede that of closed injuries.

Designated ICD-9-CM codes are recognized as comorbidities by certain third-party payors such as Medicare. For inpatient admissions, these comorbid conditions may increase the amount of reimbursement received by the provider. Comorbidities among traumatic conditions are represented by the following ICD-9-CM code numbers:

800.00	800.01	800.03
800.04	800.05	800.06
800.09	800.10	800.11
800.12	800.13	800.14
800.15	800.16	800.19
800.20	800.21	800.22
800.23	800.24	800.25
800.26	800.29	800.30
800.31	800.32	800.33
800.34	800.35	800.36
800.39	800.40	800.41
800.42	800.43	800.44
800.45	800.46	800.49
800.50	800.51	800.52
800.53	800.54	800.55
800.56	800.57	800.58

800.59	800.60	800.61
800.62	800.63	800.64
800.65	800.66	800.69
800.70	800.71	800.72
800.73	800.74	800.75
800.76	800.79	800.80
800.81	800.82	800.83
800.84	800.85	800.86
800.89	800.90	800.91
800.92	800.93	800.94
800.95	800.96	800.99
801.01	801.02	801.03
801.04	801.05	801.06
801.09	801.10	801.11
801.12	801.13	801.14
801.15	801.16	801.19
801.20	801.21	801.22
801.23	801.24	801.25
801.26	801.29	801.30
801.31	801.32	801.33
801.34	801.35	801.36
801.39	801.40	801.41
801.42	801.43	801.44
801.45	801.46	801.49
801.50	801.51	801.52
801.53	801.54	801.55
801.56	801.59	801.60
801.61	801.62	801.63
801.64	801.65	801.66
801.69	801.70	801.71
801.72	801.73	801.74
801.75	801.76	801.79
801.80	801.81	801.82
801.83	801.84	801.85
801.86	801.89	801.90
801.91	801.92	801.93
801.94	801.95	801.96
801.99	802.1	802.20
802.21	802.22	802.23
802.24	802.25	802.26
802.27	802.28	802.29
802.30	802.31	802.32
802.33	802.34	802.35
802.36	802.37	802.38
802.39	802.4	802.5
802.6	802.7	802.8
802.9	803.00	803.01
803.02	803.03	803.04
803.05	803.06	803.09

803.10	803.11	803.12
803.13	803.14	803.15
803.16	803.19	803.20
803.21	803.22	803.23
803.24	803.25	803.26
803.29	803.30	803.31
803.32	803.33	803.34
803.35	803.36	803.39
803.40	803.41	803.42
803.43	803.44	803.45
803.46	803.49	803.50
803.51	803.52	803.53
803.54	803.55	803.56
803.59	803.60	803.61
803.62	803.63	803.64
803.65	803.66	803.69
803.70	803.71	803.72
803.73	803.74	803.75
803.76	803.79	803.80
803.81	803.82	803.83
803.84	803.85	803.86
803.89	803.90	803.91
803.92	803.93	803.94
803.95	803.96	803.99
804.00	804.01	804.02
804.03	804.04	804.05
804.06	804.09	804.10
804.11	804.12	804.13
804.14	804.15	804.16
804.19	804.20	804.21
804.22	804.23	804.24
804.25	804.26	804.29
804.30	804.31	804.32
804.33	804.34	804.35
804.36	804.39	804.40
804.41	804.42	804.43
804.44	804.45	804.46
804.49	804.50	804.51
804.52	804.53	804.54
804.55	804.56	804.59
804.60	804.61	804.62
804.63	804.64	804.65
804.66	804.69	804.70
804.71	804.72	804.73
804.74	804.75	804.76
804.79	804.80	804.81
804.82	804.83	804.84
804.85	804.86	804.89
804.90	804.91	804.92

804.93	804.94	804.95
804.96	804.99	805.01
805.02	805.03	805.04
805.05	805.06	805.07
805.08	805.10	805.11
805.12	805.13	805.14
805.15	805.16	805.17
805.18	805.2	805.3
805.4	805.5	805.6
805.7	805.8	805.9
806.00	806.01	806.02
806.03	806.04	806.05
806.06	806.07	806.08
806.09	806.10	806.11
806.12	806.13	806.14
806.15	806.16	806.17
806.18	806.19	806.20
806.21	806.22	806.23
806.24	806.25	806.26
806.27	806.28	806.30
806.31	806.32	806.33
806.34	806.35	806.36
806.37	806.38	806.39
806.4	806.5	806.60
806.61	806.62	806.69
806.70	806.71	806.72
806.79	806.8	806.9
807.04	807.05	807.06
807.07	807.08	807.09
807.10	807.11	807.12
807.13	807.14	807.15
807.16	807.17	807.18
807.19	807.2	807.3
807.4	807.5	807.6
808.0	808.1	808.2
808.3	808.43	808.49
808.51	808.52	808.53
808.59	808.8	808.9
850.0	850.1	850.2
850.3	850.4	850.5
850.9	851.00	851.01
851.02	851.03	851.04
851.05	851.06	851.09
851.10	851.11	851.12
851.13	851.14	851.15
851.16	851.19	851.20
851.21	851.22	851.23
851.24	851.25	851.26
851.29	851.30	851.31

851.32	851.33	851.34
851.35	851.36	851.39
851.40	851.41	851.42
851.43	851.44	851.45
851.46	851.49	851.50
851.51	851.52	851.53
851.54	851.55	851.56
851.59	851.60	851.61
851.62	851.63	851.64
851.65	851.66	851.69
851.70	851.71	851.72
851.73	851.74	851.75
851.76	851.79	851.80
851.81	851.82	851.83
851.84	851.85	851.86
851.89	851.90	851.91
851.92	851.93	851.94
851.95	851.96	851.99
852.00	852.01	852.02
852.03	852.04	852.05
852.06	852.09	852.10
852.11	852.12	852.13
852.14	852.15	852.16
852.19	852.20	852.21
852.22	852.23	852.24
852.25	852.26	852.29
852.30	852.31	852.32
852.33	852.34	852.35
852.36	852.39	852.40
852.41	852.42	852.43
852.44	852.45	852.46
852.49	852.50	852.51
852.52	852.53	852.54
852.55	852.56	852.59
853.00	853.01	853.02
853.03	853.04	853.05
853.06	853.09	853.10
853.11	853.12	853.13
853.14	853.15	853.16
853.19	854.00	854.01
854.02	854.03	854.04
854.05	854.06	854.09
854.10	854.11	854.12
854.13	854.14	854.15
854.16	854.19	860.0
860.1	860.2	860.3
860.4	860.5	861.01
861.02	861.03	861.10
861.11	861.12	861.13

861.22	861.30	861.31
861.32	862.1	861.21
862.22	862.29	862.31
862.32	862.39	862.9
863.1	863.30	863.31
863.39	863.50	863.51
863.52	863.53	863.54
863.55	863.56	863.59
863.90	863.91	863.92
863.93	863.94	863.95
863.99	864.00	864.01
864.02	864.03	864.04
864.05	864.09	864.10
864.11	864.12	864.13
864.14	864.15	864.19
865.00	865.01	865.02
865.03	865.04	865.09
865.10	865.11	865.12
865.13	865.14	865.19
866.00	866.01	866.02
866.03	866.10	866.11
866.12	866.13	867.0
867.1	867.2	867.3
867.4	867.5	867.6
867.7	867.8	867.9
868.00	868.01	868.02
868.03	868.04	868.09
868.10	868.11	868.12
868.13	868.14	868.19
869.0	869.1	870.3
870.4	870.8	870.9
871.0	871.1	871.2
871.3	871.4	871.9
872.72	872.73	872.74
900.00	900.01	900.02
900.03	900.1	900.81
900.82	900.89	900.9
901.0	901.1	901.2
901.3	901.41	901.42
901.83	902.0	902.10
902.11	902.19	902.20
902.22	902.23	902.24
902.25	902.26	902.27
902.29	902.31	902.34
902.39	902.40	902.41
902.42	902.49	902.50
902.51	902.52	902.53
902.54	902.59	902.87
904.0	925.1	925.2

929.0	952.01	952.02
952.03	952.04	952.05
952.06	952.07	952.08
952.09	952.10	952.11
952.12	952.13	952.14
952.15	952.16	952.17
952.18	952.19	952.2
952.3	952.4	952.8
952.9	953.0	953.1
953.2	953.3	953.4
953.5	953.8	953.9
958.0	958.1	958.2
958.3	958.4	958.5
958.7	995.4	996.00
996.01	996.02	996.03
996.04	996.09	996.1
996.2	996.30	996.39
996.4	996.51	996.52
996.53	996.54	996.59
996.60	996.61	996.62
996.63	996.64	996.65
996.66	996.67	996.69
996.70	996.71	996.72
996.73	996.74	996.75
996.76	996.77	996.78
996.79	996.80	996.81
996.82	996.83	996.84
996.85	996.86	996.89
996.90	996.91	996.92
996.93	996.94	996.95
996.96	996.99	997.0
997.1	997.2	997.3
997.4	997.5	997.62
997.9	998.0	998.1
998.2	998.3	998.4
998.5	998.6	998.7
998.8	998.9	999.1
999.2	999.3	999.4
999.5	999.6	999.7
999.8		

Under the Medicare prospective payment system, diagnosis related groups (DRG's) are assigned to major diagnostic categories (MDC's). The DRG's associated with injuries and poisonings are assigned to MDC 21, Injuries, Poisonings, and Toxic Effects of Drugs (Table 11–3). The DRG's associated with major trauma are assigned to MDC 24, Multiple Significant Trauma (Table 11–4).

Reporting code numbers for nonspecific or unspecified diagnoses or procedures related to trauma should be avoided, if possible. Personnel responsible for coding and billing should attempt to ascertain and report the most specific code not only for reimbursement purposes but

TABLE 11–3

Diagnosis Related Groups for Injuries and Poisonings

DRG 439, Skin Grafts for Injuries
DRG 440, Wound Debridements for Injuries
DRG 441, Hand Procedures for Injuries
DRG 442, Other Operating Room Procedures for Injuries with Comorbidity or Complication
DRG 443, Other Operating Room Procedures for Injuries without Comorbidity or Complication
DRG 444, Traumatic Injury, Age Greater than 17 with Comorbidity or Complication
DRG 445, Traumatic Injury, Age Greater than 17 without Comorbidity or Complication
DRG 446, Traumatic Injury, Age 0–17
DRG 447, Allergic Reactions, Age Greater than 17
DRG 448, Allergic Reactions, Age 0–17
DRG 449, Poisoning and Toxic Effects of Drugs, Age Greater than 17 with Comorbidity or Complication
DRG 450, Poisoning and Toxic Effects of Drugs, Age Greater than 17 without Comorbidity or Complication
DRG 451, Poisoning and Toxic Effects of Drugs, Age 0–17
DRG 452, Complications of Treatment with Comorbidity or Complication
DRG 453, Complications of Treatment without Comorbidity or Complication
DRG 454, Other Injury, Poisoning, and Toxic Effect Diagnoses with Comorbidity or Complication
DRG 455, Other Injury, Poisoning, and Toxic Effect Diagnoses without Comorbidity or Complication

also to generate meaningful data for statistical and research purposes. Accurate, complete, and timely documentation in the patient medical record may alleviate the necessity of reporting codes for unspecified diagnoses and procedures related to traumatic conditions.

PLASTIC SURGERY REPORTING FOR BILLING

The generic coding and reporting principle applicable to all clinical services defines the principal diagnosis as the condition that was responsible for the admission of the patient, and defines the principal procedure as the procedure that was most closely associated with the diagnosis for that specific admission. Cases involving plastic or reconstructive procedures often entail multiple diagnoses of varying clinical significance and resource intensity. With certain exceptions, diagnostic conditions involving an extensive series of procedures should be sequenced with priority over procedures treated less complexly. For instance, the coding and reporting of a third-degree burn necessitating multiple skin grafts should be sequenced to precede that of a laceration sutured and observed simply in the course of two patient encounters.

TABLE 11–4

Diagnosis Related Groups for Multiple Trauma

DRG 484, Craniotomy for Multiple Significant Trauma
DRG 485, Limb Reattachment, Hip, and Femur Procedures for Multiple Significant Trauma
DRG 486, Other Operating Room Procedures for Multiple Significant Trauma
DRG 487, Other Multiple Significant Trauma

However, in particular circumstances regarding a patient in an acute care facility, major complications of greater resource intensity might unexpectedly result during the course of an admission for a lesser condition. For example, a patient admitted in stable status for extensive scar revision might develop a serious postoperative abscess requiring intensive therapeutic endeavors.

Insurance claim regulations ordinarily limit coding and reporting only to those diagnoses specifically assessed or treated during the specific admission or encounter. The principal diagnosis and procedure should always be sequenced first, and followed by all relevant secondary or additional diagnoses and procedures reported in descending order of clinical significance and resource intensity. To exemplify, the reporting of infected or complicated injuries should always sequentially precede that of superficial injuries.

Designated ICD-9-CM codes are recognized as comorbidities by Medicare and certain other third-party payors. For inpatient admissions, these comorbid conditions may increase the amount of reimbursement received by the provider. Comorbidities among traumatic conditions commonly cared for by practitioners specializing in plastic and reconstructive surgery are represented by the following ICD-9-CM code numbers:

873.33	873.9	874.00
874.01	874.02	874.10
874.11	874.12	874.3
874.5	875.0	875.1
887.0	887.1	887.2
887.3	887.4	887.5
887.6	887.7	896.0
896.1	896.2	896.3
897.0	897.1	897.2
897.3	897.4	897.5
897.6	897.7	

Within the Medicare prospective payment system, diagnosis related groups (DRG's) are distributed into major diagnostic categories (MDC's). Many of the DRG's associated with plastic surgery are among the integumentary system diseases and disorders that are assigned to MDC 9, Diseases and Disorders of the Skin, Subcutaneous Tissue, and Breast (Table 11–5). The DRG's associated with burns are assigned to MDC 22, Burns (Table 11–6).

Reporting code numbers for nonspecific or unspecified diagnoses or procedures related to plastic and reconstructive surgery should be avoided, if possible. All personnel responsible for coding and billing should attempt to determine to report the most specific code not only for reimbursement purposes but also to generate meaningful and reliable data for statistical research uses. Accurate, complete, and timely documentation in the patient medical record may alleviate the necessity of reporting codes for unspecified diagnoses and procedures related to plastic and reconstructive surgery.

ICD CODING OF EXTERNAL CAUSES

The ICD-9-CM diagnostic tabular Volume 1 includes a Supplementary Classification of External Causes of Injury and Poisoning (category range E800–E899), containing entities commonly known as the E codes. This supplement is provided to permit the classification of environmental events and circumstances as the cause of injury, poisoning, and other adverse effects. These supplementary codes may be accessed through a special index in Volume 1 entitled the Alphabetic Index to External Causes of Injury and Poisoning.

T A B L E 11–5

Diagnosis Related Groups for Diseases and Disorders of the Skin, Subcutaneous Tissue, and Breast

DRG 263, Skin Graft and/or Debridement for Skin Ulcer or Cellulitis with Comorbidity or Complication
DRG 264, Skin Graft and/or Debridement for Skin Ulcer or Cellulitis without Comorbidity or Complication
DRG 265, Skin Graft and/or Debridement except for Skin Ulcer or Cellulitis with Comorbidity or Complication
DRG 266, Skin Graft and/or Debridement except for Skin Ulcer or Cellulitis without Comorbidity or Complication
DRG 268, Skin, Subcutaneous Tissue, and Breast Plastic Procedures
DRG 269, Other Skin, Subcutaneous Tissue, and Breast Procedures with Comorbidity or Complication
DRG 270, Other Skin, Subcutaneous Tissue, and Breast Procedures without Comorbidity or Complication
DRG 271, Skin Ulcers
DRG 272, Major Skin Disorders with Comorbidity or Complication
DRG 273, Major Skin Disorders without Comorbidity or Complication
DRG 277, Cellulitis, Age Greater than 17 with Comorbidity or Complication
DRG 278, Cellulitis, Age Greater than 17 without Comorbidity or Complication
DRG 279, Cellulitis, Age 0–17
DRG 280, Trauma of Skin, Subcutaneous Tissue, and Breast, Age Greater than 17 with Comorbidity or Complication
DRG 281, Trauma to Skin, Subcutaneous Tissue, and Breast, Age Greater than 17 without Comorbidity or Complication
DRG 282, Trauma to Skin, Subcutaneous Tissue, and Breast, Age 0–17
DRG 283, Minor Skin Disorders with Comorbidity or Complication
DRG 284, Minor Skin Disorders without Comorbidity or Complication

In recent years, the emphasis placed on maintaining trauma registries increased substantially. Trauma registries utilize E codes in the compilation of statistics concerning injuries. The supplementary classification of external causes enhances the data collected through diagnostic and procedural coding and reporting.

Applicable codes from this supplementary classification, however, should be reported only as a secondary adjunct to a code selected and assigned from one of the main chapters of Volume 1 of ICD-9-CM. The code classified in the main chapters (Chapter 1 through Chapter 17) should be selected and assigned to indicate the nature of the condition documented.

T A B L E 11–6

Diagnosis Related Groups for Burns

DRG 456, Burns, Transferred to Another Acute Care Facility
DRG 457, Extensive Burns without Operating Room Procedure
DRG 458, Nonextensive Burns with Skin Graft
DRG 459, Nonextensive Burns with Wound Debridement or Other Operating Room Procedure
DRG 460, Nonextensive Burns without Operating Room Procedure
DRG 472, Extensive Burns with Operating Room Procedure

TABLE 11-7

Sections in the E Code Supplement to ICD-9-CM

1. Railway Accidents (category range E800–E807)
2. Motor Vehicle Traffic Accidents (category range E810–E819)
3. Motor Vehicle Nontraffic Accidents (category range E820–E825)
4. Other Road Vehicle Accidents (category range E826–E829)
5. Water Transport Accidents (category range E830–E838)
6. Air and Space Transport Accidents (category range E840–E845)
7. Vehicle Accidents, Not Elsewhere Classifiable (category range E846–E848)
8. Accidental Poisoning by Drugs, Medicinal Substances, and Biologicals (category range E850–E858)
9. Accidental Poisoning by Other Solid and Liquid Substances, Gases, and Vapors (category range E860–E869)
10. Misadventures to Patients During Surgical and Medical Care (category range E870–E876)
11. Surgical and Medical Procedures as the Cause of Abnormal Reaction of Patient or Later Complication, without Mention of Misadventure at the Time of Procedure (category range E878–E879)
12. Accidental Falls (category range E880–E888)
13. Accidents Caused by Fire and Flames (category range E890–E899)
14. Accidents Due to Natural and Environmental Factors (category range E900–E909)
15. Accidents Caused by Submersion, Suffocation, and Foreign Bodies (category range E910–E915)
16. Other Accidents (category range E916–E928)
17. Late Effects of Accidental Injury (category E929)
18. Drugs, Medicinal and Biological Substances Causing Adverse Effects in Therapeutic Use (category range E930–E949)
19. Suicide and Self-Inflicted Injury (category range E950–E959)
20. Homicide and Injury Purposely Inflicted by Other Persons (category range E960–E969)
21. Legal Intervention (category range E970–E978)
22. Injury Undetermined Whether Accidentally or Purposely Inflicted (category range E980–E989)
23. Injuries Resulting from Operations of War (category range E990–E999)

The supplementary classification for reporting external causes of injury, poisoning, and adverse effects consists of twenty-three sections of E code listings that are summarized in the table above (Table 11–7).

ICD CODING OF TRANSPORTATION ACCIDENTS

Seven of the sections in the supplementary classification of external causes involve listings for reporting transportation accidents. Transportation accidents, particularly motor vehicle accidents, are the leading causative factor of trauma service admissions to acute healthcare facilities.

The group of categories with listings to supplement the reporting of railways accidents is comprised of codes and titles for railway incidents involving: collisions with rolling stock or other objects; derailments without antecedent collision; explosion, or fire; falls in, on, or from a railway train; as well as other railway mishaps. This listings in this section are excluded from supplementing the reporting of accidents involving a railway train and an aircraft, a motor vehicle, or a watercraft.

The group of categories with listings to supplement the reporting of motor vehicle traffic accidents contains codes and titles for vehicular incidents involving: collision with a train; collisions or re-entrant collision with another motor vehicle or other type of vehicle; collision with a pedestrian; loss of control without a collision; as well as noncollision motor vehicle traffic accidents that occurred while boarding or alighting from the vehicle. The listings in this section are excluded from supplementing the reporting of accidents involving a motor vehicle with an aircraft.

The group of categories with listings to supplement the reporting of motor vehicle nontraffic accidents encompasses codes and titles for nontraffic accidents involving: motor driven snow vehicles or other off-the-road vehicles; collisions with moving objects; collisions with stationary objects; as well as nontraffic vehicular accidents that occurred while boarding or alighting. These categories also include listings to supplement the reporting of accidents involving motor vehicles used in recreational or sporting activities and other noncollision vehicular accidents occurring on private property. The listings in this section are excluded from supplementing the reporting of accidents involving a motor vehicle with an aircraft or a watercraft, or accidents involving a motor vehicle with agricultural machinery or construction machinery.

The group of categories with listings to supplement the reporting of other road vehicle accidents comprises codes and titles for a variety of mishaps such as pedal cycle accidents, animal drawn vehicle accidents, and accidents involving an animal being ridden. These categories also include listings to supplement the reporting of these types of mishaps if the incident occurred during recreational or sporting activities. The listings in this section are excluded from supplementing the enumerated accidents if the mishap entailed a collision with an aircraft, a motor vehicle, or a railway train.

The group of categories with listings to supplement the reporting of water transport accidents encompasses codes and titles for: accidents to watercraft causing submersion or other injury; accidental submersion or drowning in water transport accidents; falls on stairs or ladders in water transport; falls from one level to another or other types of falls in water transport; machinery accidents in water transport; and explosions or fires in watercraft. These categories also include listings to supplement the reporting of watercraft accidents in the course of recreational activities, but are excluded from supplementing the reporting of watercraft accidents involving an aircraft or objects set in motion by an aircraft.

The group of categories with listings to supplement the reporting of air and space transport accidents contains codes and titles for: accidents involving powered aircraft at takeoff or landing or otherwise; accidents involving unpowered aircraft; falls in, on, or from an aircraft; as well as accidents involving spacecraft. The group of categories with listings to supplement the reporting of vehicle accidents, not elsewhere classifiable, is comprised of codes and titles for various mishaps such as accidents involving powered vehicles used solely within the confines or premises of industrial or commercial establishments, or mishaps involving suspended cable cars not running on rails.

ICD CODING OF OTHER ACCIDENTS

Within the supplementary classification of external causes, category range E880 through E888 is comprised of listings of codes and titles to supplement the reporting of injuries sustained from accidental falls. This section contains listings for supplementary reporting of: falls on or from stairs or steps; falls on or from ladders or scaffolding; falls from or out of a building or other structure; falls into a hole or other opening in the surface; falls from one level to another; falls on a level surface from slipping, tripping, or stumbling; as well as falls on the same level resulting from collision, pushing, or shoving, by or with another person.

The listings in this section are excluded from supplementing the reporting of: falls in or from a burning building; falls into fire; falls into water; falls in or from machinery; falls on an edged, pointed, or sharp object; falls in or from a transport vehicle; or falls in or from a vehicle not elsewhere classifiable.

Category range E890 through E899 is comprised of codes and titles to supplement the reporting of injuries caused by fire and flames. This section contains listings for supplementary reporting of asphyxia or poisoning due to conflagration or ignition, burns caused by fire, and injuries sustained from secondary fires resulting from an explosion.

This section of the classification of external causes encompasses listings for supplementary reporting of various types of accidents caused by fire and flames including: injuries caused by conflagration or controlled fire either inside or outside of a private dwelling or another building or structure; injuries resulting from the ignition of clothing; and injuries sustained from the ignition of any highly inflammable material. The listings in this section are excluded from supplementing the reporting of injuries incurred as a consequence of: fire due to arson, fire in or on machinery, fire in or on a transport vehicle other than a stationary vehicle, or fire in or on a vehicle not elsewhere classifiable.

Category range E900 through E909 is comprised of codes and titles to supplement the reporting of accidents due to natural and environmental factors. This section includes listings for supplementing the reporting of conditions due to: excessive heat (such as sunstroke); excessive cold (such as frostbite); high or low air pressure and changes in air pressure (such as barotrauma); exposure to humidity; lightning; cataclysmic rainstorms, hurricanes, tornados, or blizzards; floods resulting from storms; as well as cataclysmic earthquakes, avalanches, or volcanic eruptions. This section also contains listings for supplementing the reporting of conditions due to: travel and motion; hunger; thirst; venomous animals, insects, and plants as the cause of poisoning and toxic reactions; and bites or other injuries inflicted by animals.

The listings in category *E905, Venomous animals and plants as the cause of poisoning and toxic reactions,* may be used to supplement the reporting of adverse effects generated from chemicals released by animals, insects, or plants. Listings in this category are excluded from supplementing the reporting of adverse effects of ingestion of this venom, however.

Listings in category *E906, Other injury caused by animals,* are excluded from supplementing the reporting of road vehicle accidents involving animals as well as the reporting of mishaps involving tripping or falling over animals.

Category *E907, Lightning,* is excluded from supplementing the reporting of injuries sustained from the fall of a tree or other object struck by lightning, and this category also is excluded from supplementing the reporting of injuries sustained from a fire caused by lightning.

Within the supplementary classification of external causes, category range E910 through E915 is comprised of listings of codes and titles to supplement the reporting of injuries incurred from accidents caused by submersion, suffocation, or foreign bodies. The listings in this section are designated for supplementing the reporting of: accidental drowning or submersion; inhalation and ingestion of food or other objects that results in obstruction of the respiratory tract or suffocation; accidental mechanical suffocation; and the effects of a foreign body that accidentally entered the eye and its adnexa or that entered any other bodily orifice. These listings, however, are excluded from supplementing the reporting of aspiration or inhalation of a foreign body.

The listings encompassed within category *E910, Accidental drowning and submersion,* are designated for supplementing the reporting of accidents due to immersion. However, these listings are excluded from supplementing the reporting of: diving accidents; drowning or submersion due to a natural or environmental cataclysm, a machinery accident, or a transport accident; drowning or submersion as the consequence of air pressure or changes in air pressure; as well as any injury sustained from striking against objects while in running water.

The supplementary classification of external causes contains a residual section with listings of codes and titles for other accidents. These listings in category range E916 through E928 are intended for supplementing the reporting of: injuries incurred as a result of being struck accidentally by a falling object or as a result of striking against objects or persons; injuries sustained as a consequence of being caught accidentally in or between objects; injuries resulting from accidents caused by machinery; and injuries resulting from accidents caused by cutting or piercing instruments or objects.

The listings in this residual section for external causes of accidents are also intended for supplementing the reporting of injuries sustained in an accident caused by explosion of a pressure vessel; injuries sustained in an accident caused by a firearm missile; injuries resulting from an accident caused by explosive material; injuries resulting from an accident caused by a hot substance, a hot object, caustic material, corrosive material, steam, or electric current; injuries sustained as a consequence of exposure to radiation; and injuries sustained as a consequence of overexertion or strenuous movements.

Listings of codes and titles encompassed within category *E923, Accident caused by explosive material,* are designated for supplementary reporting of flash burns and other injuries resulting from an explosion or from an ignition of explosive material. The listings in this category, however, are excluded from supplementary reporting of injuries sustained from an explosion in or on machinery or in or on any transport or stationary motor vehicle. These listings are also excluded from supplementary reporting of injuries sustained from an explosion with conflagration as well as any injuries incurred as a consequence of secondary fires resulting from explosion.

The listings of codes and titles contained within category *E924, Accident caused by hot substance or object, caustic or corrosive material, and steam,* are excluded from supplementary reporting of: chemical burns that resulted from swallowing a corrosive substance; burns sustained from a fire caused by such substances and objects; radiation burns, and similar injuries incurred as a consequence of therapeutic misadventures.

Listings of codes and titles comprised within category *E925, Accident caused by electric current,* are designated for supplementary reporting of injuries as a result of electric current from an exposed wire, a faulty appliance, high voltage, a cable, a live rail, or an open electric socket. Such injuries encompass a wide spectrum of diagnoses including burn, cardiac fibrillation, convulsion, electric shock, electrocution, puncture wound, or respiratory paralysis. These listings in this category are excluded from the supplementary reporting of burns resulting from heat by an electrical appliance and injuries sustained as a consequence of lightning.

The listings of codes and titles contained within category *E926, Exposure to radiation,* are excluded from the supplementary reporting of an abnormal reaction to or complication of treatment, with or without mention of misadventure to the patient in a surgical, medical, or other clinical procedure. These listings also are excluded from the supplementary reporting of any injury due to the use of radiation in war operations.

Accidents involving machinery may be coded and reported in greater detail through the utilization of the listings in category *E919, Accidents caused by machinery.* The fourth-digit subcategories enable the reporting of a supplementary code to indicate the type of machinery involved in the mishap. Codes reporting the injury and the cause of the injury retain sequencing priority over the codes listed in category E919.

In addition, the listings of codes and titles within category *E849, Place of occurrence,* may be used to denote the location of occurrence of an injury or poisoning that is categorized elsewhere in the supplementary classification. For example, an accident occurring on a baseball field or a golf course may be reported with supplementary code *E849.4,* and an accident in a prison or in a reformatory may be reported with supplementary code *E849.7.* Codes reporting the injury and the cause of the injury always retain sequencing priority over the codes listed in category *E849,* however.

Essentially, listings comprised within categories E849 and E919 are supplements to the supplementary codes that indicate external causes. They represent a tertiary reporting scheme to enhance the statistical tabulation of diagnostic entities related to trauma.

A unique section comprised with the supplementary classification of external causes consists of merely one category. The listings of codes and titles encompassed within category *E929, Late effects of accidental injury,* are designated to supplementarily indicate tabulation of accidental injury as the cause of death or disability from late effects that are classifiable elsewhere in the tabular.

These late effects include conditions reported as such or conditions that occurred as sequelae due to accidental injury. The listings in this category are excluded from the supplementary reporting of late effects resulting as a consequence of surgical, medical, or other clinical procedures, as well as late effects that were a consequence of the therapeutic use of pharmaceuticals and medicinal substances.

Other late effects of external causes are classified within specific sections of this supplement to the diagnostic tabular of ICD-9-CM. Categories for supplementary reporting of late effects are: category E959 for late effects of self-inflicted injury; category E969 for late effects of injury purposely inflicted by another person; category E977 for late effects of injuries due to legal intervention; category E989 for late effects of injury that are undetermined whether accidentally or purposely inflicted; and category E999 for late effects of injury due to war operations. All of these categories are designated for supplementary reporting of documented late effects or sequelae occurring after the related injury and resulting in morbidity or mortality.

ICD CODING OF SUICIDE AND HOMICIDE

The section of the supplementary classification of external causes consisting of category range E950 through E959 is comprised of listings of codes and titles to supplement the reporting of suicide (or attempted suicide) and intentional self-inflicted injury. This section includes categorization for: poisonings by solid or liquid substances; poisonings by gases in domestic use as well as other gases and vapors; injuries by hanging, strangulation, or suffocation; injuries by submersion or drowning; injuries from firearms and explosives; injuries from cutting or piercing instruments; and injuries by jumping from high places.

Category range E960 through E969 in the supplementary classification of external causes encompasses listings of codes and titles to supplement the reporting of homicide (or attempted homicide) and injury purposely inflicted by other persons. This section includes categorization of injuries inflicted with the intent to injure or kill by a variety of means.

The listings in this section include codes and titles for entities such as: fights, brawls, or rapes; and for assaults by poisoning, hanging, strangulation, submersion, drowning, firearms, explosives, cutting, piercing, battering, and other methods. The listings in these categories exclude the supplementary reporting of injuries due to legal intervention or operations of war.

The listings in category range E970 through E978 in the supplementary classification of external causes are comprised of codes and titles to supplement the reporting of injuries inflicted by the police or other law enforcing agents, including military personnel on duty, in the course of arresting or attempting to arrest alleged violators of the law, and in the course of suppressing disturbances or maintaining order. This section also includes a category for the reporting of legal execution.

Categorization in this section enables the classification of injuries from legal intervention according to the means used to inflict the injury, such as firearms, explosives, gas, blunt objects, or cutting or piercing instruments. Injuries resulting from civil insurrections are not classified in this section, but are incorporated in the subsequent section that lists injuries resulting from the operations of war.

The section of the supplementary classification of external causes consisting of category range E980 through E989 is comprised of listings of codes and titles to supplement the reporting of injuries that were undetermined whether accidentally or purposefully inflicted. These codes are primarily designated for reporting mortality tabulation if, after a thorough investigation, determination cannot be made whether the injuries sustained were accidental, suicidal, or homicidal.

The categorization in this section includes listings for the supplementary reporting of: poisoning by solid or liquid substances; poisoning by gases in domestic use or by other gases; hanging, strangulation, or suffocation; submersion or drowning; injury caused by firearms and explosives; injury caused by cutting or piercing instruments; and falls from high places.

The listings in category range E990 through E999 in the supplementary classification of external causes are comprised of codes and titles to supplement the reporting of injuries to military personnel or civilians caused by war and civil insurrections, and occurring during the time of war or insurrection. The listings within these categories exclude the supplementary reporting of accidents during the training of military personnel, or during the manufacture of war material and transport, unless the injury was directly attributable to enemy action.

This section for supplementary reporting of injuries resulting from the operations of war is comprised of listings of codes and titles for injuries sustained as a consequence of: fires or conflagrations; bullets or fragments; explosion of marine weapons or other explosions; destruction of aircraft; all forms of conventional warfare; nuclear weapons and other forms of unconventional warfare; as well as injuries resulting from war operations that occurred after the formal cessation of hostilities.

KEY CONCEPTS

adverse effect _____	nonspecific procedure _____
closed injury _____	old injury _____
combination category _____	open injury _____
combination code _____	poisoning _____
comorbidity _____	primary diagnosis _____
complicated wound _____	principal diagnosis _____
complication _____	principal procedure _____
current injury _____	prospective payment system _____
diagnosis related group _____	reimbursement _____
external causes _____	resource intensity _____
iatrogenic complications _____	sequelae _____
late effect _____	superficial injury _____
major diagnostic category _____	supplementary classification _____
multiple coding _____	toxicity _____
multiple trauma _____	unspecified diagnosis _____
nonspecific diagnosis _____	unspecified procedure _____

REVIEW QUESTIONS

1. Which sections of the injury and poisoning chapter are divided into subsections? _____
_____
_____

2. Describe the purpose of the fifth-digit subclassification for the coding of intracranial injury.
_____
_____

3. Explain the distinction provided in the ICD-9-CM classification system between the coding of current orthopedic injuries and the coding of old orthopedic injuries. _____
_____
_____

4. Explain the significance of the various modifiers essential in the coding of fractures. _____
_____
_____

5. Describe the purpose of the fifth-digit subclassification for the coding of internal injuries. ___
_____
_____

6. Describe the purpose of the fifth-digit subclassification for the coding of open wounds. _____
_____
_____

7. Describe the purpose of the fifth-digit subclassification for the coding of burns. _____
_____
_____

8. Prioritize (rank in order of importance) the following traumatic injuries:

   A. fracture of the distal radius, cerebral concussion, abrasion of abdomen _____
   _____

   B. fracture of mandible, laceration of forehead, dislocation of shoulder _____
   _____

   C. hematuria, fracture of occipital bone, anxiety _____
   _____

   D. second-degree burn of thigh, third-degree burn of forearm, laceration of chest _____
   _____

9. Identify at least ten codes and narrative titles that represent traumatic injury conditions which are recognized by Medicare as complications or comorbidities.

   _____   _____
   _____   _____
   _____   _____
   _____   _____
   _____   _____

10. Assign precise, accurate code numbers from the ICD-9-CM volume for the following trauma diagnoses:

    A.   closed skull vault fracture with cerebral contusion _____
    _____

B.   open fracture of clavicle _____

C.   closed pertrochanteric fracture, intertrochanteric section _____

D.   open dislocation of jaw _____

E.   sprained rotator cuff capsule _____

F.   brain injury _____

G.   laceration of kidney _____

H.   open wound of buttock _____

I.   amputation of lower right arm _____

J.   gunshot wound of the thigh with tendon damage _____

K.   injury of the internal jugular vein _____

L.   infected abrasion of the right cheek _____

M.   contusion of the ear _____

N.   corneal foreign body _____

O.   chemical burn of the eyelids _____

P.   visual cortex injury _____

Q.   penicillin poisoning _____

R.   lobeline poisoning _____

S.   accidental alcohol poisoning _____

T.   radiation sickness _____

U.   fracture of the fourth cervical vertebra _____

V.   closed Bennett's fracture _____

W.   open fracture of the heel bone _____

X.   open dislocation of hip _____

Y.   ankle sprain _____

Z.   prolonged concussion with loss of consciousness _____

AA. traumatic hemothorax _____

BB. laceration of the ocular adnexa _____

CC. wound of the scapular region with tendon involvement _____

DD. partial amputation of the toes of the left foot _____

EE. late effect of skull fracture _____

FF. blister of the left ring finger _____

GG. crushed larynx _____

HH. foreign body in the stomach _____

II. second-degree burn of the lower legs _____

JJ. injury to the radial nerve _____

KK. heroin poisoning _____

LL. dextromethorphan poisoning _____

MM. poisoning by death-cap mushrooms _____

NN. giant urticaria _____

OO. closed fracture of rib _____

PP. complications due to breast implant _____

QQ. tear of lateral cartilage of right knee _____

RR. Volkmann's ischemic contracture _____

SS. cerebral compression due to injury _____

TT. foreign body in the auditory canal _____

UU. punctured eardrum _____

VV. splinter in the palm of left hand _____

WW. stab wound of left hand _____

XX. late effects of radiation _____

        _____

11. Assign precise, accurate E codes for the following transportation accidents.

    A. train conductor who sustained a fractured hip when injured in collision with another train

        _____

    B. pedestrian who sustained a concussion when hit by ascending railway crossing gates ____

        _____

    C. eighty-year-old woman who fell while boarding a train and injured her ankle _____

        _____

    D. fifty-year-old man crushed by rolling boxcar at railroad siding _____

        _____

    E. unidentified youth found dead on railroad tracks _____

        _____

    F. twenty-six-year-old female who injured her right leg during collision while riding as passenger in automobile _____

        _____

    G. pedestrian who suffered a fractured pelvis when hit by a car while crossing the street ____

        _____

    H. elderly man who fell while alighting from bus and fractured his left wrist _____

        _____

    I. man who suffered severe facial lacerations from explosion of motor vehicle engine ____

        _____

    J. driver who experienced mild concussion after failing to negotiate a curve on the interstate highway _____

        _____

    K. sixteen-year-old who suffered a fractured right radius when his arm became caught by door of motor vehicle _____

        _____

    L. twenty-year-old who dislocated her left ankle when thrown from horse _____

        _____

    M. man who fell from pedal cycle while riding with friend and fractured his right index finger _____

        _____

    N. woman who sprained her right ankle while riding in horse drawn carriage _____

        _____

    O. pedestrian knocked down by sled pulled by dogs _____

        _____

    P. girl who suffered facial contusions when thrown from horse during polo practice _____

        _____

    Q. man who sustained a fractured femur from fall while boarding a streetcar _____

        _____

    R. toddler cyclist who suffered bilateral tibial fractures when his legs became entangled in the wheels _____

        _____

    S. man who drowned when boat overturned accidentally _____

        _____

    T. water skier who sustained an intertrochanteric hip fracture due to collision with another motorboat _____

        _____

U.   crew member who experienced second degree forehead burns due to a fire on board the ship _____

V.   passenger of yacht who suffered head injuries when thrown overboard by turbulent motion of vessel _____

W.   passenger who sustained a fractured humerus after slipping on the deck of a cruise ship _____

X.   crew member who suffered third-degree burns to both arms when the ship kitchen caught fire _____

Y.   woman admitted with accidental poisoning by gas on private boat _____

Z.   military officer who suffered multiple internal injuries when his aircraft exploded on takeoff _____

AA. emergency medical staff member who sustained head injuries when helicopter crashed during attempted rescue effort _____

BB. hang glider who experienced leg lacerations after landing on aircraft wing _____

CC. ground crew member who suffered rope burn abrasions when hot-air balloon became entangled with propeller of aircraft waiting take-off permission _____

DD. pedestrian who sustained mild concussion when object thrown from passing helicopter struck him on the head _____

EE. woman who suffered a fractured fibula after falling from a chair lift _____

FF. man who sustained a sprained ankle when his riding lawnmower overturned _____

GG. injuries to driver when his car was struck by another auto that crossed the median of a four-lane highway _____

HH. passenger injured when her car struck a deer _____

II.   steward who suffered broken ankle in fall on stairs during a storm at sea _____

JJ.   miner who suffered scrapes and bruises when mine tram jumped the tracks _____

KK. operator injured when wind gust overturned ice boat _____

LL. explosion of boiler causing steam burns on crewman _____

MM. rodeo clown who suffered fractured leg when stepped on by a bronco _____

NN. driver injured when tire blowout caused van to overturn _____

OO. passenger injured when train derailed _____

PP.   passenger injured when windshield was hit and broken by brick dropped from overpass

_____

QQ.   snowmobile overturned and driver suffered dislocated wrist _____

_____

RR.   stevedore injured when struck by debris dropped by crane _____

_____

SS.   ground crewman who suffered chemical burns _____

_____

TT.   passenger who suffered smoke inhalation when fire broke out in ship kitchen _____

_____

UU.   rider whose pantleg caught in chain of bicycle causing her to fall and suffer a fractured
       radius _____

_____

VV.   driver who suffered neck injuries when his vehicle was struck from behind at stop sign

_____

WW. hobo found injured on railway right-of-way _____

_____

XX.   passenger who suffered cut on leg in fall caused by air turbulence _____

_____

12. Assign precise, accurate E codes for the following external causes of injury.

A.   ten-year-old girl who ran into stationary porch railing and sustained a fractured nose

_____

B.   swimmer admitted with multiple injuries to his torso after being crushed by a boat ___

_____

C.   child who experienced food poisoning while visiting her grandparents at their farmhouse

_____

D.   elderly female admitted with accidental poisoning from ingesting codeine _____

_____

E.   intentional poisoning with tranquilizers by depressed teenager _____

_____

F.   accidental poisoning with unknown quantity of tranquilizers ingested by five-year-
      old child _____

_____

G.   overdose of antidepressants by middle-aged woman _____

_____

H.   assault by LSD surreptitiously placed in beverage of partygoer _____

_____

I.   accidental poisoning by incorrect dosage of anti-convulsant drug with an anti-
      parkinsonism drug _____

_____

J.   administration of incorrect dosage of local anesthetic _____

_____

K.   poisoning by accidental ingestion of small quantity of atropine _____

_____

L.   poisoning resulting from deliberate ingestion of drugs with effects upon the autonomic
      nervous system _____

_____

M. accidental poisoning by overdose of synthetic hormone substitute _____

N. accidental ingestion of scented dishwashing liquid by three-year-old child _____

O. accidental puncture of liver during colon surgery _____

P. foreign body left in thoracic cavity during surgery _____

Q. incorrect dilution of fluid during therapeutic infusion _____

R. amputation of right lower extremity by mistake (left lower extremity was gangrenous)
_____

S. young man suffering from accidental overdose of heroin _____

T. teenage girl overdosed on phenobarbital _____

U. six-year-old child poisoned by eating chips of lead-based paint _____

V. woman who suffered carbon monoxide poisoning due to furnace malfunction _____

W. patient who contracted HIV due to contaminated blood transfusion _____

X. patient injured during electroshock therapy _____

Y. elderly resident in nursing home who fell while getting out of bed and injured her arm
_____

Z. child burned when pajamas caught on fire while playing with a lighter _____

AA. man splitting logs for firewood who was bitten by a brown recluse spider _____

BB. child who fell into unattended swimming pool and drowned _____

CC. man who was burned when fireworks exploded prematurely _____

DD. death due to late effects of accidental fall _____

EE. patient who suffered hives caused by allergy to penicillin _____

FF. suicide caused by motor vehicle exhaust _____

GG. child who sustained cracked ribs after being struck by her father _____

HH. victim who experienced gunshot wound to shoulder while confronting police during
robbery attempt _____

II. man who was injured in fall from billboard _____

JJ. pilot who was injured when plane was shot down _____

KK. sterile precautions that failed during kidney dialysis _____

LL. cardiac arrest during insertion of cardiac pacemaker _____

MM. football player whose left knee was hyperextended during tackle _____

NN. woman burned at picnic while standing too close to bonfire _____

OO. golfer struck by lightning during thunderstorm _____

PP. child who placed marble in nose _____

QQ. astronaut subjected to prolonged stay in space _____

RR. driver who suffered blackouts caused by late effects of prior accident _____

SS. administration of measles vaccine causing an adverse reaction in child _____

TT. person who committed suicide by jumping from railing of bridge _____

UU. teenager shot in abdomen by assault rifle during a drive-by shooting _____

VV. legal execution by lethal injection _____

WW. poisoning by lye, undetermined if accidental _____

XX. patient injured by fragments from hand grenade _____

CODING OF CLINICAL DOCUMENTATION

Read the following clinical reports and assign precise, accurate diagnostic and procedural code numbers from the appropriate sections of the ICD-9-CM volumes.

PATIENT: Feldhaus, Douglas   **MR#:** 99-11-01

SURGEON: Hernandez   **ASSISTANT:** Jezik

Preoperative Diagnosis:
Right zygomatic arch fracture.

Postoperative Diagnosis:
Right zygomatic arch fracture.

Operation:
Open reduction of right zygomatic arch fracture.

Indications and Clinical History:
This young male has a history of assault approximately ten days ago resulting in a depressed right zygomatic arch fracture. He has no trismus, but desires elevation of the arch fracture for cosmetic purposes.

Operative Procedure:
The patient was brought to the OR and placed in the supine position on the operating table. After adequate induction of general endotracheal anesthesia, the right face was prepped and draped in the usual sterile fashion and hair was clipped from the right frontotemporal region. A small horizontal incision was made in the hairline and carried down until the temporalis fascia was reached. Hemostasis was achieved with Bovie electrocautery. Next the temporalis fascia was transected with a #15 blade and a Goldman elevator was passed under the fascia down to the zygomatic arch. The zygomatic arch was raised with a Goldman and a Gilles elevator until adequate contour was achieved. Multiple fragments were present and the arch did collapse somewhat after elevation. The fragments were considered to be stable and the procedure was terminated. The skin incision was closed using 3-0 Vicryl. The subcutaneous tissue was closed with 5-0 Prolene. Polysporin was applied to the wound and a styrofoam cup cut in half was placed over the zygoma for protection in the postoperative field.

Codes: _____

PATIENT: McCormick, Wanda   **MR#:** 99-11-02

ADMITTING PHYSICIAN: Billingsley

History of Present Illness and Hospital Course:
This 46-year-old white female was admitted from the emergency room following a fall in a parking lot. The patient suffered a comminuted fracture of the left femur. The patient was admitted and was seen in consultation by Dr. Fraser because of the history of asthma and obesity. She was cleared for surgery and on the evening of admission, the patient was taken to the operating room. Open reduction and internal fixation were performed under spinal anesthesia using a compression screw and fixation plate. Hemovac tubes were inserted. Due to the patient's size and immobility, she was started on Coumadin postoperatively. The hemovac was removed at 48 hours, and the patient began physical therapy. She made slow but progressive

improvement. The patient was self-sufficient on crutches. She was discharged on a regular diet with condition improved.

Discharge Diagnoses:
Comminuted fracture left femur.

Obesity.

Asthma.

Operations:
Open reduction and internal fixation of femur.

Discharge Medications:
Premarin .625 mg daily; Albuterol MDI 4 puffs q.i.d.; Vicodin q. 6 hours p.r.n. for pain.

Codes: _____

PATIENT: Sutton, Ann   **MR#:** 99-11-03

ADMITTING PHYSICIAN: Lowery   **CONSULTANT:** Fleming

History of Present Illness:
This 30-year-old white female with an unremarkable past medical history except for alcohol and cocaine abuse, was brought to the ER following electromechanical dissociation arrest. The patient was at home drinking alcohol and smoking crack Cocaine when she suddenly collapsed with her eyes rolled back in her head, a stiffening of her jaw, and no movement of her extremities. She stopped breathing. Her sister called the EMS, who arrived to find her in arrest. The patient was resuscitated and brought to the ER where she arrested twice more. She was twice more resuscitated and intubated in the right main stem bronchus. Initial arterial blood gases were 7.04, 44, and 95. She received Narcan three times and remained unresponsive and hypotensive until she was put on Levophed and Dopamine drips. The time from the initial collapse to arrival in the ER was thirty minutes.

Medications on Admission:
Antibiotics for urinary tract infection. No known drug allergies.

Past Medical History:
Urinary tract infection and a cesarean section.

Family History:
Father has coronary artery disease.

Social History:
She smokes and drinks daily and uses crack Cocaine. She does not use IV drugs.

Physical Examination:
On admission, an obese black female, intubated. *Pulse:* 102; *BP:* 90/50; *Resp:* 19; and afebrile.
Neck: supple.
Chest: sounds decreased with scattered rhonchi on the left side.
Heart: S-1 and S-2, regular rate and rhythm; no S-3, no S-4, no murmurs.
Abdomen: bowel sounds positive.
Neurological: no response to voice or pain; eyes partially opened; doll's eyes negative; and gag negative.

Extremities: flaccid, no movement with pain. The examination revealed no evidence of brain function and the absence of brainstem reflexes. Her prognosis was extremely poor. The initial event may have been a myocardial infarction, an arrhythmia, a tamponade, or a subarachnoid or intraparenchymal hemorrhage leading to severe hypoxic ischemic brain damage. The initiating factor was probably Cocaine use.

Laboratory Data:

WBC was 2300, hemoglobin was 12.6, and hematocrit was 37.6. Arterial blood gases indicated a pH of 7.35, PCO2 of 40, and a PO2 of 467. The chest X ray revealed no cardiomegaly and no infiltrates. The electrocardiogram indicated left ventricular hypertrophy with second degree and ST-T wave changes. A head CT scan revealed subarachnoid hemorrhage and massive cerebral edema with obliteration of ventricles. On admission, SMA-12 indicated albumin of 2.8, total protein of 5.9, total bilirubin of 0.4, ALT of 54, AST of 90, alkaline phosphatase of 56, calcium of 7.0, phosphate of 2.5, cholesterol of 141, triglycerides of 86, uric acid of 5.4, LD of 290, magnesium of 1.5, and CK of 183. Lactic acid was 2.1. The first set of cardiac enzymes indicated total CK of 143, CK MB of 3.1, CK MB index of 2.2, total MB of 326, and LD/LD-2 ratio of 0.58. Urine drug screen revealed Cocaine and Cocaine metabolites, Lidocaine, Nicotine, and Cotinine. Urine osmolarity was 113 millimoles per Kg. At admission, sodium was 141, potassium was 3.0, chloride was 102, CO2 was 15, BUN was 10, creatinine was 1.2; and glucose was 399.

Urology consultation was obtained and concluded that her urine output was increased tremendously at 500 cc's an hour, suggestive of diabetes insipidus. The patient was examined by neurology attending physicians and pronounced dead at 5:15 p.m. As a candidate for organ donation, she was kept on the ventilator with FIO2 of 100% and PEEP of 5. She was administered Pitressin 5 units and Magnesium Sulfate 2 grams in 100 cc's of normal Saline solution for four hours and Sodium phosphate 15 millimoles in 100 cc's of normal Saline for six hours until she was moved from the ICU.

Final Diagnosis:

Brain death due to Cocaine abuse.

Probable cause of death was myocardial infarction, arrhythmia, and tamponade, or subarachnoid hemorrhage and massive cerebral edema.

Codes: _____

PATIENT: Hampton, Michael   **MR#:** 99-11-04

ADMITTING PHYSICIAN: Chandler

History:

The patient is a 22-year-old black male who returned to the emergency room in the afternoon after being discharged from his tonsillectomy that morning. He complained of pain, fever, myalgias, and chills. He denied nausea, vomiting, bleeding, breathing difficulties, or coughing.

Physical Examination:

Vital Signs: Temp: 38.5; *Pulse:* 110; *Resp:* 24; *BP:* 140/58.
HEENT: pupils equal, round, and reactive to light and accommodation; extraocular movements intact; visual fields and acuity grossly normal; right tympanic membrane demonstrated a dry, persistent perforation; external auditory canal was clear; left tympanic membrane was

clear; boggy turbinates in the nose, no drainage; oral cavity was clear; oropharynx demonstrated status post Bovie tonsillectomy without bleeding or pus; airway was clear; no adenopathy in neck; no focal tenderness.

Chest: clear to auscultation.

Heart: regular rate and rhythm.

Abdomen: soft; nontender; nondistended; bowel sounds positive.

Neurological: nonfocal.

Hospital Course:
The patient was admitted and placed on intravenous Clindamycin. He immediately defervesced and was afebrile for the remainder of his hospital stay. The patient had no complaints of bleeding or respiratory difficulties.

Diagnoses:
Postoperative fever.

Status post tonsillectomy.

Discharge Diet:
The patient was instructed to avoid hard or sharp foods.

Discharge Medications:
Clindamycin 300 mg p.o. q. 6 hours; Tylenol number 3 Elixir 12.5 to 25 cc's p.o. q. 4 hours p.r.n.

Follow-up:
The patient was instructed to follow-up in the ENT clinic. He was also instructed to return to the emergency room in the event of recurrent fever, bleeding, or worsening sore throat.

Codes: _____

PATIENT: Dixon, Vincent   **MR#:** 99-11-05

ATTENDING PHYSICIAN: Dexter

Diagnoses:
Assault.

Perforation of left tympanic membrane.

Lip laceration.

Procedures:
Suturing of lip laceration.

Audiogram.

History:
The patient is a 36-year-old black male who was assaulted by five unknown assailants at approximately 2 a.m. on the morning of admission. The patient waited approximately ten hours before coming to the hospital because of his fear of physicians. He reports a loss of consciousness for 30 to 45 seconds after being hit by a bottle in the back of his head; he was also hit multiple times with fists. The patient complains of swelling and pain in the left occipital area, decreased hearing in his left ear, an echo in his left ear, and occasional vertigo. He denies otalgia or otorrhea.

Physical Examination:
Temp: 36.8; ***Pulse:*** 96; ***Resp:*** 18; ***BP:*** 128/74.

HEENT: His right ear was clear. His left ear demonstrated a perforation of approximately 40% from the 6 o'clock position to the 10 o'clock position. There was slight bleeding at the superior aspect of his tympanic membrane. His Weber lateralized to the left and his Rinne demonstrated air conduction greater than bone conduction bilaterally. His nose was tender and there was a 1-cm laceration on his right anterior nasal septum. There was no septal hematoma or active nasal bleeding noted. Oropharynx and oral cavity were clear. His face demonstrated a 2-cm laceration on the lower lip with a small amount of dried blood and necrotic tissue at the commissure. Cranial nerves V and VII were intact.

Eyes: pupils equal, round, and reactive to light and accommodation. Extraocular movements intact. There was some positive end gaze lateral nystagmus.

Neck: Supple.

Heart: Regular rate and rhythm.

Lungs: Clear to auscultation.

Abdomen: Soft and nontender; nondistended; bowel sounds positive.

Extremities: No clubbing; cyanosis; or edema.

Neurological: Alert and oriented times three; nonfocal; cranial nerves intact; gait normal.

Hospital Course:

The patient was admitted and begun on Decadron. The patient's lip was sutured. He was given Corticosporin drops to his left ear t.i.d. The patient underwent an audiogram, which demonstrated a severe conductive hearing loss, possibly consistent with ossicular chain disruption. There was no evidence of a neurosensory component to his hearing loss. Discharge activity is unrestricted with the exception of keeping the left ear dry.

Discharge Medications:

Keflex 500 mg p.o. q.i.d.; Dakin's 1/4 strength t.i.d. to the lip; Tylenol 3, one to two, p.o. q. 4 hours p.r.n.

Follow-up:

The patient was instructed to follow-up in the ENT clinic in three weeks. He was also instructed to follow-up in the ophthalmology clinic as soon as possible for complaints of blurry vision.

Codes: _____

PATIENT: Straub, Curtis   **MR#:** 99-11-06

ADMITTING PHYSICIAN: Powers   **CONSULTANT:** Fisher

History:

The patient is a 25-year-old, right-handed white male who lost control of his car and was involved in a motor vehicle accident. He was brought to the emergency room where he was seen and evaluated by Dr. Kraus. He has a fracture involving his mandible and also a fracture involving his left clavicle. He complained of pain in these regions in addition to pain in the thoracic region of his back.

Examination of his left shoulder revealed a large area of ecchymosis over the clavicle. The area is tender but the skin is intact. X rays taken of the left clavicle revealed undisplaced fracture involving the left clavicle. He has full passive range of motion involving the left shoulder. All muscle tendon units in the left upper extremity were tested and found to be intact. Examination of his neck revealed some tenderness in the region of the left sternocleidomastoid muscle and left pericervical muscles. He put his chin on his chest without any difficulty. He has full rotation of his cervical spine.

Examination of his back revealed tenderness without swelling over the region of the dorsal spinous process T6. X rays taken of the thoracic spine revealed no fractures or dislocations.

Impression:
Undisplaced fracture involving the left clavicle.

Fracture involving the mandible.

Multiple abrasions and contusions.

The care of the fractured clavicle as well as potential complications were discussed with the patient and his wife in detail. He is currently in a figure-of-eight clavicular strap, which may be removed for hygiene following his discharge. He will be followed in the office regarding this particular fracture.

Codes: _____

PATIENT: Grossberg, Walter   **MR#:** 99-11-07

ADMITTING PHYSICIAN: Ballard   **CONSULTANT:** Stewart

History:
The patient is a 35-year-old white male who was transported to the emergency room by the police after smoking Cocaine while the police were observing. When he arrived at the emergency room, he was very delirious, diaphoretic, twitching, and tachycardic. He complained of chest pain and became apneic for about 25 seconds. He was given Narcan, Thiamine, and Valium. He was also given Metoprolol 50 mg and was taken to the intensive care unit.

Family History, Social History, and Drug History:
All of these histories are unavailable.

Physical Examination:
The patient's blood pressure was 135/90, his pulse was 160, and his respirations were 30. The physical examination revealed jerky movements all over his body. His pupils were dilated, his neck was supple, and his heart was tachycardic without gallop or murmurs. His lungs had mild crackles, his abdomen was soft and nontender, and his extremities revealed no edema. He was drowsy and his mental status was not judged, but he was disoriented to place and person. Later he became delirious and euphoric. He had generalized muscle twitching without any focal signs and without any sensory or motor deficits.

Laboratory Data:
The electrocardiogram showed ST depression in leads V-2, V-3, V-4 and V-5. The chest X ray was clear.

Initial Impression:
Cocaine overdose.

Hospital Course:
The patient was admitted to the intensive care unit and was given intravenous Valium for restlessness and agitation. His blood pressure and pulse were reduced. He was afebrile. Metoprolol and intravenous fluids were given to reduce tachycardia and hypertension. He was acidotic at first, but with intravenous fluids and oxygen, his acidosis was corrected. His initial CK MB was 238 with an MB of 2.8, a subsequent CK MB was 1,313 with an MB of 26.3, and

the last CK MB was 6,607 with an MB of only 2.0. Therefore, a myocardial infarction was ruled out. He did not have any chest pain or any electrocardiogram changes to suggest a myocardial infarction. The Metoprolol was discontinued and the intravenous fluids were discontinued. The patient was stable at the time of discharge.

Discharge Medications:
None.

Procedures:
None.

Discharge Instructions:
The patient was advised to abstain from Cocaine.

Discharge Diagnosis:
Cocaine overdose.

Codes: _____

12 CHAPTER

CPT Coding: Evaluation and Management Services

LEARNING OBJECTIVES

Upon completion of this chapter the learner should be able to:

1. State the criteria for differentiating a new patient from an established patient.
2. Define the concept of time-based billing.
3. Define the concept of procedure-based billing.
4. Define the concept of intra-service time.
5. Define the concept of variable intensity of service.
6. Define the concept of a referral.
7. Define the concept of a transfer.
8. Define the concept of critical care.
9. Define the concept of preventive medicine.
10. Define the concept of case management.
11. Explain the function of key components and contributory factors in code number and descriptor selection for evaluation and management services.
12. Explain the function of time in code number and descriptor selection for evaluation and management services.
13. Explain the types of inpatient services and their principal differentiating attributes.
14. Explain the types of clinical consultations and their principal differentiating attributes.
15. Explain the types of nursing facility services and their principal differentiating attributes.
16. Discuss the diverse types of patient histories and their impact on code number and descriptor selection for evaluation and management services.
17. Discuss the diverse types of patient physical examinations and their impact on code number and descriptor selection for evaluation and management services.
18. Discuss the diverse types of clinical decision making and their impact on code number and descriptor selection for evaluation and management services.
19. Discuss the disparate levels of presenting problems acknowledged in the reporting of evaluation and management services.

20. Discuss the usefulness of modifiers for supplementing the codes reporting evaluation and management services.

21. Apply knowledge of coding principles by assigning accurate and precise codes to report evaluation and management services.

CATEGORIES AND SUBCATEGORIES

The evaluation and management services code numbers and descriptors were introduced into the CPT coding system in 1992 in order to balance the recognition of cognitive skills with the recognition of technical skills. The section of the CPT volume designated for evaluation and management services comprises sixteen subsections titled as categories:

1. Office or Other Outpatient Services (codes *99201–99215*)
2. Hospital Observation Services (codes *99218–99220*)
3. Hospital Inpatient Services (codes *99221–99238*)
4. Consultation Services (codes *99241–99275*)
5. Emergency Department Services (codes *99281–99288*)
6. Critical Care Services (codes *99291–99292*)
7. Neonatal Intensive Care Services (codes *99295–99297*)
8. Nursing Facility Services (codes *99301–99313*)
9. Domiciliary, Rest Home, or Custodial Care Services (codes *99321–99333*)
10. Home Care Services (codes *99341–99353*)
11. Prolonged Services (codes *99354–99360*)
12. Case Management Services (codes *99361–99373*)
13. Care Plan Oversight Services (codes *99375–99376*)
14. Preventive Medicine Services (codes *99381–99429*)
15. Newborn Care Services (codes *99431–99440*)
16. Special Evaluation and Management Services (codes *99450–99456*)
17. Other Evaluation and Management Services (code *99499*)

Many of these categories of evaluation and management services are additionally partitioned into two or more subcategories, which are typically divided into levels of service that delineate the type of service, the place of service, and the status of the patient.

The general guidelines for the Evaluation and Management Services section define key words and key phrases commonly used in this section. The categories and subcategories within the Evaluation and Management Services section contain assorted notes that direct the process of code selection for services detailed within that division of the section. These guidelines and notations are designed to alleviate or minimize divergent interpretation of terms and to enable consistent reporting of services rendered by physicians regardless of specialty.

The basic format of the evaluation and management services code numbers and descriptors is comparable to the code numbers and descriptors of the other five sections in the CPT volume, although the content and substance of the descriptors in the Evaluation and Management Services section is dissimilar from the content and substance of the descriptors in the other sections of the CPT manual. The descriptors in the Evaluation and Management Services section usually define the type of service as well as the place of service and specify the nature of the problem. And in certain instances, these descriptors for evaluation and management services indicate time factors.

Listings in the categories for Office or Other Outpatient Services, Custodial Care Services, Home Services, and Preventive Medicine Services differentiate between evaluation and management services code numbers and descriptors for new patients and evaluation and management services code numbers and descriptors for established patients. A new patient is one who has not received professional services in any setting within the past three years from a physician or another physician (of the same specialty) of the same group practice (with the same billing number). If a physician is on call or covering for another physician, the service is classified as it would be for the physican who is not available. An established patient is one who has received professional services within the last three years from a physician (or another physician of the same specialty) of the same group practice (with the same billing number).

LEVELS OF SERVICE

Each category and subcategory of the Evaluation and Management Services section of the CPT volume includes precise directives regulating the utilization of evaluation and management services code numbers and descriptors. As a rule, three, four, or five levels of service are delineated in most of the categories or subcategories of evaluation and management services (examples: codes *99201* through *99205*; and codes *99211* through *99215*).

Hospitals do not account for levels of service in coding and reporting, regardless of the complexity of clinical decision making or the nature of the presenting problem. Hospitals need report only code *99201* for outpatient services or emergency department services provided to new patients, and code *99211* for outpatient services or emergency department services provided to established patients. Each patient encounter for a hospital outpatient service or a hospital emergency department service is deemed as one unit of service, each of which may be coded and reported separately.

Hospitals may not report evaluation and management services code numbers and descriptors from the categories of: Hospital Inpatient Services; Nursing Facility Services; Domiciliary, Rest Home, or Custodial Care Services; Home Services; Prolonged Services; Case Management Services; Care Plan Oversight Services; or Preventive Medicine Services.

The levels of service in the Evaluation and Management Services section of the CPT volume report the type of service, the place of service, and the status of the patient explicitly for that category or subcategory and do not interchange or correlate within or among the levels of service in alternate categories or subcategories. For example, the first level of service for office visit, new patient, is not defined identically as the first level of service for office visit, established patient. Nor is the first level of service for office visit, new patient, defined identically as the first level of service for an office consultation. The levels of service in the Evaluation and Management Services section therefore annotate the extensive variations in

T A B L E   12–1

Key Components and Contributory Factors

Patient history	Key component
Physical examination	Key component
Medical decision making	Key component
Counseling	Contributory factor
Coordination of care	Contributory factor
Nature of presenting problem	Contributory factor

the requisite effort, skill, time, responsibility, and clinical knowledge of the physician that are applied in the prevention, diagnosis, and treatment of disease or injury and in the promotion of optimal health.

Seven components—the patient history, the patient physical examination, medical decision making, counseling, coordination of care, the nature of the presenting problem, and time—are established as the fundamental or intrinsic elements of evaluation and management services (Table 12–1). All of these components, with the exception of time, are integral in differentiating the level of an evaluation and management service.

Three of these components—the history, the physical examination, and medical decision making—are stipulated as key factors in the selection and reporting of the level of an evaluation and management service. An additional three components—counseling, coordination of care, and the nature of the presenting problem—are stipulated as contributory factors in the selection and reporting of the level of an evaluation and management service.

Counseling of patients and family and the coordination of patient care are optional components of evaluation and management services, and are not factors in every patient encounter. Coordination of care without a patient encounter is coded and reported with case management code numbers and descriptors. If counseling or coordination of care exceeds more than fifty percent of the physician–patient encounter or the physician–family encounter, then time becomes a determinate component or factor in the selection and reporting of a particular level of an evaluation and management service.

In designated categories and subcategories of the Evaluation and Management Services section of the CPT volume, all three of the key components—patient history, patient physical examination, and medical decision making (which in this section are virtually the key factors in code number and descriptor selection)—must equal or surpass the expressed specifications in the category or subcategory notations for an evaluation and management service to qualify for assignment to that level of service (Table 12–2). This stipulation is applicable to evaluation and management services listed in the following categories and subcategories: Office Services, New Patient (subcategory); Hospital Observation Services (category); Initial Hospital Care (subcategory); Office Consultations (subcategory); Initial Inpatient Consultations (subcategory); Confirmatory Consultations (subcategory); Emergency Department Services (category); Comprehensive Nursing Facility Assessments (subcategory); Domiciliary Care, New Patient (subcategory); and Home Care, New Patient (subcategory).

TABLE 12–2

Three of Three Key Components Required

Service	Patient Type
Office services	New
Hospital observation services	Any
Initial hospital care	Any
Office consultations	Any
Initial inpatient consultations	Any
Confirmatory consultations	Any
Emergency department services	Any
Comprehensive nursing facility assessments	Any
Domiciliary care	New
Home care	New

T A B L E   12–3

Two of Three Key Components Required

Service	Patient Type
Office services	Established
Subsequent hospital care	Any
Follow-up inpatient consultations	Any
Subsequent nursing facility care	Any
Domiciliary care	Established
Home care	Established

In other designated subcategories of the Evaluation and Management Services section of the CPT volume, two of the three key components or key factors—patient history, patient physical examination, and medical decision making—must equal or surpass the expressed specifications in the subcategory notations for an evaluation and management service to qualify for assignment to that level of service (Table 12–3). This stipulation is applicable to evaluation and management services listed in the following subcategories: Office Services, Established Patient; Subsequent Hospital Care; Follow-up Inpatient Consultations; Subsequent Nursing Facility Care; Domiciliary Care, Established Patient; and Home Care, Established Patient.

Actual physician performance of diagnostic tests or studies is not intrinsic or inferred in the levels of service delineated in the Evaluation and Management Services section. Both diagnostic and therapeutic procedures should be coded and reported separately with appropriate code numbers and descriptors from other sections of the CPT volume, supplemental to the code number and descriptor selected and reported from the Evaluation and Management Services section.

Clinical supplements (Appendix D of the CPT manual) for the Evaluation and Management Services section of the CPT volume demonstrate examples of the factors or constituents incorporated in each of the levels of service. These clinical supplements or synopses present diverse types of patient histories, physical examinations, medical decision making, counseling, coordination of care, and presenting problems. Each of the scenarios outlined in the clinical supplements is intended to facilitate accurate and precise as well as valid and reliable selection and reporting of code numbers and descriptors for evaluation and management services.

The levels of evaluation and management services acknowledge four types of patient history (Table 12–4) defined as:

1. Problem-focused—documentation of the chief complaint with a brief history of the present illness or current problem (examples: skin rash or minor laceration or mild upper respiratory infection).

2. Expanded problem-focused—documentation of the chief complaint with a brief history of the present illness or current problem and a pertinent review of systems (examples: urinary tract infection or joint dislocation).

3. Detailed—documentation of the chief complaint with an extended history of the present illness or current problem, a pertinent past family history and social history, and an extended review of systems (examples: epistaxis or menorrhagia).

TABLE 12–4

Types of Patient Histories

Chief Complaint	History of Present Illness	System Review
Problem-focused	Brief	
Expanded problem-focused	Brief	Pertinent
Detailed	Extended	Extended
Comprehensive	Extended	Complete

4. Comprehensive—documentation of the chief complaint with an extended history of the present illness or current problem, a complete past family history and social history, and a complete review of systems (examples: syncopal episodes or unexplained weight loss).

The levels of evaluation and management services acknowledge four types of physical examinations (Table 12–5) defined as:

1. Problem-focused—a physical examination limited to the affected body area or organ system (examples: examination of knee abrasion or examination of fecal impaction).

2. Expanded problem-focused—a physical examination of the affected body area or organ system as well as a physical examination of other symptomatic or associated organ systems (examples: examination of deviated nasal septum or examination of aphthous stomatitis).

3. Detailed—an extended physical examination of the affected body area or organ system as well as an extended physical examination of other symptomatic or associated organ systems (examples: examination of perineal edema or examination of intermittent claudication).

4. Comprehensive—a complete single system specialty physical examination or a complete multi-system physical examination (examples: a complete neurological examination for left-sided weakness or a cardiopulmonary examination for severe dyspnea).

The levels of evaluation and management services acknowledge four types of medical decision making, whereby medical decision making refers to the complexity of discerning a diagnosis and determining a clinical management option (Table 12–6). To be labeled as a

TABLE 12–5

Types of Physical Examinations

Problem-focused	Affected body area or organ system
Expanded problem-focused	Affected and symptomatic or associated body area or organ system
Detailed	Extended affected and symptomatic or associated body area or organ system
Comprehensive	Complete single system specialty or complete multi-system

T A B L E   12–6

Types of Medical Decision Making

Number of Diagnoses or Management Options	Amount or Complexity of Data To Be Reviewed	Risk of Complications and Morbidity or Mortality	Type of Decision Making
Minimal	Minimal or none	Minimal	Straightforward
Limited	Limited	Low	Low complexity
Multiple	Moderate	Moderate	Moderate complexity
Extensive	Extensive	High	High complexity

designated type of medical decision making, two of the three elements in Table 12–6 must be applicable. These four types of medical decision making are:

1. Straightforward medical decision making with a minimal number of diagnoses or management options, a minimal amount or no complex data to review, and a minimal risk of complications and morbidity or mortality (examples: suture removal or prescription refills).

2. Low complexity medical decision making with a limited number of diagnoses or management options, a limited amount of complex data to review, and a low risk of complications and morbidity or mortality (examples: benign hypertension or tibial fracture).

3. Moderate complexity medical decision making with multiple number of diagnoses or management options, a moderate amount of complex data to review, and a moderate risk of complications and morbidity or mortality (examples: alcoholic cirrhosis of the liver or carcinoma of the prostate).

4. High complexity medical decision making with extensive diagnoses or management options, an extensive amount of complex data to review, and a high risk of complications and morbidity or mortality (examples: intracranial hemorrhage or sustained ventricular tachycardia).

Comorbidities (coexisting or secondary underlying diseases) are not considered or reflected in the selection and reporting of a level of an evaluation and management service, unless the presence of these conditions significantly intensifies the complexity of medical decision making.

NATURE OF PRESENTING PROBLEM

A presenting problem is defined in the CPT volume as a disease, condition, illness, injury, symptom, sign, finding, complaint, or reason for patient encounter that is existent with or without an established diagnosis at the time of the patient encounter. Five types of presenting problems are acknowledged in the levels of evaluation and management services (Table 12–7) and are labeled as:

1. Minimal—a problem with treatment provided under the supervision of a physician but not necessitating physician presence (examples: flu vaccine inoculation or dressing change).

2. Self-limited or minor—a transient problem with a definite and prescribed course and with a good prognosis or a low probability of permanently affecting health status (examples: acute laryngitis or viral gastroenteritis).

3. Low severity—if untreated, a problem with a low probability of morbidity and no probability of mortality and with the expectation of full recovery without functional impairment (examples: otitis media or olecranon bursitis).

4. Moderate severity—if untreated, a problem with a moderate probability of morbidity and a moderate probability of mortality and with an uncertain prognosis and an increasing probability of functional impairment (examples: labile hypertension or fracture of the femur).

5. High severity—if untreated, a problem with a high probability of morbidity and a high probability of mortality and with a high probability of functional impairment (examples: myocardial infarction or acute renal failure).

TIME FACTORS

Since the publication of CPT-1992, the component of time is embraced as a variable factor in the selection and reporting of the most appropriate level of service from the Evaluation and Management Services section of the CPT volume. The explicit time specified in the listing of a descriptor is simply an average that indicates a range of times, which are contingent or dependent upon the actual clinical circumstances, and that may be higher or lower than the time specified in the descriptor listing.

Statistical surveys of practicing physicians generated the data utilized to establish the amount of time typically associated with the rendering of each evaluation and management service that is listed in the CPT volume. These estimations yielded a variable that is indicative of the level of service, both within and across clinical specialties.

Time is not a definitive component for the level of service delineated among the evaluation and management services rendered in the emergency department, however. Services in the emergency department are customarily provided on a variable intensity basis, involving multiple encounters with several patients during an extended time period. Therefore, this distinctive nature of clinical situations in most emergency departments impedes physicians in the accurate estimation of time expended with an individual patient.

The concept of intra-service time, instead of actual time, is denoted and clarified in the guidelines of the Evaluation and Management Services section. Intra-service time offers and extends a suitable criterion or standard of measurement, both through its relative ease of

TABLE 12–7

Types of Presenting Problems

	Prognosis	Probability of Morbidity or Mortality
Minimal	Good	None
Self-limited or minor	Good	None
Low severity	Good	Low
Moderate severity	Fair	Moderate
High severity	Poor	High

measurement and by its logical correlation with measurement of the actual time that is associated with the rendering of routine evaluation and management services. Intra-service time is differentiated as face-to-face time for office and outpatient encounters, and as unit or floor time for hospital and inpatient encounters.

Face-to-face time includes and encompasses the time allocated by the physician to obtain the patient history, to conduct the patient physical examination, and to counsel the patient during the patient encounter. Tasks such as reviewing medical records and test results, ordering procedures, and communicating with colleagues or ancillary healthcare personnel are accomplished either before this face-to-face time with the patient (during what is termed pre-encounter time), or after this face-to-face time with the patient (during what is termed post-encounter time).

The physician endeavors accomplished outside the bounds of face-to-face time, however, are additionally factored into the determinants of the level of service on the basis of aggregate data obtained from documentation of typical patient encounters. This aggregate data also is calculated and accounted for in establishing levels of service that are comparable for reimbursement purposes.

Unit or floor time includes and encompasses the time allocated by the physician to review or update the patient's chart, to examine the patient, to order tests or procedures, and to communicate with the patient or with the patient's family as well as with colleagues and ancillary healthcare personnel while the physician is present on the unit or floor. Tasks such as the assessment of test results, which are performed not on the unit or floor, but elsewhere in the healthcare facility (such as in the laboratory department or in the radiology department), are accomplished during what is termed pre-visit time or post-visit time.

The physician endeavors relating to a patient, which are accomplished outside the bounds of unit or floor time, however, are additionally factored into the determinants of the level of service on the basis of aggregate data obtained from documentation of typical visits on the unit or floor. This aggregate data also is calculated and accounted for in establishing levels of service that are comparable for reimbursement purposes.

As explained heretofore, if counseling or coordination of care exceeds more than fifty percent of the physician–patient encounter or the physician–family encounter, then time becomes a determinate component or factor in the selection and reporting of a particular level of an evaluation and management service. Obviously, the amount of face-to-face time and the amount of unit or floor time accounted for on a stated date should not exceed the time feasible for one workday.

EVALUATION AND MANAGEMENT SERVICES MODIFIERS

To signify special clinical circumstances or exceptional clinical situations, the listed code numbers for evaluation and management services should be properly appended with modifiers. Several of the CPT code modifiers specifically relate to evaluation and management services.

Modifier *-21* is an indicator of a protracted evaluation and management service that extends in time and effort beyond the attributes ascribed to the highest level of service listed in that distinctive evaluation and management service category or subcategory.

Modifier *-24* is an indicator of an evaluation and management service that is unrelated to an operative procedure but that is rendered either during a normal pre-operative period or during a normal post-operative period.

Modifier *-25* is an indicator of a significant and separately identifiable evaluation and management service that is rendered either during a normal pre-operative period or during a normal post-operative period.

Modifier -*32* is an indicator of consultations and/or related services required by an agency or a third-party payor.

Modifier -*52* is an indicator of a reduced or diminished evaluation and management service that does not merit or fulfill the attributes of time and effort ascribed to the lowest level of service listed in that distinctive evaluation and management service category or subcategory.

Modifier -*57* is an indicator of an evaluation and management service that results in an initial decision to perform surgery.

OFFICE OR OTHER OUTPATIENT SERVICES CODING

The initially positioned Office or Other Outpatient Services category of the section for Evaluation and Management Services contains detailed and elongated descriptors among the listings of code numbers for reporting patient services provided either in a physician's office, in an ambulatory care center, or in any other variety of outpatient facility. A patient is classified as an outpatient until he or she is admitted to a healthcare facility.

Alternate subcategories differentiate listings of office or other outpatient evaluation and management services for new patients from such listings for established patients including codes for follow-up care and periodic reevaluations. A patient initially examined by a physician in the hospital is an established patient at his or her first visit to that physician's office.

HOSPITAL OBSERVATION SERVICES CODING

The Hospital Observation Services category of the Evaluation and Management Services section encompasses two subcategories (*Observation Care Discharge Services* and *Initial Observation Care*). The listings of code numbers and descriptors in this category report hospital patient observation services provided by the admitting physician either to new patients or to established patients.

These code numbers and descriptors are designated for reporting initial observation care or observation care discharge day management rendered to patients admitted to an observation unit of the hospital, to an observation area of the hospital, or to any location within the hospital where observation care is rendered. Regardless of the exact site of provision, all evaluation and management services (with the exception of postoperative observation) that are provided on the date of admission to observation care should be reported with code numbers and descriptors for initial observation care.

HOSPITAL INPATIENT SERVICES CODING

The Hospital Inpatient Services category of the Evaluation and Management Services section comprises two subcategories (*Initial Hospital Care* and *Subsequent Hospital Care*) of listings of code numbers and descriptors for reporting hospital inpatient services provided either to new patients or to established patients. These code numbers and descriptors are also designated for reporting evaluation and management services provided to patients treated in a partial hospital setting.

Regardless of the site of provision, all evaluation and management services (including office services or other outpatient services) provided by the admitting physician on the date of admission to inpatient care should be reported with code numbers and descriptors for initial hospital care. Code numbers and descriptors for initial inpatient evaluation and management services may be reported exclusively by the admitting physician. Initial inpatient evaluation and management services rendered by physicians other than the admitting physician should be reported with code numbers and descriptors from the appropriate inpatient consultation subcategory.

Code numbers and descriptors for subsequent hospital care are designated for reporting all evaluation and management services provided by the attending physician on a specified day in conjunction with the hospital stay. These services involve reviewing and updating the patient's medical record, evaluating the results of diagnostic studies, and observing changes in the patient's clinical status. The sub-subcategory, *Hospital Discharge Services,* contains a listing for hospital discharge day management that includes examination of the patient, review and discussion of the hospital stay, instruction for continuity of care, and preparation of the discharge summary.

CONSULTATION SERVICES CODING

The Consultation Services category of the Evaluation and Management Services section contains assorted definitions and explanations for the detailed and elongated descriptors in the listings of code numbers for reporting consultations rendered by physicians. A consultation is a service providing opinion and advice regarding the evaluation and management of a select clinical problem.

A consultation is presented by a physician in response to a request from another physician, in response to a request from the patient, in response to a request from a family member of the patient, or in response to a request from a third-party payor. A consultation by a physician that is not initiated by another physician is labeled as a confirmatory consultation. Time factors are not specified in the descriptors for confirmatory consultations.

The request for a consultation and the necessity for this service must be documented in the patient's medical record. The physician consultant's opinion and advice as well as any services that were ordered or performed must also be documented in the patient's medical record.

Codes and descriptors for consultation services are grouped into four subcategories: *Office or Other Outpatient Consultations; Initial Inpatient Consultations; Follow-Up Inpatient Consultations;* and *Confirmatory Consultations.* The listings of code numbers and descriptors in each of these subcategories are designated for reporting consultation services provided either to new patients or to established patients.

Code numbers and descriptors for office or outpatient consultations are designated for the reporting of physician consultations provided in a physician's office, in an outpatient center, in an ambulatory care facility, in a hospital observation area, in a private residence, in a rest home, in a custodial care facility, or in an emergency department. Each documented request for opinion or advice that culminates in a consultation should be coded and reported separately.

Code numbers and descriptors for initial inpatient consultations are designated for the reporting of physician consultations provided in hospitals (including partial hospital settings) as well as in nursing facilities. Only one initial consultation per each patient admission may be reported by a physician consultant.

Code numbers and descriptors for follow-up inpatient consultations are designated for the reporting of a subsequent physician consultation. The subsequent consultation essentially is a reevaluation of an inpatient whom the physician previously evaluated during the same hospital stay (including also an inpatient in a partial hospital setting), or the reevaluation of a patient in a nursing facility. This subcategory of consultation is provided in response to a request by the attending physician.

A follow-up consultation involves monitoring progress of the patient and adjusting care plans in reaction to changes in the patient's clinical status. If the physician consultant initiates treatment and assumes primary responsibility for the care of a patient, or if the physician consultant together with another physician assumes concurrent care (joint care) of the patient, then henceforth the services of this physician cease to be consultations, and the code numbers and descriptors for consultations must not be reported. Instead, these evaluation and management services rendered by this physician to the patient must be coded and reported with code numbers and descriptors for subsequent hospital care.

Code numbers and descriptors for confirmatory consultations are designated for reporting physician consultations provided in response to a request from the patient, in response to a request from a family member of the patient, in response to a request from a third-party payor, or in response to a mandate from a governing or regulating agency. The code number reported for a mandated consultation service should be appended with modifier -32. Confirmatory consultations equate with second opinions or third opinions and consist of recommendations and advice only; any other procedures or services should be coded and reported separately.

Many insurance carriers require confirmatory consultations in the process of preapproval (termed as precertification) for stipulated procedures and services. Confirmatory consultations may be provided in any appropriate setting either to new patients or to established patients.

A referral is defined as the transfer or assignment of the complete and total care of a patient or of a specifically designated portion of the care of a patient from one physician to another physician. A referral (such as a referral to a specialist) is not a consultation. The word "referral" should never be used in a consultation report since the term implies or connotates the transfer of patient care.

EMERGENCY DEPARTMENT SERVICES CODING

The Emergency Department Services category of the Evaluation and Management Services section contains listings of code numbers and descriptors for reporting patient services provided either to new patients or to established patients in the emergency department as well as physician direction of emergency medical systems. An emergency department is defined as any organized hospital-based facility that is accessible twenty-four hours per day to provide unscheduled episodic services for patients necessitating urgent care. The code numbers and descriptors for emergency services are designated only for reporting services rendered by physicians assigned to the emergency department.

Time is not a determinate component for establishing the level of service among the evaluation and management services provided in the emergency department. The clinical services of the emergency department are principally rendered on a variable intensity basis, involving several encounters with multiple patients during an extended time period. Therefore, clinical situations in the emergency department hinder physicians from precisely estimating the time accorded to an individual patient.

CRITICAL CARE SERVICES CODING

The brief Critical Care Services category of the Evaluation and Management Services section encompasses merely two listings of code numbers and descriptors for reporting critical care services provided at any site (location of services is not a factor) to critically afflicted patients or critically injured patients during various clinical emergencies (such as cardiac arrest, shock, internal hemorrhage, or respiratory failure). These code numbers and descriptors are designated for reporting care that requires the constant attention of the physician, and the listings specifically include the performance and interpretation of the following procedures: cardiac output measurement; chest X ray; electrocardiogram; blood gas assay; blood pressure assessment; hematologic data review; gastric intubation; temporary transcutaneous pacing; ventilator management; and vascular catheterization. Procedures that are not expressly delineated in the listings should be coded and reported separately.

Time factors are included in both of the descriptors in this category. Code *99291* accounts for the first hour of critical care services rendered on any specific day (the time expended need not be continuous), and code *99292* (appropriately repeated as necessary) accounts for each additional thirty minutes, or any concluding duration of fifteen minutes or more of critical care services rendered on that day (example: three and one-half hours of critical care services may be reported with code *99291* to represent the first hour and code *99292* repeated five times to represent the additional one hundred and fifty minutes).

NEONATAL INTENSIVE CARE SERVICES CODING

The Neonatal Intensive Care Services category of the Evaluation and Management Services section comprises listings of code numbers and descriptors for reporting neonatal intensive care services provided by physicians. These code numbers and descriptors are designated for reporting the care of a newborn infant in a neonatal intensive care unit and should be reported only once per day per neonate patient. If the neonate is not deemed as critically ill, then code numbers and descriptors for subsequent hospital care should be utilized.

The listings of code numbers and descriptors in this category include the performance and assessment of the following services and procedures: patient case management (including nutritional maintenance, metabolic maintenance, and hematologic maintenance); parental counseling; direct supervision of the healthcare team; vascular catheterization; endotracheal intubation; lumbar puncture; bladder aspiration; as well as explicit procedures and services (for example, mechanical ventilation) that are indicated in the notation accompanying a specific code number and descriptor. Services and procedures not expressly delineated in the listings of this category should be coded and reported separately.

NURSING FACILITY SERVICES CODING

The Nursing Facility Services category of the Evaluation and Management Services section contains listings of code numbers and descriptors for reporting evaluation and management services provided by a physician in any healthcare facility (including a psychiatric institution) that renders convalescent, rehabilitative, or long-term patient care. These nursing care facilities or institutions are differentiated as any skilled care nursing facilities or any intermediate care nursing facilities that maintain continual professional staffing, as well as support comprehensive, accurate, standardized, and reproducible assessments of the functional capacity of each patient or resident, and formulate care plans that are revised as needed to enhance the physical and psychosocial functioning of each patient or resident. Skilled care nursing facilities principally focus on patient rehabilitation, whereas intermediate care nursing facilities generally focus on resident sustenance.

Within this category delineated for nursing facility services, subcategories are incorporated for *Comprehensive Nursing Facility Assessments* and *Subsequent Nursing Facility Care.* The code numbers and descriptors in these subcategories are designated for reporting comprehensive patient assessment or subsequent patient care provided either to new patients or to established patients.

Comprehensive assessment includes the evaluation and management services rendered by a physician in conjunction with admission to a nursing facility, even if these services are performed in a site other than the nursing facility. If justified, a comprehensive assessment may be repeated (and coded and reported separately as a distinct unit of service) whenever necessary during the confinement of the patient. Subsequent care includes the evaluation and management services rendered in a nursing facility by a physician to patients or residents not necessitating a comprehensive assessment and not presenting with a major change of status.

The evaluation and management services provided by the physician to a patient admitted to a nursing facility through an encounter on the same date in another location (such as the physician's office or the hospital emergency department) are regarded as a portion of the initial nursing facility care and should be considered and represented in the level of service selected for coding and reporting. Hospital discharge services, however, may be coded and reported separately as a distinct unit of service.

CUSTODIAL CARE SERVICES CODING

The Custodial Care Services category of the Evaluation and Management Services section encompasses listings of code numbers and descriptors for reporting custodial care services provided by a physician in a domiciliary, in a rest home, in a boarding home, or in any custodial care setting.

These code numbers and descriptors are designated for reporting evaluation and management services rendered either to new patients or to established patients in a facility that typically offers room, board, and personal assistance (but not clinical care) on a long-term basis.

HOME CARE SERVICES CODING

The Home Care Services category of the Evaluation and Management Services section comprises listings of code numbers and descriptors for reporting home care services rendered by a physician.

These code numbers and descriptors are designated for reporting evaluation and management services provided either to new patients or to established patients in a private residence (home, apartment, or other dwelling).

PROLONGED SERVICES CODING

The Prolonged Services category of the Evaluation and Management Services section contains three subcategories: *Prolonged Physician Service With Direct (Face-to-Face) Patient Contact; Prolonged Physician Service Without Direct (Face to Face) Patient Contact;* and *Physician Standby Services.* Listings of code numbers and descriptors in these subcategories may be used for reporting a prolonged service that entails direct patient contact either in an inpatient setting or in an outpatient setting. These code numbers and descriptors may be reported in addition to other evaluation and management services that are rendered.

Time factors are included in the seven code descriptors of this category. Code *99354* accounts for the first hour of a prolonged office or other outpatient evaluation and management service that is provided on a specific day, and code *99355* (appropriately repeated as necessary) accounts for each additional thirty minutes, or any concluding duration of fifteen minutes or more, of a prolonged office or other outpatient evaluation and management service on that day. Code *99356* accounts for the first hour of a prolonged inpatient evaluation and management service provided on a specific day, and code *99357* (appropriately repeated as necessary) accounts for each additional thirty minutes, or any concluding duration of fifteen minutes or more, of a prolonged inpatient evaluation and management service on that day.

To exemplify the coding of services listed in this category, two and one-half hours of prolonged evaluation and management services in an office setting may be reported with code *99354* to represent the first hour, and sequentially followed with code *99355* repeated three times to represent the additional ninety minutes. Four and one-half hours of prolonged evaluation and management services in a hospital inpatient setting may be reported with code *99356* to represent the first hour, and sequentially followed with code *99357* repeated seven times to represent the additional 210 minutes.

This category also comprises listings of code numbers and descriptors for prolonged physician evaluation and management services without direct patient contact as well as for physician standby service, which should be reported solely in thirty-minute increments. The time expended on a specific day for prolonged evaluation and management services to an individual patient need not be continuous. The time reported should refer to the aggregate of time accorded to evaluation and management in the care of a patient on a specific day.

CASE MANAGEMENT SERVICES CODING

The Case Management Services category of the Evaluation and Management Services section contains listings of code numbers and descriptors for reporting case management services under two subcategories, *Team Conferences* and *Telephone Calls*.

Case management is the process in which the attending physician conducts and coordinates patient healthcare services. A clinical conference with an interdisciplinary team of healthcare practitioners exemplifies a case management service. Many insurance carriers do not accept the reporting of case management services.

CARE PLAN OVERSIGHT SERVICES CODING

The Care Plan Oversight Services category of the Evaluation and Management Services section is comprised of two listings of code numbers and descriptors for reporting physician supervision of the care of a patient confined to a nursing facility or a patient served by a home healthcare agency.

Time factors are included in the two descriptors of this category. Code *99375* accounts for care plan oversight services totaling thirty to sixty minutes per patient within a thirty-day period, and code *99376* accounts for care plan oversight services totaling more than sixty minutes per patient within a thirty-day period. Care plan oversight services totaling less than thirty minutes per patient within a thirty-day period should not be coded and reported separately.

PREVENTIVE MEDICINE SERVICES CODING

The Preventive Medicine Services category of the Evaluation and Management Services section encompasses listings of code numbers and descriptors for reporting preventive medicine services. Code numbers and descriptors are designated for reporting routine assessments of adults or children provided in the absence of patient symptoms or patient complaints.

A subcategory, *Counseling and/or Risk Factor Reduction Intervention,* includes code numbers and descriptors for reporting counseling or intervention rendered to healthy persons with the intention of preventing illness. Ancillary studies requiring laboratory tests or radiologic examinations are not included and should be coded and reported separately.

NEWBORN CARE SERVICES CODING

The Newborn Care Services category of the Evaluation and Management Services section comprises listings of code numbers and descriptors for the physical examination and initial care of the normal newborn infant as well as for the subsequent care of a normal newborn infant.

This concise category also comprises a listing of a code number and descriptor *(99440 Newborn resuscitation . . .)* to report care of a high-risk newborn at the time of delivery. Hospital discharge services for a newborn infant should be reported with code number *99238.*

SPECIAL EVALUATION AND MANAGEMENT SERVICES CODING

The Special Evaluation and Management Services category of the Evaluation and Management Services section encompasses listings of code numbers and descriptors to report patient evaluations performed either for the preparation of life insurance certificates or of disability insurance certificates.

The codes in this category report simply the evaluation of the patient and do not include active management of a patient problem. If additional evaluation and management services are rendered to the patient on the same date as the insurance evaluation or the disability evaluation, then these additional services may be coded and reported separately.

EVALUATION AND MANAGEMENT SERVICES REPORTING FOR BILLING

Selecting the correct evaluation and management services code number and descriptor to report is a nine stage process:

1. Identify the category of evaluation and management services (for example, hospital observation services or neonatal intensive care services).
2. Identify the subcategory of evaluation and management services (for example, new patient or established patient).
3. Determine the extent of the patient history that is obtained by the physician (problem-focused, expanded problem-focused, detailed, or comprehensive).
4. Determine the extent of the physical examination of the patient that is performed by the physician (problem-focused, expanded problem-focused, detailed, or comprehensive).
5. Determine the complexity of the medical decision making that is accomplished by the physician (straightforward, low complexity, moderate complexity, or high complexity).
6. Verify the approximate amount of intra-service time that is expended by the physician.
7. Verify compliance with the established guidelines for coding and reporting of evaluation and management services (for example, codes for initial observation care, initial hospital care, and initial inpatient consultation should be reported by a physician only once per patient admission).

8. Verify the accuracy and completeness of the clinical documentation in the patient record, which substantiates the coding and reporting of evaluation and management services.

9. Assign the precise code for the evaluation and management services rendered by the physician.

The fee for rendering an evaluation and management service that is submitted by the physician to the third-party payor is termed the "actual charge" for the service. The amount of this actual charge generally is greater than the amount of reimbursement from the third-party-payor or the "allowed charge" for that evaluation and management service.

As third-party payors, insurance carriers usually rationalize or justify the allowed charge with its lessened amount of reimbursement as reasonable on the basis of a "customary charge" (also termed a "prevailing charge") that is compiled from the average charges of similar physicians for that evaluation and management service. Additionally, this disparity between the actual charge and the allowed charge may be rationalized and justified by reason of balance billing, which is billing the patient for the difference between the actual charge and the allowed charge. This disparity may also be rationalized and justified by reason of the co-payment, which is the portion of the actual charge that is paid by the patient directly to the healthcare provider, contingent upon a provision or clause that permits such co-payment.

Healthcare providers who render services to Medicare recipients must bill the patient for the deductible and co-payment amounts. Medicare participating providers are subject to reimbursement based upon the Medicare fee schedule. Medicare non-participating providers may or may not accept assignment but are subject to a fee limitation.

Healthcare providers who render services to Medicaid recipients must accept the Medicaid reimbursement as full payment. These healthcare providers cannot bill the Medicaid patient for the difference between the actual charge and the allowed charge.

Healthcare providers who render services to worker's compensation recipients also must accept the established or authorized fee as full payment and cannot bill the patient for the difference between that fee and the actual charge. Codes reported for worker's compensation cases should reflect solely the condition or problem treated and not any other conditions or problems of the patient.

If a patient has basic or supplemental insurance coverage through a commercial insurance carrier in addition to insurance coverage under Medicare, CHAMPUS, or CHAMPVA, then Medicare, CHAMPUS, or CHAMPVA become the secondary insurance carrier that is billed upon receipt of an explanation of benefits from the commercial insurance carrier. Medicaid is always a secondary insurance carrier if the patient has any alternate insurance coverage.

Stipulated insurance carriers may sanction or authorize either the option of time-based billing or the option of procedure-based billing with respect to the reporting of a specific evaluation and management service. If services are tallied through time-based billing, the amount of time accounted for on a stated date should not surpass the amount of work time reasonably achievable in one workday. Prudent and judicious calculation of time factors for a prolonged office or other outpatient service, for a prolonged inpatient service, and for physician standby service is advisable.

As a rule, if procedure-based billing is favored by a stipulated insurance carrier, reimbursement for emergency department services may be substantially maximized through billing by procedure in lieu of billing by time. Reimbursement for critical care services likewise may be substantially maximized by billing for each procedure performed in lieu of billing by hourly or half-hourly increments of time.

PHYSICIAN SERVICES DATA

A statistical frequency distribution of evaluation and management services codes is beneficial for planning and review in all healthcare settings (office, clinic, nursing home, and so forth). Physician group practices especially should compile code frequency distributions specifically for each physician in the group as well as comparatively, both among all physicians within the practice and in relation to announced code frequency distributions of similar practices within the same clinical specialty.

Analysis of tabulated code frequency distributions endows the group practice with useful, convenient, and worthwhile data. Such data perhaps could include the ratio of new patients to established patients accordingly by each physician in the group practice, or perhaps could include the average length of stay of their hospitalized patients accordingly by each physician in the group practice.

K E Y   C O N C E P T S

actual charge _____

allowed charge _____

average charge _____

balance billing _____

category _____

clinical scenario _____

clinical supplement _____

comprehensive assessment _____

comprehensive history _____

comprehensive physical examination _____

confirmatory consultation _____

consultation _____

contributory component _____

contributory factor _____

co-payment _____

customary charge _____

detailed history _____

detailed physical examination _____

established patient _____

expanded problem-focused history _____

expanded problem-focused physical
   examination _____

face-to-face time _____

floor time_____

frequency distribution of codes _____

high complexity medical decision making _____

high severity presenting problem _____

intra-service time _____

key component _____

key factor _____

level of service _____

low severity presenting problem _____

low complexity medical decision making _____

low severity presenting problem _____

management options _____

medical decision making _____

minimal presenting problem _____

moderate complexity medical decision
   making _____

moderate severity presenting problem _____

new patient _____

physical examination _____

post-encounter time _____

post-visit time _____

precertification _____

pre-encounter time _____

presenting problem _____

problem-focused history _____

problem-focused physical examination _____

procedure _____

procedure-based billing _____

referral _____

self-limiting presenting problem _____

service _____

straightforward medical decision making _____

subcategory _____

subsequent care _____

time-based billing _____

time factor _____

transfer _____

unit time _____

variable intensity of service _____

REVIEW EXERCISES

1. Explain the criteria that differentiate a new patient from an established patient. _____

   _____

   _____

2. Explain the key components (key factors) and the contributory components (contributory factors) in the selection and reporting of a level of service. _____

   _____

   _____

3. In each of the following clinical examples, identify the type of patient history that is ordinarily obtained by the physician:

   A. minor laceration of the forearm _____

   _____

   B. severe and recurrent low back pain _____

   _____

   C. acute maxillary sinusitis _____

   _____

   D. chest pain and dyspnea on exertion _____

   _____

4. In each of the following clinical examples, identify the type of patient physical examination that is ordinarily performed by the physician:

   A. painless rectal bleeding _____

   _____

   B. confusion, agitation, and memory loss _____

   _____

   C. poison oak exposure _____

   _____

   D. stable chronic asthma _____

   _____

5. In each of the following clinical examples, identify the type of medical decision making that is ordinarily accomplished by the physician:

   A. osteoporosis _____

   _____

   B. acute subarachnoid hemorrhage _____

   _____

   C. acute respiratory distress _____

   _____

   D. external hemorrhoids _____

   _____

6. In each of the following clinical examples, identify the type of presenting problem:

   A. aspiration pneumonia _____

   _____

   B. abrasion of the knee _____

   _____

    C. acute renal failure _____

    _____

    D. fracture of the ulna _____

    _____

    E. open wound of lung _____

    _____

7. Explain the two types of intra-service time that are acknowledged in the Evaluation and Management Services section of the CPT volume. _____

_____

_____

8. Select and indicate the appropriate modifier to append to the code number in each of the following clinical examples of evaluation and management services:

    A. patient consulting surgeon for a second opinion required by the patient's insurance carrier

    _____

    B. pre-employment physical for a massively obese patient _____

    _____

    C. near-sighted patient stumbles on stairs while exiting eye center following a vision exam and is reexamined by the physician for a periorbital contusion _____

9. Explain the significant aspects of each of these types of consultations:

    A. the office consultation _____

    _____

    B. the initial inpatient consultation _____

    _____

    C. the follow-up inpatient consultation _____

    _____

    D. the confirmatory consultation _____

    _____

10. Describe the factors that constitute a patient referral. _____

_____

_____

11. Express the meaning of the term "variable intensity of service." _____

_____

_____

12. Detail the advantages as well as the disadvantages of time-based reporting of services versus procedure-based reporting of services. _____

_____

_____

13. Describe the utility of evaluation and management services code frequency distributions in the context of the physician office environment and in the context of alternate healthcare environments. _____

_____

_____

14. Express the effect of the evaluation and management services section on balancing or equating the value of the cognitive efforts of physicians with the value of the technical procedural endeavors of physicians. _____

_____

_____

15. Assign precise, accurate code numbers from the CPT volume for these subsequent evaluation and management services:

A. office medical service for emergency care _____

_____

B. hospital visit for initial care of a normal newborn _____

_____

C. evaluation and management of observation discharge _____

_____

D. patient counseling rendered in a group setting for thirty minutes _____

_____

E. home visit for an established patient with expanded problem-focused history and expanded problem-focused physical examination _____

_____

F. office visit of new patient with detailed history, detailed physical examination, and medical decision making of low complexity _____

_____

G. initial inpatient consultation with comprehensive history, comprehensive physical examination, and medical decision making of moderate complexity _____

_____

H. comprehensive patient assessment in a nursing facility with detailed interval history, comprehensive physical examination, and medical decision making of moderate complexity __

_____

I. case management with a sixty-five minute medical conference _____

_____

J. prolonged outpatient service of three hours _____

_____

K. critical care service of ninety minutes _____

_____

L. emergency department visit with problem-focused history, problem-focused physical examination, and straightforward medical decision making _____

_____

M. domiciliary visit of an established patient with detailed history, detailed physical examination, and medical decision making of high complexity _____

_____

16. Read the following patient histories and determine the type of patient history obtained by the physician. Note the differences in format and content of these similar clinical reports.

PATIENT: Taylor, Lillian

PHYSICIAN: Edwards

Chief Complaint:
"Fell and cut my chin"

History of Present Illness:

Patient experienced dizziness and fell, striking chin on coffee table, resulting in small laceration; no associated loss of consciousness, nausea, vomiting, headache, or angina; no previous history of loss of consciousness, seizures, cerebrovascular accident, or transient ischemic attack; status post mitral valve replacement, on Coumadin; adult type diabetes mellitus on insulin; chronic obstructive pulmonary disease for twenty years requiring nasal O_2.

Past Medical History:

Positive for measles; mumps; and rheumatic fever with three months in the hospital at age 14; total right hip replacement in 1989, after a fall on the ice; gravida 3, para 3, vaginal delivery $\times$ 3; no known allergies.

Medications:

Coumadin 10 mg q.d. p.o.; NPH insulin 80 units subq. q.d. at breakfast; nasal O_2 at 2L/min; ASA 500 mg t.i.d. p.r.n. for arthritis pain; vitamin pill q.d. p.o.

Review of Systems:

Multiple age spots on hands; crepitus both hands; decreased hearing both sides; sleeps better on three pillows.

Family Medical History:

Father died of heart attack at age 67; mother died of old age; sister died in childbirth; three children alive and well.

Social History:

Lives in nursing home with few visitors; husband died two years ago; smoked three packs per day for 30 years.

A. **Type of patient history:** _____

_____

PATIENT: Whitfield, Hunter

PHYSICIAN: Sparks

Chief Complaint:

"Pain in my stomach and just feeling sick"

History of Present Illness:

Patient came to the hospital this morning with a three-day history of intermittent episodes of "crampy" pain in the right upper quadrant; this pain is diffuse without radiation and is related to eating of meals; this morning after the patient's breakfast, the pain worsened and became associated with nausea and vomiting; he is a sickle cell trait heterozygote diagnosed in 1970 after a prolonged ill feeling; he is hypertensive, well controlled on diuretic Furosemide 80 mg twice daily.

History of Past Illness:

Measles without complications, 1959; mumps with unilateral right sided orchitis, 1964; prolonged ill feeling diagnosed as anemia with etiology of sickle cell trait, 1970; hypertension diagnosed on routine physical for work, 1976; right-sided wrist fracture from a racquetball accident, 1985.

Review of Systems:

No history of weight loss; no change of diet or appetite; no changes in sleep patterns; no changes in skin, nails, or hair; no enlarged lymph nodes; no pain in joints; no recent bleeding; no recent dizziness; no changes in bowel or bladder function or habits.

Family Medical History:
Mother and father still living; mother had gallbladder removed three years ago; father has high blood pressure and chronic anemia, and had a stroke in 1983; one older brother and a sister alive and well; children, three boys, alive and well; no family history of diabetes or cardiovascular disease.

Social History:
Patient is a full-time salesman, which involves travel across the country, but not into foreign countries; eats regular meals, low salt and balanced three times per day; exercises regularly four times per week, running five miles in approximately 35–40 minutes; he is a non-smoker, and drinks socially approximately three beers per week.

B. **Type of patient history:** _____

_____

PATIENT: Mullins, Todd

PHYSICIAN: Koenig

Chief Complaint:
Motor Vehicle Accident

History of Present Illness:
Patient was passenger (without seat belt on) in automobile that crossed median and struck another car head on; patient was brought in by ambulance comatose, with neck collar, intubated, and bagged; field vitals pulse 140, blood pressure 80/40.

Past Medical History:
No known allergies; no medications.

Review of Systems:
Non-contributory.

Family Medical History:
Mother has diabetes mellitus.

Social History:
Lives with mother, father, and one sister; freshman in high school.

C. **Type of patient history:** _____

_____

PATIENT: Cooper, Paula

PHYSICIAN: Young

Chief Complaint:
"Pain in my stomach, then vomiting blood"

History of Present Illness:
Patient first noted pain in her stomach three days ago and attributed it to spicy foods, she took antacids and the pain dissipated; this morning before breakfast she felt similar pain more severely so she again took antacids and ate her breakfast; after breakfast she became

nauseous and vomited approximately one cup of bright red blood with food; about one hour later she again vomited approximately one cup of blood; no history of dizziness, shortness of breath, diarrhea, previous hematemesis, or melena.

History of Past Illness:
No major injuries or illnesses; no hospitalizations other than normal vaginal deliveries; gravida 4, para 4; no known allergies.

Medications:
Antacid tablets, p.o. p.r.n. for stomach pain; ASA occasionally for headache.

Review of Systems:
Wears glasses; deviated septum; initial insomnia without daytime sleepiness.

Family Medical History:
Negative for ulcers, coagulopathies, diabetes, or cardiovascular disease; father has colon Ca with polyposis.

Social History:
Homemaker with children 12, 10, 8, and 5 years old; does not smoke; rarely drinks alcohol.

D. **Type of patient history:** _____

_____

17. Read the following physical examination notes and determine the type of patient physical examination performed by the physician. Note the differences in format and content of these similar clinical reports.

PATIENT: Higgins, Thomas

PHYSICIAN: Caldwell

Physical Examination:
Age: 47; *Sex:* male; *Weight:* 138 lbs; *Temp:* 100.2; *Pulse:* 62; *Resp:* 14; *BP:* 138/88.
General: well-developed, well-nourished white male appearing younger than stated age; supine in pain with legs drawn up.
Skin: without erythema or edema; normal male hair distribution.
Eyes: pupils equal, round, responsive to light and accommodation; no hypertensive changes; extraocular movements intact.
Ears: air conduction greater than bone conduction; both tympanic; both membranes clear; normal wax.
Nose: without inflammation, swelling, or blood.
Mouth: upper dentures; no inflammation or masses.
Neck: range of motion is intact; no lymph nodes palpable; thyroid not palpable.
Chest: lungs clear to auscultation and percussion; symmetrical diaphragm movement by percussion.
Heart: regular rate and rhythm; first and second heart sounds present; normal physiological splitting of second heart sound without murmur, gallop, or rub.
Pulses: (Scale 1+ to 4+) carotid++, radial++, ulnar+, brachial++, femoral++, popliteal+, dorsalis pedis++, posterior tibial+, symmetrically; no bruits carotid or femoral.
Abdomen: bowel sounds normoactive; tenderness to deep palpation in right upper quadrant without rebound; no palpable masses; liver 12 cm by percussion with a smooth edge; spleen not felt.

Extremities: range of motion intact; no femoral or axillary lymph nodes noted; without cyanosis, clubbing, or edema.

Genitourinary: normal male uncircumcised; bladder not distended; right testicle smaller than normal.

Rectal: prostate not enlarged; uniform density without local areas of hardness; no masses felt; stool present in anal vault; occult and gross blood not present.

Neurological: awake, alert, oriented to time, person, and place; good muscular strength; cranial nerves II through XII intact; normal sensory perception to pain and vibration; finger-to-nose test and heel-to-shin test intact; superficial long tract reflex responds in a plantar direction.

Diagnosis:
Pain due to cholangitis, probably associated with cholecystitis and cholelithiasis.

A. **Type of patient physical examination:** _____

_____

PATIENT: Koch, Ella

PHYSICIAN: Hauser

Physical Examination:
Age: 70; *Sex:* female; *Weight:* 98 lbs; *Temp:* 96.8; *Pulse:* 96; *Resp:* 8; *BP:* 164/104.

General: frail, elderly lady in no acute distress, laying supine and relaxed.

Skin: pink, warm, without edema; laceration 2 cm right chin, 1 cm from midline.

Eyes: pupils equal and reactive to light and accommodation; extraocular movements intact.

Ears: decreased hearing both sides; air conduction greater than bone conduction both sides; tympanic membranes clear.

Nose: without inflammation; dry mucosa; deviation to left.

Mouth: edentulous with dentures; no inflammation.

Neck: limited range of motion with crepitus; no nodes; thyroid firm.

Chest: bibasalar rales 1+; very resonant to percussion.

Heart: regular rate and rhythm; S-1 clicks (mechanical); S-2 normal; slight systolic flow; murmur II/IV.

Pulses: carotid+, radial+, ulnar−, brachial+, femoral+, popliteal−, dorsalis pedis+, posterior tibial− both sides; no bruits carotid or femoral.

Abdomen: protuberant with normoactive bowel sounds; transmitted heart sounds; liver palpable, 10 cm by percussion; spleen not felt.

Extremities: limited range of motion left with crepitus; right without crepitus but painful; no ulcers.

Genitourinary: normal female; dry mucosa; no masses.

Rectal: no masses; no stool; heme+.

Neurological: awake, but at times distant; oriented × 2; good strength but motion limited on left; cranial nerves II through XII intact; decreased sensory on left; finger-to-nose and heel-to-shin tremorous but grossly intact; speech at times slurred.

Diagnosis:
Transient ischemic attack secondary to emboli formed on mitral valve.

B. **Type of patient physical examination:** _____

_____

PATIENT: Aubuchon, Lynn

PHYSICIAN: Perez

Physical Examination:

Age: 32; *Sex:* female; *Weight:* 124 lbs; *Temp:* 101.2; *Pulse:* 86; *Resp:* 18; *BP:* 132/82.

General: well-developed, well-nourished white female looking tired and older than her stated age.

Skin: pale but warm; normal female hair.

Eyes: pupils equal and reactive to light and accommodation; extraocular movements intact; fundi orange.

Ears: excessive wax occluding both tympanic membranes; air conduction greater than bone conduction both sides.

Nose: without hemorrhage; without inflammation.

Mouth: without inflammation; teeth in good repair.

Neck: range of motion intact; submandibular nodes 2 cm diameter.

Chest: diaphragm symmetrical; right dull to percussion.

Heart: regular rate and rhythm; S-1 and S-2 normal.

Pulses: carotid++, brachial++, radial++, ulnar+, femoral++, popliteal++, dorsalis pedis++, posterior tibial+, symmetrical; no bruits carotid or femoral.

Abdomen: bowel sounds hyperactive; pain sub xiphoid.

Extremities: range of motion intact; warm hands; cold feet.

Rectal: good sphincter tone; occult blood+.

Neurological: awake, alert, oriented × 3; good speech; strength good; gait good; cranial nerves II through XII intact; normal sensory; plantar response.

Diagnoses:

Gastric ulcer, rule out ETOH gastritis; Pneumonia secondary to aspiration.

C. **Type of patient physical examination:** _____

_____

PATIENT: Porter, Larry

PHYSICIAN: Vogel

Physical Examination:

Age: 12; *Sex:* male; *Weight:* 135 lbs; *Temp:* 95.6; *Pulse:* 120; thready; *Resp:* 20; bagged; *BP:* 90/50.

General: well-developed, well-nourished white male adolescent of adult proportion; multiple lacerations on face; displaced right shoulder; right rib fractures with indentation; head covered with blood.

Skin: pale; shrunken with bleeding from multiple sites.

Eyes: right pupil fixed and dilated; left pinpoint pupil; no extraocular movement; positive for corneal reflex both sides.

Ears: blood in external canal.

Nose: displaced to left grossly with blood in vestibule.

Mouth: jaw displaced to left without fracture of mandible.

Throat: endotracheal tube in place.

Neck: cervical collar; no deviation of trachea; no deformity; jugular vein distention.

Chest: lungs clear to auscultation.

Heart: weak beat; S-1 and S-2 muffled.

Abdomen: absent bowel sounds; no masses.

Pulses: carotid+, femoral+, radial−, ulnar−, dorsalid pedis−, posterior tibial−.

Extremities: right humeral head displaced.

Rectal: heme negative; no masses.

Neurological: comatose; not responsive to pain; decorticate posture; Babinski left; plantar response right.

Diagnoses:

Hemorrhage with hypovolemic hypotension; cranial damage, possibly epidural or subdural; pericardiac tamponade.

D. **Type of patient physical examination:** _____

_____

CODING OF CLINICAL DOCUMENTATION

Read the following clinical scenarios and assign precise, accurate code numbers from the Evaluation and Management Services section of the CPT volume.

PATIENT: Gibbs, Terry   **MR#:** 99-12-01

ATTENDING PHYSICIAN: O'Brien

Follow-up office visit was made by a 50-year-old male patient with a diagnosis of cervical spondylosis. The patient has responded well to physical therapy and intermittent cervical traction. He now requests evaluation and a release to return to work.

(problem-focused history and problem-focused examination with straightforward medical decision making and self-limited presenting problem)

Codes: _____

PATIENT: Clay, Gloria   **MR#:** 99-12-02

ATTENDING PHYSICIAN: Larson

Initial assessment and formulation of management plans for a 25-year-old female admitted to a rehabilitation facility. The patient is status post a diving accident with resulting C4-5 quadriplegia.

(comprehensive history and comprehensive examination with medical decision making of moderate complexity and self-limited presenting problem)

Codes: _____

PATIENT: McDonald, Kevin   **MR#:** 99-12-03

ATTENDING PHYSICIAN: Helfrich   **CONSULTANT:** Jamil

Initial emergency room consultation was provided for a 10-year-old male in status epilepticus due to a recent closed head injury. The patient is an out-of-town visitor on a school field trip and information regarding his medical history and medications is not immediately available.

(comprehensive history and comprehensive examination with medical decision making of high complexity and presenting problem of moderate severity)

Codes: _____

PATIENT: Sykes, Charles   **MR#:** 99-12-04

ATTENDING PHYSICIAN: Weinstein

An emergency room assessment was provided for an 85-year-old male with a history of arteriosclerotic cardiovascular disease. The patient is severely dehydrated, disoriented, and is experiencing auditory hallucinations.

(comprehensive history and comprehensive examination with medical decision making of high complexity and presenting problem of high severity)

Codes: _____

PATIENT: Jimenez, Felicia   **MR#:** 99-12-05

ATTENDING PHYSICIAN: Kovarik

An emergency room assessment was provided for an 8-year-old female with reported acciden-tal caustic ingestion. The patient now has fever, dyspnea, and a dropping hemoglobin.

(comprehensive history and comprehensive examination with medical decision making of high complexity and presenting problem of high severity)

Codes: _____

PATIENT: Hoffmann, Albert   **MR#:** 99-12-06

ATTENDING PHYSICIAN: Warner

An initial hospital visit was made for an 89-year-old male nursing facility patient who is trans-ported to the emergency room and then admitted to the intensive care unit. The patient re-portedly had anuria and sepsis for twenty-four hours prior to admission with two syncopal episodes, high fever, increasing confusion, chest pain, and ventricular arrhythmias. The pa-tient has complete heart block and congestive heart failure.

(comprehensive history and comprehensive examination with medical decision making of high complexity and presenting problem of high severity)

Codes: _____

PATIENT: Steinberg, Bruce   **MR#:** 99-12-07

ATTENDING PHYSICIAN: Haas   **CONSULTANT:** Molinaro

An initial hospital orthopedic consultation was rendered in the emergency room for a 35-year-old male multiple trauma patient with complex pelvic fractures sustained in a motorcycle accident. The orthopedic surgeon evaluated the patient and formulated management plans for the fractures. The patient also has a subarachnoid hemorrhage revealed by angiogram.

(comprehensive history and comprehensive examination with medical decision making of high complexity and presenting problem of high severity)

Codes: _____

PATIENT: Flynn, Arnold   **MR#:** 99-12-08

ATTENDING PHYSICIAN: Wells   **CONSULTANT:** Stuttgardt

An initial emergency room consultation was provided for a 23-year-old male patient in acute abdominal pain with guarding. The patient is febrile and has unstable vital signs.

(comprehensive history and comprehensive examination with medical decision making of high complexity and presenting problem of moderate severity)

Codes: _____

PATIENT: Snyder, Glenda   **MR#:** 99-12-09

ATTENDING PHYSICIAN: Morris

An initial office visit was made by a 52-year-old female with complaints of acute weakness of all four extremities and shortness of breath. The patient received an influenza vaccination at a community health clinic one week ago.

(comprehensive history and comprehensive examination with medical decision making of high complexity and presenting problem of moderate severity)

Codes: _____

PATIENT: Murphy, Gilbert   **MR#:** 99-12-10

ATTENDING PHYSICIAN: Schneider

An office visit was made by this 68-year-old male established patient subsequent to outpatient biopsy of the rectum. Treatment options were discussed (for seventy-five minutes) concerning his biopsy-proven adenocarcinoma of the rectum.

(expanded problem-focused history and detailed examination with medical decision making of moderate complexity and presenting problem of low complexity)

Codes: _____

PATIENT: Schaeffer, Hilda   **MR#:** 99-12-11

ATTENDING PHYSICIAN: Walsh   **CONSULTANT:** Buchanan

An initial hospital consultation was rendered by an anesthesiologist regarding pain control for this 82-year-old female with intractable chest wall pain due to metastatic carcinoma of the breast with metastases to the femoral neck and thoracic vertebrae.

(detailed history and detailed examination with medical decision making of moderate complexity and presenting problem of moderate severity)

Codes: _____

PATIENT: Wilcox, Pamela   **MR#:** 99-12-12

ATTENDING PHYSICIAN: Graves

An initial office visit was made by a 49-year-old female patient with a unilateral painful bunion.

(expanded problem-focused history and expanded problem-focused examination with straight-forward medical decision making and self-limited presenting problem)

Codes: _____

PATIENT: Tran, Hong   **MR#:** 99-12-13

ATTENDING PHYSICIAN: Dubois

An initial oral surgery office visit was made by an 18-year-old male who was referred by his orthodontist for advice regarding his impacted maxillary cuspids.

(expanded problem-focused history and expanded problem-focused examination with medical decision making of moderate complexity and self-limited presenting problem)

Codes: _____

PATIENT: Reinhardt, Eric   **MR#:** 99-12-14

ATTENDING PHYSICIAN: Baker   **CONSULTANT:** O'Connell

An office visit and a subsequent initial office consultation were provided for this 8-year-old patient referred by his pediatrician. The child has multiple systemic complaints and a recent onset of behavioral discontrol in elementary school.

(comprehensive history and comprehensive examination with medical decision making of moderate complexity and presenting problem of moderate severity)

Codes: _____

PATIENT: Delmonico, Victor   **MR#:** 99-12-15

ATTENDING PHYSICIAN: Glaser

Outpatient visit was made by this 77-year-old male established patient with hypertension, who presents with complaint of a three-month history of episodic substernal chest pain on exertion.

(detailed history and comprehensive examination with medical decision making of moderate complexity and presenting problem of moderate severity)

Codes: _____

PATIENT: Meyer, Kenneth   **MR#:** 99-12-16

ATTENDING PHYSICIAN: Theil

A follow-up office visit was made by a 27-year-old male established patient treated previously for deep follicular and perifollicular inflammation. The patient is unable to tolerate the systemic antibiotics previously prescribed due to gastrointestinal side effects and requires change of medications.

(detailed history and detailed examination with medical decision making of moderate complexity and presenting problem of low severity)

Codes: _____

PATIENT: Elkins, Rhonda   **MR#:** 99-12-17

ATTENDING PHYSICIAN: Magruder

A follow-up office visit was made by a 42-year-old female patient with resolving cellulitis of the foot.

(expanded problem-focused history and expanded problem-focused examination with straight-forward medical decision making and minimal presenting problem)

Codes: _____

PATIENT: Arnovitz, Theodore   **MR#:** 99-12-18

ATTENDING PHYSICIAN: Lorentz

An extended routine follow-up office visit was made by this 60-year-old renal dialysis patient who has an access infection as well as oral ulcerations (aphthous stomatitis). The patient is taking antibiotics and is afebrile. The patient received his regularly scheduled administration of erythropoietin.

(detailed history and detailed examination with medical decision making of moderate complexity and presenting problem of moderate severity)

Codes: _____

PATIENT: Bradshaw, Marvin   **MR#:** 99-12-19

ATTENDING PHYSICIAN: Walker

A postoperative office visit was made by this 66-year-old male patient who now has a low-grade fever eight days status post a myocutaneous flap to close a pharyngeal fistula. The patient also received dressing changes.

(expanded problem-focused history and detailed examination with medical decision making of moderate complexity and presenting problem of low severity)

Codes: _____

PATIENT: Eisele, Randy   **MR#:** 99-12-20

ATTENDING PHYSICIAN: Kaiser

Regular office visit was made by this 3-year-old established pediatric patient who has atopic dermatitis and food hypersensitivity. A routinely scheduled quarterly follow-up evaluation was performed. The patient is on topical lotions and steroid creams as well as oral antihistamines.

(expanded problem-focused history and detailed examination with medical decision making of moderate complexity and presenting problem of low severity)

Codes: _____

PATIENT: Lewis, Dorothy

MR#: 99-12-21

ATTENDING PHYSICIAN: Upton

CONSULTANT: Partridge

An initial inpatient consultation was provided for this 78-year-old female who was admitted to the intensive care unit in acute respiratory distress. The patient is hypertensive, has moderate metabolic acidosis, and has a rising serum creatinine.

(comprehensive history and comprehensive examination with medical decision making of moderate complexity and presenting problem of high severity)

Codes: _____

PATIENT: Driscoll, Neal

MR#: 99-12-22

ATTENDING PHYSICIAN: Ryan

CONSULTANT: Bellamy

An office visit for this 68-year-old established patient with myopia resulted in a referral for an initial office consultation. The patient is a diabetic and has a one-week history of multiple flashes and floaters and partial retinal detachment with progressive visual field loss, advanced optic disc cupping, and neovascularization of retina.

(expanded problem-focused history and expanded problem-focused examination with medical decision making of moderate complexity and presenting problem of moderate severity)

Codes: _____

PATIENT: Hollis, Craig

MR#: 99-12-23

ATTENDING PHYSICIAN: Lang

CONSULTANT: Trumbull

An initial hospital consultation was rendered for this 2-day-old male infant with single ventricle physiology and subaortic obstruction. Ninety minutes of counseling with family of the patient followed patient evaluation for multiple, staged surgical procedures.

(comprehensive history and comprehension examination with medical decision making of high complexity and presenting problem of high severity)

Codes: _____

PATIENT: Schultz, Harry

MR#: 99-12-24

ATTENDING PHYSICIAN: Marshall

CONSULTANT: Bialchak

A follow-up hospital consultation was rendered for a complete review and discussion of previously unavailable radiologic studies. The patient is a 26-year-old male who sustained severe facial fractures in an assault.

(expanded problem-focused history and expanded problem-focused examination with medical decision making of moderate complexity and presenting problem of moderate severity)

Codes: _____

PATIENT: Wagner, Daniel   **MR#:** 99-12-25

ATTENDING PHYSICIAN: Lammert

An initial hospital assessment in the emergency room was made for a 42-year-old male prior to admission for observation following a fall from a scaffold. Radiographs revealed a fracture of the mandible. The patient also has a contusion and an abrasion of the left lower leg.

(expanded problem-focused history and expanded problem-focused examination with medical decision making of low complexity and presenting problem of low severity)

Codes: _____

PATIENT: Caruso, Angela   **MR#:** 99-12-26

ATTENDING PHYSICIAN: Evers   **CONSULTANT:** Gaston

An initial office consultation was provided to this 66-year-old female secretary with complaints of wrist and hand pain as well as numbness of the finger tips. The patient was diagnosed with suspected median nerve compression by carpal tunnel syndrome.

(expanded problem-focused history and expanded problem-focused examination with medical decision making of low complexity and presenting problem of low severity)

Codes: _____

PATIENT: Hayden, David   **MR#:** 99-12-27

ATTENDING PHYSICIAN: Kawasaki

Urgent unscheduled office visit was made by this 36-year-old established patient who is three months status post renal transplant. The patient now complains of new onset peripheral edema, increased blood pressure, and progressive fatigue.

(comprehensive history and comprehensive examination with medical decision making of moderate complexity and presenting problem of low severity)

Codes: _____

PATIENT: Butler, Joyce   **MR#:** 99-12-28

ATTENDING PHYSICIAN: Riordan

Emergency room visit was made by a 28-year-old female with right lower quadrant abdominal pain, fever, and anorexia.

(detailed history and detailed examination with medical decision making of moderate complexity and presenting problem of moderate severity)

Codes: _____

PATIENT: Gates, Monica   **MR#:** 99-12-29

ATTENDING PHYSICIAN: Berman   **CONSULTANT:** Rao

Initial psychiatric office consultation was rendered for a 45-year-old female upon the referral of her internist. The patient complains of a three-month history of headaches, insomnia, and anxiety.

(detailed history and detailed examination with medical decision making of moderate complexity and presenting problem of moderate severity)

Codes: _____

PATIENT: Ladd, Barry   **MR#:** 99-12-30

ATTENDING PHYSICIAN: Wade

Initial hospital emergency room visit made for a healthy 12-year-old patient with a laceration of the upper eyelid involving the lid margin and superior canaliculus. Subsequent to evaluation, a decision was made to admit the patient for plastic repair surgery and to begin IV antibiotic therapy.

(detailed history and expanded problem-focused examination with medical decision making of low complexity and presenting problem of low severity)

Codes: _____

PATIENT: Mitchell, Roy   **MR#:** 99-12-31

ATTENDING PHYSICIAN: Beiser

Initial and subsequent hospital visits were made for this 61-year-old male admitted to the intensive care unit through the emergency room with acute chest pain and diagnostic electrocardiograph changes indicative of an acute anterior myocardial infarction. The patient also experienced frequent premature ventricular contractions. On the second day after admission, the patient complained of shortness of breath and new chest pain and was noted to have recurrent and sustained ventricular tachycardia, which was subsequently converted on medical therapy.

(comprehensive history and comprehensive examination with medical decision making of moderate complexity and presenting problem of high severity)

Codes: _____

PATIENT: Turner, Cynthia   **MR#:** 99-12-32

ATTENDING PHYSICIAN: McCarthy   **CONSULTANT:** Buckley

An office visit was made by this 28-year-old female, established patient, following recent arthrogram and magnetic resonance imaging performed as an outpatient to evaluate temporomandibular joint pain. She was referred to a specialist and had an initial office consultation due to the progressive symptomatology of the chronic arthralgia of the temporomandibular joint with painful swelling.

(expanded problem-focused history and expanded problem-focused examination with medical decision making of moderate complexity and presenting problem of low severity)

Codes: _____

PATIENT: Carey, Phyllis   **MR#:** 99-12-33

ATTENDING PHYSICIAN: Hubbard   **CONSULTANT:** Kumar

An initial inpatient consultation was rendered for this 64-year-old female, status post aortic aneurysm resection with nonresponsive coagulopathy, and a rather massive evolving lower gastrointestinal bleeding. The next day a follow-up inpatient consultation was rendered for this patient with lower gastrointestinal hemorrhage that has stabilized.

(detailed history and detailed examination with medical decision making of high complexity and presenting problem of high severity)

Codes: _____

PATIENT: Gavin, Brett   **MR#:** 99-12-34

ATTENDING PHYSICIAN: Landgraf

An emergency office visit was made by this 15-year-old male established patient with acute status asthmaticus unresponsive to recent outpatient therapy. The patient was taken to the hospital and admitted. Initial and subsequent hospital visits were made and the patient was stabilized on medication.

(expanded problem-focused history and expanded problem-focused examination with medical decision making of high complexity and presenting problem of moderate severity)

Codes: _____

PATIENT: Valencia, Fernando   **MR#:** 99-12-35

ATTENDING PHYSICIAN: Legrand

An initial office visit was made by a 63-year-old laborer with bilateral degenerative joint disease of the knees. The patient had no prior treatment for this condition.

(expanded problem-focused history and expanded problem-focused examination with medical decision making of low complexity and presenting problem of low severity)

Codes: _____

PATIENT: Fairbanks, Audrey   **MR#:** 99-12-36

ATTENDING PHYSICIAN: Doyle

A postoperative follow-up office visit was made by a 73-year-old female patient for the partial removal of antibiotic gauze from the operative wound site.

(problem-focused history and problem-focused examination with straightforward medical decision making and minimal presenting problem)

Codes: _____

PATIENT: Blake, Eileen   **MR#:** 99-12-37

ATTENDING PHYSICIAN: Hyatt

An initial office visit to a urologist was made by this 52-year-old female after an outpatient radiograph revealed a large obstructing stone midway in the left ureter. Management options were discussed with the patient during the office visit. These options included urethroscopy with stone extraction and electroshock wave lithotripsy. Before reaching a decision regarding surgery, the patient spontaneously passed the left ureteral calculus and was seen again in the office for a follow-up visit.

(detailed history and detailed examination with medical decision making of low complexity and presenting problem of low severity)

Codes: _____

PATIENT: Givens, Myra   **MR#:** 99-12-38

ATTENDING PHYSICIAN: Barker   **CONSULTANT:** Brenner

This 70-year-old established patient was previously maintained on low-dose corticosteroids for rheumatoid arthritis. During her regularly scheduled quarterly office visit a decision was made to proceed with joint replacement surgery as a result of incapacitating knee pain. She was admitted to the hospital and underwent the surgery without complications. Initial and subsequent hospital visits were made by the surgeon. On the third postoperative day, she experienced nocturnal confusion and visual hallucinations, and an initial inpatient psychiatric consultation was obtained.

(detailed history and detailed examination with medical decision making of moderate complexity and presenting problem of moderate severity)

Codes: _____

PATIENT: Boyer, Melissa   **MR#:** 99-12-39

ATTENDING PHYSICIAN: Stukowski

An initial office visit was made by this 9-year-old patient with an erythematous, grouped, vesicular eruption of the lip of three days duration. One week later another office visit was made by this patient requesting a release to return to school.

(expanded problem-focused history and expanded problem-focused examination with straightforward medical decision making and self-limited presenting problem)

Codes: _____

PATIENT: Hess, Barney   **MR#:** 99-12-40

ATTENDING PHYSICIAN: Duffy

Office visit was made by this 65-year-old male established patient seeking reassurance about an isolated seborrheic keratosis on his upper back. The patient is eight months status post excision of basal cell carcinoma of the nose with a nasolabial flap.

(expanded problem-focused history and expanded problem-focused examination with medical decision making of low complexity and presenting problem of low severity)

Codes: _____

PATIENT: Dickinson, Maynard   **MR#:** 99-12-41

ATTENDING PHYSICIAN: Hahn   **CONSULTANT:** Becker

Initial and subsequent hospital visits were made for this previously healthy 24-year-old male construction worker with a sudden onset of acute low back pain following a lifting injury. An initial hospital consultation was obtained for this patient who has developed progressive back and pelvic pain as well as bilateral progressive calf and thigh tightness and is unable to walk.

(comprehensive history and comprehensive examination with medical decision making of high complexity and presenting problem of moderate severity)

Codes: _____

PATIENT: Portell, Lance   **MR#:** 99-12-42

ATTENDING PHYSICIAN: Grant

Initial and follow-up hospital visits were made for this 32-year-old patient admitted through the emergency room for a corneoscleral laceration sustained in an industrial accident. The patient experienced a slight loss of vision.

(expanded problem-focused history and expanded problem-focused examination with medical decision making of low complexity and presenting problem of moderate severity)

Codes: _____

PATIENT: Bollinger, Zachary   **MR#:** 99-12-43

ATTENDING PHYSICIAN: Mikawa   **CONSULTANT:** Bauer

This 18-year-old male patient was transported to the emergency room after a motor vehicle accident. The patient suffered a fractured tibia and fibula as well as lacerations of the forehead and nose, which were sutured in the emergency room. He was apparently driving following a substantial drug overdose. Initial and subsequent hospital visits were made and suture removal was performed on the fourth subsequent visit. On the fifth day of hospitalization, the patient pulled out IVs and disconnected traction in a failed attempt to elope from the hospital. An initial inpatient psychiatric consultation revealed a sullen and subdued adolescent with six-month history of declining school performance, increasing self-endangerment, and resistance to parental expectations. The patient continues to insist on signing out against medical advice.

(comprehensive history and comprehensive examination with medical decision making of high complexity and presenting problem of high severity)

Codes: _____

PATIENT: Osterholt, Virgil   **MR#:** 99-12-44

ATTENDING PHYSICIAN: Crowder

Office visit was made by this 62-year-old male, established patient, nine months post-op emergency vena cava shunt for variceal bleeding, now with complaints of two episodes of dark bowel movements, an increase in stooling frequency, and tightness in his abdomen.

(comprehensive history and comprehensive examination with medical decision making of high complexity and presenting problem of moderate severity)

Codes: _____

PATIENT: Dalton, Ambrose   **MR#:** 99-12-45

ATTENDING PHYSICIAN: Hartmann

Office visit for a 50-year-old male salesman from out-of-town who requests prescription refills for a non-steriodal anti-inflammatory drug for bursitis and an anal skin preparation for hemorrhoids.

(problem-focused history and problem-focused examination with straightforward medical decision making and minimal presenting problem)

Codes: _____

PATIENT: Wentworth, Coleman   **MR#:** 99-12-46

ATTENDING PHYSICIAN: Hamilton

Subsequent nursing facility visit was made for this 50-year-old male quadriplegic patient with acute autonomic hyperreflexia, and pain and spasm below the lesion.

(detailed history and detailed examination with medical decision making of high complexity and presenting problem of low severity)

Codes: _____

PATIENT: Buford, Penelope   **MR#:** 99-12-47

ATTENDING PHYSICIAN: Dillon

Initial office visit was made by this 10-year-old girl for determination of visual acuity but not for determination of refractive error. The vision examination was rendered to fulfill part of a qualifying requirement for participation in a summer camp.

(problem-focused history and problem-focused examination with straightforward medical decision making and minimal presenting problem).

Codes: _____

PATIENT: Schilling, Gladys   **MR#:** 99-12-48

ATTENDING PHYSICIAN: Bartz

Routine office visit was made by this 65-year-old female established patient with primary glaucoma. An interval determination of intraocular pressure was performed and medication dosage was adjusted.

(expanded problem-focused history and expanded problem-focused examination with medical decision making of low complexity and self-limited presenting problem)

Codes: _____

PATIENT: Daly, Maurice   **MR#:** 99-12-49

ATTENDING PHYSICIAN: Gaines

Office visit was made by this 65-year-old male, established patient, with benign prostatic hyperplasia and severe bladder outlet obstruction. Surgical management options such as transurethral resection of prostate were discussed. The patient also received a routine blood pressure check for benign hypertension controlled by medication.

(expanded problem-focused history and expanded problem-focused examination with medical decision making of low complexity and presenting problem of low severity)

Codes: _____

PATIENT: Jorgensen, Bradley   **MR#:** 99-12-50

ATTENDING PHYSICIAN: Casey   **CONSULTANT:** Flannigan

Initial office visit for a 3-month-old infant with bilateral hip dislocations and bilateral club feet. The patient was admitted to the hospital and received initial and subsequent hospital visits. Traction was instituted for the congenital (developmental) dislocation of the hips after an initial hospital consultation requested by the pediatrician.

(detailed history and detailed examination with medical decision making of moderate complexity and presenting problem of low severity)

Codes: _____

PATIENT: Soras, Burton   **MR#:** 99-12-51

ATTENDING PHYSICIAN: Palestrino

Initial office visit for this 30-year-old male involved an evaluation of rhinophyma and an evaluation of a progressive saddle nose deformity of unknown etiology. Treatment options for both problems were discussed.

(expanded problem-focused history and expanded problem-focused examination with medical decision making of moderate complexity and presenting problem of low severity)

Codes: _____

PATIENT: Mainridge, Courtney   **MR#:** 99-12-52

ATTENDING PHYSICIAN: Zentgraf

An initial office visit was made by this 15-year-old patient with a four-year history of moderate comedopapular acne of the face, chest, and back with early scarring and unresponsive to over-the-counter medications. A topical desquamating agent was prescribed.

(expanded problem-focused history and expanded problem-focused examination with straightforward medical decision making and self-limited presenting problem)

Codes: _____

PATIENT: Bridges, Loraine   **MR#:** 99-12-53

ATTENDING PHYSICIAN: Gannon

Regularly scheduled monthly office visit for this 82-year-old female, established patient with a long-standing documented Vitamin B12 deficiency. She receives a Vitamin B12 injection and a routine blood pressure check by the registered nurse.

(problem-focused history and problem-focused examination with straightforward medical decision making and self-limited presenting problem)

Codes: _____

PATIENT: Vandergriff, Beverly   **MR#:** 99-12-54

ATTENDING PHYSICIAN: DiLorenzo

An initial office visit was made by this 50-year-old female new patient with symptoms of rash, swellings, diarrhea, lymphadenopathy, and arthritic complaints. The patient experienced a twenty-pound weight loss during the last month. She is an anthropologist who has just returned from field study in the Amazon.

(comprehensive history and comprehensive examination with medical decision making of high complexity and presenting problem of high severity)

Codes: _____

PATIENT: Jalinski, Bart   **MR#:** 99-12-55

ATTENDING PHYSICIAN: Swain

Office visit was made by this 10-year-old male established pediatric patient who was swimming in a lake and now presents with a one-day history of left ear pain with purulent drainage.

(expanded problem-focused history and expanded problem-focused examination with medical decision making of low complexity and self-limited presenting problem)

Codes: _____

PATIENT: Salmon, Libby   **MR#:** 99-12-56

ATTENDING PHYSICIAN: Moler   **CONSULTANT:** Campbell

Follow-up consultation was provided for this 78-year-old female nursing home resident for the evaluation of the medical management of pruritus ani by the attending physician.

(expanded problem-focused history and expanded problem-focused examination with medical decision making of low complexity and presenting problem of low severity)

Codes: _____

PATIENT: Conway-Greer, Elaine   **MR#:** 99-12-57

ATTENDING PHYSICIAN: Ashley

Initial and subsequent hospital visits were made for this 35-year-old female with history of poly-substance abuse and a history of schizophrenia. The patient appeared to be psychotic with markedly elevated vital signs. An initial hospital consultation was obtained due to nephrolithiasis that required extensive opioid analgesics, resulting in elevated vital signs. She initially denied any drug use, but later gave a recent history of multiple substance abuse, including opioids. A week after discharge, this established patient made her regular bimonthly office visit complaining of auditory hallucinations. Medications were adjusted with a new prescription, provided along with brief supportive psychotherapy.

(detailed history and expanded problem-focused examination with medical decision making of moderate complexity and presenting problem of moderate severity)

Codes: _____

PATIENT: Grabowski, Sandor   **MR#:** 99-12-58

ATTENDING PHYSICIAN: Brewer

Initial office visit was made by a 24-year-old male soccer player with complaint of painful, unilateral anterior knee pain following an injury during a game.

(expanded problem-focused history and expanded problem-focused examination with medical decision making of low complexity and presenting problem of low severity)

Codes: _____

PATIENT: Donovan, Loretta   **MR#:** 99-12-59

ATTENDING PHYSICIAN: Randolph

Initial plastic and reconstructive surgery office visit was made by a 25-year-old female who is two years status post burn injuries with hypertrophic facial burn scars, near absence of left breast, and burn syndactyly of both hands. Treatment options were discussed for eighty-five minutes.

(comprehensive history and comprehensive examination with medical decision making of high complexity and presenting problem of moderate severity)

Codes: _____

PATIENT: Barlow, Lester   **MR#:** 99-12-60

ATTENDING PHYSICIAN: Sanfillipo

Initial emergency room assessment was provided for this unfortunate 2-year-old male victim of child abuse. The patient has central nervous system depression, skull fracture, and retinal hemorrhage.

(comprehensive history and comprehensive examination with medical decision making of high complexity and presenting problem of high severity)

Codes: _____

PATIENT: Benecke, Vivian   **MR#:** 99-12-61

ATTENDING PHYSICIAN: Hoover   **CONSULTANT:** Rasmussen

An initial office consultation with a urologist was rendered for this highly functional 75-year-old female with urinary incontinence. Preliminary results of an outpatient diagnostic evaluation were reviewed.

(detailed history and detailed examination with medical decision making of moderate complexity and presenting problem of low severity)

Codes: _____

PATIENT: Heaton, Eunice   **MR#:** 99-12-62

ATTENDING PHYSICIAN: Brinkmann

Follow-up office visit was provided for a 60-year-old female with a three-year history of intermittent ticlike unilateral facial pain. The patient had constant pain for the past two weeks without relief by adequate Carbamazepine dosage.

(expanded problem-focused history and expanded problem-focused examination with medical decision making of moderate complexity and presenting problem of low severity)

Codes: _____

PATIENT: Cunningham, Lois   **MR#:** 99-12-63

ATTENDING PHYSICIAN: Schroeder

Initial office visit was made by a 37-year-old female with primary infertility. The patient received evaluation and counseling.

(comprehensive history and comprehensive examination with medical decision making of moderate complexity and self-limited presenting problem)

Codes: _____

PATIENT: Fernandez, Pedro   **MR#:** 99-12-64

ATTENDING PHYSICIAN: Manuel

Outpatient visit at an ambulatory clinic was made by a 16-year-old new patient with complaints of sore throat, fever, and headache.

(detailed history and detailed examination with medical decision making of low complexity and presenting problem of low severity)

Codes: _____

PATIENT: Dolan-Miles, Heather   **MR#:** 99-12-65

ATTENDING PHYSICIAN: Raines

Initial and subsequent hospital observation unit visits were made for this 31-year-old primigravida of 16 weeks gestation with severe hyperemesis gravidarum. The patient responded well to intravenous fluids.

(expanded problem-focused history and expanded problem-focused examination with medical decision making of low complexity and presenting problem of moderate severity)

Codes: _____

PATIENT: Montgomery, Nicholas   **MR#:** 99-12-66

ATTENDING PHYSICIAN: Klein

Emergency room assessment was provided for a 44-year-old male patient with electrical burns to the left arm.

(expanded problem-focused history and expanded problem-focused examination with straightforward medical decision making and presenting problem of low severity)

Codes: _____

PATIENT: Burns, Serina   **MR#:** 99-12-67

ATTENDING PHYSICIAN: Gallagher

Initial office visit was made by an 18-year-old female with a two-day history of acute conjunctivitis of unknown etiology.

(expanded problem-focused history and expanded problem-focused examination with medical decision making of moderate complexity and presenting problem of low severity)

Codes: _____

PATIENT: Harrell-Fields, Jill   **MR#:** 99-12-68

ATTENDING PHYSICIAN: Cullen   **CONSULTANT:** Aschmann

Subsequent hospital anesthesia consultation was rendered for a 27-year-old female two days after open reduction and internal fixation for a fracture of the lateral malleolus. The patient has a fractured upper incisor post-intubation.

(problem-focused history and problem-focused examination with straightforward medical decision making and self-limited presenting problem)

Codes: _____

PATIENT: Kaufman, Fritz   **MR#:** 99-12-69

ATTENDING PHYSICIAN: Branson   **CONSULTANT:** Pirogi

Subsequent inpatient postoperative anesthesia visit for a 56-year-old male patient, status post gastrectomy, to plan maintenance of analgesia using an intravenous Dilaudid infusion.

(expanded problem-focused history and expanded problem-focused examination with medical decision making of moderate complexity and self-limited presenting problem)

Codes: _____

PATIENT: Carlisle, Sylvia   **MR#:** 99-12-70

ATTENDING PHYSICIAN: Lockhart   **CONSULTANT:** Guerra

Upon the referral of her private physician, an initial psychiatric office consultation was provided for a 38-year-old female patient who reports progressive panic attacks and agoraphobia.

(detailed history and detailed examination with medical decision making of high complexity and presenting problem of moderate severity)

Codes: _____

PATIENT: Kincaid, Cecilia   **MR#:** 99-12-71

ATTENDING PHYSICIAN: Faulkner

A postoperative office visit was made by this 81-year-old patient with a red, painful eye due to endophthalmitis. The patient is four days status post uncomplicated cataract surgery.

(expanded problem-focused history and expanded problem-focused examination with medical decision making of moderate complexity and presenting problem of low severity)

Codes: _____

PATIENT: Archer, Vera   **MR#:** 99-12-72

ATTENDING PHYSICIAN: Haeffner

Initial emergency room assessment was rendered for this 85-year-old female with an acute onset of a thrombotic cerebrovascular accident with contralateral paralysis and aphasia.

(comprehensive history and comprehensive examination with medical decision making of high complexity and presenting problem of high severity)

Codes: _____

PATIENT: Hurst, Reba   **MR#:** 99-12-73

ATTENDING PHYSICIAN: Bischoff

A fifth subsequent hospital visit was provided for a 57-year-old female patient who remains on antibiotics for bacterial endocarditis and who continues to be slightly febrile but otherwise stable.

(expanded problem-focused history and expanded problem-focused examination with medical decision making of moderate complexity and presenting problem of moderate severity)

Codes: _____

PATIENT: Brooks, Inez   **MR#:** 99-12-74

ATTENDING PHYSICIAN: Ferguson

An initial emergency room assessment was provided for a 13-month-old child with a thirty-six hour history of spasmodic cough, respiratory distress, and fever. The patient was transported to the emergency room after a sudden onset of lethargy, photophobia, and nuchal rigidity.

(comprehensive history and comprehensive examination with medical decision making of high complexity and presenting problem of high severity)

Codes: _____

PATIENT: Harmon, Alicia   **MR#:** 99-12-75

ATTENDING PHYSICIAN: Biedermann

Initial and two subsequent hospital visits were provided for this 4-year-old pediatric patient admitted for treatment of acute viral gastroenteritis and dehydration. The patient originally required intravenous hydration and became afebrile with stable vital signs.

(detailed history and detailed examination with medical decision making of moderate complexity and presenting problem of moderate severity)

Codes: _____

PATIENT: Boston, Wesley   **MR#:** 99-12-76

ATTENDING PHYSICIAN: Nakamura

Outpatient ambulatory clinic visit was made by an 18-year-old male who was diagnosed with suppurative sialoadenitis, infectious mononucleosis, and dehydration.

(detailed history and detailed examination with medical decision making of moderate complexity and presenting problem of low severity)

Codes: _____

PATIENT: Sherman, Helen   **MR#:** 99-12-77

ATTENDING PHYSICIAN: Ward

Initial office visit was made by a 51-year-old female who is new to the area. The patient complains of pain in the lateral aspect of the forearm and requests rheumatologic care. The patient is on disability due to progressive systemic sclerosis (scleroderma).

(comprehensive history and comprehensive examination with medical decision making of moderate complexity and presenting problem of low severity)

Codes: _____

PATIENT: Cavanaugh, Spencer   **MR#:** 99-12-78

ATTENDING PHYSICIAN: Bernardi

A visit to a mental health clinic was made by a 58-year-old male with cirrhosis of liver. The patient is a previously abstinent alcoholic with occasional paranoid delusions. He has relapsed and readily accepts and consents to the need for further treatment.

(detailed history and detailed examination with medical decision making of moderate complexity and presenting problem of low severity)

Codes: _____

PATIENT: Moore, Howard   **MR#:** 99-12-79

ATTENDING PHYSICIAN: Patterson

An initial office visit was made by a 72-year-old male who complains of increasing leg pain, progressive limp, and progressive varus of both knees. The patient also has venous stasis ulcers with red streaks adjacent to the ulcers.

(detailed history and detailed examination with medical decision making of moderate complexity and presenting problem of moderate severity)

Codes: _____

PATIENT: Crawford, Frances   **MR#:** 99-12-80

ATTENDING PHYSICIAN: Gilmore

Emergency room visit was made by this 35-year-old female diagnosed one year ago with severe systemic disseminated lupus erythematosus and maintained on corticosteroids. The patient presents with fever, chills, rash, chest pain, and profound thrombocytopenia.

(detailed history and detailed examination with medical decision making of moderate complexity and presenting problem of high severity)

Codes: _____

13

CHAPTER

CPT Coding: Anesthesia and Surgery

LEARNING OBJECTIVES

Upon completion of this chapter the learner should be able to:

1. Define the concept of personally furnished anesthesia services.
2. Define the concept of supervisory anesthesia services.
3. Define the concept of anesthesia time.
4. Discuss the utility of physical status modifiers in the reporting of anesthesia services.
5. Discuss the usefulness of modifiers for supplementing the codes reporting anesthesia services.
6. Apply knowledge of coding principles by assigning accurate and precise codes to report anesthesia services.
7. Explain the consequence of documentation by the surgeon on the reporting on anesthesia services.
8. Define the concept of a professional component of a procedural service.
9. Define the concept of a technical component of a procedural service.
10. Define the concept of a surgical package.
11. Define the concept of a separate procedure.
12. Explain the usefulness of modifiers for supplementing the codes reporting surgical procedures.
13. Interpret and report the message conveyed by the star symbol in the listings of the Surgery section.
14. Apply knowledge of coding principles by assigning accurate and precise codes to report surgical procedures.

CPT CODING OF ANESTHESIA

The procedures requiring the administration of general, regional, or alternate modes of anesthesia services are reported with a selected code number and descriptor from the Anesthesia section of the CPT volume (codes *00100* through *01999*). Topical and local anesthesia infiltration are incorporated within the surgical procedure code number and descriptor listing and thus are not coded and reported separately. Headings within the Anesthesia section of the CPT volume are delineated for: *Head; Neck; Thorax (Chest Wall and Shoulder Girdle); Intrathoracic; Spine and Spinal Cord; Upper Abdomen; Lower Abdomen; Perineum; Pelvis (Except Hip); Upper Leg (Except Knee); Knee and Popliteal Area; Lower Leg (Below Knee); Shoulder and Axilla; Upper Arm and Elbow; Forearm, Wrist, and Hand; Radiological Procedures;* and *Other Procedures.*

The codes reported for anesthesia services frequently are supplemented with an appropriate modifier (modifiers for the codes that report anesthesia services are discussed in another section of this chapter). Code numbers and descriptors for anesthesia procedures are referenced under the main term *Anesthesia* in the index to the CPT volume. Anesthesia supplies and materials should be coded and reported with HCPCS codes and descriptors, if necessary.

Anesthesia services may be personally furnished by a physician anesthesiologist or may be dispensed under the supervision of the physician anesthesiologist by either an anesthesia resident physician or a certified registered nurse anesthetist. Listings in the anesthesia section include any customary intraoperative care and treatment such as the administration of fluids and the standard or routine intraoperative patient monitoring, as well as the usual preoperative and postoperative visits.

An anesthesiologist making a patient visit that is not associated either with an antecedent anesthesia procedure or with a subsequent anesthesia procedure should be coded and reported as a physician consultation with a code number and descriptor from the Evaluation and Management Services section of the CPT volume. Extraordinary or unconventional patient monitoring should be coded and reported with an additional code number and descriptor from the Medicine section of the CPT volume. Any extraordinary or unconventional monitoring in conjunction with anesthesia services should be detailed in a special report that outlines all diagnostic and therapeutic factors and any unusual circumstances that impacted the administration of anesthesia in that particular case.

ANESTHESIA TIME

Anesthesia time commences when the anesthesiologist or anesthetist initiates preparation of the patient for induction of anesthesia in the operating room or in a comparable area. Anesthesia time concludes when the anesthesiologist or anesthetist ceases to be in personal attendance with the patient.

Reporting of anesthesia time impacts reimbursement, which occasionally varies by region or by locality. Anesthesia time should be reported in units of minutes on the claim form submitted by the provider to the third-party payor. For instance, an anesthesia time of two and one-half hours should be reported on the claim form as one hundred and fifty minutes.

ANESTHESIA MODIFIERS

Anesthesia services involving noteworthy circumstances or complex situations should be reported with the procedural code number supplemented by a modifier. Modifier *-47,* anesthesia by surgeon, is not deemed as an appropriate modifier for codes reporting anesthesia procedures. Modifier *-23* reports the administration of general anesthesia during a procedure typically performed under local anesthesia. Commonly appended modifiers of codes for anesthesia services include:

Modifier *-22,* unusual procedural services
Modifier *-23,* unusual anesthesia

Modifier -*32*, mandated services

Modifier -*51*, multiple procedures

Modifier -*53*, discontinued procedure

Modifier -*59*, distinct procedural service

Anesthesia services dispensed amid risk factors or complications are coded and reported in the accepted method, but the codes reporting anesthesia procedures are supplemented with an additional code in its entirety. These corollary code numbers and descriptors in the CPT volume are:

99100 Anesthesia for patient of extreme age, under one year or over seventy.

99116 Anesthesia complicated by utilization of total body hyperthermia.

99135 Anesthesia complicated by utilization of controlled hypotension.

99140 Anesthesia complicated by emergency conditions.

Physical status modifiers categorize the physical status of the patient into six severity levels, which differentiate the complexity and intricacy of anesthesia administration in accord with criteria authorized and established by the American Society of Anesthesiologists (ASA). These six physical status modifiers for anesthesia services are:

1. P1—a healthy, normal patient.
2. P2—a patient with mild systemic disease.
3. P3—a patient with severe systemic disease.
4. P4—a patient with severe systemic disease that is a constant threat to life.
5. P5—a moribund patient who is not expected to survive without the operation.
6. P6—a declared brain-dead patient whose organs are being removed for donor purposes.

Utility and applicability of anesthesia modifiers is contingent upon the standard policies of a particular healthcare facility or physician practice. Utility and applicability of anesthesia modifiers is also relative to the disparate stipulations of various insurance carriers.

ANESTHESIA REPORTING FOR BILLING

If billing Medicare, anesthesiologists report the services rendered with code numbers and descriptors from the Anesthesia section of the CPT volume (example: anesthesia for primary repair of ruptured Achilles tendon with graft, code number *01472*). If billing the majority of other third-party payors, anesthesiologists report the services rendered with code numbers and descriptors from the Surgery section of the CPT volume (example: anesthesia for primary repair of ruptured Achilles tendon with graft, code number *27652*).

Therefore, anesthesia coders frequently must rely on the accuracy, timeliness, and completeness of the operative report prepared by the surgeon in order to facilitate precise code number and descriptor selection for the process of reporting anesthesia services. Inadequate or deficient operative report preparation often hinders expeditious reimbursement for anesthesia services.

CPT CODING OF SURGERY

The section of the CPT volume designated for listings of surgical procedures is the most lengthy and most technical section of the entire CPT volume. The Surgery section consists of seventeen subsections:

1. Integumentary System (codes *10040–19499*)

2. Musculoskeletal System (codes *20000–29909*)

3. Respiratory System (codes *30000–32999*)

4. Cardiovascular System (codes *33010–37799*)

5. Hemic and Lymphatic System (codes *38100–38999*)

6. Mediastinum and Diaphragm (codes *39000–39599*)

7. Digestive System (codes *40490–49999*)

8. Urinary System (codes *50010–53899*)

9. Male Genital System (codes *54000–55899*)

10. Intersex Surgery (codes *55970–55980*)

11. Laparoscopy/Peritoneoscopy (codes *56300–56399*)

12. Female Genital System (codes *56405–58999*)

13. Maternity Care and Delivery (codes *59000–59899*)

14. Endocrine System (codes *60000–60699*)

15. Nervous System (codes *61000–64999*)

16. Eye and Ocular Adnexa (codes *65091–68899*)

17. Auditory System (codes *69000–69979*)

The basic guidelines for the Surgery section define key words and key phrases routinely used in this section and itemize relevant codes for unlisted procedures (for example, the Berev procedure is an unlisted procedure) or unlisted services (for example, a missed appointment is an unlisted service). Innovative surgical procedures as well as surgical procedures involving variable protocols ordinarily necessitate the preparation of a special report that indicates the diagnostic and therapeutic factors affecting the decision to render the procedure in the manner performed.

The subsections within the Surgery section as well as the headings within the subsections typically include inserted notations that direct the process of code selection for procedures listed within that unique division of the section. These guidelines and notations are designed to alleviate disparate or incongruous interpretation of terms and to enable consistent reporting of services rendered by physicians.

Every surgical procedure descriptor listed in the Surgery section implies the inclusion, when essential, of the infiltration of local or topical anesthesia (but not regional or general anesthesia). All surgical procedure descriptors listed in the Surgery section also imply the inclusion of routine, uncomplicated postoperative follow-up care. These included services, collectively with the procedure performed, comprise a "surgical package." If a code number for a postoperative visit is necessary solely for documentation purposes, then code number *99024* should be used for that function.

Medicare carriers acknowledge a somewhat dissimilar concept of surgical package (also termed a global fee package). The Medicare surgical package encompasses preoperative care commencing the day prior to the surgery, and postoperative care ordinarily concluding ninety days after the surgery or concluding either zero days after the surgery or ten days after the surgery for explicitly specified procedures. The Medicare surgical package also encompasses any nonsurgical postoperative care associated with complications of the surgery.

The surgical package concept is principally applicable to therapeutic surgical procedures (tonsillectomy, hysterectomy) and is normally not applicable to diagnostic surgical procedures (arthroscopy, endoscopy) except during recovery from the actual procedure. Follow-up care subsequent to diagnostic surgical procedures should be coded and reported separately.

Furthermore, the surgical package concept is generally not applicable to treatment of complications, late effects, or exacerbations of conditions emanating from the surgical procedure. Such treatment should appropriately be coded and reported separately.

A code number and descriptor for a surgical procedure reported by a hospital implicitly includes the provision of supplies. For instance, the provision of an intraocular lens that is implanted subsequent to intracapsular cataract extraction is inherently included in the reporting of the code number and descriptor for that surgical procedure. Encounters for hospital services provided after discharge but within the standard postoperative period may be coded and reported separately. For example, treatment of complications of surgery rendered in the hospital emergency department as well as any required outpatient services (radiological or laboratory) provided after discharge but during the conventional postoperative period may be billed separately by the hospital.

Comparatively minor surgical procedures entailing variable preoperative or postoperative services are symbolized with a small black star or asterisk printed to the right of the code number. These procedures, sometimes termed "starred procedures," occur only in the Surgery section of each CPT volume and denote that the surgical package concept (that is, the inferred inclusion of stipulated preoperative care and routine postoperative care in the reported procedure code number and descriptor) is not applicable for surgical procedures reported with codes symbolized with a star or asterisk. Starred procedures do not affect the coding and reporting of surgical procedures billed by the hospital.

The starred procedures have an indefinite protocol for preoperative and postoperative services and enable flexibility for separate reporting of preoperative and postoperative care. Examples of code numbers for starred procedures are *43760** and *62270**. If two procedures (one starred and one not starred) are performed concurrently, the surgical package concept is applicable, and the preoperative and postoperative care should not be coded and reported separately. Code number *99025* may be reported in addition to the code number for a starred procedure, if a starred procedure constitutes the primary reason for the encounter of a new patient.

A surgical procedure that is regularly performed as an integral component of a total service does not warrant separate coding or reporting (examples: code number and descriptor *44312, Revision of ileostomy, simple;* or code number and descriptor *69210, Removal impacted cerumen, one or both ears*). However, if the surgical procedure is rendered with a definite rationale, independent of and not associated with a total service, separate coding and reporting is warranted (examples: code number and descriptor *31505 Laryngoscopy, indirect; diagnostic;* or code number and descriptor *50900 Ureterorrhaphy, suture of ureter*).

SURGERY MODIFIERS

Surgical procedures that involve variable or complex protocols or that involve unique circumstances should be reported with a modifier supplementing the CPT code for the surgical procedure. The guidelines for the Surgery section of the CPT volume cite the following modifiers frequently used in reporting surgical services:

Modifier *-20,* microsurgery

Modifier *-22,* unusual procedural services

Modifier *-26,* professional component

Modifier *-32,* mandated services

Modifier *-47,* anesthesia by surgeon

Modifier *-50,* bilateral procedure

Modifier -51, multiple procedures

Modifier -52, reduced services

Modifier -53, discontinued procedure

Modifier -54, surgical care only

Modifier -55, postoperative management only

Modifier -56, preoperative management only

Modifier -57, decision for surgery

Modifier -58, staged or related procedure or service by the same physician during the postoperative period

Modifier -59, distinct procedural service

Modifier -62, two surgeons

Modifier -66, surgical team

Modifier -76, repeat procedure by same physician

Modifier -77, repeat procedure by another physician

Modifier -78, return to the operating room for a related procedure during the postoperative period

Modifier -79, unrelated procedure or service by the same physician during the postoperative period

Modifier -80, assistant surgeon

Modifier -81, minimum assistant surgeon

Modifier -82, assistant surgeon, when qualified resident surgeon not available

Modifier -90, reference (outside) laboratory

Modifier -99, multiple modifiers

Microsurgery requires the application of an operating microscope and not simply the utilization of a magnifying surgical loupe on a headband or attached to the eyeglasses. The code number for the microsurgical procedure should be augmented with the microsurgery modifier, modifier -20, unless the descriptor listed for a procedure stipulates microsurgical technique. Otherwise, usage of the microsurgery modifier is redundant and inappropriate. For example, code 31576-20 represented by descriptor *Laryngoscopy, flexible fiberoptic, diagnostic with biopsy* should be supplemented with modifier -20 to indicate that the procedure was performed with an operating microscope. However, code 31531 represented by descriptor *Laryngoscopy, direct, operative, with foreign body removal; with operating microscope* should not be supplemented with modifier -20 because the descriptor denotes that the procedure was performed with an operating microscope.

Numerous surgical procedures combine or consolidate both a physician component and a technical component (examples: code number and descriptor *32405 Biopsy, lung or mediastinum, percutaneous needle;* or code number and descriptor *47530 Revision and/or reinsertion of transhepatic tube*). Modifier -26 indicates the separate reporting of the physician component (termed the "professional component") of the procedure (examples: code number 32405-26; or code number 47530-26). Hospitals must report the code for the technical component of the procedure or service.

In operative cases in which the surgeon dispenses general or regional anesthesia, the unmodified code number for the operative procedure (examples: code number 32405; or code number 47530) should be coexistently reported with and followed by that identical code number for the operative procedure supplemented with modifier -47 (examples: code number

32405-47; or code number *47530-47).* In addition, the code number for the operative procedure should be repeatedly reported and supplemented with any other applicable modifier as necessary (examples: code number *32405-26;* or code number *47530-26).* Modifier *-47* appended to the repeated code simply indicates that general or regional anesthesia administration was dispensed by the attending surgeon.

A bilateral surgical procedure performed within the same operative session should be coexistently reported with the unmodified code number for the counterpart unilateral procedure reported with and followed by that identical code number for the operative procedure supplemented with modifier *-50.* In addition, the code number for the operative procedure should be repeatedly reported and supplemented with any other applicable modifier as necessary. Modifier *-50* appended to the repeated code simply indicates that the reported operative procedure was performed bilaterally and not solely unilaterally (examples: code number *27052* reported with code number *27052-50* represented by descriptor *Arthrotomy, with biopsy, hip joint, bilateral;* or code number *50974* reported with code number *50974-50* represented by descriptor *Ureteral endoscopy through ureterotomy, . . . with biopsy, bilateral).*

Hospital coders must not augment CPT codes with modifiers, but instead should account for bilateral procedures by repeating the code number for the counterpart unilateral procedure. As examples, *27052* and *27052* denote the code numbers for reporting *Arthrotomy, with biopsy, hip joint, bilateral* as a hospital outpatient procedure; whereas *50974* and *50974* denote the code numbers for reporting *Ureteral endoscopy through ureterotomy, . . . with biopsy, bilateral* as a hospital outpatient procedure.

For both clinical and economic rationalizations, more than one surgical procedure may be performed on a patient during the same operative session. Multiple surgical procedures performed on a patient during the same operative session (or in separate operative sessions on the same date) should be reported with the major (primary or principal) procedure or service itemized first, followed by the minor (secondary or additional) procedures or services itemized next.

Each of the code numbers for the secondary or additional procedures or services are augmented with modifier *-51* (example: code number *15824* represented by descriptor *Rhytidectomy, forehead,* reported both with code number *15820-51* represented by descriptor *Blepharoplasty, lower eyelid,* and code number *15822-51* represented by descriptor *Blepharoplasty, upper eyelid).* Usage of modifier *-51* typically signals third-party payors to diminish reimbursement for the secondary or additional procedures or services.

Hospital coders, however, must not augment codes with modifiers, but instead should simply report each applicable code number. In the previous example, code number *15824* represented by descriptor *Rhytidectomy, forehead,* should be reported by the hospital both with code number *15820* represented by descriptor *Blepharoplasty, lower eyelid,* and with code number *15822* represented by descriptor *Blepharoplasty, upper eyelid.*

Modifier *-52* designates reduced or limited services, inferring that a segment of a procedure or service was not performed or rendered (example: code number and descriptor *42145-52 Palatopharyngoplasty* procedure terminated due to intraoperative myocardial infarction). This modifier is not intended to denote a lessened fee (as in care of the indigent).

Occasionally the surgeon performing an operative procedure does not also render preoperative care or postoperative care. A modifier supplementing the code for the operative procedure should be appended to signify any such fragmentation of services.

Modifier *-54* denotes the provision of surgical care exclusively. For example, code number *49587-54* represented by descriptor *Repair umbilical hernia . . . ; incarcerated,* would be appropriate for reporting this procedure if a patient was admitted to an out-of-town acute care facility for surgery, but received preoperative care and postoperative care from a local physician.

Modifier *-55* denotes solely the physician provision of postoperative patient management. For example, code number *49587-55* represented by descriptor *Repair umbilical hernia . . . ; incarcerated,* would be appropriate for reporting this procedure if the surgeon who performed the operation embarked on a vacation the day after the surgery.

Modifier *-56* denotes solely the physician provision of preoperative patient management. For example, code number *49587-56* represented by descriptor *Repair umbilical hernia . . . ; incarcerated,* would be appropriate if a patient received preoperative care from a local physician but was admitted to an out-of-town acute care facility for surgery, and convalesced there at the home of a relative.

Modifier *-57* is an indicator of an evaluation and management service resulting in an initial decision to perform surgery. Modifier *-58* is an indicator of a procedure or service rendered during the postoperative period that was planned prospectively (staged) with the original procedure, or rendered as therapy subsequent to a diagnostic surgical procedure. This modifier should not be used to report the treatment of a complication that necessitated performing a surgical procedure.

The two surgeon modifier, modifier *-62,* should be utilized to indicate that two surgeons, typically with disparate skills, were both primary surgeons performing distinct aspects of a complex operative procedure, or were each a primary surgeon performing diverse surgical procedures during the same operative session. For instance, code number *58240-62* represented by descriptor *Pelvic exenteration for gynecologic malignancy . . . ,* should be reported if this surgery was performed by a gynecologist and a urologist, or if this surgery was performed by a gynecologist and a colorectal surgeon.

Complicated or intricate operative procedures that require a surgical team comprised of several physicians should be signified with modifier *-66* supplementing the code number for the operative procedure (example: code number and descriptor *47135-66 Liver allotransplantation . . .*). Assistant surgeon services should be indicated by modifier *-80* (or by modifier *-82* when a qualified surgical resident is not available), and minimal assistant surgeon services should be indicated by modifier *-81.*

The treatment of a surgical patient may necessitate the performance of associated yet minor surgical procedures during the postoperative period. These procedures or services should be signified with modifier *-78* (example: code number and descriptor *35905-78 Excision of infected graft; thorax*). Surgical procedures or services unrelated to and not associated with other procedures or services but rendered during a postoperative period, should be signified with modifier *-79.* For instance, code number *52204-79* represented by descriptor *Cystourethroscopy with biopsy,* is applicable for reporting this diagnostic surgical procedure performed during the postoperative period following inguinal hernia repair.

Occasionally, two or more distinct modifiers must supplement a solitary code number for a surgical procedure. Thus modifier *-99* functions to signal that multiple modifiers augment this code, and should be the first modifier cited among multiple modifiers. For consistency and uniformity, multiple modifiers of a solitary code number should be reported in descending numerical order.

CPT CODING OF INTEGUMENTARY SYSTEM SURGICAL PROCEDURES

The Integumentary System subsection, the initial subsection of the CPT Surgery section, contains listings of procedures performed on the skin and on the subcutaneous tissue as well as on the accessory structures of this system. This subsection also contains listings of procedures performed on the nails and listings of procedures performed on the breast.

Headings and subheadings within this subsection are delineated by anatomic site (such as nails or breast), by diagnostic condition (such as pressure ulcers or burns), or by procedural modality (such as biopsy or repair). Table 13–1 lists the headings and subheadings within the Integumentary System subsection. The heading *Nails* is followed by a disconnected subheading entitled *Introduction* that encompasses listings of miscellaneous procedures, and thus that subheading is not included in the subsequent table.

Cross-references within the listings of the Integumentary System subsection guide code number and descriptor selection to listings elsewhere in this subsection (example: note the cross-reference for code number and descriptor *11201 Removal of skin tags . . . ; each additional ten lesions*), or to listings in other subsections of the Surgery section (example: note the cross-reference for code number and descriptor *15845 Graft for facial nerve paralysis; regional muscle transfer*), or even to listings in other sections of the CPT volume. To exemplify, radiologic supervision and interpretation of a percutaneous breast procedure should be correctly

TABLE 13–1

Headings and Subheadings in the Integumentary System Subsection

Heading	Subheadings
Skin, Subcutaneous, and Accessory Structures	Incision and Drainage
	Excision—Debridement
	Paring or Curettement
	Biopsy
	Removal of Skin Tags
	Shaving of Epidermal or Dermal Lesions
	Excision—Benign Lesions
	Excision—Malignant Lesions
Repair (Closure)	Repair—Simple
	Repair—Intermediate
	Repair—Complex
	Adjacent Tissue Transfer or Rearrangement
	Free Skin Grafts
	Flaps (Skin and/or Deep Tissues)
	Other Flaps and Grafts
	Other Procedures
	Pressure Ulcers (Decubitus Ulcers)
	Burns, Local Treatment
Destruction	Destruction, Benign or Premalignant Lesions
	Destruction, Malignant Lesions, Any Method
	Mohs' Micrographic Surgery
	Other Procedures
Breast	Incision
	Excision
	Introduction
	Repair and/or Reconstruction
	Other Procedures

reported with a code listed in the Radiology section of the CPT volume (example: note the cross-reference for code number and descriptor *19290 Preoperative placement of needle localization, wire, breast*).

Assorted notes in this subsection for integumentary system procedures encompass definitions of procedural terms such as shaving, excision, and destruction, and encompass explanations regarding the documentation and reporting of procedural techniques such as simple repair, intermediate repair (layer closure), and complex repair (plastic or reconstructive repair). Additional notations in this subsection present special instructions, such as those relating to specific documentation. For instance, these instructions indicate that the percentage of the body surface burned and depth of these burns should be documented in the medical record of the patient treated for burns.

Notations among the listings in the Integumentary System subsection enable a means to standardize the coding and reporting of surgical procedures performed on the skin and subcutaneous tissue. For instance, the diameter of lesions (benign or malignant) and the length of open wounds, regardless of shape (curvilinear, angular, or stellar), should always be measured in centimeters and documented likewise in the patient medical record.

The repair of more than one wound amid the same grouping of wounds (example: the anatomic sites of face, ears, eyelids, nose, and lips are in the same grouping of wounds) should be reported by summing the total or aggregate lengths of all of the wounds in this grouping that are repaired, and jointly reporting these repairs as one procedure (example: selection of a solitary code from the code range *12051–12057* represented by the descriptor *Layer closure of wounds of face, ears, eyelids, nose, lips, and / or mucous membranes*).

The repair of more than one wound from different groupings of wounds (example: repair of a wound from the grouping represented by code number and descriptor *13100 Repair, complex, trunk,* and repair of a wound from the grouping represented by code number and descriptor *13120 Repair, complex, scalp, arms, and / or legs*) should be coded and reported separately with the modifier *-51* attached to the code number for each of the additional repair procedures (example: concurrent reporting of code number *13100* with code number *13120-51*).

Simple ligation of blood vessels in an open wound or simple exploration of blood vessels, nerves, or tendons in an open wound is an ordinary component of the treatment and should not be coded and reported separately. Debridement of skin and subcutaneous tissue should not be coded and reported as a separate procedure unless gross contamination necessitated protracted cleansing, substantial devitalization impeded skin or subcutaneous tissue removal, or debridement was rendered without contiguous primary closure.

An adjacent tissue transfer procedure should be coded and reported only if the tissue rearrangement was intentional and not merely coincidental. Secondary repair of the donor site for a skin graft may be coded and reported as a separate procedure. A body site specified in the descriptor of a skin graft procedure refers to the recipient site in flap attachment procedures, and a body site specified in the descriptor of a skin graft procedure refers to the donor site in tube formation procedures. To exemplify, code number *15572* represented by descriptor *Formation of direct or tubed pedicle, with or without transfer; scalp, arms, or legs,* refers to these sites as the donor area; and code number *15734* represented by descriptor *Muscle, myocutaneous, or fasciocutaneous flap; trunk,* refers to this site as the recipient area.

Destruction of multiple benign or premalignant lesions within the same operative session should be coded and reported through a unit count method. For example, code number and descriptor *17100 Destruction by any method, including laser, of benign skin lesions . . .* represents the unit count of one lesion. Successive code number and descriptor listings within the same subheading represent an increased count of lesions as *17001 second lesion* and *17102 over two lesions, each additional lesion, up to 15 lesions.* For example, if twelve benign skin lesions were destroyed by laser in a single session, code number *17100* should be reported to indicate the destruction of the first lesion, code number *17101* is reported to indicate the destruction of the second lesion, and code number *17102* should be reported ten times to report the destruction of ten additional lesions.

A comparable unit count approach should be used to report the specimens obtained through chemosurgery. For instance, code number and descriptor *17304 Chemosurgery (Mohs' micrographic technique) . . . ; first stage, . . .* reports up to five specimens. If eight specimens were obtained, code number *17304* should be reported twice. Micrographic chemosurgery techniques are grouped in a distinct subheading within the Integumentary System subsection. The codes in this subheading may be reported if an individual physician functioned in two integrated yet diverse capacities, such as surgeon and pathologist. The codes in this subheading should not be reported, however, if two physicians were involved in dispensing this service.

CPT CODING OF MUSCULOSKELETAL SYSTEM SURGICAL PROCEDURES

The Musculoskeletal System subsection, the most elongated subsection of the CPT Surgery section, comprises listings of procedures performed on the bones, the joints, the tendons, and the muscles. Headings within this subsection are organized either with generic subheadings or with definitive subheadings arranged by body site or by procedural modality.

Headings within the Musculoskeletal System subsection are delineated for the body sites of head, neck and thorax, back and flank, spine, shoulder, upper arm and elbow, forearm and wrist, hand and fingers, pelvis and hip, thigh and knee, leg and ankle, and foot, and also are delineated for the services of cast application and arthroscopy. Further division of these headings into subheadings is mainly organized by procedural modality, such as incision, excision, repair, reconstruction, or arthrodesis, or organized by diagnostic indicator such as fracture, dislocation, scoliosis, or kyphosis. Table 13–2 lists the headings and subheadings within the Musculoskeletal System subsection.

TABLE 13–2

Headings and Subheadings in the Musculoskeletal System Subsection

Heading	Subheadings
General	*Incision*
	Excision
	Introduction or Removal
	Replantation
	Grafts (or Implants)
	Other Procedures
Head	*Incision*
	Excision
	Introduction or Removal
	Repair, Revision, and/or Reconstruction
	Other Procedures
	Fracture and/or Dislocation
	Other Procedures
Neck (Soft Tissues) and Thorax	*Incision*
	Excision
	Repair, Revision, and/or Reconstruction

T A B L E 13–2

Headings and Subheadings in the Musculoskeletal System Subsection—cont'd

Heading	Subheadings
Neck (Soft Tissues) and Thorax—cont'd	Fracture and/or Dislocation
	Other Procedures
Back and Flank	Excision
Spine (Vertebral Column)	Excision
	Osteotomy
	Fracture and/or Dislocation
	Manipulation
	Arthrodesis (with sub-subheadings *Anterior or Anterolateral Approach Technique; Posterior, Posterolateral or Lateral Transverse Process Technique; Spine Deformity (Scoliosis, Kyphosis);* and *Other Procedures*)
	Spinal Instrumentation
	Other Procedures
Abdomen	Excision
	Other Procedures
Shoulder	Incision
	Excision
	Introduction or Removal
	Repair, Revision, and/or Reconstruction
	Fracture and/or Dislocation
	Manipulation
	Arthrodesis
	Amputation
	Other Procedures
Humerus (Upper Arm) and Elbow	Incision
	Excision
	Introduction or Removal
	Repair, Revision, and/or Reconstruction
	Fracture and/or Dislocation
	Arthrodesis
	Amputation
	Other Procedures
Forearm and Wrist	Incision
	Excision
	Introduction or Removal
	Repair, Revision, and/or Reconstruction
	Fracture and/or Dislocation
	Arthrodesis
	Amputation
	Other Procedures
Hand and Fingers	Incision
	Excision
	Introduction or Removal
	Repair, Revision, and/or Reconstruction
	Fracture and/or Dislocation

T A B L E 13–2

Headings and Subheadings in the Musculoskeletal System Subsection—cont'd

Heading	Subheadings
Hand and Fingers—cont'd	*Arthrodesis*
	Amputation
	Other Procedures
Pelvis and Hip Joint	*Incision*
	Excision
	Introduction or Removal
	Repair, Revision, and/or Reconstruction
	Fracture and/or Dislocation
	Manipulation
	Arthrodesis
	Amputation
	Other Procedures
Femur (Thigh Region) and Knee Joint	*Incision*
	Excision
	Introduction or Removal
	Repair, Revision, and/or Reconstruction
	Fracture and/or Dislocation
	Manipulation
	Arthrodesis
	Amputation
	Other Procedures
Leg (Tibia and Fibula) and Ankle Joint	*Incision*
	Excision
	Introduction or Removal
	Repair, Revision, and/or Reconstruction
	Fracture and/or Dislocation
	Manipulation
	Arthrodesis
	Amputation
	Other Procedures
Foot and Toes	*Incision*
	Excision
	Introduction or Removal
	Repair, Revision, and/or Reconstruction
	Fracture and/or Dislocation
	Arthrodesis
	Amputation
	Other Procedures
Application of Casts and Strapping	*Body and Upper Extremity* (with sub-subheadings *Casts; Splints;* and *Strapping—Any Age*)
	Lower Extremity (with sub-subheadings *Casts; Splints;* and *Strapping—Any Age*)
	Removal or Repair
	Other Procedures
Arthroscopy	

The heading *Head* incorporates listings of procedures for the skull, the facial bones, and the temporomandibular joint. The heading *Spine (Vertebral Column)* incorporates listings of procedures for the cervical spine, the thoracic spine, and the lumbar spine. The heading *Shoulder* encompasses listings of procedures for the clavicle, the scapula, the humerus head and neck, the sternoclavicular joint, the acromioclavicular joint, and the shoulder joint. The heading *Humerus (Upper Arm)* and *Elbow* encompasses listings of procedures for the elbow area including the head and neck of the radius and the olecranon process. The heading *Forearm and Wrist* encompasses listings of procedures for the radius, the ulna, and the carpal bones or joints.

The heading *Pelvis and Hip Joint* comprises listings of procedures for the pelvis and for the head and neck of the femur. The heading *Femur (Thigh Region) and Knee Joint* comprises listings of procedures for the femur, the patella, and the tibial plateaus. The heading *Application of Casts and Strapping* comprises listings of procedures for the application, the removal, or the repair of casts, splints, and strapping.

Scores of cross-references among the listings in the Musculoskeletal System subsection direct code number and descriptor selection to listings elsewhere in this subsection (example: note the cross-reference for code number and descriptor *23660 Open treatment of acute shoulder dislocation*), or to listings in other subsections of the Surgery section (example: note the cross-reference for code number and descriptor *27035 Hip joint denervation ...*), or even to listings in other sections of the CPT volume. To exemplify, radiologic supervision and interpretation of a percutaneous musculoskeletal procedure should be properly reported with a code listed in the Radiology section of the CPT volume (example: note the cross-reference for code number and descriptor *27095 Injection procedure for hip arthrography with anesthesia*).

Extensive notes at the forefront of the Musculoskeletal System subsection encompass definitions of select orthopedic procedural terms, for example, closed treatment, open treatment, and percutaneous skeletal fixation. Notations in this subsection also encompass instructions for the proper coding and reporting of procedures. For instance, the listing for a surgical arthroscopy includes a diagnostic arthroscopy, which should not be coded and reported separately in addition to the coding and reporting of the surgical arthroscopic procedure. Also, the listing of spinal arthrodesis includes either an allograft or an autograft. If an autograft was harvested through a separate incision, code number *22820* should be reported in addition to the code number for the arthrodesis procedure.

Notations within the Musculoskeletal System subsection enable a means to standardize the coding and reporting of surgical procedures performed on the bones, the joints, the tendons, and the muscles. The descriptors of code numbers for reporting the treatment of fractures, and the descriptors of code numbers for reporting the treatment of dislocations do not differentiate between closed injuries and open injuries. A repeated fracture reduction performed by the same physician or a repeated reduction of a dislocation performed by the same physician should be reported with modifier *-76*, the repeat procedure modifier, supplementing the code for the reduction procedure.

Codes for casting or strapping may be reported solely if the cast application or traction device application was either a replacement procedure performed during or after the period of follow-up care. The initial casting procedure or the initial strapping procedure is implicitly included in the code number and descriptor listing for the treatment of the fracture or the treatment of the dislocation. The removal of casts or the removal of traction devices should be coded and reported only if the application of the cast or the traction device was performed by another physician.

Insurance carriers generally reimburse a provider for the application and removal of one cast per fracture or one traction device per dislocation. Casting or strapping materials and supplies should be coded and reported with HCPCS codes and descriptors for Medicare reimbursement.

CPT CODING OF RESPIRATORY SYSTEM SURGICAL PROCEDURES

The Respiratory System subsection of the CPT Surgery section contains listings of procedures performed on the nose, the sinuses, the larynx, the trachea, the bronchi, the lungs, and the pleura. Headings within this subsection are arranged according to anatomic sites of the respiratory system. Further division of these headings into subheadings is principally organized by procedural modality, encompassing endoscopic, incisional, excisional, reparative, and other procedures. Table 13–3 lists the headings and subheadings within the Respiratory System subsection.

T A B L E 13–3

Headings and Subheadings in the Respiratory System Subsection

Heading	Subheadings
Nose	Incision
	Excision
	Introduction
	Removal of Foreign Body
	Repair
	Destruction
	Other Procedures
Accessory Sinuses	Incision
	Excision
	Endoscopy
	Other Procedures
Larynx	Excision
	Introduction
	Endoscopy
	Repair
	Destruction
	Other Procedures
Trachea and Bronchi	Incision
	Endoscopy
	Introduction
	Repair
	Other Procedures
Lungs and Pleura	Incision
	Excision
	Endoscopy
	Repair
	Lung Transplantation
	Surgical Collapse Therapy, Thoracoplasty
	Other Procedures

Dozens of cross-references among the listings of the Respiratory System subsection guide code number and descriptor selection to listings elsewhere in this subsection (example: note the cross-reference for code number and descriptor *30140 Submucous resection turbinate, partial or complete*), or to listings in other subsections of the Surgery section (example: note the cross-reference for code number and descriptor *30920 Ligation arteries; internal maxillary artery, transantral*), or furthermore to listings in other sections of the CPT volume. To exemplify, radiologic supervision and interpretation of a percutaneous pulmonary procedure should be correctly reported with a code listed in the Radiology section of the CPT volume and prolonged services should be correctly reported with a code listed in the Medicine section of the CPT volume (example: note the cross-reference for code number and descriptor *31715 Transtracheal injection for bronchography*).

Notations amid the listings in the Respiratory System subsection provide explanations and instructions that supply a means to standardize the coding and reporting of surgical procedures performed on the nose, the sinuses, the larynx, the trachea, the bronchi, the lungs, and the pleura. Each of the major anatomic sites examined through endoscopic procedures should be coded and reported separately (example: laryngotracheobronchoscopy should be coded and reported separately as laryngoscopy, tracheoscopy, and bronchoscopy). However, the listing for a surgical sinus endoscopy always includes a sinusotomy as well as a diagnostic sinus endoscopy, and the listing for surgical thoracoscopy always includes a diagnostic thoracoscopy. Reporting of a sinus endoscopy infers the inspection of the interior of the nasal cavity, the middle and superior meatus, the turbinates, and the sphenoethmoidal recess. Code numbers for nasal endoscopy report unilateral procedures unless otherwise specified in the descriptor.

Numerous descriptors in the listings of the Respiratory System subsection indicate the diagnostic condition in the terminology of the descriptor (examples: code number and descriptor *32005 Chemical pleurodesis for recurrent or persistent pneumothorax;* or code number and descriptor *32540 Extrapleural enucleation of empyema*).

CPT CODING OF CARDIOVASCULAR SYSTEM SURGICAL PROCEDURES

The relatively prolonged Cardiovascular System subsection of the CPT Surgery section comprises listings of procedures performed on the heart, the pericardium, the cardiac valves, the arteries, and the veins. Headings within this subsection are organized by the major anatomic sites in the cardiovascular system. Further division of these headings into subheadings is also predominantly arranged either by anatomic site (examples: pericardium or cardiac valves), diagnostic indicator (examples: septal defect or aortic anomalies), or procedural modality (examples: thromboendarterectomy or repair of arteriovenous fistula). Table 13–4 lists the headings and subheadings within the Cardiovascular System subsection.

Cross-references amid the listings of the Cardiovascular System subsection direct code number and descriptor selection to listings elsewhere in this subsection (example: note the cross reference for code number and descriptor *33788 Reimplantation of an anomalous pulmonary artery*), or to listings in other subsections of the Surgery section (example: note the cross reference for code number and descriptor *37606 Ligation; internal or common carotid artery . . .*), or furthermore to listings in other sections of the CPT volume. To exemplify, radiologic supervision and interpretation of a percutaneous cardiovascular procedure (such as an angioplasty, an embolization, an infusion, or a stent placement) should be properly reported with a code listed in the Radiology section of the CPT volume (example: note the cross-reference for code number and descriptor *35476 Transluminal balloon angioplasty, percutaneous; venous*).

T A B L E 13–4

Headings and Subheadings in the Cardiovascular System Subsection

Heading	Subheadings
Heart and Pericardium	Pericardium
	Cardiac Tumor
	Pacemaker or Defibrillator
	Wounds of the Heart and Great Vessels
	Cardiac Valves (with sub-subheadings *Aortic Valve; Mitral Valve; Tricuspid Valve;* and *Pulmonary Valve*)
	Coronary Artery Anomalies
	Venous Grafting Only for Coronary Artery Bypass
	Combined Arterial-Venous Grafting for Coronary Bypass
	Arterial Grafting for Coronary Artery Bypass
	Coronary Endarterectomy
	Single Ventricle and Other Complex Cardiac Anomalies
	Septal Defect
	Sinus of Valsalva
	Total Anomalous Pulmonary Venous Drainage
	Shunting Procedures
	Transposition of the Great Vessels
	Truncus Arteriosus
	Aortic Anomalies
	Thoracic Aortic Aneurysm
	Pulmonary Artery
	Heart/Lung Transplantation
	Cardiac Assist
	Other Procedures
Arteries and Veins	Embolectomy/Thrombectomy (with sub-subheadings *Arterial, With or Without Catheter;* and *Venous, Direct or With Catheter*)
	Venous Reconstruction
	Direct Repair of Aneurysm or Excision (Partial or Total) and Graft Insertion for Aneurysm, False Aneurysm, Ruptured Aneurysm, and Associated Occlusive Disease
	Repair Arteriovenous Fistula
	Repair Blood Vessel Other Than for Fistula, With or Without Patch Angioplasty
	Thromboendarterectomy
	Transluminal Angioplasty (with sub-subheadings *Open* and *Percutaneous*)
	Transluminal Atherectomy (with sub-subheadings *Open* and *Percutaneous*)
	Bypass Graft (with sub-subheadings *Vein; In-Situ Vein;* and *Other Than Vein*)
	Arterial Transposition
	Exploration
	Vascular Injection Procedures (with sub-subheadings *Intravenous; Intra-Arterial—Intra-Aortic; Venous; Arterial;* and *Intraosseus*)
	Intravascular Cannulization or Shunt
	Portal Decompression Procedures
	Transcatheter Therapy and Biopsy
	Ligation and Other Procedures

Various descriptors among the assorted listings in the Cardiovascular System subsection indicate the diagnostic condition in the terminology of the descriptor (examples: code number and descriptor *33647 Repair of atrial septal defect and ventricular septal defect, with direct or patch closure;* or code number and descriptor *35180 Repair, congenital arteriovenous fistula; head and neck*). Notations throughout the listings of this subsection provide explanations and instructions that supply a means to standardize the coding and reporting of surgical procedures performed on the heart, the pericardium, the cardiac valves, the arteries, and the veins.

Each code number and descriptor for a selective vascular catheterization procedure inherently includes all lesser order selective catheterization procedures performed in the approach (from the site of the initial puncture and to the ultimate site of the catheterization). For example: catheterization of the right middle cerebral artery includes both the catheterization of the right common carotid artery and that of the right internal carotid artery.

Every catheterization procedure performed in a distinct vascular grouping should be coded and reported separately (example: catheterization of thoracic artery branches and that of brachiocephalic artery branches should be coded and reported separately).

The code number and descriptor listing for a vascular injection procedure encompasses any requisite injection of local anesthesia, any requisite introduction of needles or catheter, or any requisite injection of contrast media (with or without automatic power injection), as well as all preinjection and postinjection care associated with the injection procedure. Catheters, contrast media, and essential pharmaceuticals are not included in the code listing for the vascular injection procedure, but may be reported with HCPCS codes, if necessary.

The code number and descriptor listing for a vascular procedure incorporates both the establishment of inflow and outflow through any procedures necessary, and this listing also incorporates any segment of an operative arteriogram that was performed by the surgeon. Sympathectomy, if performed, is included in the listing for a procedure on the aorta.

The code number and descriptor listing for a cardiac pacemaker procedure includes all pacemaker repositioning and replacement procedures performed within the first fourteen days after the cardiac pacemaker insertion procedure.

Special instructions guide code number and descriptor selection for a coronary artery bypass grafting procedure with regard to the use of venous grafts, arterial grafts, or a combination of venous grafts and arterial grafts. Reporting of a combined arterial-venous coronary bypass graft procedure requires the selection of two codes as directed by the notation in the listings. Code number and descriptor listings for the arterial grafts include the reporting of internal mammary artery grafts, gastroepiploic artery grafts, epigastric artery grafts, radial artery grafts, as well as arterial conduits harvested from other sites.

Code number and descriptor listings for the repair of an aneurysm by graft report also the preparation of the artery for anastomosis, including any necessary endarterectomy. Venous injection procedure listings include percutaneous venipuncture and the insertion of any needles or catheter for diagnostic study or intravenous therapy.

CPT CODING OF HEMIC AND LYMPHATIC SYSTEMS SURGICAL PROCEDURES

The Hemic and Lymphatic Systems subsection of the CPT Surgery section contains listings of procedures performed on the spleen, the bone marrow, and the lymph nodes. Within this concise subsection, three headings are delineated: *Spleen, Bone Marrow or Stem Cell Transplantation,* and *Lymph Nodes and Lymphatic Channels.*

The heading *Spleen* incorporates listings of procedures within subheadings for *Excision, Repair,* and *Introduction.* The heading *Lymph Nodes and Lymphatic Channels* incorporates listings of procedures within subheadings for *Incision, Excision, Limited Lymphadenectomy for Staging, Radical Lymphadenectomy (Radical Resection of Lymph Nodes), Introduction,* and *Other Procedures.*

Surgical procedures performed on the lymph nodes and on the lymphatic channel are often accomplished in conjunction with additional surgical, radiological, or laboratory services. Thus, all codes should be reported in accordance with the notations provided among the listings of the Hemic and Lymphatic Systems subsection (examples: observe the notation for code number and descriptor *38562 Limited lymphadenectomy for staging; pelvic and para-aortic;* and observe the notation for code number and descriptor *38790 Injection procedure for lymphangiography*).

CPT CODING OF MEDIASTINUM AND DIAPHRAGM SURGICAL PROCEDURES

The brief Mediastinum and Diaphragm subsection of the CPT Surgery section encompasses listings of procedures performed on the mediastinum and the diaphragm. Within this compact subsection, two headings are delineated. The heading *Mediastinum* incorporates listings of procedures within subheadings for *Incision, Excision, Endoscopy,* and *Other Procedures.* The heading *Diaphragm* incorporates listings of procedures within subheadings for *Repair* and *Other Procedures.*

Cross-references throughout the listings of the Mediastinum and Diaphragm subsection direct code number and descriptor selection to listings in other subsections of the Surgery section (examples: note the cross-reference for code number and descriptor *39220 Excision of mediastinal tumor;* and note the cross-reference for code number and descriptor *39503 Repair, neonatal diaphragmatic hernia . . .*).

CPT CODING OF DIGESTIVE SYSTEM SURGICAL PROCEDURES

The Digestive System subsection of the CPT Surgery section comprises listings of procedures performed on the alimentary tract and on the accessory organs of digestion. Numerous headings within this subsection are organized by anatomic site including the mouth, the tongue, the palate, the uvula, the salivary structures, the pharynx, the adenoids, the tonsils, the esophagus, the stomach, the intestines, the mesentery, the appendix, the rectum, the anus, the liver, the biliary tract, the pancreas, the peritoneum, and the omentum.

Many subheadings within these headings are organized by procedural modality (endoscopic, incisional, excisional, reparative, and other procedures). Table 13–5 lists the headings and subheadings within the Digestive System subsection. The heading *Vestibule of Mouth* contains listings of procedures for the portion of the oral cavity apart from the dentoalveolar structures including the mucosal and submucosal tissues of the lips and cheeks.

Cross-references throughout the listings of the Digestive System subsection direct code number and descriptor selection to listings elsewhere in this subsection (example: note the cross-reference for code number and descriptor *45020 Incision and drainage of deep supralevator, pelvirectal, or retrorectal abscess*), or to listings in other subsections of the Surgery section (example: note the cross-reference for code number and descriptor *42806 Biopsy; nasopharynx, survey for unknown primary lesion*), as well as to listings in other sections of the CPT volume. To exemplify, radiologic supervision and interpretation of either an endoscopic gastrointestinal procedure or a percutaneous procedure performed at a site within the digestive system should be correctly reported with a code listed in the Radiology section of the CPT volume (example: note the cross-reference for code number and descriptor *47490 Percutaneous cholecystostomy*).

T A B L E 13–5

Headings and Subheadings in the Digestive System Subsection

Heading	Subheadings
Lips	Excision
	Repair (Cheiloplasty)
	Other Procedures
Vestibule of Mouth	Incision
	Excision, Destruction
	Repair
	Other Procedures
Tongue and Floor of Mouth	Incision
	Excision
	Repair
	Other Procedures
Dentoalveolar Structures	Incision
	Excision, Destruction
	Other Procedures
Palate and Uvula	Incision
	Excision, Destruction
	Repair
	Other Procedures
Salivary Glands and Ducts	Incision
	Excision
	Repair
	Other Procedures
Pharynx, Adenoids, and Tonsils	Incision
	Excision, Destruction
	Repair
	Other Procedures
Esophagus	Incision
	Excision
	Endoscopy
	Repair
	Manipulation
	Other Procedures
Stomach	Incision
	Excision
	Introduction
	Other Procedures
Intestines (Except Rectum)	Incision
	Excision
	Enterostomy—External Fistulization of Intestines
	Endoscopy, Small Bowel and Stomal
	Introduction
	Repair
	Other Procedures

T A B L E 13–5

Headings and Subheadings in the Digestive System Subsection—cont'd

Heading	Subheadings
Meckel's Diverticulum and the Mesentery	Excision
	Suture
	Other Procedures
Appendix	Incision
	Excision
Rectum	Incision
	Excision
	Destruction
	Endoscopy
	Repair
	Manipulation
	Other Procedures
Anus	Incision
	Excision
	Introduction
	Endoscopy
	Repair
	Destruction
	Suture
	Other Procedures
Liver	Incision
	Excision
	Repair
	Other Procedures
Biliary Tract	Incision
	Introduction
	Endoscopy
	Excision
	Repair
	Other Procedures
Pancreas	Incision
	Excision
	Introduction
	Repair
	Pancreas Transplantation
	Other Procedures
Abdomen, Peritoneum, and Omentum	Incision
	Excision, Destruction
	Introduction, Revision, and/or Removal
	Repair Hernioplasty, Herniorrhaphy, and Herniotomy
	Suture
	Other Procedures

Notations among the listings in the Digestive System subsection provide explanations and instructions that furnish a means to standardize the coding and reporting of surgical procedures performed on the alimentary tract and on the accessory organs of digestion. Each anatomic site examined through endoscopic procedures should be coded and reported separately (example: esophagogastroduodenoscopy should be coded and reported separately as esophagoscopy, gastroscopy, and duodenoscopy). However, the listing for a surgical endoscopy always includes diagnostic endoscopy, and thus diagnostic endoscopy in such circumstances does not warrant separate coding and reporting. Incidental appendectomy performed during intra-abdominal surgery also does not warrant separate coding and reporting.

For coding and reporting purposes, proctosigmoidoscopy is defined as the examination of the rectum and the sigmoid colon, sigmoidoscopy is defined as the examination of the rectum and the sigmoid colon as well as a portion of the descending colon, and colonoscopy is defined as the examination of the entire colon from the rectum to the cecum as well as a portion of the terminal ileum. Coding and reporting of an incomplete colonoscopy (subsequent to full preparation for a colonoscopy) should be augmented with modifier -52.

Hernia repair code numbers and descriptors in this subsection are principally classified according to the type of hernia, such as inguinal hernia, femoral hernia, incisional hernia, epigastric hernia, or umbilical hernia. These hernias are secondarily subclassified as initial or recurrent and also subclassified as reducible, incarcerated, or strangulated. Furthermore, the age of the patient is another variable among the listings for hernia repair.

The excision or repair of incarcerated or strangulated organs or structures (such as the testicles, the intestines, or the ovaries) should be coded and reported separately via the appropriate code number for the excision or repair, in addition to the code number reported for the repair of the incarcerated or strangulated hernia. With the exception of incisional hernia repairs, the use of mesh or other prostheses should not be coded and reported separately.

CPT CODING OF URINARY SYSTEM SURGICAL PROCEDURES

The Urinary System subsection of the CPT Surgery section contains listings of procedures performed on the organs of the excretory system, namely the kidneys, the ureters, the bladder, and the urethra. Headings within this subsection are arranged by anatomic site and subheadings within these headings are arranged by procedural modality (diagnostic, endoscopic, incisional, excisional, reconstructive, and other procedures). Table 13–6 lists the headings and subheadings within the Urinary System subsection.

Cross-references among the listings of the Urinary System subsection guide code number and descriptor selection to listings elsewhere within this subsection (example: note the cross-reference for code number and descriptor *50120 Pyelotomy; with exploration*), or to listings in other subsections of the Surgery section (example: note the cross-reference for code number and descriptor *53520 Closure of urethrostomy or urethrocutaneous fistula, male*) as well as to listings in other sections of the CPT volume. To exemplify, radiologic supervision and interpretation of either an endoscopic genitourinary procedure or a percutaneous procedure performed at a site within the excretory system should be properly reported with a code listed in the Radiology section of the CPT volume (example: note the cross-reference for code number and descriptor *51610 Injection procedure for retrograde urethrocystography*).

Notations amid the listings in the Urinary System subsection provide explanations and instructions that furnish a means to standardize the coding and reporting of surgical procedures performed on the kidneys, the ureters, the bladder, and the urethra. For example, certain codes for urodynamics should be reported separately, whereas other codes for urodynamics should be reported in varied combinations. Code number *51725* represented by descriptor *Simple cystometrogram,* should not be reported with code number *51726* represented by

T A B L E 13–6

Headings and Subheadings in the Urinary System Subsection

Heading	Subheadings
Kidney	Incision
	Excision
	Renal Transplantation
	Introduction
	Repair
	Endoscopy
	Other Procedures
Ureter	Incision
	Excision
	Introduction
	Repair
	Endoscopy
Bladder	Incision
	Excision
	Introduction
	Urodynamics
	Repair
	Endoscopy—Cystoscopy, Urethroscopy, Cystourethroscopy
	Transurethral Surgery (with sub-subheadings Urethra and Bladder; Ureter and Pelvis; and Vesical Neck and Prostate)
Urethra	Incision
	Excision
	Repair
	Manipulation
	Other Procedures

descriptor *Complex cystometrogram,* but may be reported with code number *51741* represented by descriptor *Complex uroflowmetry.* Items used in the provision of these urodynamic services such as the instruments, the equipment, the medications, and any additional supplies or materials are generally included in the code utilized to report these entities.

Descriptors for cystoscopy procedures and descriptors for urethroscopy procedures are listed in a manner that facilitates identification of the major (primary or principal) procedure without specifying all of the minor (secondary or additional) procedures that were performed during the same procedural session (example: note the format and content of the descriptor for a cystourethroscopy that was performed prior to a transurethral resection of the prostate). These minor procedures, which are encompassed in the listed code number and descriptor, may be augmented with modifier -22 if substantial additional time or effort was expended in rendering these procedures. For example, code number *52601* represented by descriptor *Transurethral electrosurgical resection of prostate, including control of postoperative bleeding, complete,* may be reported along with code number *52204-22* represented by descriptor *Cystourethroscopy, with biopsy,* if rendering these procedures required substantial additional time or effort. The insertion of a ureteral stent, however, should not be coded and reported separately.

Multiple major procedures performed on the urinary system during a single diagnostic session or during a single operative session should be supplemented with modifier *-51*. For example, code number *52601* represented by descriptor *Transurethral electrosurgical resection of prostate, including control of postoperative bleeding, complete* should be reported along with code number *52276-51* represented by descriptor *Cystourethroscopy with direct vision internal urethrotomy* if both of these procedures were performed during a single session.

CPT CODING OF MALE GENITAL SYSTEM SURGICAL PROCEDURES

The Male Genital System subsection of the CPT Surgery section comprises listings of procedures performed on the penis, the testes, the epididymis, the scrotum, the vas deferens, the spermatic cord, the seminal vesicles, the prostate, and all related structures. Headings within this subsection are arranged by anatomic site, and subheadings within these headings are arranged by procedural modality (incisional, excisional, reconstructive, and other procedures). Table 13–7 lists the headings and subheadings within the Male Genital System subsection.

T A B L E   13–7

Headings and Subheadings in the Male Genital System Subsection

Heading	Subheadings
Penis	*Incision*
	Destruction
	Excision
	Introduction
	Repair
	Manipulation
Testis	*Excision*
	Repair
Epididymis	*Incision*
	Excision
	Repair
Tunica Vaginalis	*Incision*
	Excision
	Repair
Scrotum	*Incision*
	Excision
	Repair
Vas Deferens	*Incision*
	Excision
	Introduction
	Repair
	Suture
Spermatic Cord	*Excision*
Seminal Vesicles	*Incision*
	Excision
Prostate	*Incision*
	Excision
	Other Procedures

Cross-references among the listings of the Male Genital System subsection direct code number and descriptor selection to listings elsewhere within this subsection (example: note the cross-reference for code number and descriptor *54505 Biopsy of testis, incisional*), or to listings in other subsections of the Surgery section (example: note the cross-reference for code number and descriptor *55041 Excision of hydrocele, bilateral*), or sometimes to listings in other sections of the CPT volume. To exemplify, radiologic supervision and interpretation of a percutaneous procedure performed on the male genital system should be correctly reported with a code listed in the Radiology section of the CPT volume (example: note the cross-reference for code number and descriptor *55300 Vasotomy for vasograms, seminal vesiculograms,* or *epididymograms, unilateral or bilateral*).

Modifier *-20* should supplement a code for a male genital system procedure that was performed with the assistance of an operating microscope. For example, code number *54901-20* represented by descriptor *Epididymovasotomy, anastomosis of epididymis to vas deferens; bilateral* should be reported if this procedure was performed with the assistance of an operating microscope.

CPT CODING OF LAPAROSCOPY/PERITONEOSCOPY PROCEDURES

The Laparoscopy/Peritoneoscopy subsection of the CPT Surgery section contains listings of procedures involving these endoscopic approaches. Code numbers and descriptors in this subsection are applicable regardless of whether cautery, laser, or other technique was utilized in rendering the procedure.

Descriptors for procedures involving laparoscopy or peritoneoscopy are listed in a manner that expedites identification of the major (primary or principal) procedure without designating all of the minor (secondary or additional) procedures that were performed during the same session (example: note the format and content of the descriptor for a lysis of adhesions that was performed with a fulguration transection of the oviducts). These minor procedures, which are encompassed in the code number and descriptor listing, may be augmented with modifier *-22* if significant additional time or effort was expended in rendering these procedures. For example, code number *56301* represented by descriptor *Laparoscopy, surgical; with fulguration of oviducts* may be reported along with code *56304-22* represented by descriptor *Laparoscopy, surgical; with lysis of adhesions* if rendering these procedures required substantial additional time or effort.

CPT CODING OF FEMALE GENITAL SYSTEM SURGICAL PROCEDURES

The Female Genital System subsection of the CPT Surgery section comprises listings of procedures performed on the vulva, the perineum, the vagina, the cervix, the uterus, the oviducts, the ovaries, and all related structures. Headings within this subsection are organized by anatomic sites, and subheadings within these headings are organized by procedural modality (laparoscopic, incisional, excisional, reconstructive, and other non-obstetrical procedures). Table 13–8 lists the headings and subheadings within the Female Genital System subsection.

Cross-references among the listings of the Female Genital System subsection guide code number and descriptor selection to listings elsewhere within this subsection (example: note the cross-reference for code number and descriptor *56810 Perineoplasty, repair of perineum, non-obstetrical*), or to listings in other subsections of the Surgery section (example: note the cross-reference for code number and descriptor *56640 Vulvectomy, radical, complete with*

T A B L E   13–8

Headings and Subheadings in the Female Genital
   System Subsection

Heading	Subheadings
Vulva, Perineum, and Introitus	*Incision*
	Destruction
	Excision
	Repair
Vagina	*Incision*
	Destruction
	Excision
	Introduction
	Repair
	Manipulation
	Endoscopy
Cervix Uteri	*Excision*
	Repair
	Manipulation
Corpus Uteri	*Excision*
	Introduction
	Repair
Oviduct	*Incision*
	Excision
	Repair
Ovary	*Incision*
	Excision
In Vitro Fertilization	*Other Procedures*

inguinofemoral, iliac, and pelvic lymphadenectomy), or sometimes to listings in other sections of the CPT volume. To exemplify, radiologic supervision and interpretation of a percutaneous procedure performed on the female genital system should be correctly reported with a code listed in the Radiology section of the CPT volume (example: note the cross-reference for code number and descriptor *58340* Injection procedure for hysterosalpingography*).

Notations amid the listings of the Female Genital System subsection offer explanations and instructions that enable a means to standardize the coding and reporting of surgical procedures performed on the vulva, the perineum, the vagina, the cervix, the uterus, the oviducts, the ovaries, and all related structures.

For coding and reporting purposes, a simple vulvectomy is defined as the removal of skin and superficial subcutaneous tissues, a radical vulvectomy is defined as the removal of skin and deep subcutaneous tissues, a partial vulvectomy is defined as the removal of less than eighty percent of the vulvar area, and a complete vulvectomy is defined as the removal of more than eighty percent of the vulvar area.

CPT CODING OF MATERNITY CARE AND DELIVERY

The unique Maternity Care and Delivery Services subsection of the CPT Surgery section contains listings of obstetrical services including antepartum care, delivery care, and postpartum care. Subheadings are delineated for *Incision; Excision; Introduction; Repair; Vaginal Delivery, Antepartum and Postpartum Care; Cesarean Delivery; Abortion;* and *Other Procedures.*

Antepartum care typically consists of an initial history and physical examination as well as nine to eleven routine visits per patient. Additional visits or services may be coded and reported separately. Non-routine antepartum visits associated with high-risk pregnancy or treatment of complications during pregnancy should be reported with codes from the listings of the Evaluation and Management Services section.

Delivery care typically consists of hospital admission processes, an admission history and physical examination, and management of labor and vaginal delivery (with or without forceps and with or without episiotomy), or management of labor and cesarean delivery. Additional resources or services may be coded and reported separately. Complications of labor and delivery should be reported separately either with codes from the listings in other subsections of the Surgery section or with codes from the listings in other sections of the CPT volume.

Postpartum care typically consists of hospital visits and office visits subsequent to either vaginal or cesarean delivery. Complications during the puerperium should be reported separately either with codes from the listings in other subsections of the Surgery section or with codes from the listings in other sections of the CPT volume. Applicable codes from the listings of the Evaluation and Management Services section should be reported if a physician renders merely a portion of a patient's maternity care.

CPT CODING OF ENDOCRINE SYSTEM SURGICAL PROCEDURES

The brief Endocrine System subsection of the CPT Surgery section is comprised of two headings that encompass listings of surgical procedures. The first heading, *Thyroid Gland,* incorporates procedures performed on the thyroid within two subheadings *Incision* and *Excision.* The second heading, *Parathyroid, Thymus, Adrenal Glands, and Carotid Body,* incorporates procedures performed on the parathyroid, the thymus, the adrenals, and the carotid body within two subheadings *Excision* and *Other Procedures.* Code numbers and descriptors for procedures performed on the pituitary gland or on the pineal gland are listed in the Nervous System subsection of the CPT Surgery section.

Cross-references amid the listings of the Endocrine System subsection lead code number and descriptor selection to listings in other sections of the CPT volume. To exemplify, radiologic supervision and interpretation of a percutaneous procedure performed on a component of the endocrine system should be appropriately reported with codes listed in the Radiology section or the Pathology and Laboratory section of the CPT volume (example: note the cross-reference for code number and descriptor *60100* Biopsy thyroid, percutaneous core needle).*

CPT CODING OF NERVOUS SYSTEM SURGICAL PROCEDURES

The lengthy Nervous System subsection of the CPT Surgery section contains listings of surgical procedures performed on the skull, the meninges, the brain, the spine, the spinal cord, and the nerves. Headings within this subsection are organized by anatomic sites, and subheadings within these headings are organized by procedural modality (such as puncture, aspiration, injection, exploration, decompression, excision, resection, or repair), or by diagnostic indicator (such as arteriovenous malformation or herniated disk). Table 13–9 lists the headings and subheadings within the Nervous System subsection.

Cross-references amid the listings of the Nervous System subsection lead code number and descriptor selection to listings elsewhere within this subsection (example: note the cross-reference for code number and descriptor *61571 Craniectomy or craniotomy; with treatment of penetrating wound of brain*), or to listings in other subsections of the Surgery section (example: note the cross-reference for code number and descriptor *61708 Surgery of aneurysm, vascular malformation or carotid-cavernous fistula, by intracranial electrothrombosis*), as well as to listings in other sections of the CPT volume. To exemplify, radiologic supervision and interpretation of a percutaneous procedure performed on a component of the nervous system should be appropriately reported with a code listed in the Radiology section of the CPT volume (example: note the cross-reference for code number and descriptor *62291* Injection procedure for diskography, each level; cervical*).

Many of the descriptors in the listings of the Nervous System subsection indicate the diagnostic condition in the terminology of the descriptor (examples: code number and descriptor *61680 Surgery of intracranial arteriovenous malformation; supratentorial; simple;* or code number and descriptor *62120 Repair of encephalocele, skull vault, including cranioplasty*).

Surgery on the skull base typically necessitates the skills of surgeons from different clinical specialties. If one surgeon performed an approach procedure and another surgeon performed a definitive procedure during an operative session, each surgeon should report only the code for the specific aspect of the procedure that he or she performed. If a sole surgeon performed both the approach procedure and the definitive procedure, he or she may report the codes for both aspects of the procedure, with modifier *-51* appended to the code for the approach procedure.

For coding and reporting purposes, definitions are instituted for approach procedure, definitive procedure, and repair/reconstruction procedure. An approach procedure is necessary to obtain adequate exposure to the lesion or pathologic entity, and is described according to the anatomical area involved, such as the anterior cranial fossa, the middle cranial fossa, the posterior cranial fossa, the brain stem, or the upper spinal cord. A definitive procedure is necessary to biopsy, excise, or otherwise treat the lesion or pathologic entity, and is described by the repair, biopsy, resection, or excision of a lesion or pathologic entity, and if applicable, is described by primary closure of the dura, the mucous membranes, and the skin. A repair/reconstruction procedure remediates the defect present subsequent to the definitive procedure, and should be coded and reported separately if extensive dural grafting was needed, if cranioplasty was needed, if local or regional myocutaneous pedicle flaps were needed, or if extensive skin grafts were needed.

The listings of code numbers and descriptors to report surgery for aneurysm, arteriovenous malformation, or vascular disease include craniotomy, if applicable for that procedure. For coding and reporting purposes, neuroplasty is defined as the decompression or releasing of intact nerve from scar tissue. The listings of code numbers and descriptors to report neuroplasty include external neurolysis and/or transposition, if applicable for that procedure.

CPT CODING OF EYE AND OCULAR ADNEXA SURGICAL PROCEDURES

The Eye and Ocular Adnexa subsection of the CPT Surgery section comprises listings of surgical ophthalmological procedures performed on the cornea, the anterior chamber, the sclera,

T A B L E 13–9

Headings and Subheadings in the Nervous System Subsection

Heading	Subheadings
Skull, Meninges, and Brain	Injection, Drainage, or Aspiration
	Twist Drill, Burr Hole, or Trephine
	Craniectomy or Craniotomy
	Surgery of Skull Base
	Approach Procedures (with sub-subheadings *Anterior Cranial Fossa; Middle Cranial Fossa;* and *Posterior Cranial Fossa*)
	Definitive Procedures (with sub-subheadings *Base of Anterior Cranial Fossa, Base of Middle Cranial Fossa;* and *Base of Posterior Cranial Fossa*)
	Repair and/or Reconstruction of Surgical Defects of Skull Base
	Endovascular Therapy
	Surgery for Aneurysm, Arteriovenous Malformation, or Vascular Disease
	Stereotaxis
	Neurostimulators (Intracranial)
	CSF Shunt
Spine and Spinal Cord	Injection, Drainage, or Aspiration
	Posterior Extradural Laminotomy or Laminectomy for Exploration/ Decompression of Neural Elements or Excision of Herniated Intervertebral Disks
	Transpedicular or Costovertebral Approach for Posterolateral Extradural Exploration/Decompression
	Anterior or Anterolateral Approach for Extradural Exploration/ Decompression
	Incision
	Excision by Laminectomy of Lesion Other Than Herniated Disk
	Excision, Anterior or Anterolateral Approach, Intraspinal Lesion
	Stereotaxis
	Neurostimulators (Spinal)
	Repair
	Shunt, Spinal CSF
Extracranial Nerves, Peripheral Nerves, and Autonomic Nervous System	Introduction/Injection of Anesthetic Agent (Nerve Block), Diagnostic or Therapeutic (with sub-subheadings *Somatic Nerves* and *Sympathetic Nerves*)
	Neurostimulators (Peripheral Nerves)
	Destruction by Neurolytic Agent (Chemical, Thermal, Electrical, Radiofrequency) (with sub-subheadings *Somatic Nerves* and *Sympathetic Nerves*)
	Neuroplasty (Exploration, Neurolysis, or Nerve Decompression)
	Transection or Avulsion
	Excision (with sub-subheadings *Somatic Nerves* and *Sympathetic Nerves*)
	Neurorrhaphy
	Neurorrhaphy with Nerve Graft
	Other Procedures

the iris, the ciliary body, the lens, the vitreous, the retina, the choroid, the extraocular muscles, the orbit, the eyelids, the conjunctiva, and the lacrimal system.

Headings within the Eye and Ocular Adnexa subsection are mainly arranged by anatomic site, and subheadings within these headings are mainly arranged by either anatomic sites (cornea, lens, or vitreous) or by procedural modality (such as incision, excision, destruction, repair, or probing). Code numbers and descriptors for medical ophthalmological diagnostic and therapeutic services are listed in a subsection of the Medicine section of the CPT volume. Table 13–10 lists the headings and subheadings within the Eye and Ocular Adnexa subsection.

Cross-references among the listings of the Eye and Ocular Adnexa subsection direct code number and descriptor selection to listings elsewhere within this subsection (example: note the cross-reference for code number and descriptor *65175 Removal of ocular implant*), or to listings in other subsections of the Surgery section (example: note the cross-reference for code number and descriptor *67938 Removal of embedded foreign body, eyelid*), as well as to

T A B L E   13–10

Headings and Subheadings in the Eye and Ocular Adnexa Subsection

Heading	Subheadings
Eyeball	*Removal of Eye*
	Secondary Implant Procedures
	Removal of Foreign Body
	Repair of Laceration
Anterior Segment	*Cornea* (with sub-subheadings *Excision; Removal or Destruction; Keratoplasty;* and *Other Procedures*)
	Anterior Chamber (with sub-subheadings *Incision* and *Other Procedures*)
	Anterior Sclera (with sub-subheadings *Excision* and *Repair or Revision*)
	Iris, Ciliary Body (with sub-subheadings *Incision; Excision; Repair;* and *Destruction*)
	Lens (with sub-subheadings *Incision; Removal Cataract;* and *Other Procedures*)
Posterior Segment	*Vitreous*
	Retina or Choroid (with sub-subheadings *Repair; Prophylaxis;* and *Destruction*)
	Sclera (with sub-subheadings *Repair* and *Other Procedures*)
Ocular Adnexa	*Extraocular Muscles*
	Other Procedures
	Orbit (with sub-subheadings *Exploration, Excision, Decompression* and *Other Procedures*)
	Eyelids (with sub-subheadings *Incision; Excision; Tarsorrhaphy; Repair (Brow Ptosis, Blepharoptosis, Lid Retraction, Ectropion, Entropion); Reconstruction;* and *Other Procedures*)
Conjunctiva	*Incision and Drainage*
	Excision and/or Destruction
	Injection
	Conjunctivoplasty
	Other Procedures
	Lacrimal System (with sub-subheadings *Incision; Excision; Repair; Probing and/or Related Procedures; Other Procedures*)

listings in other sections of the CPT volume. To exemplify, certain procedures should be correctly reported with a code listed in the Medicine section of the CPT volume (example: code number and descriptor *92018 Ophthalmological examination and evaluation, under general anesthesia* . . .).

Detailed notations amid the listings of the Eye and Ocular Adnexa subsection supply explanations and instructions that enable a means to standardize the coding and reporting of surgical ophthalmological procedures. As examples, the inclusion of incisions and injections of pharmacologic agents in the code number and descriptor listing for cataract removal, the incorporation of multiple therapeutic sessions for retinal detachment within one service code number and descriptor listing, and the inclusion of fresh grafts or preserved grafts as well as the preparation of donor material in the code number and descriptor listing for corneal transplant are stipulated in such notations. For coding and reporting purposes, an ocular implant is an implant inside of muscular cone, and an orbital implant is an implant outside of muscular cone.

Various descriptors in the listings of the Eye and Ocular Adnexa subsection indicate the diagnostic condition in the terminology of the descriptor (examples: code number and descriptor *66625 Iridectomy, with corneoscleral or corneal section; peripheral for glaucoma;* or code number and descriptor *66930 Removal of lens material; intracapsular, for dislocated lens*).

CPT CODING OF AUDITORY SYSTEM SURGICAL PROCEDURES

The Auditory System subsection, the concluding subsection of the CPT Surgery section, contains listings of surgical procedures performed on the external ear, the middle ear, the inner ear, and the temporal bone. Headings within the Auditory System subsection are mostly organized by anatomic sites, and subheadings within these headings are mostly organized by procedural modality (incision, excision, and repair). Code numbers and descriptors for medical otologic diagnostic and therapeutic services are listed in a subsection of the Medicine section of the CPT volume. Table 13–11 lists the headings and subheadings within the Auditory System subsection.

A few cross-references within the listings of the Auditory System subsection guide code number and descriptor selection to listings elsewhere within this subsection (example: note the cross-reference for code number and descriptor *69535 Resection temporal bone, external approach*), or to listings in other subsections of the Surgery section (example: note the cross-reference for code number and descriptor *69605 Revision mastoidectomy; with apicectomy*), as well as to listings in other sections of the CPT volume. To exemplify, certain procedures should be properly reported with a code listed in the Medicine section of the CPT volume (example: code number and descriptor *92502 Otolaryngologic examination under general anesthesia*).

Several notations within the listings of the Auditory System subsection supply explanations and instructions that enable a means to standardize the coding and reporting of surgical procedures performed on the external ear, the middle ear, the inner ear, and the temporal bone.

SURGERY REPORTING FOR BILLING

The principal procedure is the procedure most closely associated with the patient's principal diagnosis for that specific encounter or episode of service. The primary procedure is the procedure that is the most resource intensive in the context of time, skill, and overhead expense, among those rendered during that encounter or episode of service. The major procedure is the

TABLE 13–11

Headings and Subheadings in the Auditory System Subsection

Heading	Subheadings
External Ear	Incision
	Excision
	Removal of Foreign Body
	Repair
	Other Procedures
Middle Ear	Introduction
	Incision
	Excision
	Repair
	Other Procedures
Inner Ear	Incision and/or Destruction
	Excision
	Introduction
	Other Procedures
Temporal Bone, Middle Fossa Approach	Other Procedures

procedure performed that poses the greatest risk to the health status of the patient during that encounter or episode of service.

As a rule, the procedure posing the greatest risk to the patient is the most resource-intensive procedure and is also the procedure most closely associated with the patient's principal diagnosis for that specific encounter or episode of service. However, under exceptional circumstances involving a hospitalized patient, the most resource-intensive procedure or the procedure posing the greatest risk to the patient may be unrelated to that patient's principal diagnosis for that episode of inpatient care.

Insurance claim forms ordinarily mandate the coding and reporting of each procedure billed, the principal (or primary or major) procedure as well as all of the additional (or secondary or minor) procedures. An additional procedure is subordinate to the principal procedure, a secondary procedure is subordinate to the primary procedure, and a minor procedure is subordinate to the major procedure.

These multiple procedure codes should preferably be entered in descending order ranked by the associated or correlating fee. Thus, the procedure with the highest fee may be entered first, the procedure with the second highest fee may be entered next, followed by the procedure with third highest fee, and so forth.

If multiple procedures were performed within the same session or on the same date, the entire fee may be entered for each procedure reported on the claim form, by reason that many insurance carriers customarily or automatically reduce the allowable reimbursement for the charges billed for each of the additional procedures (with the exception of bilateral procedures). For example, these procedures should be sequenced in the following order, code number and descriptor *24575 Open treatment of humeral epicondylar fracture . . .;* then code number and descriptor *13100 Repair, complex, trunk . . . ;* and then code number and descriptor *12001 Simple repair of superficial wounds of scalp . . .*).

Reporting of code numbers for unlisted procedures should be avoided, if possible. The utilization of unlisted procedure codes usually demands the preparation and submission of a special report to the third-party payor and this task increases the workload of the organization. Accurate, complete, and timely documentation in the patient medical record may alleviate the necessity of reporting codes for unlisted procedures.

The time and effort essential for the rendering of all aspects of a particular service or a particular procedure are typically consistent with each performance of the service or the procedure. Therefore, the predictability of this time and effort enables the use of package billing or global billing.

Medicare carriers acknowledge with global billing the inclusion of postoperative care for either ten days or ninety days (conditional upon the procedure performed). Although preoperative care technically is not surmised or regarded as a constituent of the surgical package, numerous physicians additionally include this service of routine preoperative care in the fee charged for the surgical (or global fee) package.

If the listing of a surgical procedure encloses in parentheses the expression "separate procedure" adjacent to the descriptor terminology, then this procedure may be reported and billed exclusively:

1. If no other procedure was performed on the patient during the same session.
2. If no other procedure was performed on the patient on the same date.
3. If this listed procedure is not associated with any other procedures performed on the patient either during the same session or on the same date.

For example, observe the applicability of the foregoing directive concerning a separate procedure with regard to code number and descriptor *56300 Laparoscopy, diagnostic.*

If the listing of a surgical procedure is denoted with the star symbol (the asterisk symbol), then this starred procedure should be reported and billed separately in view of the potential variability of preoperative services or postoperative services for such a procedure. For example, observe the applicability of this preceding directive with regard to code number and descriptor *42300 Drainage of abscess; parotid, simple.* The fee entered in the reporting and billing of a starred procedure should reflect the charge for the procedure only, and should not be indicative either of any preoperative or postoperative services rendered.

All postoperative examinations of a patient, for instance, may or may not constitute a distinct service. Likewise each distinct surgical incision, for instance, may or may not constitute a distinct procedure.

Separate reporting of the component factors of a total surgical service or separate reporting of the component factors of an entire surgical procedure is termed "unbundling" of a surgical package, and is deemed to be an unethical and fraudulent act. For example, code number *58262* represented by descriptor *Vaginal hysterectomy, with removal of tube and ovary,* should be reported in lieu of reporting code number *58260* represented by descriptor *Vaginal hysterectomy,* separately in addition to code number *58720* represented by descriptor *Salpingo-oophorectomy, complete or partial, unilateral or bilateral.*

Similarly, package billing or global billing for a total service if a portion of the service was not performed or rendered, or package billing or global billing for an entire procedure if a portion of the procedure was not performed or rendered, is considered to be unscrupulous conduct. For example, code number *58951* should not be reported if a lymphadenectomy was not performed. Reporting and billing processes should be planned to legitimately optimize reimbursement.

KEY CONCEPTS

additional procedure _____

anesthesia time _____

assistant surgeon _____

global billing _____

major procedure _____

minor procedure _____

personally furnished anesthesia service _____

physical status modifier _____

physician component of procedure _____

primary procedure _____

principal procedure _____

professional component of procedure _____

reduced service _____

related procedure _____

repeat procedure _____

secondary procedure _____

separate procedure _____

starred procedure _____

star symbol _____

supervisory anesthesia service _____

surgical package _____

surgical team _____

technical component of procedure _____

two-surgeon modifier _____

unlisted procedure _____

unrelated procedure _____

REVIEW EXERCISES

1. Explain and differentiate personally furnished anesthesia services and supervisory anesthesia services. _____

_____

_____

2. Clarify situations in which an anesthesiologist properly reports the services provided with a code for a physician consultation. _____

_____

_____

3. Describe the parameters used to formulate anesthesia time. _____

_____

_____

4. Select and indicate the appropriate modifier to supplement the code number in each of the following clinical examples:

A. dental surgery for profoundly retarded patient _____

_____

B. exploratory surgery for postoperative hemorrhage (on the same date) _____

_____

C. thyroid surgery complicated by intra-operative cerebrovascular accident _____

_____

5. Select and indicate the appropriate physical status modifier to append to the code number in each of the following clinical examples:

A. patient with severe peripheral vascular disease _____

_____

B. patient with open wound of myocardium _____

C. patient with mild diabetes mellitus _____
_____

6. Discuss the importance and consequence of clinical documentation by the surgeon on anesthesia billing. _____
_____
_____

7. Assign precise, accurate code numbers from the CPT volume for the following anesthesia procedures and services. Presume the carrier is either Medicare or non-Medicare or both Medicare and non-Medicare.

A. anesthesia for partial pancreatectomy _____
_____

B. anesthesia for corneal transplant _____
_____

C. anesthesia for vulvectomy _____
_____

D. anesthesia for lithotripsy _____
_____

E. anesthesia for needle biopsy of thyroid _____
_____

F. anesthesia for arthroscopic repair of lateral meniscus of knee _____
_____

G. anesthesia for cesarean delivery _____
_____

H. anesthesia for biopsy of clavicle _____
_____

I. anesthesia for vaginal hysterectomy _____
_____

J. anesthesia for transurethral resection of prostate _____
_____

K. anesthesia for open reduction and internal fixation of ulnar fracture _____
_____

L. anesthesia for ventral hernia repair of upper abdomen _____
_____

M. anesthesia for femoral artery embolectomy _____
_____

8. Explain the services included in the typical "surgical package." _____
_____
_____

9. Describe the circumstances in which the separate coding and reporting of a surgical procedure are not warranted. _____
_____
_____

10. Explain the meaning of the following terms:

    A. professional component of a procedure _____

    _____

    B. technical component of a procedure _____

    _____

11. Select and indicate the appropriate modifier to supplement the code number in each of the following clinical examples:

    A. closure of vesicouterine fistula concurrently performed by Dr. Ackerman, a urologist, and Dr. Kusura, a gynecologist _____

    _____

    B. postpartum care by Dr. Dole after cesarean delivery performed by Dr. Hall _____

    _____

    C. neuroplasty of brachial plexus performed by Dr. Han with the use of an operating microscope _____

    _____

12. Prioritize (rank in order for reporting purposes) the following clusters of surgical procedures:

    A. cardiopulmonary bypass, coronary artery bypass with four coronary venous grafts, temporary transvenous pacemaker

    _____

    _____

    _____

    _____

    B. pelvic lymph node biopsy, bilateral salpingo-oophorectomy, total abdominal hysterectomy, partial vaginectomy

    _____

    _____

    _____

    _____

    C. ureteral catheterization, removal of ureteral calculus, cystourethroscopy

    _____

    _____

    _____

    _____

    D. open reduction and internal fixation of medial malleolus fracture, application of short leg cast, layer closure (intermediate repair) of laceration of knee, complex repair of laceration of thigh

    _____

    _____

    _____

    _____

13. Describe and summarize the notations concerning the reporting of the following surgical procedures located in the Integumentary System subsection of the Surgery section of the CPT volume:

    A. open wound repair _____

    _____

    B. debridement _____

    C. skin grafting _____

14. Describe and summarize the notations concerning the reporting of the following surgical procedures located in the Musculoskeletal System subsection of the Surgery section of the CPT volume:

    A. reduction of fracture _____

    B. reduction of dislocation _____

    C. application of cast _____

    D. application of traction device _____

15. Ascertain and record at least five descriptors that include a diagnostic indicator in the terminology of the descriptor among the listings of the Respiratory System subsection of the Surgery section of the CPT volume.

_____

_____

_____

_____

_____

16. Ascertain and record at least five descriptors that include a diagnostic indicator in the terminology of the descriptor among the listings of the Cardiovascular System subsection of the Surgery section of the CPT volume.

_____

_____

_____

_____

_____

17. Describe and summarize the notations regarding the reporting of the following surgical procedures located in the Cardiovascular System subsection of the Surgery section of the CPT volume:

    A. vascular catheterization _____

    B. vascular injection _____

18. Describe and summarize the notations regarding the reporting of the following surgical procedures located in the Urinary System subsection of the Surgery section of the CPT volume:

    A. urodynamics _____

    B. cystoscopy and urethroscopy _____

19. Explain the standard components of the following services:

    A. antepartum care _____

    _____

    B. delivery care _____

    _____

    C. postpartum care _____

    _____

20. Differentiate between the coding and reporting of obstetrical procedures and services in the physician's office setting from the coding and reporting of obstetrical procedures and services in the hospital setting. _____

    _____

    _____

21. Ascertain and record at least five descriptors that include a diagnostic indicator in the terminology of the descriptor among the listings of the Nervous System subsection of the Surgery section of the CPT volume.

    _____

    _____

    _____

    _____

    _____

22. Ascertain and record at least five descriptors that include a diagnostic indicator in the terminology of the descriptor among the listings of the Eye and Ocular Adnexa subsection of the Surgery section of the CPT volume.

    _____

    _____

    _____

    _____

    _____

23. Describe and summarize the notations regarding the reporting of the following ophthalmological procedures located in the Eye and Ocular Adnexa subsection of the Surgery section of the CPT volume:

    A. removal of cataract _____

    _____

    B. repair of retinal detachment _____

    _____

24. Identify any fraudulent or unethical conduct in the following scenarios:

    A. Gregory Bosich, a patient of Dr. Mundy, underwent outpatient surgery with general anesthesia administered for the excision of an area of alopecia from the scalp. As a consequence of this procedure, incidental scar tissue formation resulted, and the patient returned to the outpatient surgery center eight weeks afterward for scar revision of the scalp under local anesthesia. Both procedures, the excision of alopecia and the scar revision, were reported to the insurance carrier separately, as distinct and independent surgical packages. _____

    _____

    _____

B. Succeeding a comprehensive initial evaluation, Anita Hogan, a patient of Dr. Stokes, was rendered the radial keratotomy procedure to the left eye as an outpatient at an ophthalmology center. Two weeks later, she was rendered the radial keratotomy procedure to the right eye, again as an outpatient. Ten weeks subsequent to this latter surgery, she returned to the ophthalmology center for an enhancement of the corneal incisions on the right eye. The patient was billed individually for the initial assessment as well as for each of the three surgical procedures. _____

_____

C. Lawrence Makarian was diagnosed with hyperplasia of the prostate and scheduled for a cystourethroscopy and transurethral prostate resection. In the morning of the scheduled day of admission, however, he was transported to the emergency room with acute pain and diagnosed with ureterolithiasis. He underwent cystourethroscopy and stone extraction by Dr. Sanchez, the urology resident on call. Later that day, he underwent the scheduled cystourethroscopy and transurethral prostate resection by Dr. Kuntz. The surgical procedures performed by each of these physicians were reported to the Medicare carrier as two separate surgical packages. _____

_____

25. Assign precise, accurate code numbers from the CPT volume for the following surgical procedures and services on the integumentary system:

A. layer closure of 4-cm laceration of left foot _____

B. excision of ischial pressure ulcer with skin flap closure _____

C. insertion of tissue expander of scalp _____

D. correction of inverted nipples _____

E. blepharoplasty of upper eyelid _____

F. complex repair of 2-cm open wound of nose _____

G. shaving of 3-cm diameter dermal lesion of neck _____

H. destruction of 4-cm malignant lesion of back _____

I. incision and drainage of hematoma of forearm _____

J. modified radical mastectomy _____

K. split-thickness skin graft (50 sq cm) of upper arm _____

L. manual debridement of ten toenails _____

M. facial epidermal chemical peel _____

N. electrosurgical destruction of twenty-five fibrocutaneous tags _____

O. removal of mammary implant material _____

P. single pinch graft to cover small ulcer on tip of digit _____

Q. excision of 2.5-cm benign lesion of ear _____

R. excision trochanteric pressure ulcer with primary suture _____

S. escharotomy _____

T. suction assisted lipectomy of lower extremity _____

U. treatment of superficial wound dehiscence with packing _____

V. island pedicle flap _____

W. initial treatment of first degree burn _____

X. sectioning of flap at eyelids _____

Y. cervicoplasty _____

Z. repair of nail bed _____

26. Assign precise, accurate code numbers from the CPT volume for the following surgical procedures and services on the musculoskeletal system:

A. arthrodesis of shoulder joint with bone graft _____

B. radical resection of tumor of radius _____

C. drainage of complicated finger abscess _____

D. closed treatment of carpometacarpal dislocation of thumb with manipulation _____

E. closed reduction of proximal tibial plateau fracture without manipulation _____

F. percutaneous skeletal fixation of talus fracture with manipulation _____

G. surgical arthroscopy of the elbow with limited debridement _____

H. arthrotomy with drainage of hip for infection _____

I. excision of olecranon bursa _____

J. augmentation of the mandibular body with prosthetic material _____

K. partial claviculectomy _____

L. tendon sheath incision for trigger finger _____

M. application of patellar tendon bearing cast _____

N. invasive electrical stimulation to aid bone healing _____

O. reduction of forehead with contouring and setback of anterior frontal sinus wall _____

P. impression and custom preparation of auricular prosthesis _____

Q. coracoacromial ligament release with acromioplasty _____

R. radical ostectomy for tumor of proximal phalanx of finger _____

S. hemipatellectomy _____

T. curettage of bone cyst of talus _____

U. incision and drainage of infected bursa of wrist _____

V. osteoplasty for lengthening of metacarpal _____

W. decompression fasciotomy of posterior compartment of leg _____

X. tenodesis of biceps tendon at elbow _____

Y. adductor transfer to ischium _____

Z. wedging of clubfoot cast _____

27. Assign precise, accurate code numbers from the CPT volume for the following surgical procedures and services on the respiratory system:

A. limited thoracotomy for biopsy of pleura _____

B. intranasal maxillary sinusotomy _____

C. extensive excision of nasal polyps _____

D. repair of oronasal fistula _____

E. total extranasal ethmoidectomy _____

F. direct diagnostic laryngoscopy of newborn _____

G. diagnostic thoracoscopy of pericardial sac with biopsy _____

H. excision of thoracic tracheal carcinoma _____

_____

I. secondary (minor revision) rhinoplasty _____

_____

J. partial anterovertical laryngectomy _____

_____

K. percutaneous needle biopsy of lung _____

_____

L. emergency transtracheal tracheostomy _____

_____

M. lysis of intranasal synechia _____

_____

N. epiglottidectomy _____

_____

O. surgical thoracoscopy with segmental lobectomy _____

_____

P. pleural scarification for repeat pneumothorax _____

_____

Q. transglottic catheterization _____

_____

28. Assign precise, accurate code numbers from the CPT volume for the following surgical procedures and services on the cardiovascular system:

A. arterial catheterization for prolonged infusion therapy _____

_____

B. quadruple coronary artery bypass graft _____

_____

C. percutaneous transluminal peripheral atherectomy of iliac artery _____

_____

D. exploration of postoperative hemorrhage of chest _____

_____

E. removal of implantable intravenous infusion pump _____

_____

F. percutaneous transluminal balloon angioplasty of aorta _____

_____

G. pulmonary endarterectomy with cardiopulmonary bypass _____

_____

H. direct repair of intra-abdominal blood vessel _____

_____

I. suture repair of aorta with cardiopulmonary bypass _____

_____

J. division of aberrant vessel with reanastomosis _____

_____

K. femoral-popliteal vein bypass graft _____

_____

L. excision of pericardial cyst _____

_____

M. direct thrombectomy of subclavian vein by neck incision _____

_____

N. repair of cardiac wound with cardiopulmonary bypass _____

O. relocation of skin pocket for pacemaker _____

P. repair of sinus of Valsalva aneurysm _____

Q. thrombectomy with catheter of ulnar artery by arm incision _____

R. ilioiliac bypass graft with vein _____

S. banding of pulmonary artery _____

T. introduction of catheter into aorta _____

U. exploration with lysis of popliteal artery _____

V. ligation of external carotid artery _____

W. removal of permanent pacemaker pulse generator _____

X. replacement of implantable cardioverter-defibrillator (with sensing electrodes) by thoracotomy _____

Y. insertion of dual chamber pacemaker pulse generator _____

Z. insertion of permanent pacemaker with epicardial electrodes by xiphoid approach _____

29. Assign precise, accurate code numbers from the CPT volume for the following surgical procedures and services on the hemic and lymphatic systems:

A. biopsy of deep cervical lymph node _____

B. suprahyoid lymphadenectomy _____

C. autologous bone marrow transplantation _____

D. cannulation of thoracic duct _____

E. partial splenectomy _____

F. biopsy of deep cervical lymph node _____

30. Assign precise, accurate code numbers from the CPT volume for the following surgical procedures and services on the mediastinum and the diaphragm:

A. excision of mediastinal cyst _____

B. transthoracic repair of diaphragmatic hernia _____

C. repair of laceration of diaphragm _____

_____

D. mediastinoscopy with biopsy _____

E. median sternotomy for removal of foreign body _____

_____

F. imbrication of diaphragm for eventration _____

_____

31. Assign precise, accurate code numbers from the CPT volume for the following surgical procedures and services on the digestive system:

A. biopsy of floor of mouth _____

_____

B. flexible esophagoscopy with removal of foreign body _____

C. anterior gastropexy for hiatal hernia _____

_____

D. anoscopy with biopsy _____

_____

E. repair of recurrent and incarcerated femoral hernia _____

F. flexible sigmoidoscopy with decompression of volvulus _____

_____

G. esophagojejunostomy by thoracic approach _____

_____

H. continent ileostomy _____

_____

I. proctoplasty for prolapse of mucous membrane _____

_____

J. marsupialization of cyst of liver _____

_____

K. cholecystectomy with exploration of common duct _____

_____

L. percutaneous needle biopsy of pancreas _____

_____

M. drainage of retroperitoneal abscess _____

_____

N. vermilionectomy with mucosal advancement _____

_____

O. bilateral posterior vestibuloplasty _____

_____

P. suture of laceration of pharynx _____

_____

Q. appendectomy for ruptured appendix with generalized peritonitis _____

_____

R. injection of sclerosing solution for hemorrhoids _____

_____

S. excision of ampulla of Vater _____

_____

    T. repair of recurrent reducible incarcerated incisional hernia _____

    U. revision of peritoneal venous shunt _____

    V. external drainage of pseudocyst of pancreas _____

    W. flexible sigmoidoscopy with biopsy _____

    X. division of stricture of rectum _____

    Y. percutaneous cholecystostomy _____

    Z. removal of pancreatic calculus _____

32. Assign precise, accurate code numbers from the CPT volume for the following surgical procedures and services on the urinary system:

    A. partial cystectomy _____

    B. urethral catheterization _____

    C. transvesical ureterolithotomy _____

    D. ureteroneocystostomy _____

    E. urethral pressure profile studies _____

    F. cystourethroscopy with insertion of indwelling ureteral stent _____

    G. drainage of deep periurethral abscess _____

    H. transurethral resection of postoperative bladder neck contracture _____

    I. closure of cystostomy _____

    J. ureterectomy with bladder cuff _____

    K. excision of perinephric cyst _____

    L. change of cystostomy tube _____

    M. transurethral drainage of prostatic abscess _____

    N. aspiration of bladder by trocar _____

    O. closure of vesicouterine fistula _____

    P. cystourethroscopy with bilateral ureteral meatotomy _____

Q. removal of perineal prosthesis introduced for continence _____

_____

33. Assign precise, accurate code numbers from the CPT volume for the following surgical procedures and services on the male genital system:

A. insertion of inflatable penile prosthesis _____

_____

B. excision of spermatocele _____

_____

C. radical orchiectomy by inguinal approach _____

_____

D. retropubic radical prostatectomy with lymph node biopsy _____

_____

E. drainage of scrotal wall abscess _____

_____

F. plastic operation on penis to correct angulation _____

_____

G. bilateral epididymectomy _____

_____

H. reduction of torsion of testis with fixation of contralateral testis _____

_____

I. unilateral excision of hydrocele of spermatic cord _____

_____

J. complicated vesiculotomy _____

_____

K. needle biopsy of prostate _____

_____

L. slitting of lateral prepuce for newborn _____

_____

M. radical perineal prostatectomy _____

_____

34. Assign precise, accurate code numbers from the CPT volume for the following laparoscopic and peritoneoscopic procedures and services:

A. surgical laparotomy for cholecystectomy with cholangiography _____

_____

B. peritoneoscopy with biopsy _____

_____

C. surgical hysteroscopy for removal of leiomyomata _____

_____

D. surgical laparoscopy for lysis of adhesions _____

_____

E. surgical laparoscopy for repair of recurrent inguinal hernia _____

_____

F. surgical laparoscopy for appendectomy _____

_____

35. Assign precise, accurate code numbers from the CPT volume for the following surgical procedures and services on the female genital system:

A. pelvic examination under anesthesia _____

_____

B. nonobstetrical cerclage of uterine cervix _____

_____

C. lysis of labial adhesions _____

_____

D. plastic repair of introitus _____

_____

E. bilateral ovarian cystectomy _____

_____

F. cauterization of cervix by laser ablation _____

_____

G. colpocentesis _____

_____

H. vaginal hysterectomy with bilateral removal of tubes and ovaries _____

_____

I. drainage of ovarian abscess by vaginal approach _____

_____

J. bilateral total oophorectomy _____

_____

K. nonobstetrical repair of ruptured uterus _____

_____

L. fimbrioplasty _____

_____

M. vaginoscopy with biopsy of cervix _____

_____

36. Assign precise, accurate code numbers from the CPT volume for the following maternity care and delivery procedures and services:

A. postpartum curettage _____

_____

B. hysterorrhaphy of ruptured uterus _____

_____

C. cesarean delivery including postpartum care _____

_____

D. vaginal delivery including postpartum care _____

_____

E. chorionic villus sampling _____

_____

F. insertion of cervical dilator _____

_____

G. amniocentesis _____

_____

H. uterine evacuation and curettage for hydatidiform mole _____

_____

I. delivery of placenta as separate procedure _____

_____

J. episiotomy by physician other than attending _____

_____

K. fetal scalp blood sampling _____

_____

L. intrauterine cordocentesis _____

_____

M. abdominal hysterotomy _____

_____

37. Assign precise, accurate code numbers from the CPT volume for the following surgical procedures and services on the endocrine system:

A. partial thymectomy _____

_____

B. secondary thyroidectomy _____

_____

C. excision of recurrent thyroglossal duct cyst _____

_____

D. subtotal thyroidectomy _____

_____

E. total thyroidectomy with radical neck dissection _____

_____

F. parathyroid autotransplantation _____

_____

38. Assign precise, accurate code numbers from the CPT volume for the following surgical procedures and services on the nervous system:

A. removal of prosthetic plate of skull _____

_____

B. repair of 6-cm diameter meningocele _____

_____

C. suture of posterior tibial nerve _____

_____

D. replacement of lumbosubarachnoid shunt _____

_____

E. transection of pudendal nerve _____

_____

F. craniectomy for osteomyelitis _____

_____

G. irrigation of ventricular catheter _____

_____

H. laminectomy with rhizotomy (more than two segments) _____

_____

I. injection of anesthetic agent into stellate ganglion _____

_____

J. neuroplasty of ulnar nerve at wrist _____

_____

K. second stage nerve pedicle transfer _____

_____

L. percutaneous implantation of neurostimulator electrodes into peripheral nerve _____

M. craniectomy for craniosynostosis _____

_____

N. extradural resection of neoplastic lesion of base of anterior cranial fossa _____

_____

O. stereotactic focused proton beam or gamma radiosurgery _____

P. percutaneous aspiration procedure of nucleus pulposus of lumbar intervertebral disk ___

Q. laminectomy with release of tethered lumbar spinal cord _____

R. injection of anesthetic agent into axillary nerve _____

S. cervicothoracic sympathectomy _____

T. 5-cm single-strand nerve graft to foot _____

U. stereotactic implantation of depth electrodes into cerebrum for long-term seizure monitoring _____

V. ventriculocisternostomy of third ventricle _____

W. ligation of carotid artery in petrous canal with repair by anastomosis _____

X. removal of intracranial neurostimulator electrodes _____

Y. exploration of orbit with removal of lesion _____

Z. laminectomy with drainage of intramedullary cyst to peritoneal space _____

39. Assign precise, accurate code numbers from the CPT volume for the following surgical procedures and services on the eye and ocular adnexa:

A. trabeculotomy ab externo _____

B. iridectomy by laser surgery _____

C. biopsy of conjunctiva _____

D. removal of embedded foreign body of eyelid _____

E. strabismus surgery involving repair of detached extraocular muscle _____

F. lamellar corneal transplant _____

G. repair of ectropion by thermocauterization _____

H. discission of secondary membranous cataract by laser surgery _____

I. modification of ocular implant _____

J. excision of lesion of sclera _____

K. repair of retinal detachment by diathermy _____

L. revision of aqueous shunt to extraocular reservoir _____

_____

M. bilateral probing of nasolacrimal duct with irrigation _____

_____

N. epikeratoplasty _____

_____

O. removal of intraocular foreign body from lens _____

_____

P. repair of scleral staphyloma with graft _____

_____

Q. optic nerve decompression _____

_____

40. Assign precise, accurate code numbers from the CPT volume for the following surgical procedures and services on the auditory system:

A. modified radical mastoidectomy _____

_____

B. biopsy of external auditory canal _____

_____

C. revision of fenestration operation _____

_____

D. stapes mobilization _____

_____

E. tympanic neurectomy _____

_____

F. otoplasty of protruding ear _____

_____

G. ear piercing _____

_____

H. transnasal Eustachian tube inflation with catheterization _____

_____

I. drainage of abscess of external auditory canal _____

_____

J. myringotomy with aspiration _____

_____

K. implantation of electromagnetic bone conduction hearing device in temporal bone _____

_____

L. transcanal labyrinthectomy with mastoidectomy _____

_____

M. decompression of internal auditory canal _____

_____

CODING OF CLINICAL DOCUMENTATION — SURGERY SECTION OF THE CPT VOLUME

Read the following operative reports and assign precise, accurate code numbers from the Surgery section of the CPT volume. If applicable, differentiate variations in code numbers reportable by physicians from variations in code numbers reportable by hospitals.

OPERATIVE REPORT

PATIENT: Harding, Aaron   **MR#:** 99-13-01

SURGEON: Bailey   **ASSISTANT:** Duvall

Preoperative Diagnosis:
Posttraumatic arthritis, right knee.

Postoperative Diagnosis:
Posttraumatic arthritis, right knee with partial thickness cartilaginous loss of the patella.

Operation:
Arthroscopy with patellar debridement.

Brief Clinical History:
This is a 31-year-old white male status post right femur fracture that subsequently healed in the shortened position. The patient underwent femoral lengthening procedure and has been doing well except for complaints of leg length inequality and knee pain. Radiographs revealed that there is not a significant leg length discrepancy, however, the patient's knee pain persisted. Therefore, a decision was made to perform arthroscopy on the patient.

Operative Procedure:
Following satisfactory induction of general endotracheal anesthesia, the patient was placed in the supine position on the operating table and his right lower extremity was prepped and draped in the usual sterile fashion.

The usual portals were made for arthroscopy, including medial inflow portal, superior and medial to the patella, and the lateral scope portal, just lateral to the patellar tendon at the joint line. The patellofemoral joint was then observed and the patient was noted to have partial thickness cartilage loss on the undersurface of the patella. The medial gutter was then scoped and the medial joint entered in this fashion. The medial meniscus was noted to be intact. A second medial portal was made after an initial attempt was too close to the patellar tendon. This second portal was just medial to the first. The medial meniscus was once again probed and noted to be intact. The cartilage of the medial compartment was noted to be in good shape. The lateral compartment was also scoped and the meniscus was noted to be intact and the cartilage was noted to be in fairly good condition. Attention was once again turned to the patellofemoral joint. A fourth portal was made lateral and superior to the patellar tendon for introduction of the shaver. The cartilaginous lesion was then shaved and debrided. The cartilage was noted to be quite soft. Following this, the knee was irrigated with several hundred cc's of irrigant. The knee was then injected with 80 mg of Kenalog and 10 cc of Marcaine.

Following this, the C-arm was brought in and a screw was placed in the intercondylar region to reattach the lateral collateral ligament, identified and located using biplanar fluoroscopy. A 3-cm incision was made on the lateral aspect of the knee and carried down sharply through the subcutaneous tissue and fascia lata down to the bone. The screw was localized and removed along with its washer. The wound was irrigated and closed with nylon in the skin. Sterile dressing was then applied to the knee and the patient was awakened, extubated, and taken to the recovery room in good condition.

Codes: _____

OPERATIVE REPORT

PATIENT: Feldhaus, Douglas   **MR#:** 99-13-02

SURGEON: Hernandez   **ASSISTANT:** Jezik

Preoperative Diagnosis:
Right zygomatic arch fracture.

Postoperative Diagnosis:
Right zygomatic arch fracture.

Operation:
Open reduction of right zygomatic arch fracture.

Indications and Clinical History:
This young male has a history of assault approximately ten days ago resulting in a depressed right zygomatic arch fracture. He has no trismus, but desires elevation of the arch fracture for cosmetic purposes.

Operative Procedure:
The patient was brought to the OR and placed in the supine position on the operating table. After adequate induction of general endotracheal anesthesia, the right face was prepped and draped in the usual sterile fashion and hair was clipped from the right frontotemporal region. A small horizontal incision was made in the hairline and carried down until the temporalis fascia was reached. Hemostasis was achieved with Bovie electrocautery. Next the temporalis fascia was transected with a #15 blade and a Goldman elevator was passed under the fascia down to the zygomatic arch. The zygomatic arch was raised with a Goldman and a Gilles elevator until adequate contour was achieved. Multiple fragments were present and the arch did collapse somewhat after elevation. The fragments were considered to be stable and the procedure was terminated. The skin incision was closed using 3-0 Vicryl. The subcutaneous tissue was closed with 5-0 Prolene. Polysporin was applied to the wound and a styrofoam cup cut in half was placed over the zygoma for protection in the postoperative field.

Codes: _____

OPERATIVE REPORT

PATIENT: Weber, Jane   **MR#:** 99-13-03

SURGEON: Shaw   **ASSISTANT:** Ferrara

Preoperative Diagnosis:
Vulvovaginal condyloma.

Postoperative Diagnosis:
Vulvar, perirectal, and periclitoral condyloma.

Procedure:
Laser surgery to perineum.

Brief Clinical History:
The patient is a 20-year-old white female, gravida 0, who has several month history of condyloma refractory to both Podophyllin and TCA.

Description of Procedure:
The patient was brought to the OR where she was administered a general anesthesia and then placed in the dorsal lithotomy position. The physical examination rendered at that time revealed no lesions of the cervix or the vagina. However, lesions were noted in the periclitoral area, along the right and left labia, and in the perirectal region. She was then draped with wet towels and the CO_2 laser was set on 10 continuous beam. Starting superiorly, the lesions were cauterized with the laser down to the reticular layer just beneath the epidermis. This was carried out all the way down to the perirectal area covering all lesions. No hemorrhoids were noted. Several small bleeders were noted during the procedure. The beam was simply defocused and these were easily coagulated. After they were burned, the lesions were wiped with acetic acid. All were found to be treated and beneath skin level by the end of the procedure. She was awakened from general anesthesia without difficulty.

Codes: _____

OPERATIVE REPORT

PATIENT: Shelton, Louise   **MR#:** 99-13-04

SURGEON: Winters   **ASSISTANT:** Holmes

Preoperative Diagnosis:
Peritonitis, possible free air.

Postoperative Diagnosis:
Volvulus of mid small intestine with total proximal obstruction and perforation, gross peritoneal sepsis, hemorrhage from liver surface secondary to disruption of adhesions.

Operation:
Resection small bowel and extensive adhesiolysis.

Relevant Clinical History:
The patient is a 33-year-old black female who was 17 weeks pregnant and presented to the hospital with abdominal distention. She was seen initially by the OB/GYN service on the day of admission with vague lower abdominal pain, which was paraumbilical in nature and radiated down to both lower quadrants. The examination at that time was unremarkable for a WBC of 7600. The patient was admitted to the OB/GYN service for observation and rehydration. A surgery consultation was obtained. The patient was afebrile with a temperature of 37.5. The abdominal examination revealed a distended tympanic abdomen without bowel sounds. There was bilateral minimal lower quadrant tenderness without rebound. The rectal examination revealed heme negative stool and no tenderness. Bimanual examination revealed no masses. During the following two days, the patient continued to complain of diffuse abdominal pain. The patient was prepared for surgery because of continued severe pain and a WBC elevation to 30000. A repeat WBC just prior to surgery revealed that the WBC had decreased to 14000. The patient's examination remained equivocal and the plans to take the patient to the OR for appendectomy were deferred.

The next day, the patient was feeling better. Her abdominal pain, nausea, and vomiting appeared to resolve with nasogastric suctioning. The patient continued to be followed by the Surgery service. A left upper quadrant and a right upper quadrant ultrasound were obtained in order to investigate the possibility of a pseudocyst that may have developed due to prior abdominal trauma that she has experienced. The ultrasounds were negative. The patient continued to complain of abdominal pain. The evening of that day she had a spontaneous breech delivery of a nonviable infant. The next morning, the patient became hypotensive with a blood pressure of 60/40. Her WBC was 13700, and an obstructive series was obtained which revealed the presence of free air. Given the patient's marked change in clinical status to one of diffuse pain with distention, leukocytosis, and possible free air, the patient was taken to the OR for emergency exploration.

Operative Procedure:
The patient was brought to the OR and placed on the operating table in the supine position. General endotracheal anesthesia was induced. The patient's abdomen was prepped and draped in the usual sterile fashion. The abdomen was entered through a midline incision. Immediately upon entering the abdomen, gross, foul-smelling pus was detected. Aerobic and anaerobic cultures were sent. The abdomen was thoroughly explored. There were dense adhesions between loops of small bowel. In the distal jejunum and proximal ileum, a segment of small bowel was detected with a volvulus and a perforation. This twisted loop of small bowel was totally necrotic and gelatinous. The proximal bowel was massively distended. The distal bowel was collapsed. The uterus was moderately enlarged. The tubes and ovaries appeared edematous and had a gray discoloration to them. There was also a gray discoloration on the surface of the mesentery of the right colon and on the right colon itself. The descending colon similarly had this grayish discoloration on the exposed surface. The transverse colon appeared grossly normal. The right and left colons were thoroughly mobilized. The retroperitoneal surfaces of each were noted to be pink and clearly viable. Removal of the peritoneum, which was affected by this gray discoloration, revealed underlying viable large bowel on both the right and left sides. The appendix was normal.

After an extensive adhesiolysis of the small bowel, the area of the small bowel volvulus was totally resected and submitted to pathology. A side-to-side functional end-to-end stapled anastomosis was performed between the remaining ends after the sulcus entericus of the proximal bowel had been removed by suction. The bowel was then irrigated until clear with copious amounts of sterile Saline and then with an antibiotic containing normal Saline. The abdomen was reexamined. Dense adhesions were noted between the surface of the liver and the anterior abdominal wall, which were taken down bluntly. Hemorrhage started and was difficult to control. The blood loss at this point in the operation had been 800 cc's. Bleeding was subsequently controlled using compression packs soaked with thrombin. Before adequate hemostasis was obtained, an additional 1200 cc's of blood was lost. During the period of hemorrhage, the patient's blood pressure, which had been very stable at about 120 mm of Mercury, dropped momentarily to 98 mm Mercury. The BP was quickly restored with blood transfusion, as well as with low dose Dopamine. When hemostasis appeared to be adequate, the abdomen was closed with towel clips and covered with a sterile towel and a large iodine impregnated biodrape. The patient will be brought back to the OR in two days for reexamination of her abdomen. The hematocrit at the end of the case, after transfusion of a total of eight units of blood, was 42%. The patient was taken from the OR, still intubated, with a BP of 110. The sponge and instrument count at the end of the procedure was incorrect, with the presence of three laparotomy sponges remaining in the abdomen.

Codes: _____

OPERATIVE REPORT

PATIENT: Russell, Paul   **MR#:** 99-13-05

SURGEON: Milton   **ASSISTANT:** Kirsch

Preoperative Diagnosis:
Left hemiscrotal mass.

Postoperative Diagnosis:
Left hemiscrotal mass.

Operation:
Excision of left hemiscrotal mass.

Brief Clinical History:
The patient is a 42-year-old white male with a hard, palpable left hemiscrotal mass that he noticed increasing over the past year or so. The lesion is painless. The patient had the tumor markers alpha fetoprotein and Beta HCG measured, and these are within normal limits. The patient's testicular sonogram shows the mass to be completely separate from the testicle and his physical examination indicates the same.

Procedure:
The patient was brought to the OR and had general anesthesia induced. He was prepped and draped in the usual sterile fashion for scrotal surgery.

An incision was made in the scrotum approximately 2 cm in length. The incision was carried down through the dartos layer and on down into the tunica vaginalis. The incision cut down right to the scrotal mass. The mass and testicle were both delivered out of the scrotal wound. The mass was noted to be adherent to the tail of the epididymis. The mass was removed from the epididymis using sharp and blunt dissection, and the Bovie cautery was used to control any small bleeding blood vessels. The mass was handed off the field once it was removed from the epididymis and pathology bisected it. Satisfied that there were no more bleeders along the epididymis where the dissection took place, the scrotum was closed, closing the dartos layer with a running 3-0 chromic stitch. The scrotal skin was closed with a running 3-0 chromic stitch. The scrotum was then wrapped with a turban type dressing and a scrotal support was applied.

The mass was opened by pathology in the OR and was a very well-circumscribed lesion that appeared to have a capsule around it. The inside of the mass was a fleshy, white color with a hard texture that appeared to have concentric rings. The sponge and needle counts were correct at the end of the case. The patient tolerated the procedure very well. The patient was awakened and taken to the recovery room.

Codes: _____

OPERATIVE REPORT

PATIENT: Goodman, Robert   **MR#:** 99-13-06

SURGEONS: Thompson & Fox   **ASSISTANTS:** Lemanski & McNamara

Preoperative Diagnosis:
Pituitary adenoma.

Postoperative Diagnosis:
Pituitary adenoma.

Operation:
Excision of pituitary adenoma by sublabial transphenoidal transseptal approach.

Procedure:
The patient had been previously anesthetized and placed in the neurosurgical head holder. The anterior nares were inspected and two neurosurgical Cottonoids impregnated with a 4% Cocaine solution were placed into the anterior nasal chambers bilaterally. The anterior nasal septum, floor of the nose, and premaxillary area were infiltrated with approximately 8 cc of 2% Xylocaine with Epinephrine 1:100000. The face and abdomen were then prepped and draped in the usual manner. A left anterior hemitransfixion incision was performed and an anteroposterior mucoperichondrial and mucoperiosteal tunnel were created on the left. There was marked dislocation of the quadrilateral cartilage with fragmentation and multiple dense adhesions along the floor of the nose and anteriorly along the previous septal fracture line. Using blunt and sharp dissection, the adhesions were lysed. Several small fenestrae were created along the inferior ridge and anteriorly. A right posterior mucoperiosteal tunnel was created after disarticulating the quadrilateral cartilage. An inferior floor of the nose tunnel on the left was created using a Freer elevator. Due to the extreme deformity of the nasal cartilage, essentially submucous resection of quadrilateral cartilage and radical bony septectomy was performed. Thereafter, the remaining quadrilateral cartilage could be displaced from the maxillary crest into the right nasal chamber. A retrograde dissection was performed and an inferior tunnel on the right created. There was a large maxillary crest spur that was removed with a chisel. The face of the maxilla was then dissected beneath the piriform aperture. The anterior nasal spine was identified and removed with a Jansen-Middleton. Attention was turned to the anterior gingival labial sulcus. Incision was performed from the left canine fossa to the contralateral canine fossa. Mucoperiosteum overlying the premaxilla was incised and the previously encountered dissection plane was found. Then the Hardy was placed sublabially and used to visualize the face of the sphenoid. The mucoperiosteum was cleaned off of the face of the sphenoid. The sphenoid sinus ostea was identified and small anterior fenestrae were created in the face of the sphenoid. Thereafter, Dr. Forsyth enlarged the sphenotomy and completed his portion of the procedure to be dictated separately. Following removal of the adenoma and packing of the sphenoid sinus, the wound was closed. Several fenestrae of the mucoperichondrial tunnel were closed with interrupted sutures of 3-0 chromic. The septum was quilted with interrupted sutures of 4-0 chromic. Then two interrupted sutures of Vicryl were placed in the columella and lateral alar areas to prevent collapse of the nose on the face of the premaxilla. The sublabial incision was then closed with interrupted sutures of 3-0 chromic and bilateral intranasal trumpets were placed along with Telfa packing. The patient was uneventfully awakened from general anesthesia and removed to the recovery room in stable condition.

Codes: _____

OPERATIVE REPORT

PATIENT: Gebhardt, Ruth   **MR#:** 99-13-07

SURGEON: Kelly   **ASSISTANT:** Shapiro

Preoperative Diagnosis:
Diffuse lymphadenopathy, unknown etiology.

Postoperative Diagnosis:
Lymphoma, pathology pending.

Operation:
Biopsy of right supraclavicular lymph node.

Brief Clinical History:
The patient is a 61-year-old white female who presents with a one-month history of diffuse lymphadenopathy, most prominent in the cervical and supraclavicular areas.

Operative Note:
The patient was brought to the OR and placed in the supine position on the operating room table in the usual manner. She was then prepped and draped in sterile fashion over the right supraclavicular area.

The superficial lymph node just above the right clavicle was chosen for biopsy. 1% Lidocaine was used to infuse over the lymph node and a #15 blade was used to make an approximately 3-cm incision over the node. Then the #15 blade was used to dissect down to the subcutaneous tissue and a Bovie was used for hemostasis. Dissection was carried down through the platysma muscle and tenotomy scissors were used to dissect above the lymph node. The lymph node was then pulled up into the wound with a pair of DeBakey forceps. After this was completed, a mosquito was used to grip down under the base of the lymph node, and tenotomy scissors were used to cut down on top of the mosquito. This was repeated three times until the lymph node was removed out of the wound and sent to pathology for sectioning. Next the pedicle of the lymph node was tied off with 3-0 silk. The wound was then copiously irrigated and hemostasis was maintained with electrocautery. The wound was closed with 3-0 Vicryl times three simple sutures, and the skin was closed with a running 4-0 Vicryl subcuticular. Steri-strips and a sterile dressing were applied. The patient tolerated the procedure without complications and was transferred to the postanesthesia recovery area in stable condition. Blood loss was minimal and no fluids were administered.

Codes: _____

OPERATIVE REPORT

PATIENT: Massey, Joseph   **MR#:** 99-13-08

SURGEON: Payne   **ASSISTANT:** Garrett

Preoperative Diagnosis:
Right medial meniscus tear.

Postoperative Diagnosis:
Healed medial meniscus repair with no new tear.

Operation:
Arthroscopy, right knee.

Indications:
This patient is a young male who is status post medial meniscus repair about three months ago. He has been doing well but began having recurrent pain. He has clicking and popping in his knee and pain that was similar to his original pain before the meniscal repair. A tentative diagnosis of failed meniscus repair was made and the patient was brought to the OR for exploration and treatment.

Description of Procedure:
The patient was brought to the OR and placed on the operating table in the supine position. After the satisfactory induction of general endotracheal anesthesia, a right thigh tourniquet

was placed and the patient was placed in the arthroscopy leg holder. His knee, leg, and foot were prepped and draped in the usual sterile fashion.

The old arthroscopy portal was used, making a superior medial inflow portal and then an inferior anterolateral arthroscopy portal. The patellofemoral joint was visualized and there was no fraying. The cartilage looked good. Next the medial gutter was exposed and there was no evidence of any foreign body or any abnormalities of the medial gutter. Next the medial joint and the area where the meniscal repair was made were examined. The anterior cruciate ligament and notch were examined and there were no abnormalities. The lateral meniscus also had no abnormalities upon exploration of the lateral joint compartment. A medial portal was made with an 18-gauge needle under direct visualization. The medial meniscus was probed. The meniscus could not be displaced into the joint and did not show any evidence of tear. A grabber was used to pull the meniscus into the joint and to dislodge it, and bring it into the joint. There was no evidence of any tear. The lateral meniscus was similarly probed and there was no tear. The joint was irrigated. The arthroscope was removed. The cannula for the inflow was used to extract the water out of the knee. A single 4-0 nylon stitch was made in each portal. Then 15 cc's of Marcaine and 40 mg of Kenalog were injected into the knee joint. Dry, sterile dressings were applied and he was taken to the recovery room in stable condition. The sponge, needle, and instrument counts were correct.

Codes: _____

OPERATIVE REPORT

PATIENT: Riggins, Dale   **MR#:** 99-13-09

SURGEON: Watkins   **ASSISTANT:** Graham

Preoperative Diagnosis:
Left testicular torsion.

Postoperative Diagnosis:
Same with viable testes.

Operation:
Scrotal exploration, detorsion of left testis, and bilateral orchiopexy.

Description of Procedure:
The patient was brought to the OR and general endotracheal anesthesia was induced. The patient was prepped and draped in the usual sterile fashion. A midline scrotal incision was made. The left testis was then delivered through the dartos tissue after sharp dissection, and a single torsion of the testis was noted with the typical bell clapper deformity. This was detorsed. The testis was noted to be quite viable and therefore without further delay it was pexed into place with two 2-0 silk sutures to the dartos fibers. Exploration of the contralateral testis revealed a normal testis again with bell clapper deformity. This was similarly pexed with two 2-0 sutures. They were dropped back into the cavity. The dartos was loosely approximated with 3-0 chromic sutures. The skin was approximated with 4-0 chromic sutures. Scrotal suspensory and fluff dressing were applied. The patient was taken to the floor in stable condition without apparent intraoperative complications. The final needle and sponge counts were correct. There were no drains.

Codes: _____

OPERATIVE REPORT

PATIENT: Zimmer, Margaret   **MR#:** 99-13-10

SURGEON: Bachmann   **ASSISTANT:** Novak

Preoperative Diagnosis:
Submucosal lesion, left cheek.

Postoperative Diagnosis:
Submucosal lesion, left cheek.

Operation:
Transoral excision of submucosal lesion, left cheek.

Indications:
This is a 35-year-old female who has noticed a mass in the right cheek for several months. On physical examination, the patient was found to have a 1.5-cm firm mass in the submucosal area of the left anterior buccal gingival sulcus, just distal and inferior to the left oral commissure. This mass was completely mobile and free from the mandible and the mucosa overlying the mass appeared to be normal. The skin on the outside also appeared to be normal. The patient had no other intraoral lesions. There was no adenopathy noted anywhere in the neck or the parotid gland.

Procedure:
With the patient in the supine position, the head slightly elevated, the area of the mass was injected using 1% Lidocaine and 1:100000 Epinephrine circumferentially through the transoral route. Under satisfactory anesthesia, the mucosa overlying the mass was incised. Using sharp and blunt dissection, the mass was easily excised, leaving a cuff or buccal sac overlying it. It was removed in its entirety and handed off to pathology. The area was then inspected and hemostasis obtained. While still on the table, the patient was asked to animate the mouth, both in the smiling and frowning modes, and nerve function appeared completely intact. The mucosa was then closed using locking running sutures with 4-0 chromic material. The patient was then asked to rinse her mouth out with Listerine. The patient tolerated the procedure without any incident.

Codes: _____

OPERATIVE REPORT

PATIENT: Burke, Norman   **MR#:** 99-13-11

SURGEON: Dvorak   **ASSISTANT:** Keller

Preoperative Diagnosis:
Intermittent atrial flutter and atrial fibrillation with severe ventricular bradycardia.

Postoperative Diagnosis:
Intermittent atrial flutter and atrial fibrillation with severe ventricular bradycardia.

Operation:
Implantation of permanent transvenous cardiac pacemaker (Medtronic model 5985).

Clinical History:
Patient was admitted with episodes of atrial flutter and atrial fibrillation with very slow ventricular response (in the low 40's). Patient was entirely uncooperative and combative during the course of the operation. Five staff members were needed to hold him on the cath table. In addition, his heart rate was between 140 and 180. He has very small veins in the region of the deltapectoral groove. All of these problems led to great difficulty in the insertion of this pacemaker. However, the electrode was finally positioned in the apex of the right ventricle, with an assumably satisfactory threshold. It appeared that the threshold was an MA of 0.8, voltage 0.5 with resistance of 610 ohms. R-wave sensitivity was 7.3.

Procedure:
With the patient in the supine position, the right pectoral region was prepped and draped in the usual fashion. As mentioned above, the patient was entirely combative and uncooperative, with five people needed to hold him down. After satisfactory local anesthesia and regional anesthesia were induced, a transverse incision was made and the deltapectoral groove was dissected. One vein appeared to be slightly larger than the rest of the very small venules in this area and it was cannulated with a cardiac electrode, which with some difficulty was put into the apex of the right ventricle under fluoroscopic control. As mentioned above, the patient's threshold appeared to be satisfactory, though this was not entirely certain. Electrode was ligated in place with heavy silk, after which it was attached to the Medtronic pacemaker model 5985. The unit was implanted into the subcutaneous pocket. It should be noted that the patient has practically no subcutaneous fat, so that only a very, very thin layer of subcutaneous tissue and skin overlies the pacemaker. The wound was closed in two layers. Dressings were applied, and the patient was taken back to his room.

Codes: _____

OPERATIVE REPORT

PATIENT: Fuller, Jerry   **MR#:** 99-13-12

SURGEON: Pierce   **ASSISTANT:** Shah

Preoperative Diagnosis:
Supraumbilical ventral hernia.

Postoperative Diagnosis:
Supraumbilical ventral hernia.

Operation:
Supraumbilical ventral hernia repair.

Brief Clinical History:
The patient is a 41-year-old black male with a history of alcoholic liver disease, who presented with complaint of a protruding mass above his umbilicus. He reports that the mass is especially prominent after meals. It is only slightly tender and it is always reducible. The patient also has a history of right inguinal hernia repair and still has a left inguinal hernia, which will be repaired at a later date.

Description of Procedure:

The patient was brought to the OR, and after the induction of spinal anesthesia, was placed in the supine position. His abdomen was prepped and draped. An approximately 4-cm midline incision was made just superior to the umbilicus overlying a quarter-sized midline palpable defect with a slight bulge. Once beyond the dermis, the hernia sac was evident. Bovie cautery was used to continue to complete the opening of the dermal layer. Then blunt dissection combined with Bovie cautery was used to free up the hernia sac from the surrounding fascia. With this complete, the hernia sac was incised. There were no fixed contents within the sac. A small amount of free peritoneal fluid was seen within the abdomen, but there was no free-flowing fluid exiting the opened hernia sac. The sac was put on tension and amputated. Hemostasis was achieved with Bovie cautery. The skin flaps were elevated in all directions above the fascial layer. The fascial layer was closed with four interrupted 3-0 Vicryl sutures. The wound was then irrigated and the skin was closed with vertical mattress 3-0 Nylon sutures. Betadine ointment was then applied and the wound was covered with a dry, sterile dressing. The patient was taken to the recovery room in satisfactory condition.

Codes: _____

OPERATIVE REPORT

PATIENT: Chen, Lucy **MR#:** 99-13-13

SURGEON: Vaughn **ASSISTANT:** O'Reilly

Preoperative Diagnosis:
Status post colostomy secondary to gunshot wound.

Postoperative Diagnosis:
Same.

Operation:
Take down of loop colostomy.

Description of Procedure:

The patient was brought to the OR and placed in the supine position. The abdomen was prepped with Betadine and draped in a sterile fashion. Ostomy was taken down with blunt and sharp dissection. Once the colon was mobilized, a GIA stapler was used to connect the ostomy and the mucous fistula assuring that the mesentery was not in the anastomosis site. The end of the mucous fistula and ostomy were then closed with a GIA stapler. The distal ostomy was sent to pathology. Hemostasis was assured with electrocautery and Lembert sutures inverted the anastomosis. There was no significant bleeding. The fascial opening was extended medially and laterally in order to easily pass the bowel back into the peritoneum. Hemostasis was then assured with electrocautery and the posterior fascia was reapproximated with two figure-eight 1-0 Prolene sutures. The anterior fascia was then also reapproximated with two figure-eight 1-0 Prolene sutures. The wound packed with Saline soaked fine mesh gauze. The patient tolerated the procedure well and was discharged to the floor.

Codes: _____

OPERATIVE REPORT

PATIENT: Knight, Catherine   **MR#:** 99-13-14

SURGEON: Hodges   **ASSISTANT:** Newman

Preoperative Diagnosis:
Gallstone pancreatitis.

Peripancreatic fluid collections.

Postoperative Diagnosis:
Gallstone pancreatitis.

Peritoneal adhesions.

Omental fat necrosis.

Operation:
Cholecystectomy.

Intraoperative cholangiogram.

Anesthesia:
General endotracheal.

Indications for Operation:
The patient is a 38-year-old white female with a history of intravenous drug abuse and depression, who presented six weeks ago to the medical service, febrile and with abdominal pain. Ultrasound demonstrated gallstones with a normal common bile duct. The patient began to develop a fulminant pancreatitis with an extensive pancreatic phlegmon. She was treated with intravenous antibiotics and total parenteral nutrition. She remained persistently febrile with white blood counts in the 200.0 range. Repeat CT scan demonstrated the formation of several large fluid collections. Percutaneous aspiration of this fluid remained sterile. The patient failed to improve and was therefore admitted for drainage of these fluid collections. The bilirubin was 3 and alkaline phosphatase was 250. These elevations were attributed to the presence of pancreatitis.

Description of Operative Procedure:
The patient was sterilely prepped and draped in the supine position after induction of satisfactory general endotracheal anesthesia. The abdomen was entered through an upper midline incision. There were multiple filmy adhesions between the small bowel and the anterior peritoneum, which were manually broken to develop the peritoneal cavity. In the superior aspect of the incision, anterior to the liver and stomach, there was a large fluid collection palpable. Besides the presence of the previously mentioned fresh and moist adhesions, there was also fat necrosis in the omentum and in the region of the pancreatic head.

Codes: _____

OPERATIVE REPORT

PATIENT: Pittman, Richard   **MR#:** 99-13-15

SURGEON: Collins   **ASSISTANT:** Freeman

Preoperative Diagnosis:
Gynecomastia.

Postoperative Diagnosis:
Gynecomastia.

Operation:
Bilateral simple mastectomy.

Brief Clinical History:
The patient is a 20-year-old black male with an approximate six-year history of bilateral breast enlargement, who presents now requesting simple bilateral mastectomy for removal of gynecomastia.

Description of Procedure:
The patient was brought into the OR and placed supine on the operating table. Then he was prepped and draped in the usual sterile fashion. Anesthesia was by general endotracheal.

Then an inferior circumareolar incision was made on the left side down to the subcutaneous tissue. A pair of hooks were placed on the skin inferiorly and heavy Mayos were used to dissect down to the subcutaneous tissue around the enlarged breast tissue. Allis clamps were then used to grasp the breast tissue. The upper flap was then dissected free with sharp dissection with curved heavy Mayos. After this was completed, the inferior aspect of the breast tissue over the pectoralis fascia was freed up. Once it was felt that the tissue had been adequately removed, the sample was completely dissected and sent to pathology. The wound was then irrigated with copious amounts of normal saline. Electrocautery was used for hemostasis. Then the wound was irrigated again and checked for bleeding. Once it was adequately stopped, the wound was closed with 4-0 Vicryl subcutaneous sutures, used simple, times seven, and then a running subcuticular 4-0 Vicryl.

The other side was completed with an inferior circumareolar incision. Skin hooks were then used to hold the inferior flap back as heavy Mayos were used to dissect the breast tissue free down to the superficial pectoral fascia. Then the superior flap was freed and incised down to the pectoral fascia. Once this was completed, the tissue overlying the fascia was dissected out and the sample was removed and sent to pathology. The wound was then irrigated copiously with normal saline. Electrocautery was used for hemostasis. Then the wound was probed and all the breast tissue was felt to be removed, ensuring that equal amounts of tissue were removed on both sides. After this was completed, the wound was then irrigated once more and checked for hemostasis. Once adequate hemostasis was maintained, the wound was closed with 4-0 Vicryl subcutaneous stitch, used simple, times eight, and then a running subcuticular 4-0 Vicryl. Steri-strips were then applied on both wounds. A bulky pressure dressing was applied bilaterally. The patient tolerated the procedure without complications and was transferred back to the postanesthesia recovery area in stable condition.

Estimated Blood Loss:
About 50 cc's.

Intravenous Fluids:
Approximately one liter of crystalloid was administered.

Codes: _____

OPERATIVE REPORT

PATIENT: Kohler, Ernest   **MR#:** 99-13-16

SURGEON: Reese   **ASSISTANT:** Wynn

Preoperative Diagnosis:
Balanitis.

Postoperative Diagnosis:
Balanitis.

Operation:
Circumcision.

Procedure:
The patient was brought into the OR and placed on the operating table in the supine position. He was prepped and draped in the usual sterile fashion for circumcision. A penile nerve block was injected at the level of the pubic bone. Next the base of the penis was circumferentially anesthetized with 1% Lidocaine without Epinephrine. After testing to ascertain that the entire penis was well-anesthetized, the procedure was begun.

First, the desired line of incision was indicated with the marking pen on the outer skin and on the inner prepuce skin. Next, the knife was used to incise the foreskin on its inner portion, taking care at the ventral side not to cut too deep and damage the urethra. After completely incising circumferentially on the inner prepuce, the outer foreskin was incised in the same manner. Next the foreskin, which was cut in a double sleeve fashion, was incised across its dorsal edge to completely free it from the penis. The foreskin was then completely removed from the shaft of the penis using sharp and blunt dissection with the Mayo scissors, taking care to cut as close as possible to the foreskin being removed. Great care was exercised on the ventral side of the penis to insure that there was no injury to the urethra. After the foreskin was removed, hemostasis was obtained with Bovie electrocautery. The skin edges were reapproximated with a 3-0 chromic stitch. Stay stitches were placed at the 12, 3, 6 and 9 o'clock positions to be used as traction. Once this was completed, a running stitch of 3-0 chromic was placed between these stitches. The penis was wiped clean and a bandage consisting of a wrap of Vaseline gauze and a wrap of Kerlix gauze was placed. This completed the procedure and the patient was taken back to the outpatient surgery area for discharge.

The patient was instructed to remove the dressing tomorrow and to return in a few weeks to the Genitourinary Clinic. He was instructed not to engage in any sexual activity. He was given a prescription for Keflex and a prescription for pain pills. He was also given a prescription for Amyl Nitrate to take if he should get an erection.

Codes: _____   _____

OPERATIVE REPORT

PATIENT: Wilkerson, Fred   **MR#:** 99-13-17

SURGEON: Pagano   **ASSISTANT:** Albright

Preoperative Diagnosis:
Chronic diarrhea secondary to *Cryptosporidium* infection.

Postoperative Diagnosis:
Same.

Operation:
Raaf catheter placement in left subclavian vein.

Brief Clinical History:
The patient is a white male with a several month history of chronic diarrhea, nausea, and vomiting secondary to *Cryptosporidium* gastrointestinal infection. He presents now for intravenous access for hydration.

Description of Procedure:
The patient was brought to the OR and placed in the supine position on the operating table with a shoulder roll under his scapula. He was then prepped in the usual sterile manner. Anesthesia was by 1% Lidocaine used to infuse inferiorly to the left clavicle. Then a seeker needle was used without difficulty to find the left subclavian vein. A guide wire was passed through the seeker needle and the seeker needle was removed. Then an X ray was obtained, which showed that the wire was clearly in the left subclavian vein down to the superior vena cava. After this was completed, a second incision was made just lateral to the sternum, about level with the breast, and a #15 blade was used to make the incision down through the subcutaneous tissue. Lidocaine was used to infuse the skin between the second incision and the guide wire. The guide wire incision was made at the site where it entered the skin. Both incisions were approximately 1 cm in length. A tunneler was used to enter through the first incision down to the second and the Raaf catheter was brought under the skin. After this was completed, the dilator sheath and the introducer were both placed over the wire into the vein, and the dilator and wire were removed. Subsequently, the catheter was brought down into the guide sheath in the vein and the guide sheath was peeled away and removed. After the catheter was placed in the subclavian vein, it was then aspirated per the Raaf catheter, which was found to be functioning well. The catheter was in proper position and was infused with Heparin flush. The first incision site was closed with a 3-0 subcutaneous suture times one and then the skin was closed with a 4-0 running subcuticular. At the second incision site, one stitch was thrown with 2-0 Nylon and tied, and then a locking stitch was tied around the catheter. Sterile dressings were then applied and the patient was transferred to the postanesthesia recovery area in stable condition. A postoperative X ray was ordered to again check the catheter placement.

Codes: _____

OPERATIVE REPORT

PATIENT: Ghani, Anastasia   **MR#:** 99-13-18

SURGEON: Doherty   **ASSISTANT:** Jordan

Preoperative Diagnosis:
Medial meniscus tear and grade II chondromalacia of medial patellar facet and lateral tibial plateau.

Postoperative Diagnosis:
Medial meniscus tear and grade II chondromalacia of medial patellar facet and lateral tibial plateau.

Operation:
Arthroscopic partial medial meniscectomy with shaving of lateral tibial defect and shaving of patellar defect.

Procedure:
The patient was prepped and draped in the usual sterile fashion and induced with general anesthesia. Ancef was administered in dosage of 1 gm. The skin was prepped by scrubbing with Iodophor solution. A mechanical leg holder was used to stabilize the extremity. An arthroscope approximately 3.5 mm in diameter with a lens angle of approximately 30 degrees was inserted into the knee through a superolateral portal, a medial patellar lateral portal, and a mid patellar medial portal. Thorough examination of the menisci revealed a vertical longitudinal tear in the medial meniscus. The articular surfaces were examined and articular cartilage was noted to be split or fractured. The articular surface of the patella displayed deep fissures and fragmentation. The articular surface of the lateral tibial plateau also displayed deep fissures and fragmentation. The knee was examined for ligament instability. The anterior cruciate ligament appeared completely normal and the posterior cruciate ligament appeared completely normal. The medial gutter was inspected with valgus stress applied to the knee. The medial collateral ligament was normal. The lateral gutter was inspected with varus stress applied to the knee. The lateral capsular ligaments were normal. The medial meniscus was partially excised, removing the unstable torn fragments and any adjacent degenerative tissue, leaving the free margin smoothly contoured. This procedure was accomplished entirely with arthroscopically controlled techniques. The hyaline cartilage on the lateral tibial plateau and on the patella was thoroughly washed to remove proteolytic enzymes and any small chips of cartilage debris. The articular surface of the lateral tibial plateau and patella was shaved to reduce the profile of degenerative tags of cartilage. All arthroscopic instruments were withdrawn after aspirating the remaining irrigation fluid. Passive range-of-knee motion postoperatively was from 0 degrees to at least 120 degrees. A nonabsorbable suture skin closure was performed. A sterile compressive bandage was applied to the knee. The patient was transferred to the recovery room in good condition.

Codes: _____

OPERATIVE REPORT

PATIENT: Summers, Donald   **MR#:** 99-13-19

SURGEON: Gardner   **ASSISTANT:** Morgan

Preoperative Diagnosis:
Chronic constipation.

Irritable bowel syndrome.

Postoperative Diagnosis:
Chronic constipation.

Irritable bowel syndrome.

Colonoscopy:
Instrument: Olympus CF1TL flexible colonoscope.

Procedure:

The patient was premedicated with Demerol 50 mg and Valium 20 mg and an additional 10 mg of Valium IV was given during the procedure. The colonoscope was passed to the cecum with mild difficulty.

Findings:

The patient was poorly prepped and there was some spasm in the sigmoid colon, but otherwise, there were no mucosal lesions, mass lesions, friability, or ulcerations seen throughout the colon.

Impression:

Normal examination except for some spasm in the sigmoid colon.

Recommendations:

Antispasmodics.

High-fiber diet.

Codes: _____

CODING OF CLINICAL DOCUMENTATION— ANESTHESIA SECTION OF THE CPT VOLUME

Read the preceding operative reports. For the procedures performed, assign precise, accurate code numbers from the Anesthesia section of the CPT volume.

MR#: 99-13-01

Codes: _____

_____

MR#: 99-13-02

Codes: _____

_____

MR#: 99-13-03

Codes: _____

_____

MR#: 99-13-04

Codes: _____

_____

MR#: 99-13-05

Codes: _____

_____

MR#: 99-13-06

Codes: _____

_____

MR#: 99-13-07

Codes: _____

_____

MR#: 99-13-08

Codes: _____

_____

MR#: 99-13-09

Codes: _____

_____

MR#: 99-13-10

Codes: _____

_____

MR#: 99-13-11

Codes: _____

_____

MR#: 99-13-12

Codes: _____

_____

MR#: 99-13-13

Codes: _____

_____

MR#: 99-13-14

Codes: _____

_____

MR#: 99-13-15

Codes: _____

_____

MR#: 99-13-16

Codes: _____

_____

MR#: 99-13-17

Codes: _____

_____

MR#: 99-13-18

Codes: _____

_____

MR#: 99-13-19

Codes: _____

_____

14

CHAPTER

CPT Coding: Radiology, Pathology and Laboratory, and Medicine

LEARNING OBJECTIVES

Upon completion of this chapter the learner should be able to:

1. Define the concept of a professional component of a procedural service.
2. Define the concept of a technical component of a procedural service.
3. Define the concept of supervision and interpretation of a procedural service.
4. Report the function of evaluation and management services listings in the reporting of radiological services.
5. Explain the usefulness of modifiers for supplementing the codes reporting radiological procedures and services.
6. Apply knowledge of coding principles by assigning accurate and precise codes to report radiological procedures and services.
7. Define the concept of a reference laboratory.
8. Define the concept of automated multichannel tests.
9. Define the concept of organ or disease oriented panels.
10. Define the concept of qualitative drug testing.
11. Define the concept of quantitative drug testing.
12. Discuss the levels of service for surgical pathology consultations.
13. Explain the usefulness of modifiers for supplementing the codes reporting pathology and laboratory procedures and services.
14. Discuss the warranted application of code numbers and descriptors listed in the Medicine section for the reporting of infusion therapy procedures.
15. Discuss the warranted application of evaluation and management services code numbers and descriptors in the reporting of psychiatric services as well as discuss the warranted application of psychiatric services code numbers and descriptors in the reporting of evaluation and management services.
16. Discuss the warranted application of evaluation and management services code numbers and descriptors in the reporting of dialysis services.

17. Discuss the warranted application of evaluation and management services code numbers and descriptors in the reporting of otolaryngology services.

18. Discuss the warranted application of code numbers and descriptors listed in the Medicine section for the reporting of vascular diagnostic procedures.

19. Report the disparate levels of ophthalmology services.

20. Explain the usefulness of modifiers for supplementing the codes reporting medical procedures and services.

21. Apply knowledge of coding principles by assigning accurate and precise codes to report medical procedures and services.

CPT CODING OF RADIOLOGY

The Radiology section of the CPT volume embraces subsections for:

1. Diagnostic Imaging (codes *70010–76499*)

2. Diagnostic Ultrasound (codes *76506–76999*)

3. Radiation Oncology (codes *77261–77799*)

4. Nuclear Medicine (codes *78000–79999*)

Headings within the subsections and subheadings within these headings are arranged by anatomic site (examples: *Urinary Tract* or *Endocrine System*). Each of the subsections of the Radiology section contains notations that present explanations and instructions pertinent to that subsection.

Codes from any division of the Radiology section may be reported for services or procedures rendered by or under the direction of a physician in any specialty. As a general principle, any innovative or unique radiological service or radiological procedure should be detailed in a special report that accounts for the diagnostic and therapeutic factors impacting the decision to perform the service or the procedure. Radiological supplies and materials should be reported with HCPCS codes, if necessary.

A radiological procedure that is listed as an integral component of a total service does not warrant separate coding or reporting, and the entire service should be coded and reported as a single procedure. For example, code number *73565* represented by descriptor *Radiologic examination, knee; both knees, standing, anteroposterior,* should be reported in lieu of reporting both code number *73560-50* in addition to code number *73560-52* represented by descriptor *Radiologic examination, knee; anteroposterior and lateral views,* with the code numbers augmented with modifiers indicating bilateral anteroposterior views without lateral views.

However, if a radiologic procedure was performed independently and not as a component of a total service, then the procedure may be coded and reported as a separate procedure. For example, code number *73530* represented by descriptor *Radiologic examination, hip, during operative procedure* should be reported if this procedure was performed independently and not as a component of a total service.

If a radiological procedure was mainly performed by or under the direction of two physicians (ordinarily a radiologist and a physician from another specialty), the radiologic component is generally denoted in the applicable descriptor with the terms "radiological supervision and interpretation." For example, code number *73530-26* represented by descriptor *Radiologic examination of hip, during operative procedure,* should be reported for the professional component of the procedure. Radiological supervision and interpretation of a procedure connotes the preparation of a complete and timely written or dictated report, authenticated by the responsible physician, for placement in the patient's medical record.

Every radiological procedure listing in the Radiology section of the CPT volume (with the exception of those procedures and services listed in the Radiation Oncology subsection) reports exclusively the supervision and interpretation of that procedure. The actual procedure performed should be reported with a code listed in another section of the CPT volume. For instance, code number *71060* represented by descriptor *Bronchography, bilateral, radiological supervision and interpretation* reports the radiologic component of this procedure. The bronchography injection procedure should be reported with a code from the Respiratory System subsection of the Surgery section, specifically code number *31715* represented by descriptor *Transtracheal injection for bronchography.*

If both the radiologic component of a procedure as well as the other clinical components of the procedure were performed by or under the direction of a sole physician, two distinct codes should be reported by that physician. For instance, code number *71060* together with code number *31715* reports a bilateral bronchography performed through transtracheal injection that was rendered by an individual physician.

RADIOLOGY MODIFIERS

Radiological procedures or services involving extraordinary circumstances or involving variable protocols should be reported with the code number augmented by an applicable modifier. The commonly appended modifiers of the codes for radiological procedures and services include:

Modifier *-22*, unusual procedural services

Modifier *-26*, professional component

Modifier *-32*, mandated services

Modifier *-51*, multiple procedures

Modifier *-52*, reduced services

Modifier *-53*, discontinued procedure

Modifier *-58*, staged or related procedure or service by the same physician during the postoperative period

Modifier *-59*, distinct procedural service

Modifier *-62*, two surgeons

Modifier *-66*, surgical team

Modifier *-76*, repeat procedure by same physician

Modifier *-77*, repeat procedure by another physician

Modifier *-78*, return to the operating room for a related procedure during the postoperative period

Modifier *-79*, unrelated procedure or service by the same physician during the postoperative period

Modifier *-80*, assistant surgeon

Modifier *-90*, reference (outside) laboratory

Modifier *-99*, multiple modifiers

Modifier *-22* may be properly reported with a code for computerized tomography if additional slices were completed or if more than a standard examination was performed. Modifier *-52* may be properly reported with a code for computerized tomography if limited slices were completed or if less than a standard examination was performed.

TABLE 14–1

Headings in the Diagnostic Radiology Subsection

Head and Neck	Gynecological and Obstetrical
Chest	Heart
Spine and Pelvis	Aorta and Arteries
Upper Extremities	Veins and Lymphatics
Lower Extremities	Transcatheter Procedures
Abdomen	Transluminal Atherectomy
Gastrointestinal Tract	Other Procedures
Urinary Tract	

Numerous radiological procedures encompass both a physician (professional) component involving the skill, the judgment, and the time expended by the physician, as well as a technical component involving the equipment and the supplies used in the procedure. If the physician (professional) component of a procedure is reported separately, the code number and descriptor for the procedure should be supplemented by modifier *-26* unless the descriptor explicitly designates this code for the physician (professional) component of the procedure. For example, code number *76380-26* represented by descriptor *Computerized tomography, limited or localized follow-up study,* reports the professional component of this procedure. Hospitals must report only the code for the technical component of a radiological procedure or a radiological service.

CPT CODING OF DIAGNOSTIC RADIOLOGY

This straightforward Diagnostic Radiology subsection of the CPT Radiology section is aligned with headings organized either by anatomic site or by procedural modality. Fifteen headings are delineated within this subsection (Table 14–1).

Cross-references throughout the listings of the Diagnostic Radiology subsection direct code number and descriptor selection to listings elsewhere within the subsection (example: note the cross-reference for code number and descriptor *70490 Computerized axial tomography, soft tissue neck, without contrast material followed by contrast material and further sections*), or to listings in other sections of the CPT volume (example: note the cross-reference for code number and descriptor *74742 Transcervical catheterization of fallopian tube, radiological supervision and interpretation*).

With selective angiography, a unit count method should be used to report the number of vessels examined. Code number *75774* reports the radiological supervision and interpretation of each additional vessel examined through selective angiography.

CPT CODING OF DIAGNOSTIC ULTRASOUND

This comparatively brief Diagnostic Ultrasound subsection of the CPT Radiology section commences with technical definitions and continues with headings arranged either by anatomic site or by procedural modality. Ten headings are delineated within this subsection (Table 14–2).

Several cross-references among the listings of this Diagnostic Ultrasound subsection guide code number and descriptor selection to listings in other sections of the CPT volume

T A B L E 14–2

Headings in the Diagnostic Ultrasound Subsection

Head and Neck	Genitalia
Chest	Extremities
Abdomen and Retroperitoneum	Vascular Studies
Spinal Canal	Ultrasonic Guidance Procedures
Pelvis	Other Procedures

(example: note the cross-reference for code number and descriptor *76828 Doppler echocardiography, fetal, cardiovascular system, pulsed wave and/or continuous wave with spectral display; follow-up or repeat study*).

CPT CODING OF RADIATION ONCOLOGY

This concise Radiation Oncology subsection of the CPT Radiology section contains explicit notations with definitions, explanations, and instructions relevant to the listings of Radiation Oncology services and procedures. Eight headings or subheadings are delineated within this subsection (Table 14–3).

The code number and descriptor listing of a service or a procedure in this subsection implicitly include the initial consultation, clinical treatment planning, simulation, medical radiation physics, dosimetry, treatment devices, special services, clinical treatment management procedures, and conventional follow-up care during the course of treatment as well as the customary follow-up care rendered up to three months after the completion of radiation treatment.

Preliminary consultations and preparatory evaluations preceding the course of radiation treatment should be reported with an appropriate code from the Evaluation and Management Services section of the CPT volume. For instance, code number *99244* should be reported for an office consultation that was rendered for the discussion of radiation oncology treatment options.

The clinical treatment planning process is a complex service comprising the interpretation of special testing, the localization of tumors, and the determination of treatment volume,

T A B L E 14–3

Headings and Subheadings in the Radiation Oncology Subsection

Consultation: Clinical Management
Clinical Treatment Planning (External and Internal Sources)
Medical Radiation Physics, Dosimetry, Treatment Devices, and Special Services
Radiation Treatment Delivery
Clinical Treatment Management
Hyperthermia
Clinical Intracavitary Hyperthermia
Clinical Brachytherapy

time, dosage, modality, ports, and devices, as well as the performance of various additional procedures.

Only one teletherapy isodose plan may be reported for each course of therapy to a specific treatment area. Radiation treatment delivery includes the technical component of the service and the various energy levels utilized. Weekly clinical management is based on the delivery of five fractions in one week, regardless of the time interval between the delivery of the fractions.

Listings of code numbers and descriptors for hyperthermia treatments (used as an adjunct to radiation therapy or chemotherapy) inherently include superficial and deep external, interstitial, or intracavitary therapy, as well as physics planning, interstitial insertion of temperature sensors, use of external or interstitial heat generating sources, management of the course of therapy, and the follow-up care rendered for up to three months after conclusion of the hyperthermia treatments.

Radiation therapy, even if dispensed concurrently, is not included in the code for hyperthermia treatments, and should be coded and reported separately. For instance, code number *77425* represented by descriptor *Weekly radiology therapy management, intermediate,* may be reported together with code number *77600* represented by descriptor *Hyperthermia, externally generated, superficial.*

Preparatory consultations and preliminary evaluations preceding the course of hyperthermia treatments also should be reported with appropriate codes from the Evaluation and Management Services section of the CPT volume. For instance, code number *99244* should be reported for an office consultation that was rendered for discussion of hyperthermia treatment options.

CPT CODING OF NUCLEAR MEDICINE

The Nuclear Medicine subsection of the CPT Radiology section is organized with headings arranged either by body system or by procedural modality. Listings within this subsection are delineated under two headings and eight subheadings (Table 14–4).

Notations both at the forefront of the Nuclear Medicine subsection, and throughout the listings of this subsection, provide explanations and instructions concerning the appropriate coding and reporting of nuclear medicine procedures and services.

TABLE 14–4

Headings and Subheadings in the Nuclear Medicine Subsection

Heading	Subheading
Diagnostic	Endocrine System
	Hematopoietic, Reticuloendothelial, and Lymphatic System
	Gastrointestinal System
	Musculoskeletal System
	Cardiovascular System
	Respiratory System
	Nervous System
	Genitourinary System
	Other Procedures
Therapeutic	

The codes for nuclear medicine services and procedures listed in this subsection may be reported either if rendered independently or in the course of other clinical care. The listed code number and descriptor for a nuclear medicine service or procedure, however, does not include the supply of radium or other radioelements. These materials and supplies may be reported with a HCPCS code, if necessary.

The listed code number and descriptor for a nuclear medicine service or procedure also does not include the initial diagnostic assessments or the subsequent follow-up care provided to patients; these encounters should be reported with appropriate codes from the Evaluation and Management Services section of the CPT volume. For instance, code number *99261* should be reported for a follow-up consultation that was rendered to review results of nuclear medicine studies.

RADIOLOGY REPORTING FOR BILLING

Currently, radiology coding is typically automated, whereby a computerized chargemaster program automatically assigns the code for the designated radiology procedure or service. Infrequently performed procedures and services, however, are generally coded manually.

The preponderance of radiological procedures and services incorporate both a professional component and a technical component. The professional component involves the skill, the judgment, and the time expended by the physician, whereas the technical component involves the equipment and the supplies utilized in the procedure or service. If a radiological procedure or service was procured from an outside source (an external facility), the code number representing that entity should be augmented with modifier *-26* to represent and report the professional component of the procedure or service.

Caution should be exercised in the coding and reporting of these radiological procedures or services with dual components. Many third-party payors are exceedingly prudent and vigilant to prevent duplicative reimbursement for radiological procedures or services. If two physicians (for instance, a radiologist and a physician of another specialty) both submit a claim reporting supervision and interpretation of a radiologic procedure, the third-party payor usually reimburses the fee of the radiologist and rejects the fee of the other physician.

If a radiologist administered the necessary injection prior to a procedure and also provided the supervision and interpretation of this procedure, the codes for both procedures should be reported. For example, code number *75605* represented by descriptor *Aortography, thoracic, by serialography, radiological supervision and interpretation* should be reported together with code number *36200* represented by descriptor *Introduction of catheter, aorta*.

The fee for rendering a radiological procedure or service that is submitted by the physician radiologist to a third-party payor is termed the "actual charge" for that procedure or service. The amount of this actual charge generally is greater than the amount of reimbursement from the third-party payor or the "allowed charge" for that radiological procedure or service.

As third-party payors, insurance carriers usually justify or rationalize the allowed charge with its lessened amount of reimbursement as reasonable on the basis of a "customary charge" (also termed a "prevailing charge") that is compiled from the average charges of similar radiologists for that radiological procedure or service. Additionally, this difference between the actual charge and the allowed charge may be justified and rationalized by reason of the co-payment, which is the portion of the actual charge that is paid by the patient directly to the provider of the radiological procedure or service.

CPT CODING FOR PATHOLOGY AND LABORATORY

The Pathology and Laboratory section of the CPT volume encompasses subsections for:

1. Automated Multichannel Tests (codes *80002–80019*)
2. Organ- or Disease-Oriented Panels (codes *80050–80092*)
3. Drug Testing (codes *80100–80103*)
4. Therapeutic Drug Assays (codes *80150–80299*)
5. Evocative/Suppression Testing (codes *80400–80440*)
6. Consultations (Clinical Pathology) (codes *80500–80502*)
7. Urinalysis (codes *81000–81099*)
8. Chemistry (codes *82000–84999* spanning 16 pages in length)
9. Hematology and Coagulation (codes *85002–85999*)
10. Immunology (codes *86000–86849* containing sub-subsection for *Tissue Typing*)
11. Transfusion Medicine (codes *86850–86999*)
12. Microbiology (codes *87001–87999* including bacteriology, mycology, parasitology, and virology)
13. Anatomic Pathology (codes *88000–88299* containing headings for *Postmortem Examinations, Cytopathology,* and *Cytogenic Studies*)
14. Surgical Pathology (codes *88300–88399*)
15. Other Procedures (codes *89050–89399*)

Various subsections within the Pathology and Laboratory section of the CPT volume are prefaced with notations that furnish explanations and instructions associated with the listings of that particular subsection. Additional information such as the appropriate codes for the reporting of unlisted services is also provided. Any innovative or unique pathology and laboratory service should be detailed in a special report that indicates the diagnostic and therapeutic factors affecting the decision to render that service.

Any code number and descriptor listed in the Pathology and Laboratory section may be reported by a physician from any specialty acknowledging that the reported procedure or service was provided by technologists under the direction of that physician. Every reported pathology procedure or service and certain stipulated cytopathology procedures or services, however, must be rendered exclusively by a physician.

Automated multichannel tests are grouped in combinations (profiles) accomplished with special equipment. The groups of tests listed in the subsection designated for automated multichannel tests are differentiated from multiple tests individually completed for immediate or "stat" requisitions. An example of an automated multichannel test is the SMA-12.

Organ- or disease-oriented panels are listed in a designated subsection of the Pathology and Laboratory section. These panels are presented for coding and reporting purposes and are not offered as clinical parameters. If additional tests were completed (in addition to the itemized tests), the extra tests should be coded and reported separately.

The Drug Testing subsection of the Pathology and Laboratory section contains exemplary classes of drugs that are routinely assayed with qualitative screening. A qualitative drug screening test should be coded and reported by procedure rather than by analyte or substance analyzed (example: if chromatography is used in the testing, each combination of stationary and mobile phases should be reported separately).

A quantitative drug screening test should be coded and reported with listings from either the Therapeutic Drug Assay subsection or the Chemistry subsection. Chemistry or toxicology tests of varying substances are listed alphabetically by analyte. Chemical or toxicological tests are presumably quantitative unless stipulated otherwise.

Molecular diagnostic techniques for the assessment of nucleic acids should be coded and reported by procedure rather than by analyte. Mathematical calculations derived from the resultant data of a laboratory test are regarded as a constituent part of the testing procedure, and therefore mathematical calculations should not be coded and reported separately.

The Hematology and Coagulation subsection as well as the Immunology subsection are comprised of alphabetical listings of tests, listed either by the substance tested or by the method of testing. Laboratory procedures conducted for the identification of antibodies should be coded and reported as accurately as possible. For instance, an antibody to a virus should be coded with specificity for virus, family, genus, species, or type. If multiple assays were performed for antibodies of different immunoglobulin classes, then each assay should be coded and reported separately.

Laboratory materials and supplies should be reported with HCPCS codes, if necessary. Medicare as well as many commercial insurance carriers accept HCPCS codes for the reporting of laboratory materials and supplies.

A clinical pathology consultation is a service rendered by a pathologist in response to the request of the attending physician (example: the request to a pathologist from an attending physician regarding interpretative judgment of a laboratory specimen). The clinical pathology consultation necessitates an examination of a surgical specimen and requires the compilation of a pathology report for the patient medical record.

The specimen is the unit of service for the surgical pathology consultation. Coding and reporting should account for each specimen that received individual examination and pathologic diagnosis. Gross examination should be coded and reported only once per specimen, whereas microscopic examination may be coded and reported for each separate microscopic inspection of the specimen, utilizing a unit count method for reporting the number of blocks examined. For example, a surgical pathology consultation consisting solely of gross examination should be reported with code number *88329*. However, a surgical pathology consultation with a frozen section should be reported with code number *88331,* and code number *88332* should be synchronously reported for each additional tissue block that was examined during this surgical pathology consultation.

The listings of the Surgical Pathology subsection implicitly include the examination of the specimen, the accession of the findings into the proper index or register, and the reporting of the examination findings. The surgical pathology consultation service is delineated into six levels of service that are distinguished in the CPT volume in ascending order of complexity:

1. *Level I—surgical pathology, gross examination only*
2. *Level II—surgical pathology, gross and microscopic examination*
3. *Level III—surgical pathology, gross and microscopic examination*
4. *Level IV—surgical pathology, gross and microscopic examination*
5. *Level V—surgical pathology, gross and microscopic examination*
6. *Level VI—surgical pathology, gross and microscopic examination*

PATHOLOGY AND LABORATORY MODIFIERS

A pathology or laboratory procedure or service involving extraordinary circumstances or variable techniques should be reported with a modifier supplementing the code number for the procedure or service. Commonly appended modifiers of codes for pathology and laboratory services include:

Modifier -22, unusual procedural services

Modifier -26, professional component

Modifier -32, mandated services

Modifier -52, reduced services

Modifier -53, discontinued procedure

Modifier -59, distinct procedural service

Modifier -90, reference outside laboratory

Certain pathology and laboratory procedures and services incorporate both a physician (or professional) component and a technical component. The physician component of the procedure or service encompasses the skill, judgment, and time expended by the physician. The technical component of the procedure or service encompasses the equipment and the supplies that are utilized. For instance, code number *85060* represented by descriptor *Blood smear, peripheral, interpretation by physician with written report,* includes the physician component (skill and judgment) as well as the technical component (equipment and supplies) of this laboratory test.

If the physician or professional component of a pathology or laboratory procedure or service is reported separately by reason that the procedure or service was procured from an outside source (an external facility), the code number for that procedure or service should be augmented with modifier -26 to represent and report the physician or professional component of the procedure or service. For instance, code number *85060-26* represented by descriptor *Blood smear, peripheral, interpretation by physician with written report,* reports only the physician or professional component of this laboratory test and does not report or account for the technical component. Hospitals must report only the code for the technical component of a pathology or laboratory procedure or service.

The listed code for a laboratory procedure or service provided by an external laboratory should be reported with modifier -90 supplementing the code number. For example, code number *82042-90* represented by descriptor *Albumin, urine, quantitative,* reports that this laboratory test was provided by an external reference laboratory. Medicare carriers accept codes appended with modifier -90 exclusively from laboratories.

PATHOLOGY AND LABORATORY REPORTING FOR BILLING

Currently, pathology and laboratory coding is typically automated, whereby a computerized chargemaster program automatically assigns the code for the designated pathology or laboratory procedure or service. Infrequently performed procedures and services, however, are generally coded manually.

The subsection comprising listings of automated multichannel tests contains an expanded account of tests associated with each code (example: chloride, cholesterol, creatinine, and so on). However, the subsection containing listings of organ- or disease-oriented panels deliberately omits accounts of tests associated with the listed codes, by reason that different laboratories utilize different arrays of tests. Thus, the lack of definitive tests associated with each of the listed codes in this subsection may culminate in obstacles with regard to the coding and reporting of these tests for billing to third-party payors.

The fee for rendering a pathology or laboratory procedure or service that is submitted by the physician pathologist or the clinical laboratory to a third-party payor is termed the "actual charge" for that procedure or service. The amount of this actual charge generally is greater than the amount of reimbursement from the third-party payor or the "allowed charge" for that pathology or laboratory procedure or service.

As third-party payors, insurance carriers usually justify or rationalize the allowed charge with its lessened amount of reimbursement as reasonable on the basis of a "customary charge" (also termed a "prevailing charge") that is compiled from the average charges of similar pathologists or compiled from the average charges of similar clinical laboratories for that pathology or laboratory procedure or service. Additionally, this difference between the actual charge and the allowed charge may be justified and rationalized by reason of the co-payment, which is the portion of the actual charge that is paid by the patient directly to the provider of the pathology or laboratory procedure or service.

CPT CODING OF MEDICINE

The Medicine section of the CPT volume includes twenty subsections:

1. Immunization Injections (codes *90700–90749*)
2. Therapeutic or Diagnostic Infusions (codes *90780–90781*)
3. Therapeutic or Diagnostic Injections (codes *90782–90799*)
4. Psychiatry (codes *90801–90899*)
5. Biofeedback (codes *90901–90911*)
6. Dialysis (codes *90918–90999*)
7. Gastroenterology (codes *91000–91299*)
8. Ophthalmology (codes *92002–92499*)
9. Special Otolaryngologic Services (codes *92502–92599*)
10. Cardiovascular (codes *92950–93799*)
11. Non-Invasive Vascular Diagnostic Studies (codes *93875–93990*)
12. Pulmonary (codes *94010–94799*)
13. Allergy and Clinical Immunology (codes *95004–95199*)
14. Neurology and Neuromuscular Procedures (codes *95805–95999*)
15. Central Nervous System Assessments/Tests (codes *96100–96117*)
16. Chemotherapy Administration (codes *96400–96549*)
17. Special Dermatological Procedures (codes *96900–96999*)
18. Physical Medicine and Rehabilitation (codes *97010–97799*)
19. Osteopathic Manipulative Treatment (codes *98925–98929*)
20. Special Services and Reports (codes *99000–99199*)

Most of the subsections within the Medicine section of the CPT volume are prefaced with notations intended to impart or convey explanations and instructions that are applicable to that subsection. The notations furthermore contribute additional information such as the codes for unlisted procedures and services pertinent to that particular subsection. As a rule, an innovative or unique medical procedure or service, or a medical procedure or service with a considerably variable protocol should be detailed in a special report that accounts for the diagnostic and therapeutic factors that influenced the decision to render the procedure or service.

Codes listed in any subsection of the Medicine section may be reported for procedures or services provided by or under the direction of a physician regardless of his or her specialty.

A medical procedure or service that is rendered as an integral component of a total procedure or service does not warrant separate coding or reporting, and the entire procedure or service should be coded and reported as a solitary procedure or service. For instance, code number *92511* represented by descriptor *Nasopharyngoscopy with endoscope,* does not warrant separate reporting if this diagnostic procedure was rendered in conjunction with a surgical procedure.

If a procedure or service was performed independently, and not rendered either as a component of a total procedure or total service, the procedure or service may be coded and reported separately. For instance, code number *93610* represented by descriptor *Intra-atrial pacing,* may be reported separately if this procedure was rendered independently, and was not provided either as a component of a total procedure or total service.

Multiple medical procedures or services provided on the same date may be coded and reported separately. Medical supplies should be reported with HCPCS codes, if necessary.

MEDICINE MODIFIERS

A medical procedure or a medical service that involves remarkable circumstances or diverse protocols should be reported with the code for the procedure or for the service augmented with a modifier. Commonly appended modifiers of codes for medical procedures and medical services include:

Modifier *-22,* unusual procedural services

Modifier *-26,* professional component

Modifier *-32,* mandated services

Modifier *-51,* multiple procedures

Modifier *-52,* reduced services

Modifier *-53,* discontinued procedure

Modifier *-55,* postoperative management only

Modifier *-56,* preoperative management only

Modifier *-57,* decision for surgery

Modifier *-58,* staged or related procedure or service by the same physician during the postoperative period

Modifier *-59,* distinct procedural service

Modifier *-76,* repeat procedure by same physician

Modifier *-77,* repeat procedure by another physician

Modifier *-78,* return to the operating room for a related procedure during the postoperative period

Modifier *-79,* unrelated procedure or service by the same physician during the postoperative period

Modifier *-90,* reference (outside) laboratory

Modifier *-99,* multiple modifiers

Various medical procedures and services encompass both a physician or professional component and a technical component. The physician or professional component of a procedure or service entails the skill, judgment, and time utilized by the physician. The technical component of the procedure or service entails the equipment and the supplies used in the provision of the procedure or service. For example, code number *93040* represented by descriptor

Rhythm ECG, one to three leads; with interpretation and report, reports both the professional component and the technical component of this procedure. If the physician or professional component of a medical procedure or service is reported separately, the code for that procedure or service should be appended with modifier -26. For example, code number *93040-26* represented by descriptor *Rhythm ECG, one to three leads; with interpretation and report,* reports only the physician or professional component of this procedure.

If multiple medical procedures or services were performed during the same session or on the same date, the major (primary or principal) procedure or the major (primary or principal) service should be reported first and foremost on the claim, and is followed by the minor (secondary or additional) procedures or the minor (secondary or additional) services. The codes for the secondary procedures or services should be appended with modifier -51. For example, code number *95857* represented by descriptor *Tensilon test for myasthenia gravis,* should be reported in the initial position followed with both code number *95869-51* represented by descriptor *Needle electromyography, limited study of specific muscles,* and with code number *95832-51* represented by descriptor *Muscle testing, manual; hand.*

If two or more distinct modifiers supplement a solitary code for a medical procedure or service, then modifier -99 should be the initial modifier cited and appended to that code to signify that multiple modifiers are associated with the specific code. For consistency and uniformity, multiple modifiers of a solitary code number should be reported in descending numerical order.

CPT CODING OF INJECTION AND INFUSION SERVICES

The three initial subsections of the Medicine section of the CPT volume are entitled Immunization Injections, Therapeutic or Diagnostic Infusions, and Therapeutic or Diagnostic Injections. These subsections comprise listings of code numbers and descriptors for injection procedures or services and for infusion procedures or services.

Frequently, immunization injections are dispensed in conjunction with other codable and reportable procedures or services, such as the periodic examinations of pediatric patients. The code for an immunization injection implicitly includes the supply of materials used, whereas the codes for a therapeutic injection or diagnostic injection do not. Therefore, the use of another code, generally a HCPCS national code (level II code), may be necessary to report the supply of materials used for the injection.

The codes for infusion therapy procedures report prolonged intravenous injections that require the presence of a physician during the infusion (example: intravenous infusion therapy in code range 90780–90781). These codes are not applicable either for routine injections or for chemotherapy administration.

CPT codes for injections and infusion therapy procedures or services are not appropriate for reporting therapeutic injections or therapeutic infusions on Medicare claims. Instead of CPT codes, HCPCS national codes (level II codes from section J) for therapeutic injections or infusion therapy must be reported by both physicians and hospitals on Medicare claims.

CPT CODING OF PSYCHIATRY SERVICES

The Psychiatry subsection of the Medicine section of the CPT volume is apportioned into three headings: *General Clinical Psychiatric Diagnostic or Evaluative Interview Procedures; Special Clinical Psychiatric Diagnostic or Evaluative Procedures;* and *Psychiatric Therapeutic Procedures* (a subsection that is further divided into subheadings for *Psychiatric Somatotherapy, Other Psychiatric Therapy,* and *Other Procedures*). The Psychiatry subsection is followed in the CPT volume by a brief subsection encompassing listings of code numbers and descriptors for biofeedback training.

The Psychiatry subsection contains extensive notations that incorporate definitions, explanations, and instructions relevant to the listings of this subsection. These notations include guidelines that differentiate psychiatric services appropriately reported with evaluation and management services codes from psychiatric services appropriately reported with codes from the listings in the subsection designated for psychiatry. As examples, observe the notations for code number *90845* represented by descriptor *Medical psychoanalysis;* and observe the notations for code number *90880* represented by *Medical hypnotherapy.*

Due to the mode of psychiatric inpatient therapy, the psychiatrist principally functions as the leader of a treatment team consisting of nurses, social workers, and activity therapists. Thus, if the psychiatrist rendered auxiliary procedures or services such as psychotherapy or psychometrics, these supplementary encounters may be coded and reported separately.

The codes for consultations in the Evaluation and Management Services section of the CPT volume do not include the provision of psychotherapy. An evaluation and management service code for a consultation should be reported, however, for the initial psychiatric assessment of the patient and for the follow-up psychiatric evaluation. For example, an office consultation for an adolescent with violent behavior should be reported with code number *99245.*

For coding and reporting purposes, interactive procedures are defined as specialized diagnostic procedures that utilize physical aids and nonverbal communication to overcome barriers to therapeutic interaction between the physician and a patient who lacks expressive language communication skills.

Psychiatric care may be reported either with or without time dimensions both in accordance with the characteristic routine of a practice or a facility and with the prevalent customs of a particular region or locality. A stipulated time interval may be coded and reported as a unit count of psychiatric service. A psychiatric service of either a shortened or a lengthened duration may be reported with the procedure code for the comparable or analogous service of standard duration, but with the procedure code appended with an appropriate modifier to indicate either decreased or increased time. (For examples, *Interactive medical psychiatric diagnostic interview examination* that was curtailed may be reported with code number *90820-52;* and *Interactive medical psychiatric diagnostic interview examination* that was protracted, may be reported with code number *90820-22*).

Alcohol and drug rehabilitation services may be reported by either physicians or hospitals within guidelines parallel to those guidelines that regulate the reporting of psychiatric services. Insurance carriers typically sustain special or reduced rates of reimbursement for psychiatric and rehabilitation services.

CPT CODING OF DIALYSIS SERVICES

The Dialysis subsection of the Medicine section of the CPT volume comprises listings of hemodialysis procedures and peritoneal dialysis procedures. These services are dispensed to patients with end stage renal disease. The Dialysis subsection is divided into four headings: *End Stage Renal Disease Services; Hemodialysis; Peritoneal Dialysis;* and *Miscellaneous Dialysis Procedures.*

Any evaluation and management service associated with the end stage renal disease or rendered during the dialysis session or on the same date of the dialysis session is inherently included in the dialysis procedure code listing. For instance, physician evaluation of a patient with syncope during a dialysis session is included in the code for the dialysis service and should not be coded and reported separately.

An evaluation and management service unrelated to the dialysis service, although rendered on the same date of the dialysis service (but either prior to or after the dialysis procedure), should be coded and reported separately. For instance, physician evaluation of a patient with an abrasion of the foot that was incurred after a dialysis session should be coded and reported with an appropriate code from the Evaluation and Management Services section of the CPT volume. Medicare carriers do not require HCPCS national codes (level II codes) for the reporting of dialysis procedures and services.

CPT CODING OF GASTROENTEROLOGY SERVICES

The Gastroenterology subsection of the Medicine section of the CPT volume contains various residual or miscellaneous listings of gastrointestinal procedures and services. The preponderance of procedures performed by gastroenterologists should be coded and reported from the listings within the Digestive System subsection of the Surgery section of the CPT volume (examples: code number *43202* represented by descriptor *Esophagoscopy, rigid or flexible; diagnostic, with biopsy;* or code number *43830* represented by descriptor *Gastrostomy, temporary*).

Additional consultative or assessment services dispensed by gastroenterologic physicians should be specifically coded and reported from the listings within the Evaluation and Management Services section of the CPT volume. For example, an inpatient consultation provided for a patient hospitalized with upper gastrointestinal bleeding should be reported with code number *99263*.

CPT CODING OF OPHTHALMOLOGY MEDICAL SERVICES

The Ophthalmology subsection of the Medicine section of the CPT volume is comprised of listings of both diagnostic eye services and of therapeutic eye services, which are clustered in three distinct levels of ophthalmological service: intermediate, comprehensive, and special. The Ophthalmology subsection is divided into five headings: *General Ophthalmological Services* (with subheadings for *New Patient* and *Established Patient*); *Special Ophthalmological Services,* (with subheadings for *Ophthalmoscopy* and *Other Specialized Services*); *Contact Lens Services; Ocular Prosthetics Artificial Eye;* and *Spectacle Services Including Prosthesis for Aphakia* (with subheadings for *Supply of Materials* and *Other Procedures*).

Operative procedures performed on the eye and ocular adnexa are listed in the Eye and Ocular Adnexa subsection of the Surgery section of the CPT volume (examples: code number *65771* represented by descriptor *Radial keratotomy;* or code number *66983* represented by descriptor *Intracapsular cataract extraction with insertion of intraocular lens prosthesis*).

Modifier *-52* (indicating reduced services) should supplement the code number for an eye examination or an optometric test that was applied to one eye instead of both eyes. For example, *Gonioscopy with medical diagnostic evaluation, unilateral,* should be reported as *92020-52.*

An intermediate ophthalmological service is distinguished by the evaluation of a primary diagnostic condition (a new or existing eye condition), that was concurrently complicated by a new diagnosis. An intermediate ophthalmological service is also distinguished by the evaluation of a new clinical management problem that may or may not be associated with the primary ophthalmological diagnosis (example: external examination, ophthalmoscopy, and biomicroscopy for iritis).

A comprehensive ophthalmological service is distinguished by a general evaluation of the complete visual system during one or more sessions and implicitly includes the initiation of diagnostic studies or therapeutic interventions (example: diagnosis and initiation of treatment for glaucoma).

A special ophthalmological service is distinguished by a comprehensive evaluation or by a special treatment for a segment of the visual system expanding beyond the purview or realm of services normally encompassed either within a general ophthalmological examination or within routine ophthalmological tasks (example: fluorescein angiography).

Intermediate and comprehensive ophthalmological services include the provision of integrated services in which diagnostic evaluation cannot be separated from the examining techniques (such as keratometry or retinoscopy) used to render the service. Components of the examination such as routine ophthalmoscopy should not be coded and reported separately.

Contact lens services are not regarded as a component of general ophthalmological services and thus may properly be coded and reported separately. The code number and descriptor listing for contact lens services inherently includes the prescription for the contact lenses, and the fitting and supply of the contact lenses.

The prescription of spectacles, but not the fitting or supply of the spectacles, however, is regarded as a component of general ophthalmological services and should not be coded and reported separately.

CPT CODING OF OTORHINOLARYNGOLOGY MEDICAL SERVICES

The Special Otorhinolaryngologic Services subsection of the Medicine section of the CPT volume contains listings of special diagnostic or therapeutic otorhinolaryngologic procedures and services. This subsection encompasses three headings: *Vestibular Function Tests with Observation and Evaluation by Physician Without Electrical Recording; Vestibular Function Tests with Recording and Medical Diagnostic Evaluation;* and *Audiologic Function Tests with Medical Diagnostic Evaluation.*

Operative procedures performed on the ear, nose, and throat are listed either in the Respiratory System subsection of the Surgery section or in the Digestive System subsection of the Surgery section. For example, *Nasal endoscopy, diagnostic, unilateral or bilateral,* should be reported with code number *31231* listed in the Respiratory System subsection; and *Tonsillectomy, primary or secondary; under age 12,* should be reported with code number *42825* listed in the Digestive System subsection.

Otorhinolaryngologic procedures and services ordinarily included within a comprehensive ear, nose, and throat examination in an office or outpatient setting should be reported with codes from the Evaluation and Management Services section of the CPT volume. For example, an initial office evaluation of a patient with gradual hearing loss usually should be reported with code number *99202.* Technical otorhinolaryngologic procedures implicitly included in a standard examination of the ear, nose, or throat should not be coded and reported separately.

Audiometric tests listed in this subsection delineated for special otorhinolaryngologic services presume the use of calibrated electronic equipment (example: code number *92561* represented by descriptor *Bekesy audiometry, diagnostic*). Code numbers and descriptors in the subheading designated for audiometric testing refer to the testing of both ears unless otherwise indicated (example: code number *92592* represented by descriptor *Hearing aid check, monaural*). Modifier *-52* (indicating reduced services) should supplement the code for an ear examination or an audiometric test applied to one ear instead of both ears. For example, *Tone decay test, monaural,* should be reported as *92563-52.*

CPT CODING OF CARDIOVASCULAR MEDICAL SERVICES

The Cardiovascular subsection of the Medicine section of the CPT volume is comprised of listings of numerous procedures and services rendered principally by cardiologists. These procedures and services encompass diagnostic techniques such as electrocardiogram, cardiac catheterization, and electrophysiological cardiac monitoring as well as therapeutic measures such as cardioversion and angioplasty. The Cardiovascular subsection is divided into seven headings: *Therapeutic Services; Cardiography; Echocardiography; Cardiac Catheterization; Intracardiac Electrophysiological Procedures; Other Vascular Studies;* and *Other Procedures.*

Operative procedures performed on the cardiovascular system are listed in the Cardiovascular System subsection of the Surgery section of the CPT volume. As examples, *Pericardiocentesis, initial* should be reported with code number *33010**, and *Transluminal balloon angioplasty, percutaneous* should be reported from within the code range *35470–35476.*

Office or outpatient cardiovascular procedures and services should be reported with codes from the Evaluation and Management Services section of the CPT volume. For example, an office evaluation of a new patient presenting with exertional chest pain should be reported with code number *99205.*

Three factors must be considered prior to the selection of a code to report electrocardiography (EKG). Specifically, these factors are the tracing, the interpretation of the test by the physician, and the preparation of a report conveying the test results. Accurate code number and descriptor selection for electrocardiography (EKG) hinges upon which of these three aspects of the service were provided. For instance, code number *93000* reports an EKG with interpretation and report, and code number *93005* reports an EKG without the interpretation and report.

The reporting of echocardiography services also varies, as code selection is contingent upon whether the echocardiogram was rendered as a follow-up study or as a limited study. For coding and reporting purposes, echocardiography includes obtaining ultrasonic signals from the heart and great arteries with two-dimensional image or Doppler ultrasonic signal documentation as well as the interpretation and preparation of a report for the patient health record.

The components of the cardiac catheterization procedure must be reported with two listings from the Medicine section of the CPT volume. For example, code number *93501* represented by descriptor *Right heart catheterization* should be reported together with code number *93555* represented by descriptor *Imaging supervision, interpretation and report, for injection procedure during cardiac catheterization.*

The listed code number and descriptor for a cardiac catheterization procedure inherently includes the positioning and repositioning of the catheters, the injection of contrast media, the obtaining of blood gas and cardiac output measurements as well as their interpretation and final evaluation, as well as the preparation of a report for the patient medical record. Cardiac catheterization injection procedure listings do not, however, include these components.

CPT CODING OF VASCULAR DIAGNOSTIC SERVICES

The Non-Invasive Vascular Diagnostic Studies subsection of the Medicine section of the CPT volume is divided into five headings: *Cerebrovascular Arterial Studies; Extremity Arterial Studies (Including Digits); Extremity Venous Studies (Including Digits); Visceral and Penile Vascular Studies;* and *Extremity Arterial-Venous Studies.* This subsection contains listings of code numbers and descriptors for certain examination procedures performed on the arteries and the veins (example: code number *93882* represented by descriptor *Duplex scan of extracranial arteries, unilateral or limited study*).

The listings within the Non-Invasive Vascular Diagnostic Studies subsection include the provision of requisite patient care in the course of rendering these studies, and additionally include the supervision of the test and the interpretation of the test results, encompassing both the physician's analysis of the data and appropriate documentation in the patient health record.

For coding and reporting purposes, the Duplex scan is defined as an ultrasonic scanning procedure with display of both two-dimensional structure and motion with time and Doppler ultrasonic signal documentation with spectral analysis and color flow velocity mapping or imaging.

A physical examination of the vascular system completed without an assessment of bidirectional vascular flow should not be coded and reported from the listings of the Non-Invasive Vascular Diagnostic Studies subsection. For example, an office evaluation and management of a new patient with compromised circulation to the limbs should be reported with code number *99205*.

Studies in this subsection for vascular studies are presumed to be bilateral. Therefore, if a unilateral vascular diagnostic test was performed, modifier *-52* (signifying reduced services) should supplement the code reported for the procedure rendered.

CPT CODING OF PULMONARY SERVICES

The Pulmonary subsection of the Medicine section of the CPT volume is comprised of listings of pulmonary diagnostic studies and respiratory therapy. A majority of the procedures and services usually performed by pulmonologists should be reported with codes from the Respiratory System subsection of the Surgery section (examples: code number *31625* represented by descriptor *Bronchoscopy; with biopsy;* or code number *32000** represented by descriptor *Thoracentesis, puncture of pleural cavity for aspiration, initial or subsequent*).

Office or outpatient pulmonary services are generally reported with codes from the listings in the Evaluation and Management Services section of the CPT volume. For instance, a follow-up office visit of a patient with chronic asthma should be reported with code number *99213*.

The listings of the Pulmonary subsection of the Medicine section include any associated laboratory tests or procedures as well as any related interpretations rendered by the physician regarding the findings resulting from these tests or procedures. Thus, such constituent tests or procedures should not be coded and reported separately.

CPT CODING OF ALLERGY AND CLINICAL IMMUNOLOGY SERVICES

The Allergy and Clinical Immunology subsection of the Medicine section of the CPT volume contains listings of procedures and services under two headings: *Allergy Testing* and *Allergen Immunotherapy*. The codes listed within this subsection may be reported separately or may be reported in addition to the office or outpatient evaluation and management services codes.

If additional assessment services were rendered by the physician in conjunction with these tests or therapies, applicable evaluation and management services codes should be reported. As examples, an office assessment of a new patient with allergic rhinitis usually should be reported with code number *99202,* and an office visit by an established patient for instruction in the use of a peak flow meter usually should be reported with code number *99211*. Similarly, medical conferences with a patient concerning the use of mechanical or electronic devices (such as precipitators or humidifiers), or the use of climatotherapy or physical therapy should be coded and reported from the listings in the Evaluation and Management Services section.

The notations delineated for the Allergy and Clinical Immunology subsection emphasize the prudent use of clinical acumen in dispensing the services listed within the subsection.

Insurance carriers may or may not accept the separate coding and reporting of the supply of serum used in therapeutic injections.

Notations at the beginning of the Allergy and Clinical Immunology subsection present standardized definitions for coding and reporting purposes. Allergy sensitivity tests are defined as the performance and evaluation of selective cutaneous and mucous membrane tests in correlation with the patient history, the patient physical examination, and other observations of the patient. Immunotherapy (desensitization, hyposensitization) is the parenteral administration of allergenic extracts as antigens at periodic intervals, usually on an increasing dosage scale to a dosage that was maintained as maintenance therapy.

CPT CODING OF NEUROLOGY AND NEUROMUSCULAR SERVICES

The Neurology and Neuromuscular Procedures subsection of the Medicine section of the CPT volume is comprised of listings of neurological procedures and services that may acceptably be coded and reported separately from the listings in the Evaluation and Management Services section. For instance, an office evaluation of dysphagia in an established patient with amyotrophic lateral sclerosis should be reported with code number *99215*.

Under the heading of *Sleep Testing,* notations within this subsection define procedures and services for coding and reporting purposes. Sleep studies and polysomnography refer to at least six hours of continuous and simultaneous monitoring and recording of various physiological and pathophysiological parameters of sleep (such as ventilation and respiratory effort or extremity muscle activity). Physician interpretation and preparation of a report are inherently included in the service; fewer than six hours of monitoring and recording constitutes a reduced service that should be reported with modifier *-52*. For a sleep study to be coded and reported as polysomnography, the sleep must be staged and recorded.

Many neurological services are typically consultative, and therefore accurate evaluation and management services code number and descriptor selection relies upon the level of service, the condition of the patient, and the examination skills utilized. As examples, *Muscle testing, manual,* reported from code range *95831–95834* should be reported in addition to an appropriately selected evaluation and management services code; and *Needle electromyography,* reported from code range *95860–95872* also should be reported in addition to an appropriately selected evaluation and management services code.

Distinct code numbers and descriptors for electroencephalography (EEG) services are listed in the Neurology and Neuromuscular Procedures subsection (example: *Electroencephalogram (EEG),* code range *95822–95827*). The services in these listings are presumed to include the attainment of the tracing, the interpretation of the study, and the preparation of a report. If these three aspects are not encompassed in an electroencephalography (EEG) service, modifier *-52* should be appended to the code reported to denote reduced services (example: code number *95955-52* represented by descriptor *Electroencephalogram during nonintracranial surgery,* without preparation of a report).

CPT CODING OF CHEMOTHERAPY ADMINISTRATION SERVICES

The Chemotherapy Administration subsection of the Medicine section of the CPT volume contains listings of code numbers and descriptors for chemotherapy administration procedures that are independent of and reported separately from office or other outpatient evaluation and management services. For example, an evaluation of increasing dyspnea in an established patient receiving chemotherapy for adenocarcinoma of the colon should be reported with code number *99214*.

Regional chemotherapy perfusion should be reported with codes for arterial infusion. Separate codes should be reported for each method or technique of chemotherapy administration that was utilized (examples: *Chemotherapy administration, intravenous,* should be reported from code range *96408–96414; Chemotherapy administration, intra-arterial,* should be reported from code range *96420–96425*).

The chemotherapy injection procedure codes include the preparation but exclude their supply of chemotherapeutic agents. HCPCS national codes (level II codes from section J) for chemotherapy pharmaceuticals must be reported on Medicare claims by both physicians and hospitals.

CPT CODING OF DERMATOLOGY SERVICES

The Special Dermatological Procedures subsection of the Medicine section of the CPT volume comprises various residual or miscellaneous listings of dermatologic procedures and services (example: *Actinotherapy,* code number *96900*). The preponderance of procedures and services performed by dermatologists should be coded and reported from the listings within the Integumentary System subsection of the Surgery section of the CPT volume (example: *Initial treatment, first degree burn . . . ,* code number *16000*).

Additional consultative or assessment services dispensed by dermatologic physicians should be specifically coded and reported from the listings within the Evaluation and Management Services section of the CPT volume. For example, an initial office visit provided for a patient with cystic acne should be reported with code number *99202*.

CPT CODING OF PHYSICAL MEDICINE AND REHABILITATION SERVICES

The Physical Medicine and Rehabilitation subsection of the Medicine section of the CPT volume contains listings of physical medicine procedures and services (including diagnostic tests and measurements) typically rendered by a registered physical therapist under the direction of a physician. This subsection is divided under three headings. The initial heading, *Modalities,* refers to any physical agent producing therapeutic changes to biologic tissue, including but not limited to thermal, acoustic, light, mechanical, and electric energy.

The heading, *Modalities,* encompasses two subheadings *Supervised,* for application of a modality that does not require direct patient contact with the provider, and *Constant Attendance,* for application of a modality that does require direct patient contact. To exemplify, code number and descriptor *97012 Application of a modality to one area; traction, mechanical* reports a supervised modality, whereas code number descriptor *97034 Application of a modality to one area; contrast baths . . .* reports a modality necessitating constant attendance.

The second heading, *Therapeutic Procedures,* refers to a manner of effecting change through the application of clinical skills and services that attempt to improve function. For example, code number and descriptor *97122 Therapeutic procedure to one area traction, manual* reports a therapeutic procedure. The therapist or physician is required to be in direct patient contact during a therapeutic procedure or service.

The third and last heading, *Tests and Measurements,* refers to evaluation of physical performance or the assessment of development of cognitive skills. For example, code number and descriptor *97750 Physical performance test or measurement . . .* should be utilized to report a test of musculoskeletal functional capacity.

Time factors profoundly affect proper code number and descriptor selection for physical medicine procedures and services. Therefore, adequate documentation of time dimensions for patient treatment modalities is essential. Instead of CPT codes, HCPCS national codes (level II codes) for physical medicine procedures, services, and supplies must be reported on Medicare claims by hospitals.

CPT CODING OF OSTEOPATHIC MANIPULATIVE TREATMENT SERVICES

The Osteopathic Manipulative Treatment subsection comprises a group of five listings to report manual treatment applied by a physician to ameliorate or alleviate somatic dysfunction and related disorders. Osteopathic manipulative treatment can be performed through various techniques and applied to specific body regions, namely, the head region, the cervical region, the thoracic region, the lumbar region, the sacral region, the pelvic region, the rib cage region, the abdomen and viscera region, the upper extremities, and the lower extremities.

If additional assessment services exceeding the customary preservice or postservice work associated with these procedures was rendered by the osteopathic physician in conjunction with these therapies, then applicable evaluation and management services codes should be reported.

CPT CODING OF SPECIAL SERVICES AND REPORTS

The final subsection of the Medicine section of the CPT volume, the Special Services and Reports subsection, furnishes a residual compartment for listings of numerous miscellaneous services. This subsection encompasses three headings.

The first heading, *Miscellaneous Services,* contains listings of code numbers and descriptors to denote the conveyance of specimens, to signify that services were rendered at night or on weekends, to delineate compensation for medical testimony, to indicate physician efforts with educational services, and so forth. The second heading, *Qualifying Circumstances for Anesthesia,* contains listings of code numbers and descriptors to supplement the reporting anesthesia administration in complicated surgical cases. The third and final heading of this concluding subsection of the Medicine section, *Other Services,* contains listings of code numbers and descriptors for miscellaneous medical procedures or services.

The listings of the Special Services and Reports subsection are predominantly adjunct codes or secondary codes utilized and reported with other codes to specify extraordinary effort or unusual situations, and are not codes for reporting the principal reason for a patient encounter. The codes within this subsection may be reported by physicians but may not be reported by hospitals. Diligent usage of the special services codes can positively impact physician reimbursement.

Physicians who are chosen as expert witnesses in legal or administrative proceedings should negotiate appearance or stand-by fees with the attorneys and should request payment prior to their appearance. Code number *99080* may be utilized to report the review of medical records for workers' compensation and casualty cases.

MEDICINE REPORTING FOR BILLING

Physician charges for medical services should be submitted in claims for the aggregate of services rendered to a patient on a single day, and not for each separate and individual patient encounter. Thus, to emphasize, two separate charges for medical services provided to a sole patient by a solitary physician on the same date should not be submitted on insurance claims to third-party payors. If a physician rendered services to a patient more than once on a particular day, a higher level of service may be reported, or the level of service reported may be augmented with an appropriate modifier.

The fee for rendering a medical procedure or service that is submitted by the physician to the third-party payor is termed the "actual charge" for the procedure or service. The amount of this actual charge generally is greater than the amount of reimbursement from the third-party-payor or the "allowed charge" for the medical procedure or service.

As third-party payors, insurance carriers usually rationalize or justify the allowed charge with its lessened amount of reimbursement as reasonable on the basis of a "customary charge" (also termed a "prevailing charge") that is compiled from the average charges of similar physicians for that medical procedure or service. Additionally, this difference between the actual charge and the allowed charge may be rationalized and justified by reason of the co-payment, which is the portion of the actual charge that is paid by the patient directly to the provider of the medical procedure or service.

KEY CONCEPTS

actual charge _____

allowed charge _____

automated multi-channel test _____

average charge _____

customary charge _____

disease-oriented panel _____

modifier _____

organ oriented panel _____

outside laboratory _____

physician component _____

prevailing charge _____

professional component _____

qualitative screening _____

quantitative screening _____

reference laboratory _____

reimbursement _____

separate procedure _____

technical component _____

third-party payor _____

unlisted procedure _____

unlisted service _____

unrelated procedure _____

unrelated service _____

REVIEW EXERCISES

1. Explain the meaning of the term "supervision and interpretation" with reference to the coding and reporting of a radiological procedure or service. _____

_____

2. Explain the meaning of the terms "technical component" and "professional component" with reference to the coding and reporting of a radiological procedure or service. _____

_____

3. Select and indicate the appropriate modifier to supplement the code number in each of the following clinical examples:

   A. radiological supervision and interpretation of a repeat percutaneous placement of enteroclysis tube by another radiologist _____

   B. magnetic resonance imaging of knee joint (physician supervision and interpretation) ____

   C. radiologic examination of the shoulder (two views) with radiologic examination of the elbow (three views) _____

D. computerized axial tomography of the pelvis with contrast material (detailed examination with additional slices) _____

_____

4. Assign precise, accurate code numbers from the CPT volume for the following diagnostic imaging procedures and services:

A. computerized axial tomography of orbit with contrast material _____

_____

B. complete radiological examination of scapula _____

_____

C. oral contrast cholecystography _____

_____

D. retrograde urography _____

E. cardiac magnetic resonance imaging for velocity flow mapping _____

_____

F. radiological supervision and interpretation of epidural venography _____

_____

G. single view radiologic examination of teeth _____

_____

H. radiological examination of thoracic spine (anterolateral and posterior) _____

_____

I. computerized axial tomography of thorax without contrast material _____

_____

J. radiologic supervision and interpretation of bilateral angiography of lower extremities

K. magnetic resonance imaging of brain stem without contrast material _____

_____

L. computerized tomography for bone density study _____

_____

M. radiological supervision and interpretation of lumbosacral myelography _____

_____

5. Assign precise, accurate code numbers from the CPT volume for the following diagnostic ultrasound procedures and services:

A. transrectal echography _____

_____

B. ophthalmic ultrasonic foreign body localization _____

_____

C. radiological supervision and interpretation of gastrointestinal endoscopic ultrasound

_____

D. radiological supervision and interpretation of ultrasonic guidance for endomyocardial biopsy _____

_____

E. fetal biophysical profile _____

_____

F. limited real time renal echography with image documentation _____

_____

G. follow-up B scan nonobstetric pelvic echography with image documentation _____

6. Assign precise, accurate code numbers from the CPT volume for the following radiation oncology procedures and services:

A. complex intracavitary radioelement application _____

B. deep externally generated hyperthermia _____

C. intermediate therapeutic radiology treatment planning _____

D. special medical radiation physics consultation _____

E. surface application of radioelement _____

F. hyperthermia generated by intracavitary probes _____

G. simple interstitial radioelement application _____

7. Assign precise, accurate code numbers from the CPT volume for the following nuclear medicine procedures and services:

A. parathyroid imaging _____

B. liver and spleen imaging with vascular flow _____

C. tomographic brain imaging (complete study) _____

D. intra-articular radionuclide therapy _____

E. red cell survival study _____

F. acute gastrointestinal blood loss imaging _____

G. urinary bladder residual study _____

8. Differentiate between automated multichannel tests and organ- or disease-oriented panels. _____

9. Distinguish between qualitative drug testing and quantitative drug testing. _____

10. Describe the criteria that is imperative or essential for reporting a clinical pathology consultation service. _____

11. Select and indicate the appropriate modifier to supplement the code number in each of the following clinical examples:

A. hepatitis panel performed by reference laboratory _____ _____

B. gross and microscopic necroscopy with spinal cord but not brain _____

12. Explain the meaning of the terms "technical component" and "professional component" with reference to the coding and reporting of a pathology or laboratory procedure or service. ____

13. Assign precise, accurate code numbers from the CPT volume for the following laboratory procedures and services:

A. obstetric panel _____

B. insulin tolerance test _____

C. direct measurement of lipoprotein _____

D. automated hemogram and platelet count _____

E. heparin assay _____

F. viral neutralization test _____

G. culture typing with phage method _____

H. hemagglutination inhibition test _____

I. water load test _____

J. nasal smear for eosinophils _____

K. leukocyte histamine release tent _____

L. flow cytometry reticulocyte count _____

M. arthritis panel _____

N. progesterone receptor assay _____

O. calcium-pentagastrin stimulation panel _____

P. automated urinalysis without microscopy _____

Q. platelet antibody identification _____

R. qualitative syphilis test _____

S. forensic cytopathology _____

_____

T. morphometric analysis of nerve _____

_____

U. pathology consultation during surgery _____

_____

V. complete Rh phenotyping _____

_____

W. platelet neutralization _____

_____

X. forensic examination of acid phosphatase _____

_____

Y. chlorinated hydrocarbon screen _____

_____

Z. cold agglutination screen _____

_____

14. Explain the meaning of the terms "technical component" and "professional component" with reference to the coding and reporting of a medical procedure or service. _____

_____

_____

15. Select and indicate the appropriate modifier to supplement the code number in each of the following clinical examples:

A. unilateral acoustic reflex testing _____

_____

B. esophagogastric manometric studies performed by Dr. Quigley repeated by Dr. Eustus __

_____

C. three hours of individual medical psychotherapy by Dr. Xavier including insight-oriented and behavior-modifying psychotherapy _____

_____

16. Describe the warranted application of evaluation and management services codes in the reporting of psychiatric services and describe the warranted application of psychiatric services codes in the reporting of evaluation and management services. _____

_____

_____

17. Describe the warranted application of evaluation and management services codes in the reporting of dialysis services. _____

_____

_____

18. Explain and differentiate the distinct levels of medical ophthalmology services. _____

_____

_____

19. Describe the warranted application of evaluation and management services codes in the reporting of otolaryngology services. _____

_____

_____

20. Assign precise, accurate code numbers from the CPT volume for the following injection and infusion procedures and services:

   A. immunization injection of poliomyelitis vaccine _____

   _____

   B. immunization injection of tetanus toxoid _____

   _____

   C. immunization injection of influenza virus vaccine _____

   _____

   D. intramuscular injection of antibiotic _____

   _____

   E. intra-arterial therapeutic injection _____

   _____

   F. passive immunization with human immune serum globulin _____

   _____

21. Assign precise, accurate code numbers from the CPT volume for the following psychiatry and biofeedback procedures and services:

   A. psychiatric evaluation of psychometric tests for medical diagnostic purposes _____

   _____

   B. medical psychoanalysis _____

   _____

   C. interactive group medical psychotherapy _____

   _____

   D. electroconvulsive therapy (single seizure) _____

   _____

   E. narcosynthesis for psychiatric diagnostic purposes _____

   _____

   F. family medical psychotherapy without presence of the patient _____

   _____

   G. interactive medical psychiatric diagnostic interview examination _____

   _____

   H. 45 minutes of individual medical psychotherapy _____

   _____

   I. medical hypnotherapy _____

   _____

   J. interactive individual medical psychotherapy _____

   _____

   K. biofeedback training in conduction disorder _____

   _____

   L. biofeedback training by electroencephalogram application _____

   _____

   M. biofeedback training by electromyogram application _____

   _____

22. Assign precise, accurate code numbers from the CPT volume for the following dialysis procedures and services:

   A. peritoneal dialysis with single physician evaluation _____

   _____

   B. one session of patient dialysis training _____

   C. hemodialysis procedure with single physician evaluation _____

   D. hemoperfusion _____

   E. peritoneal dialysis with single physician evaluation _____

   F. one month of end stage renal disease services for a 30-year-old patient _____

23. Assign precise, accurate code numbers from the CPT volume for the following gastroenterology procedures and services:

   A. gastric saline load test _____

   B. esophageal motility study _____

   C. anorectal manometry _____

   D. gastric analysis test with injection of stimulant of gastric secretion _____

   E. breath hydrogen test _____

   F. acid perfusion test for esophagitis _____

24. Assign precise, accurate code numbers from the CPT volume for the following medical ophthalmology procedures and services:

   A. determination of refractive state _____

   B. extended color vision examination _____

   C. repair and refitting of spectacles _____

   D. replacement of contact lens _____

   E. electroretinography with medical diagnostic evaluation _____

   F. fitting of bifocal spectacles _____

   G. fundus photography with medical diagnostic evaluation _____

   H. fluorescein angioscopy with medical diagnostic evaluation _____

   I. tonography with water provocation _____

   J. ophthalmodynamometry _____

K. dark adaptation examination with medical diagnostic evaluation _____

L. supply of contact lenses as permanent prosthesis for aphakia _____

M. comprehensive ophthalmological service for established patient _____

25. Assign precise, accurate code numbers from the CPT volume for the following medical oto-laryngology procedures and services:

A. laryngeal function studies _____

B. ear protector attenuation measurements _____

C. audiometric testing of groups _____

D. oscillating tracking test with recording _____

E. filtered speech test _____

F. electrocochleography _____

G. positional nystagmus test _____

H. Lombard test _____

I. electrodermal audiometry _____

J. diagnostic evaluation of evoked otoacoustic emissions _____

K. acoustic reflex testing _____

L. bidirectional peripheral stimulation optokinetic nystagmus test with recording _____

M. individual speech and language therapy with continuing medical supervision _____

26. Assign precise, accurate code numbers from the CPT volume for the following medical cardiovascular procedures and services:

A. total body plethysmography with interpretation and report _____

B. endomyocardial biopsy _____

C. intracardiac phonocardiogram _____

D. percutaneous balloon valvuloplasty of pulmonary valve _____

E. apex cardiography _____

    F. temporary trancutaneous pacing _____

    G. percutaneous insertion of intra-aortic balloon catheter _____

    H. induction of arrhythmia by electrical pacing _____

    I. determination of venous pressure _____

    J. left heart catheterization by left ventricular puncture _____

    K. cardiopulmonary resuscitation _____

    L. injection procedure during cardiac catheterization for aortography _____

    M. peripheral thermogram _____

    N. rhythm electrocardiogram using three leads without interpretation and report _____

    O. combined transseptal and retrograde left heart catheterization _____

    P. electronic analysis of dual chamber internal pacemaker system _____

    Q. electrophysiologic evaluation of cardioverter-defibrillator _____

27. Assign precise, accurate code numbers from the CPT volume for the following vascular diagnostic procedures and services:

    A. complete bilateral Duplex scan of lower extremity arterial bypass grafts _____

    B. Duplex scan of inferior vena cava (follow-up study) _____

    C. unilateral Duplex scan of extracranial arteries _____

    D. follow-up Duplex scan of arterial inflow and venous outflow of penile vessels _____

    E. transcranial Doppler complete study of the intracranial arteries _____

    F. Duplex scan for complete bilateral study of upper extremity arteries _____

28. Assign precise, accurate code numbers from the CPT volume for the following pulmonary procedures and services:

    A. complex pulmonary stress testing _____

    B. subsequent manipulation of chest wall _____

    C. determination of resistance to airflow by oscillatory method _____

D. initiation and management of continuous negative pressure ventilation _____

E. bronchospasm evaluation _____

F. nonpressurized inhalation treatment for acute airway obstruction _____

G. carbon dioxide expired gas determination by infrared analyzer _____

H. thoracic gas volume test _____

I. test of maximum breathing capacity and maximal voluntary ventilation _____

J. membrane diffusion capacity test _____

K. subsequent intermittent positive pressure breathing oxygen treatment with nebulized medication _____

L. test of respiratory flow volume loop _____

M. functional residual capacity test by helium method _____

29. Assign precise, accurate code numbers from the CPT volume for the following allergy and clinical immunology procedures and services:

A. ophthalmic mucous membrane test _____

B. ingestion challenge test _____

C. rapid desensitization procedure (one hour) _____

D. skin end point titration _____

E. professional allergen immunotherapy service with provision of allergenic extract for two stinging insect venoms _____

F. inhalation bronchial challenge testing with antigens _____

30. Assign precise, accurate code numbers from the CPT volume for the following neurology and neuromuscular procedures and services:

A. electroencephalogram for cerebral death evaluation _____

B. electrodiagnostic testing of orbicularis oculi reflex _____

C. sensory nerve conduction velocity study _____

D. electroencephalogram during nonintracranial surgery _____

E. two hours of intraoperative neurophysiology testing _____

F. somatosensory testing _____

G. electrocorticogram at surgery as separate procedure _____

H. one hour neurobehavioral status exam with interpretation and report _____

I. physician insertion of sphenoidal electrodes for electroencephalographic recording _____

J. one hour assessment of aphasia with interpretation and report _____

K. needle electromyography of two extremities and related paraspinal areas _____

L. neuromuscular junction testing _____

M. needle electromyographic ischemic limb exercise with lactic acid determination _____

31. Assign precise, accurate code numbers from the CPT volume for the following chemotherapy administration procedures and services:

A. refilling and maintenance of portable pump _____

B. chemotherapy administration into pleural cavity with thoracentesis _____

C. intramuscular chemotherapy administration with local anesthesia _____

D. one hour of intravenous chemotherapy administration by infusion technique _____

E. ten hours of intra-arterial chemotherapy administration by infusion technique with the use of a portable pump _____

F. subcutaneous chemotherapy administration with local anesthesia _____

32. Assign precise, accurate code numbers from the CPT volume for the following dermatology procedures and services:

A. ultraviolet light therapy _____

B. photochemotherapy with psoralens and ultraviolet A _____

33. Assign precise, accurate code numbers from the CPT volume for the following physical medicine and rehabilitation procedures and services:

A. initial thirty minutes of testing of upper extremities for strength _____

B. physical medicine whirlpool treatment to legs _____

   C. forty-five minutes of prosthetic training _____

   _____

   D. physical medicine massage treatment to arms _____

   _____

   E. physician manipulation of wrist _____

   _____

   F. one hour of training in activities of daily living _____

   _____

34. Assign precise, accurate code numbers from the CPT volume for the following osteopathic manipulative treatment services:

   A. osteopathic manipulative treatment involving five body regions _____

   _____

   B. osteopathic manipulative treatment involving ten body regions _____

   _____

35. Assign precise, accurate code numbers from the CPT volume for the following special services and reports:

   A. therapeutic phlebotomy _____

   _____

   B. medical testimony _____

   _____

   C. total body hypothermia _____

   _____

   D. office services provided on an emergency basis _____

   _____

   E. conveyance of a specimen for transfer from the physician's office to a laboratory _____

   _____

   F. anesthesia complicated by emergency conditions _____

   _____

CODING OF CLINICAL DOCUMENTATION— RADIOLOGY SECTION OF THE CPT VOLUME

Read the following radiology reports and assign precise, accurate code numbers from the Radiology section of the CPT volume. Radiology reports customarily contain a brief clinical history that is omitted from the following documentation.

RADIOLOGY REPORT

PATIENT: Allen, Mary   **MR#:** 99-14-01

ATTENDING PHYSICIAN: Woods

Portable AP Erect Chest:
An AP erect portable view of the chest shows the heart, lungs, mediastinum, and bony thorax to be within normal limits.

Impression:
Normal portable AP erect chest.

Codes: _____

RADIOLOGY REPORT

PATIENT: Griffith, Delores   **MR#:** 99-14-02

ATTENDING PHYSICIAN: Johnston

Chest:
Consolidation of the left lower lobe has increased since the previous film. There is also involvement of the left upper lobe to a lesser degree. The decubitus view shows a small mobile left pleural effusion. There is linear atelectasis in the right base.

Impression:
Increasing consolidation of the left lung. Small left pleural effusion.

Obstructive Series:
Standard supine and upright views of the abdomen demonstrate no evidence of free air under the diaphragm. Scattered bowel gas is noted in the small and large bowel without significant distention or fluid levels, and there is no radiological evidence for bowel obstruction. The bowel gas pattern is considered to be nonspecific.

Codes: _____

RADIOLOGY REPORT

PATIENT: Miller, Steven   **MR#:** 99-14-03

ATTENDING PHYSICIAN: Skaggs

Pulmonary Ventilation/Perfusion Scan:
Isotope: Tc-99m DTPA, 40 mCi; Tc-99m MAA, 5 mCi

Findings:
There is marked decrease in ventilation and perfusion of the left lung, corresponding to extensive consolidation on the chest X ray.

Impression:
Intermediate probability for pulmonary embolus.

Codes: _____

RADIOLOGY REPORT

PATIENT: Sanders, Anthony   **MR#:** 99-14-04

ATTENDING PHYSICIAN: Hughes

Chest:
The cardiac size appears within normal limits. Interstitial pneumonic infiltrates involving the right upper and lower lung fields are consistent with pneumonia. No pleural effusion is identified.

Impression:
Infiltrates, right upper and lower lobes, rule out pneumonia.

Barium Enema:
There is nonvisualization of the appendix in the filled colon X rays. However, a proximal 1-cm appendix was visualized in the post evacuation X rays. This finding is rather nonspecific for appendicitis. There are no strictures, no abnormal dilations, or no other abnormalities in the colon. There are a few fecal filling defects, limiting this examination for the detection of polypoid lesions.

Codes: _____

RADIOLOGY REPORT

PATIENT: Wallace, Barbara   **MR#:** 99-14-05

ATTENDING PHYSICIAN: Mills

Sonogram Abdomen:
Shows gallstone. There is thickening of the gallbladder wall due to edema. Common bile duct is 4.5 mm and is normal. Pancreas is normal. There is fluid density around both kidneys. No mass or abscess of kidneys is seen. Liver is normal.

Impression:
Gallstone. Edema of gallbladder wall. Perinephric fluid in both kidneys, questionable perinephritis. Recommend CT scan.

Codes: _____

RADIOLOGY REPORT

PATIENT: Hiashi, Takara   **MR#:** 99-14-06

ATTENDING PHYSICIAN: Barber

Portable Chest:
There is pulmonary vascular congestion. Questionable infiltrates are noted in the left upper lung. There are linear densities in the left mid lung that could be from linear atelectasis or fluid. Prominent left basal vascular markings are noted. There is a left chest tube. There is a left subcutaneous emphysema. There is dextroscoliosis of the thoracic spine.

Codes: _____

RADIOLOGY REPORT

PATIENT: Carpenter, Mark   **MR#:** 99-14-07

ATTENDING PHYSICIAN: Stephens

IVP:
The scout film shows a large calcification in the left pelvis measuring about 4 cm × 6 cm. There is also a calcification overlying the right kidney region. There is good excretion of contrast material bilaterally. The size and shape of both kidneys are normal. There is a dromedary hump on the left side. There is minimal dilation of the collecting system on the left, and there is moderate dilation of the left ureter. The calyceal system on the right shows partial duplication but is otherwise normal. The right ureter is normal. The bladder is also within normal limits. The distal left ureter does point right towards the stone seen on the scout film.

Impression:
Large left ureteral stone in the distal left ureter, which is causing only minimal obstructive symptoms.

Codes: _____

RADIOLOGY REPORT

PATIENT: Harris, Lee   **MR#:** 99-14-08

ATTENDING PHYSICIAN: Bommarito

Portable Chest:
Shows pulmonary edema. NG tube is seen in the stomach. Otherwise negative.

KUB:
Compared to previous examination 24 hours ago, there is no interval change. No bowel obstruction, ileus, or other anomaly.

Obstructive Series:
No evidence of bowel obstruction, ileus, free air, or mass in the abdomen.

Impression:
Negative.

Codes: _____

RADIOLOGY REPORT

PATIENT: Pappas, Ellen   **MR#:** 99-14-09

ATTENDING PHYSICIAN: Hakeem

Chest:
Anteroposterior and Lateral
   Extensive consolidation of the left lung is unchanged. No significant pleural fluid layers on the decubitus view. There is linear atelectasis at the right base.

Impression:
Extensive left lung consolidation.

Codes: _____

RADIOLOGY REPORT

PATIENT: Maxwell, Frank   **MR#:** 99-14-10

ATTENDING PHYSICIAN: Simmons

Chest:
There is a calcified nodule in the right upper lobe. There is no active cardiopulmonary disease or pleural effusion.

Impression:
No active disease.

Upper GI Series:
There is a superficial ulceration of the distal antrum, pyloric channel, and duodenal bulb.

Obstructive Series:
There is no free air under the diaphragm. No obstruction to the small or large bowel.

Impression:
Grossly negative abdomen.

Codes: _____

CODING OF CLINICAL DOCUMENTATION— LABORATORY REPORTS

Read the following laboratory reports and assign precise, accurate code numbers from the Pathology and Laboratory section of the CPT volume.

LABORATORY REPORT

PATIENT: Sullivan, John   **MR#:** 99-14-11

ATTENDING PHYSICIAN: Quinn

Chem 13

Test Result	Unit Expected Value	Graph	
Albumin	2.5 g/dL	(3.4–5.0)	(*)
Total Protein	7.6 g/dL	(6.5–8.0)	(*)
Total Bilirubin	0.2 mg/dL	(0.1–1.0)	(*)
ALT	34 IU/L	(0–40)	(*)
AST	30 IU/L	(10–37)	(*)
ALP	196 IU/L	(39–117)	( )
Calcium	8.5 mg/dL	(8.5–10.6)	(*)
Phosphate	3.6 mg/dL	(2.7–4.5)	(*)
Cholesterol	154 mg/dL	(165–280)	( )
Triglyceride	151 mg/dL	(0–150)	( )
Uric Acid	2.5 mg/dL	(3.4–7.0)	( )
LDH	146 IU/L	(85–190)	(*)

Codes: _____

LABORATORY REPORT

PATIENT: Kemp, Debra   **MR#:** 99-14-12

ATTENDING PHYSICIAN: Rizzo

Chem 20

Test Result	Unit Expected Value	Graph	
BUN	13 mg/dL	(6–19)	(*)
Sodium	140 mEq/L	(135–148)	(*)
Potassium	4.7 mEq/L	(3.5–5.3)	(*)
Chloride	105 mEq/L	(100–112)	(*)
CO_2	23 mEq/L	(23–29)	(*)
Glucose	91 mg/dL	(70–110)	(*)
Creatinine	1.1 mg/dL	(0.7–1.3)	(*)
Anion Gap	12	(4–14)	(*)

BUN/Creatinine	11.8 mg/dL	(10.0–20.0)	(*)
Albumin	3.3 g/dL	(3.4–5.0)	( )
Total Protein	7.7 g/dL	(6.5–8.0)	(*)
Total Bilirubin	0.4 mg/dL	(0.1–1.0)	(*)
ALT	65 IU/L	(0–40)	( )
AST	53 IU/L	(10–37)	( )
ALP	64 IU/L	(39–117)	(*)
Calcium	8.8 mg/dL	(8.5–10.6)	(*)
Phosphate	3.3 mg/dL	(2.7–4.5)	(*)
Cholesterol	188 mg/dL	(165–280)	(*)
Triglyceride	130 mg/dL	(0–150)	(*)
Uric Acid	6.7 mg/dL	(3.4–7.0)	(*)
LDH	212 IU/L	(85–190)	( )
CPK	157 IU/L	(24–195)	(*)

Toxicology Drug Screen
Specimen Submitted:
   Urine

Drugs Detected in Urine:
Benzodiazepine Metabolites
   The submitted specimen was screened for, but not limited to, the following drugs:

Amphetamines	Barbiturates	Volatiles
Acetaminophen	Ethchlorvynol	Acetone
Salicylate	Glutethimide	Ethanol
Antihistamines	Methaqualone	Methanol
Antidepressants	Cocaine	Isopropranol
Anticonvulsants	Phencyclidine	Lidocaine
Phenobarbital	Phenylpropanolamine	Quinidine
Primidone	Phenothiazine Metabolites	
Phenytoin	Benzodiazepine Metabolites	
Carbamazepine	Narcotics	Meprobamate

Note: Results also include any other drugs that were detected that are not in the preceding list.

Codes: _____

LABORATORY REPORT

PATIENT: Blumenthal, Wayne   **MR#:** 99-14-13

ATTENDING PHYSICIAN: Milligan

Chem 20

Test Result	Unit Expected Value	Graph	
BUN	14 mg/dL	(6–19)	(*)
Sodium	138 mEq/L	(135–148)	(*)

Potassium	4.4 mEq/L	(3.5–5.3)	(*)
Chloride	106 mEq/L	(100–112)	(*)
CO_2	30 mEq/L	(23–29)	( )
Glucose	77 mg/dL	(70–110)	(*)
Creatinine	1.4 mg/dL	(0.7–1.3)	( )
Anion Gap	2	(4–14)	( )
BUN/Creatinine	10.0 mg/dL	(10.0–20.0)	(*)
Albumin	3.6 g/dL	(3.4–5.0)	(*)
Total Protein	7.9 g/dL	(6.5–8.0)	(*)
Total Bilirubin	0.4 mg/dL	(0.1–1.0)	(*)
ALT	41 IU/L	(0–40)	( )
AST	32 IU/L	(10–37)	(*)
ALP	81 IU/L	(39–117)	(*)
Calcium	9.3 mg/dL	(8.5–10.6)	(*)
Phosphate	3.5 mg/dL	(2.7–4.5)	(*)
Cholesterol	127 mg/dL	(165–280)	( )
Triglyceride	160 mg/dL	(0–150)	( )
Uric Acid	7.4 mg/dL	(3.4–7.0)	( )
LDH	226 IU/L	(85–190)	( )

Codes: _____

LABORATORY REPORT

PATIENT: Oakley, Nancy   **MR#:** 99-14-14

ATTENDING PHYSICIAN: Palmer

PRO 8

Test Result	Unit Expected Value	Graph	
BUN	9 mg/dL	(6–19)	(*)
Sodium	144 mEq/L	(135–148)	(*)
Potassium	3.8 mEq/L	(3.5–5.3)	(*)
Chloride	104 mEq/L	(100–112)	(*)
CO_2	26 mEq/L	(23–29)	(*)
Glucose	110 mg/dL	(70–110)	(*)
Creatinine	1.2 mg/dL	(0.7–1.3)	(*)
Anion Gap	14	(4–14)	(*)
BUN/Creatinine	7.5 mg/dL	(10.0–20.0)	( )
Cholesterol	234 mg/dL	(145–240)	(*)
Triglyceride	171 mg/dL	(0–150)	( )

Toxicology Drug Screen:
Specimen Submitted:
Urine

Drugs Detected in Urine:

Ethanol

Diphenhydramine

The submitted specimen was screened for, but not limited to, the following drugs:

Amphetamines	Barbiturates	Volatiles
Acetaminophen	Ethchlorvynol	Acetone
Salicylate	Glutethimide	Ethanol
Antihistamines	Methaqualone	Methanol
Antidepressants	Cocaine	Isopropranol
Anticonvulsants	Phencyclidine	Lidocaine
Phenobarbital	Phenylpropanolamine	Quinidine
Primidone	Phenothiazine Metabolites	Meprobamate
Phenytoin	Benzodiazepine Metabolites	
Carbamazepine	Narcotics	

Note: Results also include any other drugs that were detected that are not in the preceding list.

Codes: _____

LABORATORY REPORT

PATIENT: Costello, Brian   **MR#:** 99-14-15

ATTENDING PHYSICIAN: Evans

PRO 8

Test Result	Unit Expected Value	Graph	
BUN	5 mg/dL	(6–19)	( )
Sodium	140 mEq/L	(135–148)	(*)
Potassium	3.2 mEq/L	(3.5–5.3)	( )
Chloride	107 mEq/L	(100–112)	(*)
CO_2	20 mEq/L	(23–29)	( )
Glucose	76 mg/dL	(70–110)	(*)
Creatinine	0.9 mg/dL	(0.7–1.3)	(*)
Anion Gap	13	(4–14)	(*)
BUN/Creatinine	5.6 mg/dL	(10.0–20.0)	( )

Chem 20

Test Result	Unit Expected Value	Graph	
BUN	17 mg/dL	(6–19)	(*)
Sodium	141 mEq/L	(135–148)	(*)
Potassium	4.2 mEq/L	(3.5–5.3)	(*)

Chloride	105 mEq/L	(100–112)	(*)
CO_2	30 mEq/L	(23–29)	( )
Glucose	127 mg/dL	(70–110)	( )
Creatinine	1.3 mg/dL	(0.7–1.3)	(*)
Anion Gap	6	(4–14)	(*)
BUN/Creatinine	13.1 mg/dL	(10.0–20.0)	(*)
Albumin	4.1 g/dL	(3.4–5.0)	(*)
Total Protein	6.9 g/dL	(6.5–8.0)	(*)
Total Bilirubin	0.9 mg/dL	(0.1–1.0)	(*)
ALT	8 IU/L	(0–40)	(*)
AST	15 IU/L	(10–37)	(*)
ALP	63 IU/L	(39–117)	(*)
Calcium	9.2 mg/dL	(8.5–10.6)	(*)
Phosphate	3.8 mg/dL	(2.7–4.5)	(*)
Cholesterol	182 mg/dL	(140–260)	(*)
Triglyceride	165 mg/dL	(0–150)	( )

Codes: _____

LABORATORY REPORT

PATIENT: Austin, Karen   **MR#:** 99-14-16

ATTENDING PHYSICIAN: Wexler

Chem 13

Test Result	Unit Expected Value	Graph	
Albumin	4.5 g/dL	(3.4–5.0)	(*)
Total Protein	8.0 g/dL	(6.5–8.0)	(*)
Total Bilirubin	0.4 mg/dL	(0.1–1.0)	(*)
ALT	22 IU/L	(0–40)	(*)
AST	29 IU/L	(10–37)	(*)
ALP	53 IU/L	(39–117)	(*)
Calcium	9.1 mg/dL	(8.5–10.6)	(*)
Phosphate	3.3 mg/dL	(2.7–4.5)	(*)
Cholesterol	253 mg/dL	(140–260)	(*)
Triglyceride	118 mg/dL	(0–150)	(*)
Uric Acid	7.9 mg/dL	(3.4–7.0)	( )
LDH	169 IU/L	(85–190)	(*)

Codes: _____

CODING OF CLINICAL DOCUMENTATION — SURGICAL PATHOLOGY REPORTS

Read the following surgical pathology reports and assign precise, accurate code numbers from the Pathology and Laboratory section of the CPT volume.

SURGICAL PATHOLOGY REPORT

PATIENT: Vickers, Peter   **MR#:** 99-14-17

SURGEON: Delaney

Clinical Diagnosis:
Ventral hernia.

Postoperative Diagnosis:
Ventral hernia.

Operative Procedure:
Ventral hernia repair.

Specimen:
Ventral hernia sac.

Gross:
The specimen labeled "ventral hernia sac" consists of a piece of soft tissue showing focal areas of fibrous thickening with membranous appearance measuring approximately 3.7 cm in length. A representative section is submitted in Block A.

Microscopic:
The sections of hernia sac show diffuse areas of fibrosis. Foci of mild chronic inflammatory cell infiltrates are also seen.

Diagnosis:
Soft tissue, abdominal wall, excision and repair of ventral hernia. Hernia sac with fibrosis and chronic inflammation.

Codes: _____

SURGICAL PATHOLOGY REPORT

PATIENT: Schmitt, Laura   **MR#:** 99-14-18

SURGEON: Haynes

Clinical Diagnosis:
Status Post Colostomy.

Postoperative Diagnosis:
Same.

Operative Procedure:
Colostomy takedown.

Specimen:
Distal anastomotic site of colostomy takedown.

Gross:

The specimen is labeled as "colostomy takedown" and consists of a linear piece of tissue that is 6.0 cm × 0.3 cm in greatest dimensions and is reddish brown in appearance. The specimen is totally submitted and labeled as Block A.

Microscopic:

The section of the colostomy stump shows a portion of the colonic wall, which shows chronic inflammation with fibrosis. In focal areas, foreign body giant cell reaction to suture material is also noted. No evidence of malignancy is noted.

Diagnosis:

Chronic inflammation with fibrosis of colonic wall.

Foreign body giant cell reaction to suture material.

Codes: _____

SURGICAL PATHOLOGY REPORT

PATIENT: Kramer, Dennis   **MR#:** 99-14-19

SURGEON: Owens

Specimens:

A: Right spermatic cord lipoma.
B: Right inguinal node.

Gross Examination:

A: Received is a fragment of fibromembranous and fatty tissue that measures 4.4 cm × 3.0 cm × 2.0 cm. On cut section most of the tissue appears to be fat, which is circumscribed and appears to be partially encapsulated. One representative section is submitted.
B: Received is a fragment of yellow fatty tissue measuring 1.5 cm × 1.4 cm × 0.8 cm. On cut section all of the tissue appears to be fat and appears to be partially encapsulated. No evident lymph node structure is identified grossly. One representative section is submitted.

Microscopic Diagnoses:

A: Hernia sac and lipoma.
B: Lymph node showing fatty replacement.

Codes: _____

SURGICAL PATHOLOGY REPORT

PATIENT: Baldwin, Sandra   **MR#:** 99-14-20

SURGEON: Jackson

Specimen:

Gallbladder.

Gross:

There is a single calculus that is yellow to brown 0.7 cm diameter mulberry type. The previously opened gallbladder consists of two portions, one measuring 6.0 cm × 3.5 cm × 1.2 cm showing abundant fat and multiple staples, the other portion measuring 6.0 cm × 3.0 cm × 1.5 cm is the portion of fundus that is previously opened.

Microscopic Diagnoses:
1. Chronic cholecystitis.
2. Cholelithiasis.

Codes: _____

SURGICAL PATHOLOGY REPORT

PATIENT: Tucker, Gary   **MR#:** 99-14-21

SURGEON: Mayfield

Clinical Diagnosis:
Left scrotal mass.

Postoperative Diagnosis:
Left scrotal mass.

Operative Procedure:
Excision left scrotal mass.

Specimen:
Left scrotal mass.

Gross:
The specimen labeled "rectal scrotal mass" consists of a piece of grayish tan soft tissue that is roughly ovoid in shape, measuring approximately 2.3 cm in length and 2.0 cm in greatest diameter. In cut section it is moderately firm in consistency, grayish tan in color, and slightly trabeculated. A representative section is submitted in Block A.

Microscopic:
The sections show a mass made up of groups and nests of cells with moderate amount of pink cytoplasm, round- or oval-shaped nuclei with inconspicuous nucleoli arranged in chords or glandular fashion around empty spaces that are somewhat variable in size and shape, separated from each other by strands of fibrocollagenous soft tissue. The histological features are characteristic of adenomatoid tumor.

Diagnosis:
Adenomatoid tumor.

Codes: _____

SURGICAL PATHOLOGY REPORT

PATIENT: Ewing, Carol   **MR#:** 99-14-22

SURGEON: Hudson

Clinical Diagnosis:
Partial small bowel obstruction.

Perforated viscus.

Intrauterine pregnancy of 17 weeks gestation.

Postoperative Diagnosis:
Partial small bowel obstruction.

Perforated viscus.

Complete second trimester miscarriage.

Operative Procedure:
Exploratory laparotomy and small bowel resection.

Specimens:
Small bowel, nonviable fetus, membranes, cord, placenta.

Gross:
The specimen is received in two parts.

The first part of the specimen is labeled "small bowel" and consists of a segment of bowel measuring approximately 22 cm in length and 4 cm in greatest diameter. Located approximately in the middle of the specimen there appears to be constriction of the lumen due to the specimen being twisted. In this constricted area, there is a marked softening and necrosis of the intestine, which has a grayish discoloration and is fragmented. The discoloration also extends into half of the bowel on one side. In this discolored area, the mucosal surface shows focal areas of congestion and hemorrhage with marked edema, however, the entire mucosal wall does not appear to be necrotic, except in the area of obstruction. The external surface in the other half shows yellowish white exudate. The mucosal surface is unremarkable except for edema. Also included in the same container is an irregular fragment of grayish soft tissue that appears necrotic and measures approximately 9 cm × 6 cm × 1 cm in greatest dimension. Representative sections are submitted as Block A. Sections from the discolored half of the bowel area are submitted as Block B and Block C. Sections from the relatively normal appearing bowel are submitted as Block D. A section of the separate necrotic fetus is submitted as Block E. The head is normocephalic, and no external deformities are identified. All four extremities include the usual five digits. A segment of umbilical cord measuring approximately 24 cm in length is attached to the fetus; the umbilical cord measures 8 mm in greatest diameter and appears to contain three umbilical vessels. Representative sections of the fetal liver and umbilical cord are submitted as Block F. The placenta weighs approximately 57 grams and the umbilical cord is completely separated from the placenta. The membranes are translucent. The placenta measures approximately 9.5 cm by 8.5 cm by 0.5 cm in greatest dimensions. On the maternal surface, the cotyledons appear intact. Representative sections of the placenta and membranes are submitted as Block G and Block H.

Microscopic:
In Block A, sections of the small bowel exhibit complete necrosis and hemorrhage at the site of the obstruction. These necrotic changes extend to and involve the adjacent mesentery. In Block B and in Block C there is marked congestion with focal hemorrhage in the mucosa. The submucosa is edematous and with acute inflammatory reaction on the serosal surface. Block D also exhibits edema with acute inflammatory reaction on the serosal surface that is consistent with peritonitis. Block E consists of adipose tissue with marked congestion and focal areas of hemorrhage with acute inflammation. Sections of fetal tissue exhibit partially autolyzed hepatic tissue with prominent extramedullary hematopoiesis. Sections of the placenta exhibit immature chorionic villi and decidua. The villi appear hypercellular and several blood vessels are identified. The umbilical cord contains three blood vessels.

Diagnosis:
Necrosis with a history of obstruction; Edema with acute peritonitis; Fetal demise at approximately 17 to 18 weeks of gestational age

Codes: _____

SURGICAL PATHOLOGY REPORT

PATIENT: Moran, William   **MR#:** 99-14-23

SURGEON: Reed

Clinical Diagnosis:
Mass of left cheek, inner aspect of left side of mouth.

Postoperative Diagnosis:
Same.

Operative Procedure:
Excision of mass of left mouth

Specimen:
Lesion from inner left aspect of mouth

Gross:
The specimen labeled "cyst from left side of mouth" consists of a piece of soft tissue that is irregular in shape, measuring approximately 2.0 cm × 1.5 cm × 1.2 cm in maximum dimensions. In cut section almost the entire specimen is made up of a whitish gray, slightly firm mass with somewhat glistening and mucoid lobulated appearance in the cut surface. Small amount of pinkish red soft tissue consistent with the skeletal muscle is focally noted in the periphery of the lesion. The entire surgical margin is labeled with green ink. The specimen is serially sectioned and totally submitted as Block A and Block B.

Microscopic:
The sections show a low-grade mucoepidermoid carcinoma made up primarily of glandular or cystic spaces lined by goblet cells containing large amounts of intracytoplasmic mucin. Cystic dilation of the glands containing large amounts of mucin in the lumen are also frequently seen. Extravasation of mucin into the interstitial tissue, between collagen and skeletal muscle fibers, carries with it nests and groups of tumor cells. Small groups and nests of intermediate and poorly differentiated squamous cells are occasionally seen next to mucin-producing cells lining the glandular and cystic spaces. The stroma shows fairly dense fibrosis containing foci of chronic inflammatory cell infiltrates, predominantly plasma cells. The tumor involves surgical margins labeled with green ink at multiple points.

Diagnosis:
Low-grade mucoepidermoid carcinoma.

Codes: _____

SURGICAL PATHOLOGY REPORT

PATIENT: Valentino, Billy   **MR#:** 99-14-24

SURGEON: Moss

Clinical Diagnosis:
Right cervical lymphadenopathy.

Postoperative Diagnosis:
Right cervical lymphadenopathy.

Operative Procedure:
Excisional biopsy of right cervical lymph node.

Specimen:
Right cervical lymph node.

Gross:
The specimen is labeled as "right cervical lymph node" and consists of an irregular mass of tissue, which is 1.3 cm × 1.1 cm in greatest dimensions. A lymph node is identified. On cut sections it is pale white in appearance. It is bisected, totally submitted, labeled as Block A and Block B.

Microscopic:
The section of the cervical lymph node shows partial loss of normal architecture and infiltration by polymorphous cellular infiltrate typical of Hodgkin's lymphoma. The infiltrate is mostly comprised of eosinophils, lymphocytes, and histiocytes. Several typical lacunar and multilobated giant cells are also included. Many of the cells are multilobated and have smudgy nuclei, however, several typical binucleated Reed-Sternberg cells are also identified. One lymph node included also shows increased fibrosis with tendency to nodule formation. The pattern is consistent with the nodular sclerosing type of Hodgkin's lymphoma.

Diagnosis:
Hodgkin's lymphoma, nodular sclerosing type.

Codes: _____

SURGICAL PATHOLOGY REPORT

PATIENT: Foster, Linda   **MR#:** 99-14-25

SURGEON: Rodgers

Clinical Diagnosis:
Cholelithiasis.

Postoperative Diagnosis:
Cholelithiasis.

Pancreatic pseudocyst.

Operative Procedure:
Exploratory laparotomy, cholecystectomy, biopsy.

Specimen:
Gallbladder.

Biopsy of cyst wall.

Gross:
The specimen is received in two parts.

The first part of the specimen is labeled "gallbladder" and consists of a gallbladder, which is 9.5 cm × 3.5 cm in greatest dimensions. The serosal surface of the gallbladder is discolored green. On opening the gallbladder, it contains a large amount of bile and a few small, mulberry-shaped stones are also noted. These stones range from 3 cm to 4 mm in greatest dimension. The wall of the gallbladder is thickened and the mucosa is granular and slightly speckled in appearance. Representative sections are submitted and labeled as Block A.

The second part of the specimen is labeled as "biopsy, cyst wall" and consists of an elliptical piece of tissue, which is 3.0 cm × 1.0 cm × 1.0 cm in greatest dimensions. One surface of this cyst wall is hemorrhagic in appearance. Representative sections are submitted and labeled as Block B.

Microscopic:
The sections of the gallbladder show fibromuscular thickening of the wall and the interstitium is infiltrated by chronic inflammatory cells. The overlying epithelium is secretory and no evidence of malignancy is noted.

The sections of the biopsy of the cyst wall show fibroconnective tissue in which no definite epithelial lining is noted. The wall is infiltrated by acute and chronic inflammatory cells. The inner surface of the cyst is lined by granulation tissue and a large number of acute inflammatory cells are also noted with proliferation of the fibroblasts. No evidence of malignancy is noted.

Diagnosis:
Chronic cholecystitis.

Cholelithiasis.

Pancreatic pseudocyst.

Acute and chronic inflammation of pancreatic pseudocyst wall.

Codes: _____

SURGICAL PATHOLOGY REPORT

PATIENT: Smoot, Donna   **MR#:** 99-14-26

SURGEON: Li

Clinical Diagnosis:
Mammary hyperplasia.

Postoperative Diagnosis:
Mammary hyperplasia.

Operative Procedure:
Bilateral mastectomy.

Specimen:
Left breast tissue.

Right breast tissue.

Gross:
The specimen is received in two parts.

Specimen 1, labeled "left breast tissue" consists of two irregular fragments of yellowish tan soft tissue measuring approximately 5.0 cm × 4.5 cm × 3.0 cm and 3.5 cm × 3.2 cm × 2.6 cm in greatest dimensions, respectively. The external surface is irregular. On sectioning, part of the specimen appears to be white in color and indurated. The area of induration is irregular, measuring approximately 2.2 cm × 3.5 cm. Representative sections are submitted as Block A, Block B, and Block C.

Specimen 2, labeled "right breast tissue" consists of two irregular fragments of soft tissue partly covered by fat. The fragments measure 5.5 cm × 4.5 cm × 2.7 cm and 5.5 cm × 4.4 cm × 2.8 cm in greatest dimensions, respectively. Sectioning shows focal areas of whitish induration. The bulk of the tissue consists of yellow lobulated fat. Representative sections are submitted as Block D, Block E, and Block F.

Microscopic:
Sections of the left and right breast tissue show extensive stromal fibrosis and hyalinization. Few mammary ducts are identified and some of these show slight hyperplasia. No definite periductal edema or inflammation is seen. The histologic changes, other than the stromal fibrosis, are very slight, but consistent with mammary hyperplasia.

Diagnosis:
Intraductal hyperplasia, mild, focal with stromal fibrosis.

Codes: _____

POSTMORTEM EXAMINATION

PATIENT: Szabo, Louis   **MR#:** 99-14-27

PATHOLOGIST: Abbott

External Description:
The body is that of a well-developed, well-nourished elderly Caucasian male. The head is normal in size and shape, and the scalp is partially covered with long white hair. Facial features are not remarkable. The right cornea has a cloudy, glazed appearance. The mouth is largely edentulous, and the mucosal surfaces having a pasty grayish green appearance. There is a slight degree of beard growth. The chest is slightly increased in AP diameter and the abdomen is protuberant. External genitalia are normal adult male except for reddish purple discoloration of the scrotum. Extremities are bilaterally symmetrical. There is no rigor or livor mortis.

Body Cavities:
The body is opened by the usual Y-shaped incision and the sternum removed. There is no abnormal accumulation of blood or fluid in any of the body cavities. There are a few fibrous adhesions in the apical portions of the upper lobes of both lungs.

Cardiovascular System:
The heart is of normal size and shape. Coronary arteries are in their usual distribution and show a moderate degree of arteriosclerosis with areas of up to 50% narrowing of the lumen. No thrombi or other occlusions are identified. The myocardium is firm reddish brown and of normal thickness. The valves of the heart are normally disposed and appear grossly normal except for slight fusion of the aortic cusps. The aorta and great vessels show a mild to moderate degree of arteriosclerosis.

Codes: _____

CODING OF CLINICAL DOCUMENTATION — CLINICAL DISCHARGE REPORTS

Read the successive clinical discharge reports and itemize (without codes) the evaluation and management services indicated in these reports. Assign precise, accurate code numbers from the CPT volume to completely report (without modifiers) all codable procedures and services (except evaluation and management services), but do not repeat codes for repeat procedures. Code all procedures and services rendered either by the physician or the hospital including procedures and services from the Anesthesia, Surgery, Radiology, Pathology and Laboratory, and Medicine sections, and indicate any definitive principal procedure.

DISCHARGE SUMMARY

PATIENT: Abrams, George   **MR#:** 99-14-28

ATTENDING PHYSICIAN: Ott

History of Present Illness:

This 77-year-old male with a history of exertional dyspnea recently underwent exercise stress testing. There were ST-T changes suggestive of ischemia. The patient had a mild decrease of his systolic blood pressure as well as exercise-induced Wenckebach and ventricular ectopy. This was interpreted as a positive exercise stress test and he was referred for cardiac catheterization. Details of his cardiac catheterization are contained in the previously dictated cardiac catheterization note.

Physical Examination:

The patient is a pleasant white male with a resting blood pressure of 140/80. His skin is warm and dry. The head, eyes, ears, nose, and throat are unremarkable. The chest is somewhat barreled in configuration with decreased breath sounds and scattered wheezes. Cardiac exam reveals normal PMI, regular in rate, no evidence of S-2, S-3, or S-4. The carotid artery pulses are 2+ without bruits. The extremities are normal.

Hospital Course:

The patient was admitted and underwent left and right heart catheterization with ventriculography and coronary arteriography. He was found to have normal systemic arterial hemodynamics and pulmonary arterial hypertension with pressures running 30-32/14. Cardiac output was normal. Ventricular function, systolic and diastolic, was normal; and coronary arteriography was normal. The patient experienced no difficulties from the cardiac catheterization, and by the following morning his groin was healing well without evidence of hematoma and with good distal pulse. On telemetry it was noted that he was bradycardic into the 40s and had a brief transitory period of Wenckebach type 20 A-V block. He was asymptomatic during this time. He was discharged with no ill effects from the cardiac catheterization. He is to follow up with Dr. Rivera in two weeks for pulmonary consultation and pulmonary function testing. The patient was informed that his heart is fine and that the likely reason for his dyspnea seems to be pulmonary in origin.

Discharge Diagnosis:

Dyspnea on exertion.

Pulmonary arterial hypertension.

Chronic obstructive lung disease by history.

Normal coronary arteriography.

Wenckebach A-V block, asymptomatic.

Procedures:

Left and right heart catheterization with ventriculography and coronary arteriography.

Discharge Medications:

Alupent 10 mg b.i.d.; Sloxin 400 mg b.i.d.; Dilatrate 40 mg b.i.d.

Codes: _____

DISCHARGE SUMMARY

PATIENT: Goldstein, Rose   **MR#:** 99-14-29

ATTENDING PHYSICIAN: Yaeger

Chief Complaint and History of Present Illness:

This 78-year-old white female was admitted for evaluation of abdominal pain, nausea, and vomiting with reports of coffee-ground emesis. Several weeks ago she was evaluated as an out-patient for similar symptoms and was told she has several ulcers in her distal esophagus. She was subsequently started on medications and did fairly well after the initiation of medications, but over the course of the past three days prior to admission, she had increasing left upper quadrant discomfort along with nausea, vomiting, and hematemesis. She also states a history of a 35-pound weight loss over the last 18 months. She underwent another evaluation and was found to have erosive gastritis with duodenitis as well as reflux esophagitis. She also has left upper quadrant pain, which is attributed to post herpes zoster neuritis. The patient previously had a cholecystectomy and an appendectomy.

Physical Examination on Admission:

Multiple well-healed abdominal scars are present. No masses are palpable. There is mild discomfort in the left upper quadrant on palpation. Bowel sounds are normal.

Laboratory Data on Admission:

Hemoglobin was 13.8 and WBC was 8000. Urinalysis showed 3+ protein with 1 to 3 RBC's/HPF. SMAC was normal except for a slight elevation of BUN at 38.

Hospital Course:

The patient underwent esophagogastroduodenoscopy by Dr. Mattingly with findings of some mild erythema in the prepyloric area. Otherwise the exam was unremarkable. CT scan of the abdomen was normal. Serum gastrin was slightly elevated at 256, and gastric analysis showed a quite low basal rate of 0.3 mEq/hr, an also low maximal acid output of 7.1, and a peak acid output of 10 mEq/hr. Zantac was discontinued about 24 hours prior to the gastric analysis. Barium enema was done, and was grossly normal. The patient has atrophic gastritis. She was started on Reglan and displayed marked improvement with regard to her nausea and abdominal discomfort. The patient has irritable bowel syndrome. A high-fiber diet was instituted with the continuation of Reglan and Zantac. She was instructed to continue a bland diet and to add additional foods gradually. She is to return to the office in three weeks for follow-up.

Diagnoses:

Atrophic gastritis.

Irritable bowel syndrome.

Procedures:
Esophagogastroduodenoscopy.

Discharge Medications:
Zantac 150 mg p.o. b.i.d.; Reglan 10 mg p.o. a.c and h.s.; Restoril 30 mg h.s. p.r.n. for sleep; Darvocet-N 100 1 q. 4 hours p.r.n. for pain.

Codes: _____

DISCHARGE SUMMARY

PATIENT: McCormick, Wanda   **MR#:** 99-14-30

ATTENDING PHYSICIAN: Billingsley

History of Present Illness and Hospital Course:
This 46-year-old white female was admitted from the emergency room following a fall in a parking lot. The patient suffered a comminuted fracture of the left femur. The patient was admitted and was seen in consultation by Dr. Fraser because of the history of asthma and obesity. She was cleared for surgery and on the evening of admission, the patient was taken to the operating room. Open reduction and internal fixation was performed under spinal anesthesia using a compression screw and fixation plate. Hemovac tubes were inserted. Due to the patient's size and immobility, she was started on Coumadin postoperatively. The hemovac was removed at 48 hours, and the patient began physical therapy. She made slow but progressive improvement. The patient was self-sufficient on crutches. She was discharged on a regular diet with condition improved.

Discharge Diagnoses:
Comminuted fracture left femur.

Obesity.

Asthma.

Operations:
Open reduction and internal fixation of femur.

Discharge Medications:
Premarin .625 mg daily; Albuterol MDI 4 puffs q.i.d.; Vicodin q. 6 hours p.r.n. for pain.

Codes: _____

DISCHARGE SUMMARY

PATIENT: Sutton, Ann   **MR#:** 99-14-31

ATTENDING PHYSICIAN: Lowery   **CONSULTANT:** Fleming

History of Present Illness:
This 30-year-old white female with an unremarkable past medical history except for alcohol and cocaine abuse, was brought to the ER following electromechanical dissociation arrest. The patient was at home drinking alcohol and smoking crack Cocaine when she suddenly collapsed with her eyes rolled back in her head, a stiffening of her jaw, and no movement of her extremities. She stopped breathing. Her sister called the EMS, who arrived to find her in arrest.

The patient was resuscitated and brought to the ER where she arrested twice more. She was twice more resuscitated and intubated in the right main stem bronchus. Initial arterial blood gases were 7.04, 44, and 95. She received Narcan three times and remained unresponsive and hypotensive until she was put on Levophed and Dopamine drips. The time from the initial collapse to arrival in the ER was thirty minutes.

Medications on Admission:
Antibiotics for urinary tract infection. No known drug allergies.

Past Medical History:
Urinary tract infection and a cesarean section.

Family History:
Father has coronary artery disease.

Social History:
She smokes and drinks daily and uses crack Cocaine. She does not use IV drugs.

Physical Evaluation:
On admission, an obese black female, intubated.
Pulse: 102; *BP:* 90/50; *Resp:* 19; and afebrile.
Neck: supple.
Chest: sounds decreased with scattered rhonchi on the left side.
Heart: S-1 and S-2, regular rate and rhythm; no S-3, no S-4, no murmurs.
Abdomen: bowel sounds positive.
Neurological: no response to voice or pain; eyes partially opened; Doll's eyes negative; and gag negative.
Extremities: flaccid, no movement with pain. The examination revealed no evidence of brain function and the absence of brainstem reflexes. Her prognosis was extremely poor. The initial event may have been a myocardial infarction, an arrhythmia, a tamponade, or a subarachnoid or intraparenchymal hemorrhage leading to severe hypoxic ischemic brain damage. The initiating factor was probably Cocaine use.

Laboratory Data:
WBC was 2300, hemoglobin was 12.6, and hematocrit was 37.6. Arterial blood gases indicated a pH of 7.35, PCO_2 of 40, and a PO_2 of 467. The chest X ray revealed no cardiomegaly and no infiltrates. The electrocardiogram indicated left ventricular hypertrophy with second degree and ST-T wave changes. A head CT scan revealed subarachnoid hemorrhage and massive cerebral edema with obliteration of ventricles. On admission, SMA-12 indicated albumin of 2.8, total protein of 5.9, total bilirubin of 0.4, ALT of 54, AST of 90, alkaline phosphatase of 56, calcium of 7.0, phosphate of 2.5, cholesterol of 141, triglycerides of 86, uric acid of 5.4, LD of 290, magnesium of 1.5, and CK of 183. Lactic acid was 2.1. The first set of cardiac enzymes indicated total CK of 143, CK MB of 3.1, CK MB index of 2.2, total MB of 326, and LD/LD-2 ratio of 0.58. Urine drug screen revealed Cocaine and Cocaine metabolites, Lidocaine, Nicotine, and Cotinine. Urine osmolarity was 113 millimoles per Kg. At admission, sodium was 141, potassium was 3.0, chloride was 102, CO_2 was 15, BUN was 10, creatinine was 1.2; and glucose was 399.

Urology consultation was obtained and concluded that her urine output was increased tremendously at 500 cc's an hour, suggestive of diabetes insipidus. The patient was examined by neurology attending physicians and pronounced dead at 5:15 p.m. As a candidate for organ donation, she was kept on the ventilator with FIO2 of 100% and PEEP of 5. She was administered Pitressin 5 units and Magnesium Sulfate 2 grams in 100 cc's of normal Saline solution for four hours and Sodium phosphate 15 millimoles in 100 cc's of normal Saline for six hours until she was moved from the ICU.

Final Diagnosis:

Brain death due to Cocaine abuse. Probable cause of death was myocardial infarction, arrhythmia, and tamponade, or subarachnoid hemorrhage and massive cerebral edema.

Codes: _____

DISCHARGE SUMMARY

PATIENT: Atkinson, Dana   **MR#:** 99-14-32

ATTENDING PHYSICIAN: Townsend

Chief Complaint and History of Present Illness:

The patient is a 51-year-old black male with a history of hypertension, end stage renal disease on peritoneal dialysis, and adult onset diabetes, who was in his usual state of health until four days prior to admission when on the way to a family reunion he began having abdominal cramping and sharp abdominal pain without radiation around his peritoneal dialysis catheter site. He also forgot his medications and was unable to take them as scheduled. The patient began to feel diffuse weakness and lightheadedness. In addition, he noticed that his Dialysate had been draining out as cloudy yellow fluid. Over the next three days prior to admission, he had continued weakness and abdominal pain with occasional vomiting. He denies fever, night sweats, headaches, blurred vision, or chest pain. He had chills and a slight increase in baseline dyspnea on exertion.

Past Medical History:

As above. No surgeries except peritoneal dialysis catheter placement. Admission for peritonitis three months ago. Adult onset diabetes and hypertension for ten years. No known drug allergies.

Admission Medications:

Calcium carbonate 1 gm p.o. b.i.d.; Procardia XL 90 mg p.o. q. a.m.; Lobetalol 600 mg p.o. b.i.d.; Clonidine 0.2 mg p.o. b.i.d.

Family History:

Mother with hypertension and diabetes mellitus. Father with hypertension and gout. Sister with hypertension.

Social History:

The patient is divorced, has four children. He does not drink alcohol. His last alcoholic drink was fifteen years ago. He does not smoke. His last cigarette was fifteen years ago. He smoked one pack per day for twenty years. He denies IV drug abuse and takes no medications without a prescription.

Admission Physical Examination:

In general, he is a well-developed, well-nourished, cooperative black male in mild acute distress.

Temp: 36.8; *Pulse:* 64, *Resp:* 20; *BP:* 140/80 (after receiving four liters of fluid).

HEENT examination: non-icteric sclerae; pupils equal and reactive to light and accommodation; extraocular movements intact; oral nasal mucosa slightly dry; oropharynx without exudate or erythema; neck supple without lymphadenopathy or masses; no thyromegaly.

Fundoscopic examination: AV nicking bilaterally; no hemorrhages or exudates.

Chest examination: lungs clear to auscultation bilaterally; no CVA tenderness.

Cardiovascular examination: regular rate and rhythm with a grade II/IV systolic ejection murmur along the left sternal border radiating to the apex and axillae; no S-3; but S-4 present.

Abdominal examination: abdomen slightly distended with mild diffuse tenderness, greatest by the peritoneal dialysis catheter site with plus-minus rebound and positive guarding; trace bowel sounds; no masses; no hepatosplenomegaly; shifting dullness.

Neurological examination: sensory intact to light touch; 5/5 motor strength throughout; cranial nerves II/XII grossly intact.

Extremity examination: no clubbing or cyanosis; 1+ pitting edema.

Chest X ray: no infiltrate or acute disease seen.

Obstructive series: unremarkable.

Admission Laboratory Data:

White count of 5.9; hemoglobin of 9.0; hematocrit of 27.0 with 282000 platelets; differential on CBC was 68 segs, 6 bands, 19 lymphs, and 7 monos; sodium of 137; potassium of 4.2; chloride of 102; bicarb of 27; BUN of 64; creatinine of 14; and glucose of 172.

Hospital Course:

The patient was orthostatic on admission and subsequently rehydrated. Peritoneal dialysis was continued with Vancomycin in his Dialysate. Culture of his Dialysate indicated *Pseudomonas aeruginosa* and subsequently he was given Gentamicin in his Dialysate, four exchanges per day. Over his hospital stay, his abdominal pain resolved. The patient remained afebrile throughout his hospital course.

Discharge Diagnoses:

1. Peritonitis.
2. End stage renal disease.
3. Chronic ambulatory peritoneal dialysis.
4. Hypertension.
5. Adult onset diabetes mellitus.

Discharge Medications:

Procardia XL 90 mg p.o. q. a.m.; Lobetalol 600 mg p.o. b.i.d.; Clonidine 0.3 mg p.o. b.i.d.; Gentamicin 6 mg in each bag of Dialysate.

Codes: _____

DISCHARGE SUMMARY

PATIENT: Padberg, Herbert   **MR#:** 99-14-33

ATTENDING PHYSICIAN: Bates

History of Present Illness:

This 52-year-old white male with a history of alcohol abuse and tobacco use was brought to the ER after being picked up by police while he was wandering around in the streets, confused and hallucinating. The patient resides in an apartment above a bar. According to the bartender, he is a withdrawn person who rarely leaves the apartment. He drinks heavily, and stores trash in his apartment including the 39 cases of empty beer cans found today. Supposedly he was going door-to-door today searching for a friend and conversing with imaginary persons. He was also wandering through traffic smoking an imaginary cigarette. In the ER, the patient believes he is in the bar and cannot provide a reliable history. The patient had a phone conversation with the bartender who confirmed that the patient was confused and was not at his baseline.

Medications on Admission:
Supposedly on Haldol, Cogentin, and aspirin. No known drug allergies.

Past Medical History:
Peptic ulcer disease; status post appendectomy; status post T & A; patient stated that he has a disease of the nerves for which he takes little pills in a brown bag.

Family History:
Positive for leukemia and throat cancer.

Social History:
Smokes about one pack per day; drinks about twelve beers per day. He is divorced, has five children, and was recently arrested for failure to pay child support.

Physical Examination:
Cooperative white male.
Pulse: 55; *Resp:* 28, *Temp:* 36.4; *BP:* 108/64.
HEENT: normocephalic and atraumatic; throat clear; sclerae anicteric.
Neck: supple without any abnormalities.
Chest: clear to auscultation.
Cardiovascular: regular rate and rhythm; S-1 normal; S-2 normal; no murmurs or gallops.
Abdomen: soft; nontender; hepatomegaly, which was palpable and percussible 6 cm below the costal margin.
Extremities: without clubbing, cyanosis, or edema.
Rectal: normal tone with no masses; guaiac negative.
Neurological: alert, oriented to name but not to place or time, believes the bar was turned into a doctor's office to give physical examinations; normal psychomotor activity; flow of thought was sequential with occasionally illogical thought content; actively hallucinating and delusional regarding a cigarette in his hand but denied visual or auditory hallucinations; memory was 3/3 at 5 minutes; distant memory intact; serial 3's rapid and correct; calculations intact; named Presidents Clinton to Kennedy; pupils were 4 by 4 reacting down to 2 by 3; visual fields were full to confrontation; fundi benign; extraocular movements full; end point gaze nystagmus; face symmetric; bilaterally symmetric upgoing tongue; Barre without drift; good fine finger movements; diffuse muscle without fasciculations; strength 5/5 throughout; mildly tremulous, mostly postural tremor; relatively multifocal myoclonus; deep tendon reflexes were 2+ and toes downgoing bilaterally; sensation intact to light touch, pin prick, temperature, and joint position; mild decrease in vibration in toes; finger-nose-finger and heel-shin without dysmetria; gait mildly wide-based and unsteady with increased tremulousness.

Laboratory Data:
On admission, chest X ray was clear with slight cardiomegaly. The electrocardiogram showed sinus bradycardia with minimal left ventricular hypertrophy. SMA-12 revealed low albumin of 2.8, low total protein of 5.8, ALT of 51, AST of 70, calcium of 8.2, LDH of 254, BUN of 7, sodium of 139, potassium of 3.8, chloride of 109, CO_2 of 24, glucose of 116, and creatinine of 0.7. Drug screen revealed the presence of acetone in the urine. B-12 was 320, folic acid was 12.6, and iron and total iron binding capacity were low with normal male ferritin levels. PT was 12.3, PTT was 25.7, and reticulocyte count was 0.5 with a retic index of 226.

Sedimentation rate was 30, WBC was 6100, hemoglobin was 11.1, hematocrit was 32.9, platelet count was 372000, and MCV was 94.5. Thyroid function tests were within normal limits. Glucose was 69. Blood alcohol was less than .10. RPR was non-reactive. Urinalysis was clear. Cerebrospinal fluid protein was 24. Cerebrospinal fluid routine culture was negative for any growth.

Hospital Course:

The assessment on admission was alcoholic hallucinations. He was started on Librium, Thiamine, and Multivitamins. Clonidine was also added as part of the treatment for alcohol withdrawal. He did remarkably better with this regimen, and by the second day of admission, his sensorium was clear, and he was not hallucinating further. His discharge was delayed, however, because of placement problems. He was finally discharged to a VA shelter.

Discharge Diagnoses:

Alcoholic hallucinosis and withdrawal.

Discharge Medications:

Multivitamins one tablet p.o. q.d.

Thiamine 100 mg p.o. q.d.

Codes: _____

DISCHARGE SUMMARY

PATIENT: Andrews, Elizabeth   **MR#:** 99-14-34

ATTENDING PHYSICIAN: Weiss

History of Present Illness:

The patient is a 27-year-old female admitted to the hospital with severe abdominal pain and fever. She has a significant past history of an abdominal hysterectomy with a bout of acute urinary retention approximately three months ago. The patient had a history of chronic neurogenic bladder so the acute urinary retention was not really that unexpected with the trauma of the pelvic surgery. She was advised to learn intermittent catheterization but decided that she could not handle the procedure. Therefore, as an outpatient, she had a suprapubic tube placed to allow her to open and close the tube on her own and thus to void spontaneously. The patient developed progressive abdominal discomfort last night. She was seen in the emergency room and had a WBC count of 19600 and a sed rate of 56 with severe abdominal pain, which appeared to be quite acute in nature. It was decided that the patient possibly had pelvic cellulitis or sepsis causing her pain.

Laboratory Data upon Admission:

The initial admission SMA-6 was essentially normal. Creatinine was 2.3, BUN was 18, and glucose was 24. The next day, creatinine was 1.0 and BUN was 8 and basically remained at those levels through the entire hospital course. The initial admission SMA-12 revealed a calcium of 10.6, a phosphorus of 1.6, an SGOT of 13, a total bilirubin of 1.2, with the rest of the SMA-12 essentially normal. The patient had a urinalysis upon admission showing large amount of blood (consistent with recent suprapubic tube placement), negative nitrates, moderate leukocytes, 25-30 WBC's, and 8-10 RBC's. PT and PTT were essentially normal. The patient had blood cultures that showed no growth. A urine culture showed greater than 100000 *Klebsiella oxytoca* and less than 10000 Beta hemolytic strep group B. Culture after treatment showed no growth. The patient's initial hemoglobin was 13.1, subsequently dropped down to 10, and remained at approximately that level throughout the rest of the hospital course. The admission white count was 196.0 and the discharge white count was 92.0.

Hospital Course:

The patient was started on broad-spectrum antibiotics, Ampicillin and Gentamicin. Pending the culture results, a consultation was obtained from Dr. Ross. A CT scan of the abdomen revealed evidence of a soft tissue density in the pelvis consistent with the possibility of hematoma, possibly inflammation secondary to either the vaginal hysterectomy or the suprapubic tube placement, all consistent with pelvic cellulitis. The patient continued to have abdominal discomfort with nausea and vomiting, and was seen by Dr. Alvarez in GI consultation. He concluded that the patient's known Crohn's disease would not cause the acute exacerbation of her pain. Her fever may have been related to the patient's diarrhea, which may have been related to her Crohn's disease. She has been tried on multiple medications in the past, as documented in her chart. Contrast was injected into the suprapubic tube, revealing it intact and in good position with no extravasation. The patient continued to have abdominal pain, and was seen in infectious disease consultation by Dr. Price. The patient's antibiotics were changed by adding Flagyl, continuing Gentamicin, discontinuing Unasyn, and adding Piperacillin. The patient also was seen in the gynecologic consultation by Dr. Krueger who concluded that the patient had a stable pelvis, and that she had pelvic cellulitis post abdominal hysterectomy. During the next week, the patient slowly defervesced, her white count improved, and her pain and discomfort also improved somewhat. She appeared to be having probable bladder spasms, perhaps related to the suprapubic tube in place. Repeat CT scan continued to reveal some cellulitis. The patient's suprapubic tube was removed and a Foley catheter was placed to attempt to alleviate the patient's pain. She continued with pain although the pain was not quite as severe. The patient's Foley catheter was discontinued and she voided spontaneously without problems except for some spasms during micturition. The patient's diet was advanced, her nausea improved, and she remained afebrile.

Discharge Medications:

Zantac 100 mg b.i.d.; Voltaren 75 mg b.i.d.; Soma with codeine q. 8 hours p.r.n.; Ativan 1 mg t.i.d. p.r.n.; Butibel 1 q.i.d. p.r.n.

Codes: _____

DISCHARGE SUMMARY

PATIENT: Mueller, Joan   **MR#:** 99-14-35

ATTENDING PHYSICIAN: Phillips

Chief Complaint:

This 37-year-old woman was admitted with increasing chronic anxiety and severe depressive symptoms.

Laboratory Studies:

Hemoglobin 12.8; hematocrit 38 with MCV of 101; WBC 6300; normal differential; platelets 324000; serum sodium 143; potassium 4.2; chloride 111; BUN 7; creatinine 0.9; glucose 62; cholesterol 196; SMA otherwise normal; total T4 6.8; TSH 0.6; urinalysis negative; B12 level 577; folic acid 6.4; MRI of the cervical spine negative.

Hospital Course:
The patient was given anti-anxiety medication. She was seen by Dr. Henderson, a neurosurgical consultant, whose impression was cervical strain. The consultant recommended treatment with physical therapy, heat, and ultrasound electric stimulation. She was also given Voltaren 75 mg b.i.d. The patient was additionally seen by Dr. Fitzpatrick, a neurology consultant, whose impression also was cervical strain. The neurologist agreed with the recommendation of physical therapy as well as the use of Voltaren and muscle relaxants. The patient attended psychodrama. She was continued on treatment with lithium, although this medication was discontinued prior to discharge. The patient felt that she had improved and was discharged to be followed in outpatient psychiatry. She also is to be followed up by Dr. Rubenstein, an orthopedic physician.

Discharge Diagnoses:
Major depression, recurrent.

Acute and chronic cervical strain.

Allergic rhinitis.

Chronic bronchitis.

Spastic colitis.

Duodenal ulcer by history.

Codes: _____

DISCHARGE SUMMARY

PATIENT: Hampton, Michael   **MR#:** 99-14-36

ATTENDING PHYSICIAN: Chandler

History:
The patient is a 22-year-old black male who returned to the emergency room in the afternoon after being discharged from his tonsillectomy that morning. He complained of pain, fever, myalgias, and chills. He denied nausea, vomiting, bleeding, breathing difficulties, or coughing.

Physical Examination:
Vital Signs: Temp: 38.5; *Pulse:* 110; *Resp:* 24; *BP:* 140/58.
HEENT: pupils equal, round, and reactive to light and accommodation; extraocular movements intact; visual fields and acuity grossly normal; right tympanic membrane demonstrated a dry, persistent perforation; external auditory canal was clear; left tympanic membrane was clear; boggy turbinates in the nose, no drainage; oral cavity was clear; oropharynx demonstrated status post Bovie tonsillectomy without bleeding or pus; airway was clear; no adenopathy in neck; no focal tenderness.
Chest: clear to auscultation.
Heart: regular rate and rhythm.
Abdomen: soft; nontender; nondistended; bowel sounds positive.
Neurological: nonfocal.

Hospital Course:
The patient was admitted and placed on intravenous Clindamycin. He immediately defervesced and was afebrile for the remainder of his hospital stay. The patient had no complaints of bleeding or respiratory difficulties.

Diagnoses:

Postoperative fever.

Status post tonsillectomy.

Discharge Diet:

The patient was instructed to avoid hard or sharp foods.

Discharge Medications:

Clindamycin 300 mg p.o. q. 6 hours; Tylenol number 3 Elixir 12.5 to 25 cc's p.o. q. 4 hours p.r.n.

Follow-up:

The patient was instructed to follow up in the ENT clinic. He was also instructed to return to the emergency room in the event of recurrent fever, bleeding, or worsening sore throat.

Codes: _____

DISCHARGE SUMMARY

PATIENT: Blair, Henry   **MR#:** 99-14-37

ATTENDING PHYSICIAN: Osborn

Reason for Admission:

The patient is a 68-year-old black male with a history of recently diagnosed squamous cell esophageal cancer who presented with a complaint of nausea and vomiting since the day prior to admission. One week ago, he had a previous food impaction secondary to esophageal narrowing, which required esophagogastroduodenoscopy with balloon dilation. He was doing well until yesterday when nausea and vomiting occurred with ingestion of pureed food as well as with drinking liquids. The patient admits to eating cheese curls the prior evening. He has no fever, cough, hematemesis, or melena. His last bowel movement was the morning of the day prior to admission.

Past Medical History:

The patient's history is significant for esophageal cancer without evidence of metastases. The patient refused surgery and had radiation therapy, which he currently also refuses. The tumor is located at the gastroesophageal junction and the patient has required multiple dilations as an outpatient to restore esophageal patency. Last month, a G-tube was placed through which the patient receives medications as well as four or five cans of Ensure daily. The patient has non-insulin dependent diabetes mellitus and a history of myocardial infarction in 1988. Echocardiogram obtained last month revealed right ventricular enlargement and right atrial enlargement with normal left ventricular function. The patient has a history of hypertension and a history of peptic ulcer disease. He has no known drug allergies.

Medications on Admission:

Cardizem 30 mg q.i.d.; Digoxin 0.125 mg q.d.; Tagamet 300 mg liquid q. h.s.; Nitrol Paste 1 inch q. 6 hours p.r.n.; Reglan 250 mg q. a.m.; Compazine 10 mg p.r.n.; Tylenol 3 p.r.n.; and Easy-Lax 2 mg p.r.n.

Family History:

Not significant.

Social History:
The patient lives by himself. He has a 60 pack per year history of smoking.

Review of Systems:
The patient has noticed a ten-pound weight loss within the past two months and has increased coughing while eating.

Physical Examination:
The patient is an emaciated, elderly, black male in no acute distress.
Vital Signs: Temp: 36.5; *BP:* 108/64; *Pulse:* 75. There were no orthostatic changes.
HEENT: Examination showed temporal wasting. Pupils are equal, round, and reactive to light; bilateral arcus senilis is present. Oropharynx is pink and moist without lesions. The neck is supple with no adenopathy.
Lungs: Clear to auscultation.
Heart: Regular rate and rhythm; 3/6 systolic ejection murmur at the left sternal border; no rubs or gallops.
Abdomen: Scaphoid with minimal tenderness to palpation in the right upper quadrant; decreased bowel sounds; clean, dry dressing over his G-tube.
Extremities: 2+ pulses; thin, bony extremities; no cyanosis or edema.
Rectal: Heme negative.
Neurological: Nonfocal.

Laboratory Data:
Sodium 132; potassium 4.7; chloride 93; bicarbonate 26; BUN 17; creatinine 0.8; glucose 204; amylase 48; total bilirubin 0.2; AST 930; WBC 16300; hemoglobin 8.0; hematocrit 26.7; platelet count 102400; PT 14.7; PTT 28.1; abdominal X ray showed no air fluid levels.

Condition on Discharge:
Stable.

Discharge Medications:
Tagamet 300 mg q. 8 hours; Compazine p.r.n.; Lanoxin 0.125 mg b.i.d.; Nitrol Paste one inch q. 6 hours p.r.n.; Jevity 5 to 6 cans per day via G-tube.

Discharge Diet:
Jevity 6 cans per day and pureed foods; the patient was told to avoid solid foods.

Follow-up:
Seven to ten days in GI Clinic.

Final Diagnoses:
Esophageal stricture secondary to squamous cell carcinoma.

Peptic ulcer disease.

Non-insulin dependent diabetes mellitus.

History of hypertension.

History of myocardial infarction.

Codes: _____

DISCHARGE SUMMARY

PATIENT: Dixon, Vincent   **MR#:** 99-14-38

ATTENDING PHYSICIAN: Baxter

Diagnoses:

Assault.

Perforation of left tympanic membrane.

Lip laceration.

Procedures:

Suturing of lip laceration.

Audiogram.

History:

The patient is a 36-year-old black male who was assaulted by five unknown assailants at approximately 2 a.m. on the morning of admission. The patient waited approximately ten hours before coming to the hospital because of his fear of physicians. He reports a loss of consciousness for 30 to 45 seconds after being hit by a bottle in the back of his head; he was also hit multiple times with fists. The patient complains of swelling and pain in the left occipital area, decreased hearing in his left ear, an echo in his left ear, and occasional vertigo. He denies otalgia or otorrhea.

Physical Examination:

Vital Signs: Temp: 36.8; *Pulse:* 96; *Resp:* 18; *BP:* 128/74.

HEENT: His right ear was clear. His left ear demonstrated a perforation of approximately 40% from the 6 o'clock position to the 10 o'clock position. There was slight bleeding at the superior aspect of his tympanic membrane. His Weber lateralized to the left and his Rinne demonstrated air conduction greater than bone conduction bilaterally. His nose was tender and there was a 1-cm laceration on his right anterior nasal septum. There was no septal hematoma or active nasal bleeding noted. Oropharynx and oral cavity were clear. His face demonstrated a 2-cm laceration on the lower lip with a small amount of dried blood and necrotic tissue at the commissure. Cranial nerves V and VII were intact.

Eyes: Pupils equal, round, and reactive to light and accommodation. Extraocular movements intact. There was some positive end gaze lateral nystagmus.

Neck: Supple.

Heart: Regular rate and rhythm.

Lungs: Clear to auscultation.

Abdomen: Soft and nontender; nondistended; bowel sounds positive.

Extremities: No clubbing; cyanosis; or edema.

Neurological: Alert and oriented times three; nonfocal; cranial nerves intact; gait normal.

Hospital Course:

The patient was admitted and begun on Decadron. The patient's lip was sutured. He was given Corticosporin drops to his left ear t.i.d. The patient underwent an audiogram, which demonstrated a severe conductive hearing loss, possibly consistent with ossicular chain disruption. There was no evidence of a neurosensory component to his hearing loss. Discharge activity is unrestricted with the exception of keeping the left ear dry.

Discharge Medications:

Keflex 500 mg p.o. q.i.d.; Dakin's 1/4 strength t.i.d. to the lip; Tylenol 3, one to two, p.o. q. 4 hours p.r.n.

Follow-up:

The patient was instructed to follow up in the ENT clinic in three weeks. He was also instructed to follow up in the ophthalmology clinic as soon as possible for complaints of blurry vision.

Codes: _____

DISCHARGE SUMMARY

PATIENT: Huebner, Percy   **MR#:** 99-14-39

ATTENDING PHYSICIAN: Mason

History of Present Illness:

This patient is a 49-year-old white male who was admitted to the intensive care unit as a result of chest pain. He complained of sudden chest pain that radiated to the medial aspect of the left arm. This pain lasted for about two hours, he then slept two hours, but awakened with the pain more intense. He denied shortness of breath, nausea, or back pain. The patient took Tagamet, but the pain was not relieved. Therefore, he came to the emergency room.

Past Medical History:

Hypertension, not treated; epigastric discomfort, treated by himself with Tagamet; chronic cough; and a history of alcohol abuse.

Family History:

Father has hypertension; mother died of breast cancer.

Physical Examination:

Alert and in no acute distress; **BP:** 160/100; **Pulse:** 88; afebrile.
HEENT: essentially unremarkable.
Lungs: clear.
Heart: S-1, S-2, no gallop.
Abdomen: soft; mild epigastric tenderness.
Extremities: no edema.

Laboratory Data:

CBC was unremarkable. ASTRA-8 was unremarkable. CK on admission was 157, LD was 212, PT and PTT were within normal limits. Electrocardiogram showed normal sinus rhythm, Q-wave on leads 2 and 3, AVF and inversion in lead 1, AVL in V-3 and V-6, questionable ST elevation in V-1 and V-2.

Hospital Course:

The patient was admitted to the intensive care unit and was treated medically with myocardial infarction protocol. He proved to have non-Q-wave myocardial infarction with positive enzymes. The patient improved and underwent echocardiogram, which revealed left ventricular hypertrophy, posterior basilar and anterior basilar hypokinesia, and mild decrease in left ventricular systolic function. Stress test was negative for five minutes without chest pain, and upper GI series showed superficial ulcerations of the distal antrum, the pyloric channel, and the duodenal bulb. The patient was treated with Tagamet, Cardizem, Isordil, and enteric-coated aspirin, and was discharged in stable condition.

Discharge Medications:

Tagamet 400 mg p.o. b.i.d.; Enteric-coated aspirin b.i.d.; Compazine 60 mg b.i.d.; Isordil 10 mg p.o. t.i.d.; Nitroglycerin 0.4 mg p.r.n.

Discharge Diagnosis:
Non-Q-wave myocardial infarction.

History of alcohol abuse.

Instruction on Discharge:
Wait 5 to 6 weeks for full stress Thallium scan and follow up in the office.

Codes: _____

DISCHARGE SUMMARY

PATIENT: Fletcher, Raymond   **MR#:** 99-14-40

ATTENDING PHYSICIAN: Jenkins

Admitting Diagnosis:
Supraglottitis.

Discharge Diagnosis:
Same.

History:
The patient is a 28-year-old male who experienced a gradual increase in throat soreness and difficulty swallowing on the morning of admission. The patient was eating chicken the previous evening, but the next morning he experienced a progressive increase in throat soreness with mild shortness of breath. The patient reported mild nausea during the prior two days and also had a bout of diarrhea.

Past Medical History:
Negative.

Past Surgical History:
None.

Medications on Admission:
None. No known drug allergies.

Physical Examination:
On admission, temperature was 99.5, and the other vital signs were normal. The patient was noted to have hoarseness; he had no stridor. On fiberoptic examination, he had moderate supraglottic edema with a 6-mm to 7-mm airway and erythema of the supraglottis. His vocal cords were mobile. His chest was clear, his abdomen was soft, his heart was regular, and his extremities were within normal limits. His neck was noted to have tenderness on palpation of the larynx.

Laboratory Data:
On admission, the WBC was 9700, the hematocrit was 41, and the platelet count was 227000. His SMA-6 revealed a sodium of 138, a potassium of 4.1, a chloride of 99, a bicarbonate of 27, a glucose of 109, and a creatinine of 1.2.

Hospital Course:
The patient was admitted and given IV antibiotics and three doses of Decadron. The patient was given IV Ceftazidine and remained afebrile during his hospitalization. The patient had

mild gastric discomfort and was given Tagamet as well as Maalox with subsequent resolution of these symptoms. The patient improved dramatically. The patient was discharged on Clindamycin 300 mg p.o. q. 6 hours, Tagamet, and Maalox. The patient was instructed to eat soft foods and to continue oral rinses with salt water. If any swelling, fever, or difficulty breathing occurs, he was instructed to immediately return to the emergency room.

Discharge Diagnosis:
Supraglottitis.

Follow-up:
In ENT clinic.

Codes: _____

DISCHARGE SUMMARY

PATIENT: Eastmann, Leonard   **MR#:** 99-14-41

ATTENDING PHYSICIAN: Reynolds

Reason for Admission:
Colostomy takedown.
The patient is a young male, status post gunshot wound and subsequent colostomy. He was admitted for colostomy takedown.

Past Surgical History:
Exploratory laparotomy.

Past Medical History:
Not significant.

No drug allergies known.

Medications on Admission:
None.

Physical Examination:
Benign on admission. The patient was brought to the operating room for a colostomy takedown, status post gunshot wound. He tolerated the procedure well without complications. The patient returned to the floor postoperatively. Vital signs remained stable and he was afebrile. The patient began to have bowel sounds on postoperative day three. His wound was noted to be clean, dry, and intact. The patient began to have bowel movements and tolerated clear liquid diet well. He was advanced to a regular diet and was discharged in good condition.

Discharge Medications:
Colace 100 mg p.o. b.i.d.; Tylenol p.r.n.

Discharge Instructions:
No heavy lifting or driving for six weeks.

Follow-up:
In office in one week.

Codes: _____

DISCHARGE SUMMARY

PATIENT: Ludwig, Harvey   **MR#:** 99-14-42

ATTENDING PHYSICIAN: Shea

Reason for Admission:
This gentleman was admitted for an elective cervical microdiskectomy. He underwent the procedure at the C6-7 level, with removal of a large, free fragment. Postoperatively, he did well and was discharged on the first postoperative day to be followed by Dr. Scott.

Discharge Diagnoses:
Cervical disk disease, degenerative.

Status post cervical microdiskectomy.

Operation:
As indicated.

Codes: _____

DISCHARGE SUMMARY

PATIENT: Straub, Curtis   **MR#:** 99-14-43

ATTENDING PHYSICIAN: Powers   **CONSULTANT:** Fisher

Reason for Admission:
The patient is a 25-year-old, right-handed white male who lost control of his car and was involved in a motor vehicle accident. He was brought to the emergency room where he was seen and evaluated by Dr. Kraus. He has a fracture involving his mandible and also a fracture involving his left clavicle. He complained of pain in these regions in addition to pain in the thoracic region of his back.

Examination of his left shoulder revealed a large area of ecchymosis over the clavicle. The area is tender but the skin is intact. X rays taken of the left clavicle revealed undisplaced fracture involving the left clavicle. He has full passive range of motion involving the left shoulder. All muscle tendon units in the left upper extremity were tested and found to be intact.

Examination of his neck revealed some tenderness in the region of the left sternocleidomastoid muscle and left pericervical muscles. He put his chin on his chest without any difficulty. He has full rotation of his cervical spine.

Examination of his back revealed tenderness without swelling over the region of the dorsal spinous process T6. X rays taken of the thoracic spine revealed no fractures or dislocations.

Impression:
Undisplaced fracture involving the left clavicle.

Fracture involving the mandible.

Multiple abrasions and contusions.

The care of the fractured clavicle as well as potential complications were discussed with the patient and his wife in detail. He is currently in a figure-of-eight clavicular strap, which may be removed for hygiene following his discharge. He will be followed in the office regarding this particular fracture.

Codes: _____

DISCHARGE SUMMARY

PATIENT: Grossberg, Walter

MR#: 99-14-44

ATTENDING PHYSICIAN: Ballard

CONSULTANT: Stewart

Reason for Admission:

The patient is a 35-year-old white male who was transported to the emergency room by the police after smoking Cocaine while the police were observing. When he arrived at the emergency room, he was very delirious, diaphoretic, twitching, and tachycardic. He complained of chest pain and became apneic for about 25 seconds. He was given Narcan, Thiamine, and Valium. He was also given Metoprolol 50 mg and was taken to the intensive care unit.

Family History, Social History, and Drug History:

All of these histories are unavailable.

Physical Examination:

The patient's blood pressure was 135/90, his pulse was 160, and his respirations were 30. The physical examination revealed jerky movements all over his body. His pupils were dilated, his neck was supple, and his heart was tachycardic without gallop or murmurs. His lungs had mild crackles, his abdomen was soft and nontender, and his extremities revealed no edema. He was drowsy and his mental status was not judged, but he was disoriented to place and person. Later he became delirious and euphoric. He had generalized muscle twitching without any focal signs and without any sensory or motor deficits.

Laboratory Data:

The electrocardiogram showed ST depression in leads V-2, V-3, V-4, and V-5. The chest X ray was clear.

Initial Impression:

Cocaine overdose.

Hospital Course:

The patient was admitted to the intensive care unit and was given intravenous Valium for restlessness and agitation. His blood pressure and pulse were reduced. He was afebrile. Metoprolol and intravenous fluids were given to reduce tachycardia and hypertension. He was acidotic at first, but with intravenous fluids and oxygen, his acidosis was corrected. His initial CK MB was 238 with an MB of 2.8, a subsequent CK MB was 1,313 with an MB of 26.3, and the last CK MB was 6,607 with an MB of only 2.0. Therefore, a myocardial infarction was ruled out. He did not have any chest pain or any electrocardiogram changes to suggest a myocardial infarction. The Metoprolol was discontinued and the intravenous fluids were discontinued. The patient was stable at the time of discharge.

Discharge Medications:

None.

Procedures:

None.

Discharge Instructions:

The patient was advised to abstain from Cocaine.

Discharge Diagnosis:

Cocaine overdose.

Codes: _____

DISCHARGE SUMMARY

PATIENT: Schwartz, Martha   **MR#:** 99-14-45

ATTENDING PHYSICIAN: Bennett

History of Present Illness:

The patient is a 42-year-old white female who was admitted for vomiting blood. She vomited dark blood the night before admission and in the morning of the day of admission she vomited dark blood again. She also had diarrhea with dark contents that morning. She was nauseated but had neither abdominal pain nor chest pain. She did have mild shortness of breath and did feel light-headed.

Past Medical History:

The patient has a history of manic depression for three years. She was involved in a motor vehicle accident last year. She drinks alcohol occasionally but not to excess. She has no known drug allergies.

Medications on Admission:

Thioridazine 25 mg p.o. q. h.s.; Pamelor 75 mg p.o. q. h.s.; Lithonate 300 mg p.o. t.i.d.

Physical Examination:

Temp: 95.2; *BP:* 100/70 lying down, 90/70 sitting up; *Pulse:* 100; *Resp:* 16.

General: appearance of distress from nausea and vomiting; nasogastric tube suctioning bright red blood; sweating during the examination.

HEENT: slightly pale; neck supple; no nodes.

Heart: tachycardia; normal sounds.

Lungs: clear on both sides.

Abdomen: soft; no tenderness.

Extremities: no lesions; no edema.

Neurological: alert and oriented times three; moves all extremities.

Laboratory Data:

CBC: WBC 11470; hemoglobin 10.8; hematocrit 33.4; MCV 98.0; platelet count 195000.

ASTRA-8: sodium 139; potassium 4.8; chloride 106; bicarbonate 22; BUN 24; creatinine 1.0; total bilirubin 0.8; amylase 199.

ABG: pH 7.36; PO_2 127; PCO_2 38; bicarbonate 21; oxygen saturation 98.4%.

Electrocardiogram:

Normal sinus rhythm; Q-wave in lead number 3; no ST change.

Initial Impression:

Acute upper gastrointestinal bleeding.

Manic depressive disorder.

Hospital Course:

She was admitted to the hospital and received intravenous fluid resuscitation with D5 and normal Saline 150 cc's per hour. She was typed and crossed with six units of packed red blood cells and transfused with two units packed red blood cells. She received triple lumen insertion in her right groin and a Foley catheter. Reglan 10 mg IV push q. 8 hours was given, as well as Tagamet infusion 900 mg in 24 hours, and Compazine 10 mg IM p.r.n. for nausea and vomiting. CBC check was done every six hours while she was on bed rest. She received an upper GI endoscopy, which revealed a Mallory-Weiss tear at the distal end of her esophagus. She received Vasopressin 20 units IV bolus in 20 minutes. This was followed by 0.4 units per minute IV drip. She also received Tridil drip 10 micrograms to keep systolic blood pressure higher than 130, and she received a total of 11 units of packed red blood cells and 10 units of platelets. The bleeding ceased and the hemoglobin and hematocrit remained stable. Her last CBC showed a WBC of 8200; a hemoglobin of 9.3; a hematocrit of 26.2; and a platelet count of 105000. The patient was discharged in stable condition with no restrictions on activity.

Discharge Medications:

Lithonate 300 mg p.o. t.i.d.; Pamelor 75 mg p.o. q. h.s.; Thioridazine 25 mg p.o. q. h.s.; Cimetidine 800 mg p.o. q. h.s.; Reglan 10 mg p.o. t.i.d. one hour a.c.; Ferrous Sulfate 325 mg p.o. t.i.d.; Folic Acid 1 mg p.o. q. a.m.; Multivitamin one tablet p.o. q. a.m.; Neutra-phos 250 mg 2 tablets p.o. b.i.d. for five days.

Discharge Diagnoses:

Mallory-Weiss tear at the lower end of the esophagus, which caused the upper GI bleeding.

Manic depressive disorder.

Procedures:
Upper GI endoscopy.

Operations:
None.

Codes: _____

DISCHARGE SUMMARY

PATIENT: Smith, Christopher   **MR#:** 99-14-46

ATTENDING PHYSICIAN: Wilson   **CONSULTANT:** Hsaio

History of Present Illness:

The patient is a 40-year-old white male who was diagnosed with AIDS three years ago. He was recently discharged from this hospital four days prior to this admission. During this prior admission, he had an extensive work-up for intractable nausea, vomiting, and diarrhea. He underwent endoscopy and biopsy revealed Cryptosporidium in the duodenal area. Since the patient was discharged four days ago, he has been extremely weak and has been nauseated and experiencing intermittent diarrhea. He became short of breath on exertion and so light-headed that he could not walk from his bedroom to his bathroom. These complaints necessitated that the patient return to the emergency room.

Past Medical History:

Acquired immune deficiency syndrome with Cryptosporidium infection causing diarrhea. Staphylococcus in right kidney. This patient was admitted multiple times in the past for nausea, vomiting, diarrhea, and dehydration.

Medications on Admission:

AZT 100 mg p.o. five times a day; Tagamet 300 mg b.i.d.; Lomotil one tablet p.o. t.i.d.; Reglan 10 mg q. a.c. and q. h.s.; Amitriptyline 35 mg p.o. t.i.d.; Erythromycin 200 mg q.i.d.

Social History:

The patient is a homosexual and has a history of mild tobacco and alcohol use.

Physical Examination:

General: Cachetic without acute distress.

Vital Signs: Temp 35.6; *Pulse* 122; *Resp* 24; *BP* 92/70 standing, 100/70 sitting, showing orthostasis.

HEENT: Bitemporal wasting; pupils equal, round, and reactive to light and accommodation.

Neck: Supple, no lymph nodes.

Lungs: Clear.

Cardiovascular: Regular rhythm; S-1 and S-2, no murmurs.

Abdomen: Soft; bowel sounds positive; no tenderness; and no organomegaly.

Rectal: Laxed tone; guaiac positive; liquid stools of brown color.

Extremities: No edema; no cyanosis; muscular wasting.

Skin: Rash on abdomen with maculopapular characteristics.

Laboratory Data:

WBC 6000; hemoglobin 14; hematocrit 32; platelets 456000; arterial blood gases, pH 7.47, PCO_2 25, PO_2 128; bicarbonate 21; oxygen saturation 98%; sodium 128; potassium 2.7; chloride 93; CO_2 18; BUN 44; creatinine 2.1; glucose 116; AST 65; ALT 34; total bilirubin 1; amylase 4; magnesium 1.2; calcium 9.4; phosphate 1.8. The chest X ray showed perihilar fluid and no significant infiltrate. Obstructive series revealed no obstruction, no free air, just moderate bilateral loops. Urinalysis indicated no infection.

Hospital Course:

This patient received intravenous fluids to treat his dehydration, and received Lomotil, AZT, Rocephin, Peri-Colace, Reglan, Septra, Amitriptyline, and Tagamet. Erythromycin was tried but discontinued because the patient could not tolerate the side effect of an increase in vomiting. The diarrhea was not controlled because the Cryptosporidium infection has no specific treatment. After the patient was well hydrated, a central line was placed on the left side to allow intensive nursing care at his home, including intravenous fluid administration. The patient was discharged moderately dehydrated, but requested to go home since home health nursing care could provide enough intravenous fluids through his central line. The patient was then discharged with no further work-up planned.

Discharge Medications:

AZT 100 mg five times a day; Tagamet 300 mg b.i.d.; Lomotil two tablets t.i.d.; Reglan 10 mg q.i.d.; Amitriptyline 25 mg t.i.d.; Potassium 40 mg p.o. b.i.d.; Septra DS one tablet p.o. q.d.

Discharge Diagnoses:

Acquired immunodeficiency syndrome.

Cryptosporidium infection of the intestine.

Dehydration, not well controlled.

Instructions for Care:

Regular diet plus a can of Ensure t.i.d. The patient is to have home health nursing care, especially for the administration of intravenous fluids and electrolytes.

Follow-up:

The patient is to return to the infectious disease clinic in one week.

Codes: _____

CHAPTER

HCPCS Coding: National Codes and Local Codes

LEARNING OBJECTIVES

Upon completion of this chapter the learner should be able to:

1. Define the concept of carrier discretion.
2. Explain the hierarchy implicit within the HCPCS coding system.
3. Discuss the process of updating the HCPCS coding system.
4. Explain the rationale for maintenance of the HCPCS coding system.
5. Discuss the usefulness of modifiers in the HCPCS national coding system.
6. Interpret and discuss the regular layout of entries in the index to the HCPCS national coding system.
7. Interpret and explain the columns used in the HCPCS table of drugs.
8. Demonstrate knowledge of the proper index search sequence by correctly assigning code numbers from the HCPCS Record to narrative statements of entities.
9. Discuss the usefulness of modifiers for supplementing the HCPCS national codes.
10. Interpret and explain the symbols in the fields of data within the HCPCS Record.
11. Apply knowledge of coding principles by assigning accurate and precise HCPCS national codes to report clinical services and supplies.

HCPCS CODES

HCPCS is an acronym for the Health Care Financing Administration (HCFA) Common Procedure Coding System, a classification developed by that agency in 1983. The system is designed to monitor and process billed charges with Medicare claims and with Medicaid claims in most states, in order to sustain uniform claims reporting and to support valid and reliable statistical data collection. HCPCS encompasses a three-level or three-tier coding system consisting of:

1. CPT code numbers and descriptors (level I of the HCPCS coding system).
2. National codes and descriptors (level II of the HCPCS coding system) allocated primarily for supplies, materials, injections, and select physician and nonphysician

procedures and services, the majority of which are not specifically incorporated in the CPT coding system.

3. Local codes and descriptors (level III of the HCPCS coding system) with varying content in different regions of the United States.

The HCPCS coding system is maintained by the medical coding staff of the Office of Coverage and Eligibility Policy in the Bureau of Policy Development, which is a component of the Health Care Financing Administration. However, inclusion of an entity in the listings of the HCPCS coding system is not an endorsement of that entity by HCFA nor an implication of guaranteed Medicare or Medicaid reimbursement for submitted claims that report the code for the entity. Current HCPCS hardcopy is disseminated by the Superintendent of Documents of the United States Printing Office. The HCPCS national and local codes and descriptors are published in various formats and in alternate media by various health industry organizations and by vendors of coding products. The official version of the HCPCS coding system, the HCPCS Record, is circulated by HCFA through the auspices of the United States Printing Office and does not contain coding guidelines. However, many of the reproduced versions are developed with explicit and definitive coding guidelines.

Hundreds of HCPCS codes and descriptors in the twenty sectional alpha-numeric listings as well as hundreds of entries in the index to the HCPCS national coding system are added, revised, or deleted annually to maintain general consistency with contemporary clinical patient care. Decisions with respect to additions, revisions, and deletions to the HCPCS national codes and descriptors (level II of the HCPCS coding system) are formulated by a panel of representatives from the Blue Cross and Blue Shield Association of America, the Health Insurance Association of America, and the Health Care Financing Administration. Overlap of identical entities listed in two or three different levels of the HCPCS system occurs in some instances.

NATIONAL CODES

HCPCS national codes (level II of the HCPCS coding system) include nearly three thousand codes. These national codes are five-digit alpha-numeric codes grouped in twenty sections of the HCPCS Record according to the first digit of the code. The first digit of a national code is a letter (either A, B, D, E, G, H, J, K, L, M, P, Q, R, or V) and the second, third, fourth, and fifth digit is a number (examples of national codes and descriptors: *M0075 Cellular Therapy* and *H5300 Occupational Therapy*).

The HCPCS coding system also contains one-hundred and three optional two-digit modifiers for the national codes (level II of the HCPCS coding system). These modifiers may be either alphabetic, comprised of two letters, or alpha-numeric, comprised of one letter and one number. Examples of national modifiers are -AP, *determination of refractive state was not performed in the course of diagnostic ophthalmological examination* and -Q5, *service furnished by a substitute physician under a reciprocal billing arrangement.*

HCPCS national modifiers may also be attached to CPT code numbers in the reporting of procedures and services to Medicare fiscal intermediaries. A comprehensive itemization of HCPCS national modifiers precedes the sectional tabular listings of the HCPCS level II codes and descriptors.

The vast perponderance of the HCPCS national level II listings of codes and descriptors were developed for reporting the usage of medical and surgical supplies in procedures and services rendered to Medicare patients. The CPT volume is notably generic in its sparse listings for medical and surgical supplies. Precise specification of the supplies used is realizable through selection of codes and descriptors from within the more than two thousand listings of medical and surgical supplies incorporated among the HCPCS national codes and descriptors. Such reporting is normally obligatory with the submission of Medicare claims as well as with the submission of many Medicaid claims, and is also compulsory in reporting claims to stipulated commercial insurance carriers.

HCPCS NATIONAL INDEX

Preceding the alpha-numeric listings of the HCPCS national codes and descriptors is an alphabetical index to these listings. This index contains noun and adjective main term entries printed with an initial uppercase letter (examples: *Accessories* or *Dental Procedures*) and, if applicable, indented subterm entries printed with an initial lowercase letter. The entries incorporate supplies and materials (example: *Elastic Bandage A4460*), clinical equipment (example: *Blood Pump, Dialysis E1620*), drugs and therapeutics (example: *Heparin Sodium A4800* and *J1644*), and stipulated procedures and services (examples: *Recement Inlay D2910*). Wherever possible, index entries are listed under a common noun or adjective main term.

More than one HCPCS national code may appear to be applicable for an imprecise or indefinite statement of an entity. Therefore, a code range instead of a distinct code may be specified in the alphabetical index to the national codes (examples: *Non-Emergency Transportation A0080-A0210* and *Orthopedic Footwear L3201-L3265*). Each code within the range must be examined with its total descriptor prior to finalizing code selection.

To competently utilize the alphabetical index for the selection of HCPCS national codes, the coder should always adhere to the following code search sequence:

- First, the statement of the entity to be coded should be analyzed to determine its nominative (noun) form.
- Second, the alphabetical index should be scanned to locate a main term correlating with the nominative (noun) form of this entity.
- Third, any and all subterms indicated beneath that main term entry as well as any cross-reference notations related to the entry that guide the code search to an alternative entry should be inspected and scrutinized. Noun main term entries are cross-referenced to adjective main term entries and vice versa.
- Fourth, the appropriate and suitable code or code range for the entity should be chosen.
- Fifth, and finally, the code and its entire descriptor in the alpha-numeric sectional listings should be verified for accuracy of the code selection.

As with all coding systems, HCPCS national code and descriptor selection must never be concluded solely by utilizing the alphabetical index to the national codes. Even if only one code is printed in the main term index entry for a stated entity, the code must be confirmed in the alpha-numeric sectional listings in order to assure precise and accurate code and descriptor selection.

HCPCS TABLE OF DRUGS

A comprehensive table of drugs comprising entries with codes for prescription pharmaceuticals is positioned after the HCPCS alphabetical index to the national codes. The HCPCS table of drugs is vertically arranged in exact alphabetical order by the generic name of the drug. Although the brand name or trade name of pharmaceuticals is included among the alphabetical entries in the table of drugs, such entries are always annotated with a cross-reference indicating "see generic name" (example: *Hyperstat IV, see Diazoxide*).

Vertical columns in the table of drugs are established for the drug name, the amount (the dosage), the route of administration, and the HCPCS code for the drug. A dash or hyphen (—) placed within a column of an entry in the table of drugs denotes that no data is posted for that variable within the listing for a specific pharmaceutical (example: *Chorionic Gonadotropin—IM J0725*).

The route of administration of the pharmaceutical is designated in an entry termed a "posting," which is placed in horizontal columns of the table. Abbreviations posted to signify routes of pharmaceutical administration in the HCPCS table of drugs are:

IM	for intramuscular administration
INH	for administration by inhalation
IT	for intrathecal administration
IV	for intravenous administration
ORAL	for oral administration
OTH	for other routes of administration
SC	for subcutaneous administration
VAR	for various routes of administration

With several exceptions (examples: *Methotrexate* or *Prednisolone*), the oral method of pharmaceutical administration is omitted from the postings of the route of administration column. The posting of "intravenous administration" includes gravity infusions, intravenous injections, and timed intravenous pushes. The posting of "other routes of administration" includes suppositories and catheter injections. The posting of "various routes of administration" includes parenteral and topical administration of pharmaceuticals as well as the administration of pharmaceuticals into joints, body cavities, and body tissues. If multiple routes of administration are posted, the first posting indicates the most common method of administration of the pharmaceutical.

Within the table of drugs, an entry requiring more than one line is printed with indentation of the subsequent lines of that entry. An indented line in the table of drugs is regarded as a continuation of the previous line. The name of the drug is repeated without indentation if more than one line is necessary for conveying various dosages or alternate routes of administration of the same pharmaceutical. For example, note the listing of *Methylprednisolone Sodium Succinate up to 40 mg IM, IV J2920* and the listing of *Methylprednisolone Sodium Succinate up to 125 mg IM, IV J2930*.

LOCAL CODES

HCPCS local codes (level III codes) are established by regional Medicare fiscal intermediaries with the authorization of HCFA for reporting entities for reimbursement to Medicare carriers as well as to Medicaid carriers in various states. Commercial insurance carriers generally do not utilize HCPCS local codes.

The entities that are assigned local codes (level III codes) ordinarily are already listed in either the CPT volume or among the HCPCS national codes, although occasionally local codes do represent innovative procedures, services, or supplies. The regional Medicare fiscal intermediaries may also establish local modifiers for codes in order to report special circumstances involving the coded entity.

HCPCS local codes (level III codes) include hundreds of five-digit alpha-numeric codes grouped in sections according to the first digit of the code, and listed in alpha-numeric order in these sections. The first digit of a local code is a letter (either W, X, Y, or Z) and the second, third, fourth, and fifth digit of a local code is a number. The HCPCS local modifiers consist of optional two-digit modifiers that are either alphabetic, consisting of two letters, or alphanumeric, consisting of one letter and one number. If appropriate, HCPCS local modifiers may be appended to CPT code numbers or to the HCPCS national codes.

Each regional Medicare fiscal intermediary must receive the sanction of HCFA to establish and implement local codes and local modifiers for use in the administration of the Medicare program within its geographic boundaries. HCPCS local codes are typically instituted in preference to the codes existent among either the HCPCS national codes or the codes in the CPT volume. Bulletins announcing newly activated local codes and local modifiers emanate from the regional Medicare fiscal intermediaries and are distributed to healthcare providers at periodic intervals.

The HCPCS coding system mandates a definitive ranking for selection and utilization. The HCPCS local codes and local modifiers (level III of the HCPCS coding system) retain the highest priority in this system, and maintain precedence over the HCPCS national codes and national modifiers (level II of the HCPCS coding system). Both the HCPCS local codes and local modifiers and the HCPCS national codes and national modifiers retain higher priority and maintain precedence over the CPT codes and CPT modifiers (level I of the HCPCS coding system).

Therefore, to reiterate, the HCPCS coding system supports a defined hierarchy of code selection and usage. The HCPCS local codes and local modifiers have the highest priority, the HCPCS national codes and national modifiers have a lower priority than the HCPCS local codes and local modifiers, but have a higher priority than the CPT codes and CPT modifiers, and the CPT codes and CPT modifiers have the lowest priority in the HCPCS coding system.

CARRIER DISCRETION

Coinciding with the authority and power of administration of the Medicare program on a regional basis by fiscal intermediaries is a concurring latitude (termed "carrier discretion") allowed or permitted these fiscal intermediaries in their interpretation of the federal Medicare regulations. The often dissimilar understanding and comprehension of reimbursement directives may subject healthcare providers to idiosyncratic or erratic claims processes. The assignment of HCPCS local codes and local modifiers contrasts significantly among the regional intermediaries and even the uses of HCPCS national codes and national modifiers (which presumably ought to be consistent throughout the country) differ considerably from one regional Medicare fiscal intermediary to another. Thus, providers of healthcare to Medicare patients should remain informed of the current coding and reporting guidelines, and should become aware of all corollary reimbursement policies in effect by diligently maintaining adequate communications with the Medicare fiscal intermediary in their region.

HCPCS NATIONAL MODIFIERS

HCPCS national codes (level II codes) and code modifiers are reissued annually in the HCPCS Record. A complete itemization of the HCPCS national code modifiers precedes the sectional tabular listings of the HCPCS level II codes and descriptors.

Optional two-digit alphabetic or alpha-numeric modifiers are provided to supplement various level II codes. HCPCS code modifiers listed in the HCPCS Record may also be appended to CPT code numbers (level I codes) for reporting procedures and services on claims submitted to Medicare fiscal intermediaries. Examples of HCPCS code modifiers primarily for use with the national codes are: *-AA, anesthesia services personally furnished by anesthesiologist;* or *-Q6, service furnished by a locum tenens physician.*

HCPCS FIELDS OF DATA

The mode of publication by the Health Care Financing Administration for the officially circulated itemization of HCPCS national codes and descriptors incorporates tabular listings arranged in sections. These listings are presented horizontally in relation to vertical columns that are termed "fields of data."

Currently, the listings encompass twenty-five data fields. Several of these fields, such as the spacing control code field, contain administrative information that does not warrant or merit attention in the process of selecting and reporting a HCPCS code. Most of the other data fields, however, such as the anesthesia base unit quantity field and the laboratory certification code field do warrant or merit cognizance in the process of coding and reporting billed charges for clinical procedures, services, and supplies.

Although several of these fields of data within the tabular listings of HCPCS national codes do not necessitate attention or cognizance in the process of code selection, these data fields involve factors that impact reimbursement for clinical procedures, services, and supplies. For example, the termination date field identifies the day, month, and year of the discontinuation of a listing from the <u>HCPCS Record</u>. The data fields that potentially influence reimbursement are signified with standard abbreviations (Table 15–1).

The fields of data in the listings of HCPCS national codes are:

- Field #1, the record field.
- Field #2, the common procedure coding system code field (This field defines the levels of the HCPCS coding system.).
- Field #3, the modifier code field (This field defines the use of modifiers in the three levels of the HCPCS coding system.).

T A B L E   15–1

HCPCS Abbreviations for Select Data Fields

Symbol	Description
ACTN	Action code field
BETOS	Berenson-Eggers type of service code field
CD ADD	Code added field
CIM	Coverage issues manual reference number field
CVRG	Coverage code field
LAB CRTFCTN	Laboratory certification code field
MCM	Medicare carrier manual
MDFR	Modifier code field
PRCSG	Processing note field
SQNC	Sequence number field
STATUTE	Statute number field
TOS	Type of service code field
XREF	Cross-reference code field

- Field #4, the sequence number field (This field groups procedure codes together within the tabular sections of the <u>HCPCS Record</u>.).
- Field #5, the record identification field (This field contains a number that signifies the spacing and indentation of data in the <u>HCPCS Record</u>; thus, the number "3" denotes the first line of a listing; the number "4" denotes a subsequent line of a listing, spacing before a data element; the number "7" denotes the first line of a modifier description; and the number "8" denotes the subsequent line of a modifier description.).
- Field #6, the long description field (This field yields an eighty-character space for the text of a listing.).
- Field #7, the short description field (This field yields a twenty-eight character space for an abridged text of a listing.).
- Field #8, the filler field (This field is not presently used.).
- Field #9, the coverage issues manual reference number field (This annually amended field, denoted with the abbreviation "CIM," indicates the section reference for the data stipulated in the subsequent field.).
- Field #10, the Medicare carrier manual reference number field (This annually updated field, denoted with the abbreviation "MCM," indicates the section reference for the data stipulated in the preceding field.).
- Field #11, the statute number field (This field indicates the statute reference for entities not covered under Mecicare reimbursement.).
- Field #12, the laboratory certification code field (This annually updated field, indicated with the abbreviation "LAB CRTFCTN," classifies laboratory procedures and laboratory services numerically, according to specialty certification categories such as: microbiology including bacteriology, mycology, parasitology, and virology; immunology and serology; clinical chemistry including urinalysis, endocrinology, and toxicology; hematology; immunohematology including antibody detection, antibody identification, and compatibility testing; pathology including histology and cytology; radiobioassay; or clinical cytogenetics.).
- Field #13, the cross-reference code field (This annually amended field, indicated with the abbreviation "XREF," designates a crosswalk to a five-digit numeric CPT code or to another alpha-numeric HCPCS national code to denote a procedure or a service previously or presently coded with an alpha-numeric HCPCS national code; for example, HCPCS code *D7490 Radical Resection of Mandible with Bone Graft* is referred to CPT code number *21095*.).
- Field #14, the coverage code field (refer to Table 15–2).
- Field #15, the ambulatory surgery center payment group effective date field (This annually updated field identifies the appropriate payment group from among the nine groups approved by HCFA.).
- Field #16, the ambulatory surgery center payment group effective date field (This field identifies the day, the month, and the year of approval by HCFA.).
- Field #17, the processing note number field (This field accommodates space for footnote comments selected from among the fifty footnotes situated at the conclusion of the alpha-numeric sectional tabular listings in Appendix A of the <u>HCPCS Record</u>; for examples, *0007—the laboratory should not bill for both the method and the test code,* or *0015—reimbursement is included in the basic allowance of another procedure.*).
- Field #18, the Berenson-Eggers type of service code field (This field, abbreviated

BETOS," presents an alpha-numeric designation that categorizes entities into clinically meaningful groups.).

- Field #19, the filler field (this field is not presently used.).
- Field #20, the type of service code field (This field, abbreviated "TOS," presents a single digit designation, either a number or a letter, to categorize entities for the carrier; up to five service codes may be presented for a single entity.).
- Field #21, the anesthesia base unit quantity field (This three-digit field indicates a relative value for anesthesia services.).
- Field #22, the code added field (This field signifies the year a code was added to the HCFA Common Procedure Coding System.).
- Field #23, the action effective date field (This field designates the day, month, and year of an addition or revision to a listing among the HCPCS national codes.).
- Field #24, the termination date field (This field designates the day, the month, and the year of a deletion of a listing from the HCPCS national codes.).
- Field #25, the action code field (refer to Table 15–3).

COVERAGE CODE FIELD OF DATA

The coverage code field of data is indicated by the abbreviation "CVRG" in the listings of the HCPCS national codes. This data field is updated annually (Table 15–2).

The letter "D" in the coverage code field of data indicates that coverage of the entity under Medicare reimbursement is contingent upon the diagnosis. For example, the letter "D" is posted in the coverage code field for the listing of code and descriptor *A0225 Ambulance Service, Neonatal Transport* . . . .

The letter "I" in the coverage code field of data indicates that the entity is not valid for Medicare coverage. For example, the letter "I" is posted in the coverage code field for the listing of code and descriptor *D7510 Incision and Drainage of Abscess—Intraoral Soft Tissue.*

The letter "M" in the coverage code field of data indicates that the entity is not covered under Medicare reimbursement. For example, the letter "M" is posted in the coverage code field for the listing of code and descriptor *M0302 Assessment of Cardiac Output by Electrical Bioimpedance.*

The letter "S" in the coverage code field of data indicates that the entity is not acknowledged by Medicare statute, and therefore is not covered under Medicare reimbursement. For example, the letter "S" is posted in the coverage code field for the listing of code and descriptor *E0625 Patient Lift* . . . .

T A B L E 15–2

HCPCS Coverage Code Field

Symbol	Description
D	Entity is covered contingent upon the diagnosis
I	Entity is not valid for Medicare coverage
M	Entity is not covered by Medicare
S	Entity is not acknowledged by Medicare statute
	Coverage of entity is at the discretion of carrier

If the coverage code field remains blank, coverage of the entity is at the discretion of the Medicare carrier. For example, the coverage code field is blank in the listing of code and descriptor *L0920 Torso Support, Pendulous Abdomen Support, Custom Fitted.*

ACTION CODE FIELD OF DATA

The annually amended action code field of data is signified by the abbreviation "ACTN" and by the less than symbol (>) in the listings of the HCPCS national codes. This data field denotes updates to this coding system (Table 15–3). If the less than symbol (>) is printed at the left of the listing, the transaction list or Appendix B at the end of the HCPCS Record should be consulted to determine the type of action performed on that listing since the previous publication of the HCPCS Record.

The letter "A" in the action code field of data signifies a new code listing inserted since the last publication, analogous to the symbol of the circle or the bullet in the CPT volume. For example, the letter "A" is posted in the action code field for the listing of code and descriptor *J1610 Glucagon Hydrochloride . . . .*

The letter "B" in the action code field signifies an administrative change in the long procedure description field with no effect on coding or reporting. For example, the letter "B" is posted in the action code field for the listing of code and descriptor *A4402 Lubricant, Per Ounce.*

The letter "C" in the action code field of data signifies that the descriptor terminology for that code changed since the last publication, analogous to the symbol of the triangle or the pyramid or the delta in the CPT volume. For example, the letter "C" is posted in the action code field for the listing of code and descriptor *L5667 Addition to Lower Extremity . . . .*

The letter "D" in the action code field of data signifies deletion of a code since the last publication, analogous to the symbol of parentheses in the CPT volume. For example, the letter "D" is posted in the action code field for the listing of code and descriptor *M0900 Excision, Revision, or Removal of A-V Shunt Anastomosis With or Without Graft.*

Deleted or discontinued codes and descriptors are retained in the HCPCS Record for four editions (four years) following the deletion or discontinuation. Such listings are enclosed within parentheses.

The letter "F" in the action code field of data signifies an internal change in the administrative data base with no effect on coding or reporting. For example, the letter "F" is posted in the action code field for the listing code and descriptor *V5050 Hearing Aid, Monaural . . . .*

TABLE 15–3

HCPCS Action Code Field

Symbol	Description
A	New code listing inserted since last publication
B	Administrative change in long procedure description
C	Descriptor terminology changed since last publication
D	Deletion of code since last publication
F	Internal change in administrative data base
R	Reactivation of discontinued code
S	Administrative change in short procedure description

The letter "R" in the action code field of data signifies the reactivation of a discontinued code, and the letter "S" in the action code field of data signifies an administrative change in the short procedure description field with no effect on coding or reporting.

HCPCS CODING OF TRANSPORTATION SERVICES

The CPT volume contains merely one code to report patient transportation services. However, numerous HCPCS national codes for transportation services are listed in the "A" section of the HCPCS Record. These listings incorporate assorted codes for the reporting of emergency ambulance transportation services including surface transport, air transport, and water transport. In addition, various listings in this section also incorporate assorted codes for the reporting of non-emergency transportation services by automobile, taxi, van, or bus, as well as for the reporting of the auxiliary costs of non-emergency transportation services, such as parking fees, tolls, lodging, and meals.

The listings of this section delineated for patient transportation services include sixteen distinct two-digit alphabetic modifiers for the codes reporting ambulance services. Eleven letters of the alphabet are used in two-digit modifiers to represent the origin (the first digit) and the destination (the second digit) of patient transportation. For example, the letter "H" represents the *hospital* and the letter "R" represents the *patient's residence,* thus the modifier -HR represents *ambulance trip from the hospital to the patient's residence,* and conversely, the modifier -RH represents *ambulance trip from the patient's residence to the hospital.*

A waiting timetable also is included to augment the codes for patient transportation services. The waiting timetable includes ten distinct one-digit or two-digit numeric modifiers that denote the interval of waiting time based on one-half hour increments.

Transportation services are never subjected to packaging or bundling regulations. The codes for patient transportation services may always be reported separately, unless a stipulated insurance carrier mandates an alternative method of coding and reporting these services. Reusable devices (such as backboards and splints) are considered as an inherent part of the patient transportation service and should not be reported separately.

HCPCS CODING OF CHIROPRACTIC SERVICES

Chiropractic procedures and services also are grouped among the listings of HCPCS codes and descriptors in the "A" section of the HCPCS Record. With all chiropractic procedures, appropriate documentation of each patient treatment phase of chiropractic services is exceedingly important for accurate and precise submission of claims to Medicare carriers. The treatment phase commences on the date that service was initiated. That date and the number of treatments rendered must be documented with each claim submitted to Medicare.

The principal chiropractic service is the manual manipulation of the spine for a diagnosis entailing the subluxation of the spine. These diagnoses include intervertebral disc disorders, curvatures of the spine, spondylolisthesis, and spondylosis. The level of subluxation and the diagnosis or symptoms relevant to the condition must be documented and submitted with the claim. Reporting the treatment of acute conditions may be augmented with modifier -AT; for example, *A2000-AT Manipulation of Spine by Chiropractor, acute treatment.*

If an established patient encounter for chiropractic procedures or services involved a heretofore untreated condition or a very recent injury, another treatment phase begins, and another documenting X ray (to substantiate the diagnosed condition) may usually be required by the carrier. Most insurance carriers do not reimburse providers of maintenance care without a restorative potential.

HCPCS CODING OF CLINICAL SUPPLIES

Amid the diverse listings of HCPCS codes and descriptors in the "A" section of the HCPCS Record are groups of listings of codes to report on submitted reimbursement claims for the use of clinical supplies. The supplies listed in this section include a multitude of entities such as gauze, dressings, syringes, needles, lancets, alcohol, peroxide, betadine, paraffin, surgical trays, and surgical stockings.

Headings and subheadings in this section classify listings of numerous other items such as vascular catheters, urinary catheters, incontinence appliances, enterostomy appliances, ureterostomy appliances, ostomy pouches, irrigation kits, as well as orthopedic casting materials (plastic and fiberglass), and replacement parts for canes, crutches, and walkers. Additional headings or subheadings in this section categorize listings of items used in conjunction with durable medical equipment such as replacement batteries, components of respiratory equipment (nasal cannulas, mouth pieces, face tents, and tracheostomy tubes), and components of renal dialysis equipment (dialyzers, dialysate solution, and blood tubing).

The listings of clinical supplies also includes codes and descriptors for the contrast material utilized in radiological procedures, and codes and descriptors for the iodine utilized in nuclear medicine procedures. Placed at the conclusion of this section are administrative or miscellaneous listings of codes and descriptors for non-covered entities.

HCPCS CODING OF ENTERAL AND PARENTERAL THERAPY SERVICES AND SUPPLIES

The HCPCS Record encompasses the "B" section of listings of HCPCS national codes and descriptors for enteral and parenteral services and supplies. These listings include entities such as enteral tubing, enteral or parenteral infusion pumps, enteral formulae, and parenteral nutrition solutions.

Codes for reporting enteral formulae are delineated by the variable components of the formulae such as semi-synthetic protein, natural intact protein, and hydrolized protein. For reporting purposes, 100 calories equals one unit of enteral formulae. The supply of powdered enteral formulae should be coded and reported with modifier -DD, *powdered enteral formulae,* augmenting the HCPCS level II code.

Codes for solutions in the "B" section are designated for reporting the use of solutions for parenteral nutrition therapy. If these solutions are utilized for purposes other than parenteral nutrition therapy, then this usage should be reported with codes from the "J" section of the HCPCS Record. For reporting purposes, 500 milliliters equals one unit of parenteral nutrition solution.

HCPCS CODING OF DENTAL AND ORAL SURGERY SERVICES

By reason that the CPT coding manual was developed to report the procedures and the services rendered by physicians, most of the procedures and services rendered by dentists are not included in the CPT volume. Nevertheless, dental and oral surgery procedures and services may be reported with CPT codes for unlisted procedures or unlisted services.

If the stipulated insurance carrier allows, dental procedures and services may be reported with codes from *Common Dental Terminology (CDT).* This manual is published by the American Dental Association.

The HCPCS Record contains a section of HCPCS national codes and descriptors, the "D" section, that groups both listings of dental and oral surgery procedures, and services and listings of dental supplies. This protracted section, developed under the auspices of the American

Dental Association, is comprised of listings grouped in subsections for diagnostic dentistry, preventive dentistry, restorative dentistry, endodontics, periodontics, removable prosthodontics, maxillofacial prosthetics, implants, fixed prosthodontics, oral surgery, orthodontics, and adjunctive services.

The listings in the subsection for diagnostic dentistry include codes and descriptors for clinical oral examinations (initial exams, periodic exams, and emergency exams). Emergency dental exams should be reported with the service code augmented by modifier -*ET, emergency treatment*.

The listings in the subsection for diagnostic dentistry also comprise codes and descriptors for intraoral radiographs (with a unit count method specified for reporting each film), and extraoral radiographs (also with a unit count method specified for reporting each film). If the X-ray supplier submits a separate claim to the carrier, codes on that claim should be augmented with the modifier -*TC, technical component*. This subsection for diagnostic dentistry additionally contains listings of codes and descriptors for bacteriologic studies, caries susceptibility tests, pulp vitality tests, and histopathologic studies.

The subsection for dental prophylaxis or preventive dentistry includes a variety of listings of codes and descriptors. Entities such as topical application of fluoride, nutritional counseling, oral hygiene instruction, tooth sealants, and space maintainers (unilateral or bilateral and fixed or removable) are contained within this subsection.

The listings in the subsection for restorative dentistry contain codes and descriptors for restoration procedures with amalgam, gold foil, metallic inlay, porcelain inlay, ceramic inlay, resin inlay, or composite materials. Stipulated listings delineate the number of tooth surfaces restored, whether the restoration was on the anterior surface or the posterior surface, and whether the restoration was performed on a primary tooth or a permanent tooth. This subsection also includes listings of codes and descriptors for restoration procedures with resin or porcelain crowns and veneers.

The subsection for endodontics includes listings of codes and descriptors for pulpotomy and apicoectomy. The components of root canal therapy are contained within the listings of this subsection.

The listings in the subsection for periodontics encompass codes and descriptors for operative procedures such as gingivectomy, gingivoplasty, bone grafts, and soft tissue grafts. The listings in the subsection for removable prosthodontics encompass codes and descriptors for both complete dentures and partial dentures, as well as for denture repairing, rebasing, and relining.

The subsection for maxillofacial prosthetics contains codes and descriptors for nasal, auricular, orbital, ocular, cranial, and other prostheses. The subsection for implants contains codes and descriptors for implant maintenance, removal, and repair. The subsection for fixed prosthodontics contains codes and descriptors for bridge pontics and crowns (porcelain and resin), and for retainers (metallic inlay and metallic onlay).

The listings in the subsection for oral surgery include codes and descriptors for surgical dental extraction, tooth implantation, tooth transplantation, biopsy of oral tissue, alveoloplasty, vestibuloplasty, excision of lesions and neoplasms, incision and drainage of abscess, reduction of fracture and dislocation, temporomandibular joint procedures, traumatic wound repair, and procedures on the maxilla and the mandible. The listings in the subsection for orthodontics includes codes and descriptors for appliance therapy and treatment for malocclusion, as well as post-treatment stabilization.

The subsection for adjunctive services contains listings of codes and descriptors for regional anesthesia, general anesthesia, dental consultation, and miscellaneous entities. The listings of codes for dental and oral surgery procedures and services implicitly include both the provision of local infiltration anesthesia and routine postoperative care. Therefore, local infiltration anesthesia and routine postoperative care should not be coded and reported separately in the submission of reimbursement claims for dental and oral surgery procedures and services.

The listings in the "D" section of the HCPCS national codes distinguish among dental alloys. These alloys are classified as: high noble; noble; and predominantly base. Proper code selection by categorization of the alloy relies upon accurate and precise clinical documentation.

HCPCS CODING OF DURABLE EQUIPMENT SERVICES

The HCPCS Record encompasses an elongated section of codes and descriptors, the "E" section, that groups listings of HCPCS national codes to report on submitted reimbursement claims for the use of durable equipment. Such claims (preferably electronic claims) must be submitted to the appropriate one of the four regional carriers that processes reimbursement claims for durable medical equipment.

The residence of the beneficiary determines the claim jurisdiction of the regional carrier. A carrier may deny a claim for durable medical equipment unless the cost of the equipment was altogether justified by the therapeutic benefit to the patient.

Modifiers are typically used to supplement the codes for durable medical equipment. The modifier -NU reports new durable medical equipment, and the modifier -UE reports used durable medical equipment. Other modifiers used in the coding and reporting of durable equipment include: modifier -LL, lease/rental, indicating that charges for the equipment rental fee are applied toward the purchase price; modifier -NR, new when rented, indicating the subsequent purchase of new rental equipment; modifier -RP, replacement and repair, indicating substitution or restoration of equipment, and modifier -MS, six month maintenance and servicing fee for reasonable and necessary parts and labor that are not covered under any manufacturer or supplier warranty.

The various entities incorporated among the listings of the "E" section include canes, crutches, walkers, commodes, decubitus care pads and decubitus care mattresses, heat application devices, cold application devices, bath aids, toilet aids, hospital beds, and hospital bed accessories. The numerous entities contained within the listings of the "E" section also include oxygen, oxygen concentrators, and related respiratory equipment, IPPB machines, humidifiers, nebulizers, suction pumps, room vaporizers, monitoring devices, patient lifts, pneumatic compressors and appliances, ultraviolet cabinets, safety devices, restraints, transcutaneous and neuromuscular electrical nerve stimulators, traction devices and other orthopedic devices, wheelchairs and wheelchair accessories, artificial kidney machines, and artificial kidney machine accessories.

Codes for reporting the provision of hospital beds are delineated for fixed-height beds and variable-height beds, for semi-electric beds and total electric beds, for beds with side rails and beds without side rails, and for beds with or without the inclusion of a mattress.

Codes for reporting the provision of an oxygen system are delineated for gaseous systems and liquid systems, for stationary systems and portable systems, as well as for purchased systems and rented systems. A unit count method is specified for coding and reporting the supply of oxygen. Gaseous oxygen is tallied per cubic foot and liquid oxygen is tallied per pound.

Codes for reporting the provision of IPPB machines are delineated for machines with manual valves and for those with automatic valves, and are delineated for machines with an internal power source and for those with an external power source. Codes for reporting the provision of pneumatic compressor appliances are delineated for segmental appliances and non-segmental appliances, for half-arm appliances and full-arm appliances, and for half-leg appliances and full-leg appliances.

The reporting of codes for specially sized wheelchairs or specially constructed wheelchairs should be augmented with a notation of the brand name and the model number of the wheelchair, as well as a brief explanation of the justification for the special size or the special construction.

HCPCS CODING OF REHABILITATIVE SERVICES

The "H" section of the HCPCS Record formerly contained codes and descriptors that grouped listings of HCPCS national codes to report on submitted reimbursement claims for rehabilitative services. These prior listings in the "H" section included individual psychotherapy, group psychotherapy, residential care, educational therapy, and rehabilitative evaluation.

Currently, the only reportable code in this section is *H5300 Occupational Therapy, Excluding Initial or Periodic Evaluation.* Time dimensions are not included in this listing.

HCPCS CODING OF INJECTION AND INFUSION SUPPLIES

The HCPCS Record encompasses an extended section, the "J" section of codes and descriptors, that groups listings of HCPCS national codes to report on submitted reimbursement claims for injectable pharmaceuticals and therapeutic infusions. This "J" section of the HCPCS Record incorporates four disparate subsections in alphabetical arrangements: listings of codes and descriptors for injectable drugs; listings of codes and descriptors for infusions; listings of codes and descriptors for immunosuppressive drugs, and listings of codes and descriptors for chemotherapy drugs. The HCPCS code for a chemotherapeutic drug reports merely the supply of the pharmaceutical and does not report the administration of chemotherapy.

With the exception of immunosuppressive drugs, the pharmaceuticals listed in the "J" section are drugs dispensed by methods other than oral administration. Injectable pharmaceuticals include drugs administered by subcutaneous injection, by intramuscular injection, or by intravenous injection.

Various descriptors in this section specify the unit or the dosage range reported by the corresponding code. For example, *J0695 Injection, Cefonicid Sodium, 1 gm* indicates that the unit amount reported by that code is one gram; and *J1630 Injection, Haloperidol, up to 5 mg* indicates that the dosage reported by that code ranges up to five milligrams.

Code *J0110* represented by descriptor *Administration of Injection . . .* is a generic code for reporting the administration of any injectable pharmaceutical. Stipulated carriers may sanction the use of this code for reporting injections that are reimbursed with a standard sum. Code *J3490* may be used to report the administration of unclassified drugs.

HCPCS CODING OF TEMPORARY EQUIPMENT AND SUPPLIES

The "K" section of the HCPCS Record contains listings of HCPCS national codes and descriptors that are designated by the Health Care Financing Administration (HCFA) as temporary listings. These temporary listings include codes for selected durable clinical equipment as well as codes for select supplies and other entities.

The "K" section of the current publication of the HCPCS Record contains a mixture of codes and descriptors encompassing (but not limited to) entities such as wheelchairs and wheelchair accessories, infusion pumps, spinal orthotics, immunosuppressive pharmaceuticals, recumbent ankle splints, glucose monitors, incontinence supplies and appliances, surgical dressings, and tracheostomy care supplies. Examples of codes and descriptors from the "K" section include: *K0012 Lightweight Portable Motorized/Power Wheelchair; K0031 Safety Belt/Pelvic Strap; K0065 Spoke Protectors;* and *K0129 Ankle Contracture Splint.*

The codes for entities listed in the "K" section should be used on an interim basis to report these items on submitted claims for reimbursement, as determined by the regulations of HCFA. The listings of the "K" section encompass cross-references for the previous temporary listings that were either superseded by the subsequently assigned HCPCS national alphanumeric codes in other sections of the HCPCS Record or superseded by the five-digit numeric (level I) codes, which are contained within the CPT volume.

HCPCS CODING OF ORTHOTIC AND PROSTHETIC SERVICES

The lengthy "L" section of the HCPCS Record is comprised of groups of listings of HCPCS national codes and descriptors for orthotic procedures, orthotic devices, and prosthetic supplies. These various subsections of the "L" section of listings include codes to report on submitted reimbursement claims for the provision of scores of entities and services.

Orthotic entities comprised in this section encompass cervical collars (flexible and semirigid), thoracic rib belts, dorsolumbar orthoses, lumbosacral orthoses, sacroiliac orthoses, surgical supports, torso supports, cervical halos, scoliosis correction pads, hip orthoses, knee orthoses, ankle-foot orthoses, lower extremity fracture orthoses, torsion cables, numerous orthotic additions for the lower limbs, arch supports, orthopedic shoes and footwear, heels, insoles, heel lifts and wedges, and sole lifts and wedges. Orthotic entities comprised in this section also encompass shoulder orthoses, elbow orthoses, wrist-hand-finger orthoses, shoulder-elbow-wrist-hand orthoses, upper extremity fracture orthoses, numerous orthotic additions for the upper limbs, as well as repairs to orthotic devices.

Prosthetic entities comprised in this section encompass lower limb prostheses, lower limb prosthesis fitting procedures, additions to lower limb prostheses (such as sockets, socket inserts, and other components), upper limb prostheses, upper limb prosthesis fitting procedures, addition to upper limb prostheses (such as hinges, harnesses, sockets, socket inserts, hooks, gloves, and other components), external power devices for limb prostheses, breast prostheses, prosthetic sheaths, and prosthetic implants. Other entities comprised in this section encompass elastic support stockings, trusses, and tissue expanders.

Descriptors within the "L" section commonly identify orthotic and prosthetic devices, and orthotic and prosthetic procedures by eponyms. For instance, the Benesch boot, the Hosmer prehensile actuator, the Milwaukee orthosis, and the Pavlik harness are entities listed within the "L" section.

Codes for reporting the provision of orthopedic shoes may be appended with an additional code, if applicable. Code *L3254* reports shoes of a non-standard width and code *L3255* reports shoes of a non-standard length.

Two codes may also be necessary to report an orthotic device or a prosthetic device that was modified with an addition. To exemplify, both code *L1825* represented by descriptor *Knee Orthosis Elastic Knee Cap* and code *L2810* represented by descriptor *Addition to Lower Extremity Orthosis, Knee Control, Condylar Pad* are needed to report the provision of an elastic knee cap with a condylar pad; and both code *L5200* represented by descriptor *Above Knee Molded Socket, Single Axis Constant Friction . . .* and code *L5610* represented by descriptor *Addition to Lower Extremity, Above Knee Hydracadence System* are needed to report the provision of an above knee molded socket prosthesis with single axis constant friction and a hydracadence system.

HCPCS CODING OF PHYSICIAN SERVICES

The "M" section of the HCPCS Record contains listings of HCPCS national codes and descriptors for specified physician services. The listings of this section include codes to report on reimbursement claims submitted for certain physician office services, home visits of patients by physicians, miscellaneous clinical diagnostic examination procedures, and certain podiatric services.

Many of the listings formerly in this section were replaced by the evaluation and management codes in the CPT volume. The codes for physician visits of patients that are listed in the "M" section should be reported only if required by the stipulated carrier.

HCPCS CODING OF LABORATORY SERVICES

The "P" section of the HCPCS Record is comprised of groups of listings of HCPCS national codes and descriptors for laboratory testing services. These listings include codes to report on submitted reimbursement claims for chemistry tests, toxicology tests, pathology screening tests, microbiology tests, and other laboratory services such as the supply of blood components.

Codes and descriptors for most pathology and laboratory procedures and services are listed in the CPT volume. The codes listed in the "P" section for pathology and laboratory procedures and services should be reported only if required by the stipulated carrier. Modifiers typically supplementing the codes reported from the section include *-LR, laboratory round trip,* and *-TC, technical component,* that report the institutional charges for the pathology or laboratory procedure or service.

HCPCS CODING OF TEMPORARY SERVICES AND SUPPLIES

The "Q" section of the HCPCS Record contains listings of HCPCS national codes and descriptors that are designated by the Health Care Financing Administration (HCFA) as temporary listings. These temporary listings include codes for selected clinical procedures as well as codes for select supplies and other entities.

The "Q" section of the current publication of the HCPCS Record contains a mixture of codes and descriptors encompassing (but not limited to) entities such oxygen contents, Pap smears, magnetic resonance imaging, seat lift mechanisms, chemotherapy administration, injections, and footwear for diabetics. Examples of codes and descriptors from the "Q" section include: *Q0035 Cardiokymography; Q0047 Anesthesia for Blepharoplasty; Q0074 Aqueous Shunt;* and *Q0104 Physical Therapy Re-evaluation, Periodic.*

The codes for entities listed in the "Q" section should be used on an interim basis to report these entities on submitted claims for reimbursement, as determined by the regulations of HCFA. The listings of the "Q" section encompass cross-references for the previous temporary listings that were either superseded by the subsequently assigned HCPCS national alpha-numeric codes in other sections of the HCPCS Record or superseded by the five-digit numeric (level I) codes, which are contained within the CPT volume.

HCPCS CODING OF DIAGNOSTIC RADIOLOGY SERVICES

The "R" section of the HCPCS Record is comprised of merely three listings of HCPCS national codes and descriptors for miscellaneous radiologic transportation. Radiologic procedures and services should be reported on submitted reimbursement claims with CPT codes (level I codes).

Examples of HCPCS level II codes and descriptors in the "R" section are: *R0070 Transportation of Portable X-Ray Equipment and Personnel to Home or Nursing Home, Per Trip to Facility or Location, One Patient Seen; R0075 Transportation of Portable X-Ray*

Equipment and Personnel to Home or Nursing Home, Per Trip to Facility or Location, More Than One Patient Seen, Per Patient; and *R0076 Transportation of Portable EKG to Facility or Location, Per Patient.*

HCPCS CODING OF VISION AND HEARING SERVICES AND SUPPLIES

The "V" section of the HCPCS Record contains groups of listings of HCPCS national codes and descriptors for vision services and supplies. These listings include codes to report on claims submitted for reimbursement of such entities as eyeglass frames, spectacle lenses (single vision, bifocal, and trifocal), intraocular lenses, and eye prostheses.

The "V" section of the HCPCS Record also contains groups of listings of HCPCS national codes and descriptors for hearing services and supplies. These listings include codes to report on claims submitted for reimbursement of such entities as audiometric tests and appraisal, hearing aids and devices, and speech and language evaluations and therapies.

KEY CONCEPTS

action code field _____

alphabetical index _____

alpha-numeric code _____

anesthesia base unit quantity field _____

carrier discretion _____

chiropractic treatment phase _____

code range _____

coverage code field _____

cross-reference _____

cross-reference code field _____

dash _____

dental alloy _____

HCPCS _____

hyphen _____

laboratory certification code field _____

local code _____

main term _____

national code _____

orthotic addition _____

posting _____

processing notes _____

route of administration column _____

table of drugs _____

temporary listing _____

three-level coding system _____

transaction list _____

transportation waiting timetable _____

type of service code field _____

REVIEW EXERCISES

1. Explain the three-level structure of the HCPCS coding system. _____

_____

_____

2. Discuss the overlap of listed entities among the three levels of the HCPCS coding system. __

_____

_____

3. Contrast the responsibility for maintenance of each of the three levels of the HCPCS coding system. _____

_____

_____

4. Scan the alphabetical index to the national codes of the HCPCS coding system and list at least five main terms for which cross-reference notations are designated.

_____

_____

_____

_____

_____

5. Locate within the alphabetical index to the national codes of the HCPCS coding system at least five main terms for which a code range (instead of a specific code) is designated.

_____

_____

_____

_____

_____

6. Using the alphabetical index to national codes, select accurate and precise codes for the following entities:

A.   medicine dropper _____

B.   quad cane _____

C.   cardiac output assessment _____

D.   venipuncture _____

E.   trimming of nails _____

F.   cervical pillow _____

G.   oxygen face tent _____

H.   artificial larynx _____

I.   non-emergency transport by mini-bus _____

J.   conformity hearing aid _____

K.   standard bed pan _____

L.   orthomolecular therapy _____

M.   decubitus care mattress _____

N.   hair analysis _____

O.   ostomy belt _____

P.   parenteral nutrition kit _____

Q. iodine swabs _____

R. perineal strap _____

S. hearing aid orientation _____

T. raised toilet seat _____

U. bacterial sensitivity study _____

V. tube tracheostomy _____

W. wheelchair narrowing device _____

X. dialysis storage tank _____

Y. portable hemodialyzer system _____

Z. blood icterus index test _____

AA. hemodialysis machine _____

BB. air bubble detector for dialysis _____

7. Using the HCPCS table of drugs (mindful of the columns and abbreviations in the table of drugs), select accurate and precise codes for the following pharmaceuticals:

A. Phentolamine Mesylate intravenous 5 mg _____

B. Hyoscyamine Sulfate injection 0.25 mg _____

C. Levorphanol Tartrate injection 2 mg _____

D. Tobramycin Sulfate intravenous 80 mg _____

E. Cortisone injection 50 mg _____

F. Secobarbital Sodium intramuscular 250 mg _____

G. Diazepam intravenous 5 mg _____

H. Methoxamine intramuscular 20 mg _____

I. Estradiol Valerate injection 20 mg _____

J. Kanamycin Sulfate injection 500 mg _____

K. Niacinamide injection 15 mg _____

L. Succinylcholine Chloride intravenous infusion 20 mg _____

_____

M. Hydrocortisone Acetate injection 25 mg _____

_____

N. Droperidol intravenous 5 mg _____

_____

O. Gentamicin intravenous infusion 80 mg _____

_____

P. Papaverine injection through catheter 5 ml _____

_____

Q. Vancomycin Hydrochloride intravenous 500 mg _____

_____

R. Dimercaprol injection 100 mg _____

_____

S. Prednisolone Tebutate injection 20 mg _____

_____

T. Etidronate Disodium injection 300 mg _____

_____

U. Triamcinolone Acetonide intramuscular 10 mg _____

_____

V. Nicotinamide infusion 100 mg _____

_____

W. Largon injection 20 mg _____

_____

X. Lasix intramuscular 20 mg _____

_____

Y. Oxytocin intravenous 10 units _____

_____

Z. Iron Dextran injection 5 cc _____

_____

8. Describe the priority ranking of codes in the HCPCS coding system. _____

_____

_____

9. Clarify the rationale for:

A. the augmentation of level I codes with level II modifiers _____

_____

B. the augmentation of level I codes with level III modifiers _____

_____

C. the augmentation of level II codes with level I modifiers _____

_____

D. the augmentation of level II codes with level III modifiers _____

_____

E. the augmentation of level III codes with level I modifiers _____

_____

F. the augmentation of level III codes with level II modifiers _____

_____

10. Define the term "carrier discretion." _____

_____

_____

11. Select and indicate the appropriate modifier to supplement the code in each of the following clinical examples:

A. a dental patient was treated immediately for the reimplantation of a potentially viable tooth _____

B. a Medicare patient was advised last week by a general surgeon to undergo a colon resection for Crohn's disease and subsequently sought the advice of a colorectal surgeon _____

C. a specimen was conveyed both to and from an independent laboratory by an employee of the physician's office _____

D. an obstetrical procedure was rendered by a nurse practitioner employed by the patient's attending physician _____

E. a replacement spectacle was provided for the right eye only _____

F. group counseling was conducted by a clinical psychologist for patients diagnosed with a grief reaction _____

G. a patient who has twice within the last month consulted with two different cardiothoracic surgeons concerning coronary bypass surgery (one advised for the surgery and one advised against the surgery) subsequently sought the counsel of yet another cardiothoracic surgeon _____

_____

12. Explain the message conveyed by the following symbols in the stated data fields:

A. "M" in the coverage code field _____

B. "I" in the coverage code field _____

C. "A" in the action code field

_____

D. "C" in the action code field _____

E. "T" in the type of service code field _____

F. "G" in the type of service code field _____

_____

13. Select and indicate the appropriate modifier to supplement the code number in each of the following examples of patient transportation services:

A. a paraplegic patient transported by ambulance from her apartment to a routinely scheduled appointment with her physician _____

_____

B. a patient in a persistent vegetative state transported by ambulance to a nursing home after a lengthy hospital stay _____

C. a Medicaid patient transported by ambulance from a hospital in Illinois to a hospital in Missouri _____

D. a patient stricken with a myocardial infarction during a physical examination in the office of his internist _____

E. a bicyclist struck by a car and transported by ambulance to the nearest emergency room _____

14. Describe three modes of coding and reporting dental procedures. _____
_____
_____

15. Assign precise, accurate codes from the <u>HCPCS Record</u> for the following transportation services:

A. transport by air with helicopter ambulance service _____
_____

B. nonemergency intra-city taxi transportation _____
_____

C. nonemergency transportation of social case worker (per mile) _____
_____

D. meals for nonemergency transportation escort _____
_____

16. Assign precise, accurate codes from the <u>HCPCS Record</u> for the following medical and surgical supplies:

A. one roll of non-elastic gauze _____
_____

B. one point of peroxide _____
_____

C. two-way latex indwelling Foley catheter _____
_____

D. nonsterile irrigation kit _____
_____

E. hemostatic cellulose _____
_____

F. one point of betadine _____
_____

G. irrigation syringe _____
_____

H. disposable ostomy bag _____
_____

I. one roll of elastic bandage _____
_____

J. rib belt _____
_____

K. external urethral clamp _____

L. implantable vascular access catheter _____

M. nasal cannula _____

17. Assign precise, accurate codes from the <u>HCPCS Record</u> for the following enteral and parenteral services and supplies:

A. Levine-type stomach tube _____

B. parenteral nutrition, 8% amino acid solution (homemix) _____

C. parenteral nutrition, 10% lipids solution, with administration set _____

D. nasogastric tubing without stylet _____

E. enteral nutrition infusion pump with alarm _____

F. enteral formulae, category II, intact protein or protein isolates _____

G. stationary parenteral nutrition infusion pump _____

H. parenteral nutrition solution, compounded amino acid and carbohydrates with electrolytes, trace elements, vitamins, and 80 grams of protein _____

18. Assign precise, accurate codes from the <u>HCPCS Record</u> for the following dental and oral surgery procedures, services, and supplies:

A. cast metal retainer _____

B. implantable mandibular staple _____

C. porcelain crown fused to noble metal _____

D. dental bridge repair _____

E. surgical removal of residual tooth root _____

F. dental extraction of two teeth _____

G. biopsy of soft oral tissue _____

H. incision and drainage of abscess of intraoral soft tissue _____

I. fluoride gel carrier _____

J. suturing of 2-cm oral wound _____

K.   dental radiation shield _____

L.   closed reduction of mandible _____

M.   temporomandibular arthroplasty _____

N.   sialography _____

O.   caries susceptibility test _____

P.   removable unilateral space maintainer _____

Q.   prefabricated resin crown _____

R.   molar pulpotomy excluding final restoration _____

S.   apical curettage _____

T.   mandibular staple implant _____

U.   recementing of bridge _____

V.   sialodochoplasty _____

W.   complete facial moulage _____

X.   extracoronal provisional splinting _____

Y.   fabrication of athletic mouth guards _____

Z.   rebase of lower partial denture _____

AA. transosseus implant _____

BB. open osteotomy of ramus _____

CC. temporomandibular arthroscopy _____

DD. tooth transplantation _____

EE. laboratory reline of complete upper denture _____

FF. complicated suturing of 3-cm oral wound _____

19. Assign precise, accurate code numbers from the <u>HCPCS Record</u> for the provision of the following durable equipment:

A.   adjustable folding walker _____

B.   portable negative pressure ventilator _____

C.   female jug-type urinal _____

D.   foam rubber mattress _____

E.   mobile commode chair with detachable arms _____

F.   ultrasonic nebulizer _____

G.   blood leak detector for dialysis _____

H.   tracheotomy mask _____

I.   fracture frame attachments for complex pelvic traction _____

J.   wrist restraints _____

K.   portable whirlpool _____

L.   surgically implantable osteogenesis stimulator _____

M.   high-strength lightweight wheelchair with detachable full length arms and swing-away
      detachable foot rests _____

N.   stationary volume ventilator _____

O.   hydraulic patient lift with sling _____

P.   cervical pillow _____

Q.   neuromuscular stimulator for scoliosis _____

R.   apnea monitor _____

S.   free-standing traction stand for pelvic traction _____

T.   transfer tub rail attachment _____

U.   passive motion exercise device _____

V.   postural drainage board _____

W.   synthetic sheepskin pad _____

X.   pail for use with commode chair _____

Y.   nebulizer with compressor and heater _____

Z.   wheeled walker with seat _____
_____

AA. portable hydrocollator unit _____
_____

BB. dry pressure mattress _____
_____

CC. total electric hospital bed with mattress and side rails _____
_____

DD. standard electric heat pad _____
_____

EE. air pressure pad for mattress _____
_____

FF. fully reclining wheelchair with detachable arms and swing-away detachable footrest __
_____

20. Assign precise, accurate code numbers from the HCPCS Record for the provision of the following injections and supplies:

A. injection of codeine phosphate _____
_____

B. injection of lincomycin _____
_____

C. injection of depogen _____
_____

D. injection of progesterone _____
_____

E. injection of digoxin _____
_____

F. injection of 200 mg of diazoxide _____
_____

G. injection of 0.2 mg of atropine sulfate _____
_____

H. injection of 50 mg of orphenadrine _____
_____

I. supply of 50 mg vial of cisplatin _____
_____

J. supply of 20 mg of mitomycin _____
_____

K. vitamin therapy _____
_____

L. infusion of 800 cc of Ringer's lactate _____
_____

M. injection of 100 mg of zolicef _____
_____

N. supply of 10 mg of etoposide _____
_____

O. supply of 30 mg of paclitaxel _____
_____

P. injection of 15 mg of furosemide _____
_____

Q. injection of streptokinase _____
_____

21. Assign precise, accurate code numbers from the <u>HCPCS Record</u> for the following orthotic and prosthetic devices and supplies:

A.   heel wedge _____

B.   elastic elbow orthosis with stays _____

C.   postoperative body jacket for scoliosis procedure _____

D.   custom-fitted ankle gauntlet _____

E.   semi-rigid, adjustable, plastic cervical collar _____

F.   pneumatic knee splint _____

G.   tissue expander _____

H.   mastectomy form breast prosthesis _____

I.   rotation wrist unit with cable lock _____

J.   molded distal below knee cushion _____

K.   double truss with standard pads _____

L.   prosthetic implant of distal ulna _____

M.   prosthetic implant of testicle _____

N.   halo procedure, cervical halo incorporated into jacket vest _____

O.   custom-fitted thoracic rib belt _____

P.   one pair of peroneal straps _____

Q.   elastic knee orthosis with condylar pads _____

R.   static plastic custom-fitted hip orthosis for abduction control of hip joints _____

S.   flexible custom-fabricated lumbosacral surgical support _____

T.   sternal pad addition to scoliosis orthosis _____

U.   custom-fabricated pendulous abdomen support _____

V.   thoracic-lumbar-sacral orthosis, anterior-posterior-lateral control, molded to patient model, with interface material _____

W.   wrist-hand-finger orthosis, flexion glove with elastic finger control _____

X.   replacement of pretibial shell _____

Y.   hightop orthopedic shoe (with supinator) for child _____

Z.   custom-fitted ptosis support _____

AA. thoracic-lumbar-sacral orthosis, flexible dorsolumbar surgical support, elastic type, with rigid posterior panel _____

BB. removable premolded metatarsal arch support _____

CC. Boston switch-controlled electronic elbow _____

DD. prosthetic sheath for upper limb _____

EE. complete prosthesis for passive restoration of shoulder disarticulation _____

FF. outflare wedge _____

22. Assign precise, accurate code numbers from the <u>HCPCS Record</u> for the following physician procedures and services:

A. intragastric hypothermia using gastric freezing _____

B. electrical recording of Achilles reflex response _____

C. one hour of psychological testing with written report _____

D. orthomolecular therapy _____

23. Assign precise, accurate code numbers from the <u>HCPCS Record</u> for the following laboratory procedures and supplies:

A. blood icterus index test _____

B. supply of each unit of platelet concentrate _____

C. blood cephalin flocculation test _____

D. supply of each unit of whole blood for transfusion _____

E. autogenous vaccine _____

F. supply of one unit of cryoprecipitate _____

G. hair analysis _____

H. catheterization for collection of specimen from nursing home patient _____

24. Assign precise, accurate code numbers from the <u>HCPCS Record</u> for the following vision supplies:

A. single vision spectacles with aniseikonic lens _____

B. single vision spectacles, sphere plus 10.00 diopters per lens _____

C. bifocal spectacles, sphere minus 3.00 diopters per lens _____

D. bifocal spectacles with lenticular aspheric lens _____

E. gas-permeable extended-wear contact lens _____

F. posterior chamber intraocular lens _____

G. custom glass prosthetic eye _____

H. reduction of ocular prosthesis _____

I. monaural (behind the ear) hearing aid _____

J. assessment for hearing aid _____

K. assessment for augmentative communicative system _____

L. assessment of vestibular function by electronystagmography _____

M. dysphagia screening _____

16 CHAPTER

Coding and Reimbursement

LEARNING OBJECTIVES

Upon completion of this chapter the learner should be able to:

1. State a minimum of two challenges or obstacles encountered by healthcare providers with insurance claim processors, insurance claim examiners, or electronic insurance claims systems.
2. State a minimum of two challenges or obstacles encountered by insurance claim processors, insurance claim examiners, or electronic insurance claims systems with healthcare providers.
3. State a minimum of two policies or procedures that healthcare providers might actuate to enhance communications with third-party payors.
4. State a minimum of two policies or procedures that third-party payors might actuate to enhance communications with healthcare providers.
5. State at least two advantages of coding from a fee ticket or a superbill.
6. State at least two disadvantages of coding from a fee ticket or a superbill.
7. Define the concept of up-coding.
8. Define the concept of down-coding.
9. Define the concept of a provider profile.
10. Define the concept of a code distribution graph.
11. Apply knowledge of ICD coding principles to appraise the quality of ICD coded data in the physician office setting.
12. Apply knowledge of ICD coding principles to appraise the quality of ICD coded data in the ambulatory clinic setting.
13. Apply knowledge of ICD coding principles to appraise the quality of ICD coded data in the hospital medical record department setting.
14. Apply knowledge of ICD coding principles to appraise the quality of ICD coded data in the hospital patient accounts department setting.

15. Apply knowledge of CPT coding principles to appraise the quality of CPT coded data in the physician office setting.
16. Apply knowledge of CPT coding principles to appraise the quality of CPT coded data in the ambulatory clinic setting.
17. Apply knowledge of CPT coding principles to appraise the quality of CPT coded data in the hospital medical record department setting.
18. Apply knowledge of CPT coding principles to appraise the quality of CPT coded data in the hospital patient accounts department setting.
19. Discuss the responsibility for the quality of clinical documentation.

CLAIMS PROCESSING AND CLAIMS EXAMINATION

Insurance claims processing and insurance claims examination (also termed insurance claims adjudication), as well as electronic insurance claims systems frequently elicit and provoke frustrations for healthcare providers and healthcare organizations. Each insurance carrier maintains distinctive systems and methods; for example, consider the diverse or alternative modes of coding and reporting the billed charges for a therapeutic injection in accordance with the directives of various insurance carriers. Although the enterprises of all insurance carriers are regulated by insurance commissions in each state, the insurance firms are not legally obligated to reimburse the billed charges submitted for any procedure, service, or supply listed in any coding system.

Processing of insurance claims submitted by the healthcare provider to the insurance carrier entails a multifaceted technical routine. Coverage of the patient must be confirmed. Inclusion in the policy or contract of the reported encounter or diagnosis as well the reported procedure or service must be authenticated. The appropriateness of the codes reported for procedures, services, and supplies with relation to the codes reported for the diagnosis or the encounter must be corroborated.

Databases must be searched to probe prior claims submitted by either the same healthcare provider or another healthcare provider who rendered treatment for the condition or problem of this patient with insurance coverage. Databases must also be searched to survey the coordination of benefits clauses of the policy or contract in order to limit reimbursement from exceeding the maximum coverage amount, if this patient is insured by two or more third-party payors. The allowed charge (the average charge submitted for that entity by all healthcare providers in a geographical region) and the co-payment (the portion of the charge that is the payment obligation of the patient) must be ascertained, and lastly an explanation of benefits (EOB) must be prepared.

Examination or adjudication of insurance claims is a professional technique that occurs for claims entailing special reports for any procedure or service that is unusual, variable, or new. Examination or adjudication scrutinizes the explanation of the symptoms, the physical findings, and the diagnosis, and also reviews the clinical appropriateness and the justification for the procedure or service, as well as the reported time, staff, and equipment utilized to render the procedure or the service.

Dilemmas and predicaments concerning insurance claims typically occur if an insurance claims processor or examiner does not comprehend the claims information manually submitted by the healthcare provider, or if an insurance claims system is not programmed for the claims information electronically billed by the healthcare provider. As a result of misunderstandings or inaccuracies, the insurance claims processor, examiner, or system for electronic billing may reject or disallow a legitimate claim, or may return such a claim to its originator with a request for additional information.

Healthcare providers may alleviate these dilemmas or predicaments by submitting accurate, complete, and timely claims data that is appended with brief (one or two paragraph) descriptions of extraordinary or unusual services, and supplemented with photocopies of clinical documentation. The third-party payors may alleviate the consequent misunderstandings or inaccuracies through competent training of insurance claims processors and examiners, and through adequate and efficacious design of insurance claims systems.

Training of claims processors and examiners should include instruction in medical terminology as well as instruction in both diagnostic (ICD-9) and procedural (CPT and HCPCS) coding systems. Insurance claims systems should be designed by staff who have the requisite knowledge and comprehension of clinical terminology and healthcare classification systems.

Each provider of healthcare services should formulate policies and procedures to verify that the claims data submitted to third-party payors has reliability, validity, and accuracy. Documentation in the patient medical record should substantiate and justify all codes submitted in claims data.

PROVIDER PROFILES

Third-party payors in both the public and private sectors analyze the aggregate of claims data submitted by healthcare providers as a means of establishing individual profiles based upon the claims data submitted by each of these providers. The individual profiles yield a distribution of the codes reported in the claims data submitted for reimbursement by each healthcare provider. Established profiles also generate a compilation of the mean (average) or median charges for procedures and services rendered by each provider, and indicate variances from the profiles of comparable or similar healthcare providers.

If an individual provider profile significantly deviates from the norm established through assessment of the aggregate claims data, the analysis process of the third-party payor may activate an audit of the claims data submitted by that healthcare provider. Medicare carriers, as well as other third-party payors, may solicit repayment if an audit of claims data discloses consequential overcharges made by a provider seeking reimbursement.

Therefore, each provider of healthcare services should devise and maintain a distribution graph as a log for the codes reported in the data submitted with claims for reimbursement. Analysis of this graph can furnish a comparison (proportion or ratio) of procedures performed or services rendered among either physicians on a healthcare facility staff or in a specialty group practice. Analysis of this graph can additionally furnish a comparison (proportion or ratio) of services rendered among similar healthcare organizations or among similar physician specialty groups.

Review and assessment of the distribution graph of codes reported with the data submitted with reimbursement claims moreover can reveal useful information, such as the ratio of new patients to established patients either among physicians in a practice or among practices in a specialty. Survey and evaluation of the distribution graph can also disclose practical information, such as the typical level of service in consultations rendered by physicians within a practice or by practices within a specialty. For instance, if the highest level of service is consistently reported for the bulk of the consultations rendered by an individual physician within a group practice, and if in contrast the lowest level of service is consistently reported for the majority of the consultations rendered by all of the other physicians within that group practice, this deviation from the standard by one physician may warrant further investigation.

UP-CODING

Up-coding is the process in which a healthcare provider changes or modifies the code reported with the claims data submitted to the third-party payor. The code is usually changed or modified to a code representing an entity with a higher payment rate.

In inpatient settings affected by diagnosis related groups, DRG's, a variation of up-coding is found in "DRG creep," a process by which diagnostic data is manipulated to increase reimbursement. In the example of a patient admitted in severe pain and found to have bladder calculi and prostatic cancer, two procedures were performed: extraction of the stones and resection of the prostatic tumor. DRG creep was employed, however, to sequence the diagnosis and the procedure so that no match would occur. Thus, the provider healthcare facility reasoned that the cancer condition was more life threatening and therefore was the principal diagnosis. The bladder condition, although less of a threat to life, was more painful and required more imminent surgery. Thus, the provider contended that the stone extraction was the principal procedure. This procedure was unrelated to the principal diagnosis, however, and consequently placed the care into a higher paying DRG.

Audits conducted by this author indicated that approximately forty-five percent of the diagnostic codes and approximately thirty-five percent of the procedural codes that were submitted by physician practices to third-party payors were not correct, based upon the clinical documentation in the patient record. Comparable findings were established in audits of diagnostic codes and procedural codes submitted by acute care hospitals.

The inaccurate and imprecise codes reported with the claims data submitted to third-party payors by healthcare facilities and by physician practices occasionally impeded claims processing or resulted in payment delays. However, the vast majority of these inaccurate and imprecise diagnostic and procedural codes evaded or eluded detection by the insurance carrier, and consequently a substantial sum of unmerited or unwarranted revenue was received by these healthcare facilities and physician practices.

Analogous findings from similar audits conducted in physician practices and in healthcare facilities can be located in various articles published in journals related to the healthcare field. Although many vendors advertise warnings of lost revenue from incompetent coding, scientifically documented research indicates that more revenue is garnered from fraud than is forfeited through ineptitude.

The misuse of modifier -22, the unusual services modifier, typifies fallacious up-coding in physician practices. This modifier should connote that uncommon circumstances necessitated extraordinary time or effort to render a procedure or a service. Unjustifiable reporting of this modifier throughout recent years netted vast amounts of unjustifiable revenue for physician practices, and therefore many insurance claims processors, examiners, or electronic insurance claims systems currently routinely disregard the reporting of modifier -22 by a healthcare provider.

The reporting of codes for physician consultations further exemplifies the prevalence of the impropriety of up-coding throughout recent years. Former volumes of the CPT manual defined the complex consultation as a rarely performed service. Yet during those years, sixty percent of initial consultations by physicians were coded and reported to Medicare as complex consultations.

In another unpublished audit, the administration of flu shots by a nurse practitioner was found to be routinely coded and reported as a comprehensive service. Deliberate and intentional up-coding and reporting of such routine injections as a comprehensive service constitutes not merely misrepresentation, but rather fraud and deceit.

DOWN-CODING

Down-coding is the process in which a third-party payor changes or modifies the code reported with the claims data submitted by the healthcare provider. The code is usually changed or modified to a code representing an entity with a lower payment rate.

The process of down-coding may be a consciously routine activity by the insurance claims processor or examiner, or a program design feature of the electronic insurance claims system in order to decrease the amount of reimbursement sent to the healthcare provider. The process of down-coding, however, may also occur if an insurance claims processor or examiner, or an electronic insurance claims systems program designer does not understand the complexities involved with claims information submitted by the healthcare providers.

As a result of this lack of comprehension, the insurance claims processor or examiner, or the electronic insurance claims system may change or modify claims data presumed to be duplicative, erroneous, or unjustified. For example, certain claims processors and examiners do not understand the function of the V codes in ICD-9-CM, and consequently they regularly reject all claims with V codes submitted as the principal diagnosis.

Down-coding of the codes reported for procedures performed, for services rendered, or for supplies, equipment, and pharmaceuticals provided can be minimized by submitting accurate and precise claims data. This claims data should present each ICD-9-CM, CPT, or HCPCS code number and title or descriptor reported in a manner that coincides exactly with the listing of that identical code number and title or descriptor as printed in the most recent volume of the manuals.

The numeric (or alpha-numeric) code number and its title or descriptor verifiably defines each diagnosis rendered, each encounter rendered, each procedure performed, each service rendered, and each supply or material provided. Appropriate reporting of ICD-9-CM, CPT, and HCPCS codes to insurance carriers facilitates and expedites accurate, complete, and timely reimbursement to healthcare providers.

QUALITY OF CODED DATA

The quality of data coded through the listings of the ICD-9-CM volumes, through the listings of the CPT volume, or through the listings of the HCPCS Record relies and depends on the quality of the documentation in the patient medical record. Documentation of the diagnoses determined, the procedures performed, the services rendered, and the supplies, equipment, and pharmaceuticals provided is the responsibility of the physicians, nurses, therapists, and technicians who administer or provide patient care.

These healthcare practitioners are accountable for the accuracy, completeness, legibility, and timeliness of patient health information that is collected through the endeavors of a physician practice or a healthcare organization. Unfortunately, however, clinical documentation of patient care typically is inadequate and unsatisfactory.

The policies and procedures for healthcare data collection may contribute to negligent recordkeeping practices. A fee ticket or a superbill is a printed form used by clinics and physicians to enter coded data for diagnoses and procedures as well as billed charges. This document, alternatively termed an encounter form, a routing form, a charge slip, or a routing slip, may lack sufficient clinical documentation to enable accurate, precise coding and submission of adequate, complete claims data to third-party payors.

For instance, a patient presented to a clinic with a laceration of the hand that was sutured. "Laceration of the hand" was entered by the physician as the diagnosis on the fee ticket or the superbill. A week later, the same patient returned for suture removal. Once more, "laceration of the hand" was entered by the physician as the diagnosis on the fee ticket or superbill. This diagnosis does not validly report the reason for the return patient encounter, which was not the treatment of the laceration, but instead was the removal of the sutures. Coding from these two fee tickets or superbills reported two hand lacerations sustained by an individual patient within a week, and thus furnished invalid and unreliable healthcare data.

To reiterate, the quality of coded healthcare data principally depends on the clinical documentation of the healthcare practitioners who administer and provide patient care and treatment. The proficiency and expertise of a coder is likewise a crucial element in the generation of quality healthcare data.

Coders first and foremost must be thoroughly and intensely prepared with knowledge and comprehension of the format and content of the two major coding systems in widespread use. They must be proficient in reviewing patient medical records to ascertain reportable diagnostic, procedural, and material entities. Coders must also be proficient in referencing the resources (practitioners, publications, or professional associations) essential for generating coded data of superb quality.

Excellent coding skills are cultivated and developed through disciplined practice and application of the principles of the coding systems in order to accurately and precisely code and report the diagnoses determined, the procedures performed, the services rendered, and the supplies, the equipment, and the pharmaceuticals provided. Coding skills cannot be cultivated and developed through rigid productivity standards or by threats of impending corrective action.

The productivity of the coder definitely is hindered if the clinical documentation in the patient medical record is missing, deficient, vague, or illegible. The clinical documentation of the healthcare provider is a greater determinant of the quality of healthcare data than is the competency of the coder. Accurate and precise coding averts the necessity for recoding and the potential for delays in reimbursement, and likewise upholds the process of coding as a meaningful function in the contemporary healthcare industry.

KEY CONCEPTS

allowed charge _____	insurance claim examination _____
audit of claims data _____	insurance claim processing _____
charge slip _____	insurance commission _____
coder productivity _____	maximum coverage _____
coordination of benefits _____	median charges _____
co-payment _____	overcharges _____
coverage _____	payment delay _____
database _____	payment obligation _____
data quality _____	physician practice _____
diagnosis related groups _____	physician specialty group _____
distribution graph _____	profile variance _____
down-coding _____	proportion for comparison _____
DRG creep _____	provider profile _____
encounter form _____	ratio for comparison _____
explanation of benefits _____	reimbursement _____
fee ticket _____	routing form _____
healthcare organization _____	superbill _____
healthcare provider _____	third-party payor _____
insurance carrier _____	up-coding _____
insurance claim adjudication _____	

REVIEW EXERCISES

1. Describe the challenges or difficulties often encountered by healthcare providers with insurance claim processors and examiners, and with electronic insurance claim systems. _____

_____

_____

2. Describe the challenges or difficulties often encountered by insurance claim processors and examiners, and by electronic insurance claim systems with healthcare providers. _____

_____

_____

3. Discuss policies and procedures that healthcare providers might activate to enhance communications with third-party payors. _____

_____

_____

4. Discuss policies and procedures that third-party payors might activate to enhance communications with healthcare providers. _____

_____

_____

5. Explain the concept of up-coding and its primary utilization. _____

_____

_____

6. Explain the concept of down-coding and its primary utilization. _____

_____

_____

7. Describe the content and utility of provider profiles. _____

_____

_____

8. Describe the content and utility of a code distribution graph. _____

_____

_____

9. List two advantages and two disadvantages of coding from a fee ticket or superbill. _____

_____

_____

10. Discuss methods to assure the quality of coded data in the physician office setting. _____

_____

_____

11. Discuss methods to assure the quality of coded data in the ambulatory clinic setting. _____

_____

_____

12. Discuss methods to assure the quality of coded data in the hospital medical record department setting. _____

_____

_____

13. Discuss methods to assure the quality of coded data in the hospital patient accounts department setting. _____

_____

_____

GLOSSARY

abbreviation a condensed or shortened representation of an entity

acquired condition any manifested disorder not present at birth

action code field an annually amended column of the <u>HCPCS Record</u> (indicated with the abbreviation "ACTN") that denotes updates (additions, revisions, deletions, and editorial changes) to the HCPCS national coding system

actual charge the fee for rendering a procedure or a service that is submitted by the healthcare provider to the third-party payor

additional code a secondary code used to supplement and clarify the reporting of a disease or injury condition or the reporting of a procedure or service

additional procedure a clinical service rendered secondary to another clinical service; a procedure subordinate to a principal procedure

adverse effect term used to indicate a condition resulting from the use of a drug taken as prescribed

allowed charge the amount of reimbursement from the third-party payor to the healthcare provider on a claim submitted for a procedure or service rendered

alphabetic code a mode of representation for an entity that consists entirely of letters

alphabetical index a list of entities organized by letters of the alphabet; the source of a CPT code search sequence

alpha-numeric code a mode of representation for an entity that consists both of letters and numbers

anatomic term a word or words describing a part of the body

anesthesia base unit quantity field a column of the <u>HCPCS Record</u> that identifies suggested anesthesia rates with a decimal point assumed between the second and third positions in the field

anesthesia time the interval commencing when the anesthesiologist or anesthetist initiates preparation of the patient for induction of anesthesia in the operating room or in a comparable area and concluding when the anesthesiologist or anesthetist ceases to be in personal attendance with the patient

anomaly a marked deviation from normal; a term used to refer to a defect present at birth

appendix an addendum or supplement; the ICD-9-CM Volume 1 contains five appendices; the CPT volume contains three appendices

assistant surgeon a physician subordinate to the primary surgeon during an operative session

automated multi-channel test laboratory tests accomplished with special equipment that are grouped in combinations known as profiles

braces ({ }) symbols used in ICD-9-CM to enclose a series of terms, each of which is modified by the statement printed at the right of the brace

brackets ([ ]) symbols used in ICD-9-CM to enclose synonyms, alternative wordings, or explanatory phrases

carrier discretion a latitude granted by the administration of the Medicare program to the regional fiscal intermediaries allowing these fiscal intermediaries to interpret federal Medicare regulations and that often results is dissimilar reimbursement directives to healthcare providers

category a tertiary division throughout the ICD-9-CM tabular volumes; a primary division of the Evaluation and Management Services section of the CPT volume

causal relationship a relationship between or among clinical conditions; in ICD-9-CM indices and tabular lists, the words "due to" indicate that a causal relationship between conditions is present

chapter   a primary division of the ICD-9-CM tabular volumes

chiropractic treatment phase   a series of encounters for a heretofore untreated condition

circles or bullets (o)   symbols printed at the left of CPT code numbers to indicate newly added CPT codes

classification   a categorization or arrangement of entities such as diseases or clinical procedures

classification system   an established and organized process of grouping entities, such as the ICD-9-CM system

clinical specialty   an accepted career discipline of physicians usually proficient in knowledge of a specific body system or a specific procedural modality

clinical supplement   scenarios or synopses published by the American Medical Association as Appendix D of the CPT volume to demonstrate examples of the components or factors incorporated in each of the levels of service; these scenarios or synopses present diverse types of patient histories, physical examinations, medical decision making, counseling, coordination of care, and presenting problems and are intended to facilitate accurate and precise as well as valid and reliable selection and reporting of code numbers and descriptors for evaluation and management services

closed fracture   injury in which the skin is not punctured by broken bone

closed injury   wound not exposed to the external environment

code   digits (letters or numbers) that represent an entity

code also   an instruction to report another diagnostic or procedural entity in order to supplement and clarify the information presented

code range   a numeric sequence with the first code number of the sequence and the last code number of the sequence indicated and separated with a hyphen

code series   code numbers placed in numerical order and separated with a comma from the foregoing code number

coding system   an established and organized process of grouping entities and representing each of those entities by a unique code such as CPT

colon (:)   symbol used in ICD-9-CM to indicate an incomplete term that requires one or more modifiers in order to determine code selection and assignment

combination code   a single code used to report either two diagnostic conditions or two procedures

common narrative expression   the portion of the first code title or descriptor among a group of listings that is printed once, followed by a semicolon, and is not repeated or reiterated in subsequent entries that refer back to and are dependent upon or subordinate to that portion of the first code title or descriptor

comorbidity   the simultaneous occurrence of two or more diseases in the same patient

complicated wound   a wound that is infected or that contains a foreign body

complication   a disease or injury condition concurrent with or resultant from another disease or injury condition

comprehensive assessment   a complete patient evaluation in conjunction with admission to a nursing facility and repeated if necessary during the confinement of the patient

comprehensive history   a report containing documentation of the chief complaint of the patient with an extended history of the present illness or current problem, a complete past family history and social history of the patient, and a complete review of systems

comprehensive physical examination   a documented assessment of a complete single system specialty physical examination or a complete multi-system physical examination

confirmatory consultation   a service by a physician providing opinion and advice regarding the evaluation and management of a select clinical problem with the request for this service initiated not by another physician, but rather by the patient, a family member of the patient, a third-party payor, or another agency

congenital condition   a disorder present at and existing from the moment of birth

consultation   a service by a physician providing opinion and advice regarding the evaluation and management of a select clinical problem

contributory component   any of three secondary factors (counseling, coordination of care, and nature of the presenting problem) among the seven fundamental elements of an evaluation and management service; these contributory components are subordinate to the key components in the selection of a level of an evaluation and management service

contributory factor   any of three secondary components (counseling, coordination of care, and nature of the presenting problem) among the seven fundamental elements of an evaluation and management service; these contributory factors are subordinate to the key factors in the selection of a level of an evaluation and management service

convention   an abbreviation, a symbol, or a standard notation used in a coding system

co-payment   the portion of the actual charge that is paid by the patient directly to the healthcare provider

coverage code field   an annually amended column of the HCPCS Record (indicated by the abbreviation "CVRG") that signifies whether or not an entity is covered under Medicare reimbursement and whether coverage of an entity under Medicare reimbursement is contingent upon the diagnosis or at the discretion of the Medicare carrier

CPT   an acronym for Physicians' Current Procedural Terminology, a coding and classification system for clinical procedures and services

cross-reference   a notation with direction to information elsewhere

cross-reference code field   an annually amended column of the HCPCS Record (indicated with the abbreviation "XREF") that designates a crosswalk from an alpha-numeric HCPCS national code to a five-digit numeric CPT code or to another alpha-numeric HCPCS national code to denote a procedure or a service previously or presently coded with an alpha-numeric HCPCS national code

current injury   unhealed condition resulting from trauma

customary charge   the average charge compiled from charges of similar healthcare providers for a specific procedure or service

dash   an indicator placed in a vertical column of the HCPCS table of drugs denoting that no data is posted for that variable within the listing for a specific pharmaceutical

descriptor   a narrative expression that identifies an entity

detailed history   a report containing documentation of the chief complaint of the patient with an extended history of the present illness or current problem, a pertinent past family history and social history of the patient, and an extended review of systems

detailed physical examination a documented assessment of an extended physical examination of an affected body area or organ system as well as an extended physical examination of other symptomatic or associated organ systems

diagnosis the process of identifying an illness or injury by its signs or symptoms

diagnosis related group set of diagnostic entities determined by ICD-9-CM codes reported under the Medicare prospective payment system

diagnostic term a word or words describing an illness, disease, injury, or symptom

digit an alphabetic letter or a numeral

down-coding the process in which a third-party payor changes or modifies the code reported with the claims data submitted by the healthcare provider; the code is usually changed or modified to a code representing an entity with a lower payment rate

DRG creep fraudulent manipulation of data into diagnostic related groups under the Medicare prospective payment system in order to obtain increased reimbursement

DSM-IV an acronym for <u>Diagnostic and Statistical Manual, Fourth Edition</u>, a clinical classification system used in psychiatry, mental health, and behavioral health

edition the form or version of an issued or reissued publication such as the first edition or the second edition

encounter patient service rendered by healthcare practitioners

episode of care an encounter or series of encounters by a patient for any stated condition

eponym an entity named after a person

essential modifier term that affects or alters code selection and assignment

established patient a patient who has received professional services within the past three years from a physician or from another physician of the same specialty of the same group practice with the same billing number

etiology the cause of a disease condition

exclusion note directive in ICD-9-CM leading code search elsewhere in the classification

expanded problem-focused history a report containing documentation of the chief complaint of the patient with a brief history of the present illness or current problem and a pertinent review of systems

expanded problem-focused physical examination a documented assessment of a physical examination of an affected body area or organ system as well as a physical examination of other symptomatic or associated organ systems

face-to-face time the time allocated by the physician to obtain the patient history, to conduct the patient physical examination, and to counsel the patient during the patient encounter

fee-for-service health insurance plan a contractual agreement through which the insurer pays the provider for each covered clinical service that is rendered; these fee-for-service plans include individual policyholder indemnity insurance in which each person purchases coverage from an insurance firm and group policyholder indemnity insurance (a group healthcare plan) in which an employer or an association purchases coverage for an entire group

five-digit modifier a supplement consisting of five numbers that augments the code used for reporting of entities with qualifying or additional information; in the CPT coding system this type of modifier is reported as a separate code number with three zeros as the initial three digits

floor time   the time allocated by the physician to review or update the patient's chart, to examine the patient, to order tests or procedures, and to communicate with the patient or with the patient's family, as well as to communicate with colleagues and ancillary healthcare personnel while the physician is present on the unit or floor

foreign body   artifact situated in an abnormal, improper, or unnatural place in the body

frequency distribution of codes   a statistical analysis of procedures and services rendered by physicians in a group or among all physicians within a practice and in relation to announced code frequency distributions of similar practices within the same clinical specialty

functional activity   pathophysiological action produced by a bodily process

global billing   the acknowledgment by Medicare carriers of the inclusion of postoperative care for either ten days or ninety days (conditional upon the procedure performed) with the charges for the procedure

glossary   a list of words with their definitions, such as the glossary of mental disorders contained in Appendix B of ICD-9-CM

group indemnity insurance   a fee-for-service group healthcare plan in which an employer or an association purchases coverage for an entire group of people from an insurance firm

guideline   instructional notation; rule for accurate and precise coding

HCPCS   an acronym for the Health Care Financing Administration Common Procedure Coding System, denoting a classification system developed by that agency designed to monitor and process billed charges with Medicare and Medicaid claims in order to sustain uniform claims reporting and to support valid and reliable statistical data collection

heading   a secondary division of the following sections of the CPT volume: Anesthesia; Surgery; Radiology; Pathology and Laboratory; and Medicine

health maintenance organization (HMO)   a prepaid health insurance plan under a contractual agreement in which the insurer pays the provider a fixed or predetermined sum (a capitation) for contingent services directed by a primary care physician accessible to each person (each member) insured regardless of the actual services rendered to each plan member

hierarchical level   a position or rank within a hierarchy, such as the level II national codes in the HCPCS coding system hierarchy

hierarchical structure   a classification with ranks that are subordinate to the one above

hierarchy   a progression or scale of levels increasing in rank or status such as that used with ICD-9-CM codes, CPT codes, HCPCS national codes, and HCPCS local codes

high complexity medical decision making   clinical patient assessment involving extensive diagnoses or management options, an extensive review of complex data, and an appraisal of high risks of complications and morbidity or mortality

high severity presenting problem   a patient condition that if untreated potentially has a high probability of morbidity, a high probability of mortality, and also has a high probability of functional impairment

hypertension table   a feature of the Volume 2 alphabetic index of ICD-9-CM that facilitates the coding and reporting of abnormally high arterial blood pressure

hyphen   an indicator placed in a vertical column of the HCPCS table of drugs denoting that no data is posted for that variable within the listing for a specific pharmaceutical

ICD-9-CM an acronym for <u>International Classification of Diseases, Ninth Edition, Clinical Modification</u>, a coding and classification system for diagnostic conditions or symptoms and reasons for encounters with healthcare providers

inclusion note directive in ICD-9-CM that confirms or verifies code assignment

indented code and title or descriptor a listing in the coding system that is dependent upon or subordinate to the first non-indented listing directly prior to the indented listing; the non-indented listing contains a common narrative expression that is not repeated or reiterated in the indented listing

index a list of entities; coding systems maintain alphabetic indices as the initial source of the code search sequence

individual indemnity insurance a fee-for-service healthcare plan in which a singular person purchases coverage from an insurance firm

individual practice association (IPA) a prepaid health insurance plan under a contractual agreement in which the insurer pays the provider a fixed or predetermined sum (a capitation) for contingent services opted from among individual healthcare providers and accessible to each person (each member) insured regardless of the actual services rendered to each plan member

in situ confined to the site of origin in its normal position

instructional notation guideline or directive to facilitate accurate and precise coding

insurance claim examination assessment and evaluation of billing information submitted to a third-party payor from a healthcare provider

insurance claim processing clerical and technical functions with billing information submitted to a third-party payor from a healthcare provider

intra-service time a standard of measurement rather than an actual duration; intra-service time is differentiated as face-to-face time for office and outpatient encounters and as unit or floor time for hospital and inpatient encounters

italicized code and title a convention of ICD-9-CM indicating that the listing is not intended for primary tabulation of disease and cannot be designated as a principal diagnosis

key component any of three primary factors (patient history, patient physical examination, and medical decision making) among the seven fundamental elements of an evaluation and management service; these key components are foremost and predominant to the contributory components in the selection of a level of an evaluation and management service

key factor any of three primary components (patient history, patient physical examination, and medical decision making) among the seven fundamental elements of an evaluation and management service; these key factors are foremost and predominant to the contributory factors in the selection of a level of an evaluation and management service

laboratory certification code field a column of the <u>HCPCS Record</u> that classifies laboratory procedures and laboratory services numerically according to specialty certification categories

late effect residual condition remaining after the termination of the acute phase of an illness or an injury

level of service a measure of the type of service, the place of service, and the status of the patient explicitly for a category or subcategory of Evaluation and Management Services; the level of service annotates the variations in the requisite effort, skill, time, responsibility, and clinical knowledge of the physician that is applied in the prevention, diagnosis, and treatment of disease or injury and in the promotion of optimal health

listing   an individual code or code number and its title or descriptor

local code   a level III code of the HCPCS coding system

low complexity medical decision making   clinical patient assessment involving a limited number of diagnoses or management options, a limited review of complex data, and an appraisal of low risks of complications and morbidity or mortality

low severity presenting problem   a patient condition that, if untreated, potentially has a low probability of morbidity, no probability of mortality, and also has the expectation of full recovery without functional impairment

lozenge (□)   a symbol used in ICD-9-CM to denote that a category or subcategory rubric in the classification was clinically modified for use in the United States

main term   nominative entries for entities; these entries are printed in bold type

major diagnostic category   set of diagnosis related groups under the Medicare prospective payment system

major procedure   the procedure performed that poses the greatest risk to the health status of the patient during that encounter or episode of service

manifestation   a clinical sign or symptom of a disease process

metastasis   transfer of disease (pathogenic abnormal cells) from one anatomic site to another non-contiguous anatomic site

minimal presenting problem   a patient condition with treatment provided under the supervision of a physician but not necessitating physician presence

minor presenting problem   a self-limited or transient patient condition that has a definite and prescribed course, and that has a good prognosis or a low probability of permanently affecting health status

minor procedure   a clinical service rendered ancillary to another clinical service; a procedure subordinate to a major procedure

moderate complexity medical decision making   clinical patient assessment involving multiple diagnoses or management options, a moderate review of complex data, and an appraisal of moderate risks of complications and morbidity or mortality

moderate severity presenting problem   a patient condition that, if untreated, potentially has a moderate probability of morbidity, a moderate probability of mortality, and also has an uncertain prognosis and an increasing probability of functional impairment

modifier   an appendage or supplement that limits or restricts meaning; code modifiers augment the reporting of entities with qualifying or additional information

morphology   the form and structure of a particular organism, organ, tissue, or cell

multiple coding   using general and nonspecific codes to report one or more concurrent conditions

mutual exclusion   a situation in which two entities each preclude the other

narrative   the words represented by a numeric code

national code   a level II code of the HCPCS coding system

neonatal period   the duration from the moment of birth through the twenty-eighth day of life

neoplasm   new and abnormal tumor growth, specifically cell multiplication that is uncontrolled and progressive

neoplasm table   a feature of the Volume 2 alphabetic index of ICD-9-CM that facilitates the coding and reporting of tumor conditions

new patient   a patient who has not received professional services in any setting within the past three years from a physician or another physician of the same specialty of the same group practice with the same billing number

nomenclature   a vocabulary used in a profession or vocation (such as medical terminology in the healthcare field)

nonessential modifier   term that does not affect or alter code selection and assignment

nontraumatic condition   a patient condition that was not produced by injury

notation   a directive or a guideline to facilitate code selection and assignment

numeric code   a mode of representation for an entity that consists entirely of numbers

observation   attentive perception of physical findings to monitor established or suspected conditions

old injury   healed condition resulting from trauma

open fracture   injury in which the skin is punctured by broken bone

open injury   wound exposed to the external environment

organ- or disease-oriented panel   groups of laboratory tests performed for assessment of a specific anatomic site or diagnostic condition

orthotic addition   an attachment to a support or brace for muscles or joints

package billing   the acknowledgment by a third-party payor of the inclusion of postoperative care for either ten days or ninety days (conditional upon the procedure performed) with the charges submitted for the procedure; numerous healthcare providers also include routine preoperative care in package billing

parentheses ( )   symbol enclosing modifiers and notations in the ICD-9-CM coding system; symbol enclosing a newly deleted CPT code number printed alongside a cross-reference notation to an equivalent replacement code number

perinatal period   the duration before and after birth, from the twenty-ninth week of gestation to the fourth week after birth

personally furnished anesthesia service   anesthesia administration as well as preoperative, intraoperative, and postoperative monitoring and care dispensed directly by a physician anesthesiologist

physical status modifier   an indicator that categorizes the physical condition of the patient into one of six severity levels (normal, mild disease, severe disease, severe life-threatening disease, moribund, or brain dead) that differentiate the complexity and intricacy of anesthesia administration in accord with criteria authorized and established by the American Society of Anesthesiologists

physician component of procedure   the expertise, skill, and time of the physician utilized for rendering the procedure

poisoning table   a feature of the Volume 2 alphabetic index of ICD-9-CM that facilitates the coding and reporting of drug ingestion

post-encounter time   the time after face-to-face time that is allocated by the physician to review medical records and test results, to order procedures, and to communicate with colleagues or ancillary healthcare personnel

posting   an indicator placed within a horizontal column of the HCPCS table of drugs that designates the route of administration of a pharmaceutical

post-visit time   the time allocated by the physician for tasks such as the assessment of patient test results in the laboratory department or the radiology department that are performed after departure from the unit or floor

precertification prior approval from a third-party payor before incurring charges for a procedure or service

pre-encounter time the time before face-to-face time that is allocated by the physician to review medical records and test results, to order procedures, and to communicate with colleagues or ancillary healthcare personnel

preferred provider organization (PPO) a prepaid health insurance plan under a contractual agreement in which the insurer pays the provider a fixed or predetermined sum (a capitation) for contingent services accessible from within a network of providers (physicians and facilities) to each person (each member) insured regardless of the actual services rendered to each plan member

prepaid health insurance plan a contractual agreement through which the insurer pays the provider a fixed or predetermined sum (a capitation) for contingent services accessible to each person (each member) insured regardless of the actual services rendered to each plan member; these prepaid plans include the health maintenance organization (HMO), the preferred provider organization (PPO), and the individual practice association (IPA)

pre-visit time the time allocated by the physician for tasks such as the assessment of patient test results in the laboratory department or the radiology department that are performed before arrival on the unit or floor

primary procedure the procedure which is the most resource intensive procedure (in the context of time, skill, and overhead expense) that is rendered during that encounter or episode of service

principal procedure the procedure most closely associated with the patient's principal diagnosis for that specific encounter or episode of service

problem-focused history a report containing documentation of the chief complaint of the patient with a brief history of the present illness or current problem

problem-focused physical examination a documented assessment of a physical examination limited to an affected body area or organ system

procedural term a word or words describing a diagnostic or therapeutic operation or test

procedure in the healthcare field, a term for a diagnostic or therapeutic technique rendered by a healthcare provider

procedure-based billing charges based on actual services rendered rather than on time intervals

processing notes an itemized compendium of footnotes in the HCPCS Record; Appendix A of the HCPCS Record

professional component of procedure the expertise, skill, and time of the physician utilized for rendering the procedure

prospective payment system Medicare reimbursement system for healthcare providers

prosthetic addition an attachment to an artificial device used to replace a body part

punctuation a textual mark, such as the colon that is utilized as a symbol in the ICD-9-CM coding system

qualitative screening a laboratory drug test coded and reported by procedure rather than by analyte or substance analyzed

quantitative screening a laboratory drug test coded and reported by analyte or substance analyzed rather than by procedure

reduced service   a diminished evaluation and management service that does not merit or fulfill the attributes of time and effort ascribed to the lowest level of service listed in that distinctive evaluation and management service category or subcategory

reference laboratory   an outside laboratory source at an external facility

referral   the assignment of the complete and total care of a patient or the assignment of a specifically designated portion of the care of a patient from one physician to another physician

related complex   signs, symptoms, and clinical findings associated with a pathological process

related procedure   a procedure that is associated with another procedure performed on the patient during an operative session or on a stated date

repeat procedure   a procedure that is performed more than once within an episode of care

residual category   a segment of a classification system reserved for entities not specified in the nomenclature

resource intensity   time, skill, effort, supplies, and equipment utilized to provide patient care and treatment for a specific condition

route of administration column   a vertical column in the HCPCS table of drugs denoting whether a pharmaceutical is dispensed intramuscularly, by inhalation, intrathecally, intravenously, orally, subcutaneously, or by various other means

screening   examination or testing of a group of individuals to ascertain those who are healthy and those who are inflicted with a condition or at risk of acquiring that condition

secondary procedure   a clinical service rendered auxiliary to another clinical service; a procedure subordinate to a primary procedure

section   a secondary division of the ICD-9-CM tabular volumes found in certain chapters of Volume 1; a chapter or primary division of the CPT volume: Evaluation and Management Services; Anesthesia; Surgery; Radiology; Pathology and Laboratory; and Medicine

section mark (§)   a symbol used in ICD-9-CM to denote that a footnote is applicable to the section or category as indicated

section title   the name or designation ascribed to a division of the CPT volume; sections are provided in CPT for Evaluation and Management Services, Anesthesia, Surgery, Radiology, Pathology and Laboratory, and Medicine

see   a cross-reference notation in ICD-9-CM that directs code selection to a more specific term

see also   a cross-reference notation in ICD-9-CM that directs code selection to additional codes

see category   a cross-reference notation in ICD-9-CM that directs code selection to the tabular list for specific information

self-limited presenting problem   a minor or transient patient condition that has a definite and prescribed course and that has a good prognosis or a low probability of permanently affecting health status

semicolon following descriptor   An indicator that the preceding words are not repeated or reiterated in subsequent entries that refer back to and are dependent upon or subordinate to those words

separate procedure a procedure that is the solely performed procedure on a patient during an operative session or on a stated date or a procedure that is not associated with any other procedure performed on the patient during an operative session or on a stated date

service in the healthcare field, a diagnostic or therapeutic activity rendered by a healthcare provider

service code a V code in ICD-9-CM used to report a principal or primary diagnosis for a health service encounter in which a specific service is rendered

special report a note submitted to a third-party payor to detail the charges for any procedure or any service that is unusual, variable, or new; this report should include an explanation of the patient's symptoms, physical findings, and diagnosis, and a clarification of the clinical appropriateness of the procedure or the service including a reasonable and proper description of the nature, extent, and justification for the procedure or the service, and the time, staff, and equipment necessary to render the procedure or the service

starred procedure a relatively minor surgical service listed in the CPT volume; this service involves variable and indefinite preoperative or postoperative care

stars or asterisks (*) symbols printed at the right of a CPT code number to indicate relatively minor surgical procedures that involve variable preoperative services or variable postoperative services and to indicate that the surgical package concept is not applicable for these procedures due to the indefinite nature of preoperative services and postoperative services

status code a V code in ICD-9-CM used to report a factor in the medical or surgical history of the patient

status post term referring to a previous event such as a prior illness or a prior operation

straightforward medical decision making clinical patient assessment involving a minimal number of diagnoses or management options, minimal or no review of complex data, and an appraisal of minimal risks of complications and morbidity or mortality

subcategory a quartiary division throughout the ICD-9-CM tabular volumes; a secondary division of the Evaluation and Management Services section of the CPT volume

subentry term a modifier placed and indented beneath an index entry

subheading a tertiary division of the following sections of the CPT volume: Anesthesia; Surgery; Radiology; Pathology and Laboratory; and Medicine

subsection a primary division of the following sections of the CPT volume: Anesthesia; Surgery; Radiology; Pathology and Laboratory; and Medicine

subsection title the name or designation ascribed to a primary division of a section of the CPT volume

subsequent care the evaluation and management services rendered in a nursing facility by a physician to patients or residents not necessitating a comprehensive assessment and not presenting with a major change of status

sub-subheading a quartiary division of the following sections of the CPT volume: Anesthesia; Surgery; Radiology; Pathology and Laboratory; and Medicine

sub-subterm indented nominative entries for an entity that refers to the antecedent non-indented subterm

subterm nominative entries for an entity referring to the antecedent main term; these entries are printed in normal (not bold) type

superbill a printed form used by healthcare providers to enter coded data for diagnoses and procedures as well as billed charges

supervision and interpretation   the cognitive aspects of the physician component or the professional component of a procedure

supervisory anesthesia service   anesthesia administration as well as preoperative, intraoperative, and postoperative monitoring and care dispensed by an anesthesia resident physician or a certified registered nurse anesthetist under the overall direction of a physician anesthesiologist

supplementary classification   additional tabular listings in ICD-9-CM used to report factors influencing health status and contact with health service (V codes) and external causes of injury and poisoning (E codes)

surgical package   a concept defining the inclusion of preoperative care and postoperative care in the reported procedure code

surgical team   the chief surgeon and all the assistant surgeons for an operative session

symbols   conventional printed signs that represent a quality or quantity; the ICD-9-CM classification system uses six symbols namely brackets [ ], parentheses ( ), the colon :, braces { }, the lozenge ▱, and the section mark §; the CPT classification system uses four symbols namely the circle or bullet ○, the triangle, delta, or pyramid ▲, parentheses ( ), and the star or asterisk *

symptom   a clinical sign that may be indicative of a disease process

synonym   a word that has an equivalent or identical meaning as another word

table of drugs   a feature of the <u>HCPCS Record</u> that contains comprehensive entries of codes and descriptors for prescription pharmaceuticals and which is positioned after the HCPCS alphabetical index to the national codes

technical component of procedure   the equipment and supplies utilized for rendering the procedure

temporary entry   listing in sections of the <u>HCPCS Record</u> for an entity not yet permanently assigned to another section of the <u>HCPCS Record</u>

terminology   a vocabulary or nomenclature used in a profession, occupation, or vocation

third-party payor   reimburser of healthcare claims; insurance carrier

three-level coding system   the structural organization of the HCPCS coding system: level I CPT codes; level II national codes; and level III local codes

time-based billing   charges based on time intervals rather than on actual services rendered

topography   description of an anatomic site or a body part

transaction list   a compendium of changes (additions, revisions, or deletions) in the <u>HCPCS Record</u> made since the previous publication; Appendix B of the <u>HCPCS Record</u>

transfer   the assignment of the complete and total care of a patient or the assignment of a specifically designated portion of the care of a patient from one physician to another physician

transportation waiting timetable   a tabular entry to augment the codes for patient transportation services with modifiers that denote the interval of waiting time based on one-half hour increments

trauma registry   a roster of patients treated for acute injuries

traumatic condition   a patient condition that was produced by injury

triangles, delta, or pyramid (▲)   symbols printed at the left of CPT code numbers to indicate newly revised CPT code descriptors with either modified narrative expressions or altered definitions

tumor registry   a roster of patients treated for malignant neoplasms

two-digit modifier   an appendage consisting of letters or numbers that augments the code used for reporting of entities with qualifying or additional information; in the CPT coding system this type of modifier is attached to the code number with a hyphen

two-surgeon modifier   an indicator that two operating physicians with disparate skills both functioned as primary surgeons, each performing distinct aspects of a complex operative procedure or each performing diverse surgical procedures during the same operative session

type of service code field   a column of the HCPCS Record (indicated with the abbreviation "TOS") that denotes a clinical categorization for a listed entity

uncertain behavior   in the context of neoplasms, this term is used when microscopic examination of the tumor does not disclose a clear determination indicating whether the tumor cells are benign, malignant, or in a stage of transformation

unconfirmed diagnosis   a condition stated as probable, suspected, possible, or likely; this condition should not be coded and reported for outpatient billing but could be coded and reported for inpatient billing

underlying disease   a condition responsible for a manifestation of a disease; in ICD-9-CM, this condition receives sequencing priority over the manifestation

unit time   the time allocated by the physician to review or update the patient's chart, to examine the patient, to order tests or procedures, and to communicate with the patient or with the patient's family as well as to communicate with colleagues and ancillary healthcare personnel while the physician is present on the unit or floor

unlisted procedure   a diagnostic or therapeutic technique rendered by a healthcare provider that is not represented by a specific code number and descriptor in the CPT volume

unlisted service   a diagnostic or therapeutic activity rendered by a healthcare provider that is not represented by a specific code number and descriptor in the CPT volume

unrelated procedure   a procedure that is not associated with any other procedure performed on the patient during an operative session or on a stated date

up-coding   the process in which a healthcare provider changes or modifies the code reported with the claims data submitted to the third-party payor; the code is usually changed or modified to a code representing an entity with a higher payment rate

variable intensity of service   various patient care rendered to multiple patients during an extended time interval

visit   another term for a health service encounter

volume   a book issued in a series; each book of ICD-9-CM is termed a volume; the annual publication of CPT is termed a volume

A B O U T   T H E   A U T H O R

The author, Alex Toth, has earned several credentials particularly related to the healthcare field. With successful completion of national examinations, he has been designated as an accredited record technician (A.R.T.), a certified coding specialist (C.C.S.), a certified medical assistant (C.M.A.), and a certified procedural coder (C.P.C.).

Toth has held positions in various healthcare settings specifically involving coding and billing thereby gaining experience as a technician, a coordinator, a consultant, and an instructor. His familiarity with coding and billing ranges throughout the spectrum of clinical specialties in primary, secondary, and tertiary care.

Educational sessions sponsored through two firms that were established and managed by the author as well as sessions conducted by him under the direction of other coding vendors, stress a philosophy based on the overall structure of the coding systems. This philosophy emphasizes teaching and learning of the sectional and categorical arrangement of headings and subheadings within the ICD, CPT, and HCPCS systems to expedite accurate and precise coding, accentuating the function of each nomenclature or classification to facilitate and enhance code selection and assignment.

Similar methodology is employed in this text under the premise that visualizing the coding system in a structural framework reinforces the concept that individual codes are integral to the total coding system. ICD, CPT, and HCPCS codes should not be simply regarded as randomly assigned digits, such as telephone area codes that do not correlate with other area codes in a given region. Instead, codes in these diagnostic and procedural classifications should be regarded as intentionally selected representations of entities related to the entire system, such as postal zip codes that correspond with geographical territories in a definite pattern.

RELATED TITLES

For additional reading, choose from one of these McGraw-Hill Healthcare Education Group titles. For order information, please call our toll-free number: 1-800-262-4729.

Duane C. Abbey, *ChargeMaster: Review Strategies for Improved Billing and Reimbursement.*
(ISBN: 0-7863-0997-0, $175.00, 1997)

Duane C. Abbey, *Outpatient Services: Designing, Organizing, and Managing Outpatient Resources*
(ISBN: 0-7863-1085-5, $60.00, 1998)

Cherilyn Murer, J.D., C.R.A., Michael Murer, J.D., and Lyndean Lenhoff Brick, J.D., *Post Acute Care Reimbursement Manual*
(ISBN: 0-7863-1248-3, $595.00, 1998)

Dennis M. Adams, *Diagnosis: Documentation and Coding (The Key to Reimbursement and Capitation)*
(ISBN: 0-7863-1000-6, $40.00, 1997)

INDEX